drug
information

A GUIDE FOR
PHARMACISTS

drug information

A GUIDE FOR PHARMACISTS

third edition

Editors

Patrick M. Malone, PharmD, FASHP
Professor of Pharmacy Practice
Assistant Dean
The University of Findlay
School of Pharmacy
Findlay, Ohio

Karen L. Kier, PhD, MSc, RPh
Professor of Clinical Pharmacy
Director, Drug Information
Director, NTPD Program
College of Pharmacy
Ohio Northern University
Ada, Ohio

John E. Stanovich, RPh
Assistant Professor of Clinical Pharmacy
Assistant Dean
College of Pharmacy
Ohio Northern University
Ada, Ohio

McGraw-Hill
Medical Publishing Division

New York • Chicago • San Francisco • Lisbon • London • Madrid • Mexico City • Milan
New Delhi • San Juan • Seoul • Singapore • Sydney • Toronto

The McGraw·Hill Companies

Drug Information: A Guide for Pharmacists, Third Edition

4 5 6 7 8 9 0   DOC/DOC   9 8

ISBN 0-07-143791-6

This book was set in Century Old Style by International Typesetting and Composition.
The editors were Michael Brown, Maya Barahona, and Lester A. Sheinis.
The production supervisor was Catherine H. Saggese.
Project management was provided by International Typesetting and Composition.
The cover was designed by Aimee Nordin.
The indexer was Robert Swanson.
RR Donnelley was the printer and binder.

This book is printed on acid-free paper.

Library of Congress Cataloging-in-Publication Data

Malone, Patrick M., PharmD.
  Drug information : a guide for pharmacists / Patrick M. Malone, Karen L. Kier, John E. Stanovich.—3rd ed.
    p. ; cm.
  Rev. ed. of: Drug information / Patrick M. Malone ... [et al.]. 2nd ed. c2001.
  Includes bibliographical references and index.
  ISBN 0-07-143791-6 (softcover : alk. paper)
  1. Pharmacy—Information services. 2. Drugs. I. Kier, Karen L. II. Stanovich, John E. III. Drug information.   IV. Title.
  [DNLM: 1. Drug Information Services. 2. Pharmacy Administration—methods. QV 737 M257d 2006]
  RS56.2.D78 2006
  615'.1—dc22   20004020

International Edition   ISBN: 0-07-110548-4
Copyright © 2006. Exclusive rights by The McGraw-Hill Companies, Inc., for manufacture and export. This book cannot be reexported from the country to which it is consigned by McGraw-Hill. The International Edition is not available in North America.

Contents

Chapter Six. Controlled Clinical Trial Evaluation 139
Michael G. Kendrach and Maisha Kelly Freeman

Contributors

Ann B. Amerson, PharmD
Professor
Department of Pharmacy Practice and Science
College of Pharmacy
University of Kentucky
Lexington, Kentucky
Chapter 1

H. Glenn Anderson, Jr., PharmD
Associate Professor of Pharmacy Practice
Director, Drug Information and Health Policy
School of Pharmacy
Texas Tech University Health Science Center
Amarillo, Texas
Chapter 7

Amy E. Archer, PharmD
Staff Pharmacist
Safeway
Lakewood, Colorado
Appendix 14-7

Patrick J. Bryant, PharmD, FSCIP
Director, Drug Information Center
Clinical Associate Professor, Division of
  Pharmacy Practice
University of Missouri–Kansas City, School of
  Pharmacy
Kansas City, Missouri
Chapter 7

**Karim Anton Calis, PharmD, MPH, BCPS,
BCNSP, FASHP, FCCP**
Clinical Professor
Department of Pharmacy Practice
  and Science
School of Pharmacy
University of Maryland
Baltimore, Maryland
Department of Pharmacy
School of Pharmacy
Shenandoah University
Winchester, Virginia
Clinical Specialist
Endocrinology and Women's Health
Coordinator
Drug Information Service
Warren G. Magnuson Clinical Center
National Institutes of Health
Bethesda, Maryland
Chapter 3

Nancy L. Fagan, BS, BSPharm, PharmD
Assistant Professor of Pharmacy Practice
School of Pharmacy and Health Professions
Creighton University Medical Center
Alegent Health Immanuel Medical Center
Omaha, Nebraska
Chapters 14 and 15

Maisha Kelly Freeman, PharmD, BCPS
Assistant Professor
McWhorter School of Pharmacy
Drug Information Specialist
Samford University
Birmingham, Alabama
Chapter 6

Mary Lea Gora-Harper, PharmD, FASHP
Clinical Associate Professor
College of Pharmacy
University of Kentucky
Lexington, Kentucky
Chapter 1

Philip J. Gregory, PharmD
Assistant Professor, Pharmacy Practice
Thomas J. Long School of Pharmacy & Health
    Sciences
University of the Pacific
Stockton, California
Chapter 17

Bambi Grilley, RPh, CCRA, CCRC, CIP
Instructor, Baylor College of Medicine
Director, Clinical Protocol Research and
    Regulatory Affairs
Texas Children's Cancer Center
Center for Cell and Gene Therapy
Houston, Texas
Chapter 18

Carrie J. Johnson, PharmD
Manager, Clinical Pharmacy
    Services
The Regence Group
Seattle, Washington
Chapter 7

Michael G. Kendrach, PharmD
Associate Professor
Director, Drug Information Services
McWhorter School of Pharmacy
Samford University
Birmingham, Alabama
Chapter 6

Karen L. Kier, PhD, MSc, RPh
Professor of Clinical Pharmacy
Director, Drug Information
Director, NTPD Program
College of Pharmacy
Ohio Northern University
Ada, Ohio
Chapters 2 and 10

Craig F. Kirkwood, PharmD
Associate Professor of Pharmacy
    and Pharmaceutics
School of Pharmacy
Virginia Commonwealth University
Medical College of Virginia
Associate Director of
    Pharmacotherapy Services
Department of Pharmacy Services
Medical College of Virginia Hospitals
Richmond, Virginia
Chapter 2

Elaine Lust, PharmD
Assistant Professor
School of Pharmacy and
    Health Professions
Creighton University Medical Center
Omaha, Nebraska
Chapter 4

Mark A. Malesker, PharmD
Associate Professor of Pharmacy Practice
  and Medicine
Clinical Pharmacy Specialist
School of Pharmacy and Health Professions
Creighton University Medical Center
Omaha, Nebraska

Chapters 14 and 15

Patrick M. Malone, PharmD, FASHP
Professor of Pharmacy Practice
Assistant Dean
The University of Findlay
School of Pharmacy
Findlay, Ohio

Chapters 5, 11, 14, and 15

Cydney E. McQueen, PharmD
Assistant Director, Drug Information Center
Section Head, Natural Product Information
Clinical Assistant Professor, Division of
  Pharmacy Practice
University of Missouri-Kansas City, School
  of Pharmacy
Kansas City, Missouri

Chapter 7

Kevin G. Moores, PharmD
Associate Professor (Clinical)
Director, Division of Drug Information Service
College of Pharmacy
The University of Iowa
Iowa City, Iowa

Chapter 9

Paul J. Nelson, MD
Vice-Chairman
Formulary Committee
Alegent Health
Omaha, Nebraska

Chapters 14 and 15

Mark A. Ninno, BS, PharmD
Clinical Coordinator
Drug Information Services
Orlando Regional Healthcare
Orlando, Florida

Chapter 16

Sharon Davis Ninno, PharmD
Clinical Projects Coordinator
Orlando Regional Healthcare
Orlando, Florida

Chapter 16

Karen P. Norris, PharmD
Assistant Director, Drug Information Center
Section Head, Natural Product Information
Clinical Assistant Professor, Division of
  Pharmacy Practice
University of Missouri-Kansas City, School
  of Pharmacy
Kansas City, Missouri

Chapter 7

Linda K. Ohri, PharmD
Associate Professor of Pharmacy Practice
School of Pharmacy and Health Professions
Creighton University
Omaha, Nebraska

Chapter 13

Elizabeth A. Poole, PharmD
Fellow, Natural Product Information
  Research
Drug Information Center
University of Missouri–Kansas City, School of
  Pharmacy
Kansas City, Missouri

Chapter 7

Karen L. Rascati, RPh, PhD
Professor, Pharmacy Administration Division
The University of Texas College of Pharmacy
Austin, Texas
Chapter 8

Martha M. Rumore, PharmD, JD, LLM,
  FAPhA
Attorney at Law
Scully, Scott, Murphy & Presser, P.C.
Garden City, New York
Chapter 12

Amy Heck Sheehan, PharmD
Associate Professor of Pharmacy Practice
Purdue University School of Pharmacy and
  Pharmaceutical Sciences
Drug Information Specialist
Clarian Health Partners
Indianapolis, Indiana
Chapter 3

Kelly M. Shields, PharmD
Assistant Professor of Pharmacy Practice
Assistant Director, Drug Information Center
Ohio Northern University
Ada, Ohio
Chapter 4

James P. Wilson, PharmD, PhD, FASHP
Associate Professor
Head, Pharmacy Practice
Pharmacy Practice and Administration Division
Centre for Pharmacoeconomics Study
The University of Texas College of Pharmacy
Austin, Texas
Chapter 8

Linda R. Young, PharmD
Director, Medication Use
Department of Pharmacy Services
Carilion Medical Center
Roanoke, VA 24014
Chapter 7

Preface

Over the last ten years, there has been an increasing realization of the importance of information. Much of this can be related to the increased availability of Internet information sources throughout society, along with the ease by which material can be located and used. The impact of the Internet can also been seen in this book. The first edition contained only two pages of information about the Internet, which reflected the small amount of medical information available and the little impact that it had on the profession at that time. In this new edition, it seems as if hardly a page can be found without some reference to Internet material. This increased emphasis on information has had an effect on both the health care professional, who uses the material, and the patient, who may look up material directly and even bring it in to talk about with a pharmacist or physician. The ability to obtain, manage, and use information has become an important core skill for the professional.

Unfortunately, pharmacists in practice may find it difficult to learn how to manage information, due to a lack of good, comprehensive resources to teach them proven methods for improving their skills. Students also need a source to supplement the classroom and clerkship training they receive. It is to serve those populations that this book was originally written. In this third edition, the goal of this book continues to be to educate both students and practitioners on how to efficiently research, interpret, collate, and disseminate information in the most usable form. While there is no one right method to do these things, proven methods are presented and demonstrated. Also, seldom-addressed issues are covered, such as the legal and ethical considerations of providing information.

The book begins by introducing the concept of drug information, including its history, and providing information on various places drug information specialists may be employed. The book continues on by describing the various steps for obtaining, evaluating, and providing information. As with the first edition, the "Modified Systematic Approach" to answering a question is presented. "Formulating Effective Responses" further expands on this topic by addressing problems that pharmacists experience when answering questions and providing techniques for overcoming these issues in order to reach appropriate conclusions. This section of the book is designed to teach pharmacists and students useful methods for determining what information is actually needed and how to adequately respond to requests.

Subsequent chapters allow the reader to further expand their skills in these areas. Once the pharmacist determines what information is needed using the skills outlined in the initial chapters, resources must be consulted to formulate a response. As always, a chapter discussing various resources that may be consulted for specific types of information has been provided, which has expanded coverage of electronic resources, particularly those for personal digital assistants (PDAs). New material on how to find information regarding veterinary medicine and complementary/alternative medicine has been added. A chapter on electronic information management is included, although there has been an effort to include this type of information throughout the book.

Even when information is found, pharmacists must evaluate the literature for quality and usefulness. The earlier editions of this book provided information on how to evaluate the medical literature. Those evaluation techniques are again in this edition with additional information being provided.

Two specific types of literature have been identified for even greater examination—pharmacoeconomics and evidence-based clinical practice guidelines. Information is presented on how to both perform such functions and evaluate work prepared by others. Evaluation of information resources often requires knowledge about statistical tests. The "Clinical Application of Statistical Analysis" chapter is an expansion of information provided in previous editions. The reader of this chapter will discover how to evaluate the appropriateness of statistical tests used in clinical studies.

Pharmacists may be asked to provide information in written form. The next chapter describes how this may be done. Additionally, sections describing how to prepare materials for formal presentations (platform and poster) and develop Websites are also provided.

The legal and ethical aspects of providing information always must be considered. The chapters on these topics have been updated and improved to be even more useful tham those in previous editions. In particular, additional information has been provided on new privacy regulations that have been instituted because of the Health Insurance Portability and Accountability Act of 1996 (HIPAA).

The remaining chapters deal with specialized functions that have often been the responsibility of drug information specialists but may be addressed by other pharmacists. These chapters will build upon the first part of the book. Much of the information in these chapters was covered in the Pharmacy and Therapeutics (P&T) chapter of the first edition; however, that chapter is now mostly limited to formulary management and some minor P&T functions. The formulary material also has increased information regarding third-party payer (e.g., insurance companies) formularies. New and expanded information is provided on quality assurance, adverse drug reactions and medication errors. Also, the information on how to prepare a drug evaluation monograph has been moved to a new chapter, with additional information on standards that have been prepared by the Academy of Managed Care Pharmacy (AMCP) and various governments.

Finally, the chapter on Investigation Drugs has been updated to take into account new information and procedures.

With the veritable Niagara Falls of drug or pharmacy information available, much of which is complex, pharmacists have an increasing need for information management skills. This book will assist any pharmacist or student in the improvement of his or her skills in this area and allow individuals to evolve into new roles for the advancement of both the profession and care of patients. We hope you enjoy your journey toward expertise in information management.

Acknowledgment

The authors would like to thank Dr. Kristen Wilkinson Mosdell for her major contributions to the first two editions of this book. Dr. Mosdell's work was invaluable in their preparation. We would like to recognize the enormous amount she has done to get the book to this point and to state that she has been greatly missed in preparing this current edition. We hope that it will be possible to collaborate again at some time in the future.

1

Chapter One

Introduction to the Concept of Medication Information

Mary Lea Gora-Harper • Ann B. Amerson

Objectives

After completing this chapter, the reader will be able to

- Define the term *drug information*, use it in different contexts, and relate it to the term *medication information*.
- Describe the importance of drug information centers in the evolution of pharmacy practice.
- Identify the services provided by drug information centers.
- Identify medication information functions performed by individual pharmacists.
- Describe the skills needed by pharmacists to perform medication information functions.
- Identify major factors that have influenced the ability of pharmacists to provide medication information.
- Describe practice opportunities for a medication information specialist.

Introduction

The provision of medication information is among the most fundamental responsibilities of pharmacists. The information may be either patient specific, as an integral part of pharmaceutical care, or relative to a group of patients, such as in the development of a therapeutic guideline, publishing an electronic newsletter, or updating a website. The pharmacist can serve as a resource for issues regarding cost-effective medication selection and use, medication policy decisions (drug benefits), medication information resource selection, or practice-related issues. Medication information opportunities are developing and expanding with changes in the health care environment. With national efforts to expand access to care while reducing health care costs, the advent of consumerism, and the integration of new technologies, medication information opportunities are growing in several areas including managed care organizations, pharmaceutical industry, medical and specialty care clinics, scientific writing and medical communication companies, and the insurance industry.

The term *drug information* may have different meanings to different people depending on the context in which it is used. If asked to define this term, one could describe it as printed information in a reference or verbalized by an individual that pertains to medications. In many cases, individuals use this term in different contexts by associating it with other words, which include the following:

- Specialist/practitioner/pharmacist/provider
- Center/service/practice
- Functions/skills

The first group of words implies a specific individual, the second group implies a place, and the third implies activities and abilities of individuals. The term *drug information* will be used in these different contexts to describe the beginnings and evolution of this area of practice. Relative to current practice, the term *medication information* is used in place of *drug information* to convey the management and use of information on medication therapy and to signify the broader role that all pharmacists take in information provision. These terms may refer to either the provision of information for a specific patient or in the context of addressing medication use issues for a group of patients (e.g., development of policies and procedures on medication use). The term *population* is frequently used to refer to an aggregation or group of individuals defined by a set of common characteristics.

Drug informatics is another term used to describe the evolving roles of the medication information specialist. Drug informatics emphasizes the use of technology as an integral tool in effectively organizing, analyzing, and managing information on medication use in patients. The impact of new technologies and opportunities in drug informatics in current and future practice will be discussed later in the chapter.

The goals of this chapter are to describe how the role of the pharmacist has evolved in providing medication information, to discuss factors contributing to the evolution, and to describe opportunities for use of medication information skills, either as a generalist or in a specialty practice. This chapter provides the foundation for understanding the pharmacist's need to have proficiency in the knowledge and skills discussed in this book.

The Beginning

The term *drug information* developed in the early 1960s when used in conjunction with the words *center* and *specialist*. In 1962, the first drug information center was opened at the University of Kentucky Medical Center.[1] An area separated from the pharmacy was dedicated to provide drug information. The center was to be "a source of selected, comprehensive drug information for staff physicians and dentists to evaluate and compare drugs"[1] as well as to provide for the drug information needs of nurses. The center was expected to take an active role in the education of health professional students including medicine, dentistry, nursing, and pharmacy. A stated goal was to influence pharmacy students in developing their role as drug consultants.

Several other drug information centers were established shortly thereafter. Different approaches to providing drug information services included decentralizing pharmacists in the hospital, offering a clinical consultation service, and providing services for a geographic area through a regional center. The first formal survey, conducted in 1973, identified 54 pharmacist operated centers in the United States.[2]

The individual responsible for operation of the center was called the *drug information specialist*. The expectation was that drug information would be stored in the center and retrieved, selected, evaluated, and disseminated by the specialist. Information would be disseminated to respond to specific questions, to assist in the evaluation of drugs for use in the hospital, or to inform others through newsletters of current developments related to drugs. These and other functions, as listed in Table 1–1, have evolved over a period of years and reflect the services provided in most drug information centers. Detailed information regarding these activities is provided in subsequent chapters.

To develop some perspective for the reader on why the development of drug information centers and specialists was important, consider 4 of the 15 summary points in a congressional review of a survey by the National Library of Medicine on *The Nature and Magnitude of Drug Literature* published in 1963.[3]

- "Drug literature is vast and complex. The very problem of defining what constitutes the literature is difficult."

TABLE 1–1. MEDICATION INFORMATION SERVICES

Support for clinical services
Answering questions
   Developing criteria/guidelines for medication use
Pharmacy and therapeutics committee activity
   Development of medication use policies
   Formulary management
Publications—newsletter, journal columns, websites
Education—in-services for health professionals, students, consumers
Medication usage evaluation/medication use evaluation
Investigational medication control
   Institutional Review Board activities
   Information for practitioners
Coordination of reporting programs, e.g., adverse medication reactions
Poison information

- "Drug literature is growing rapidly in size. It is also increasingly complex, i.e., inter-disciplinary and interprofessional in nature. Thus, drug information 'sprawls across' many professional journals of the most varied types."
- "Literature on clinical experience with drugs is sizable and is growing. Its effective use by the practitioner offers many difficulties."
- "Competent evaluation of masses of drug information is particularly necessary."

Interestingly, these statements still seem applicable even today when given the figures of more than 20,000 biomedical journals and approximately 17,000 new biomedical books published annually are considered.[4] Many journals are now published both in print and on the Internet (i.e., e-journal or electronic journal). Training in computer and information technology was considered one of the five core areas of focus for health professionals' education in an Institute of Medicine (IOM) report published in April 2003.[5] Drug information specialists can provide leadership in this area.

In the 1960s, the availability of new drugs (e.g., neuromuscular blockers and first-generation cephalosporins) was providing challenges for practitioners to keep abreast and make appropriate decisions for their patients. Part of the problem was finding a way to effectively communicate the wealth of information to those needing it. The information environment relied heavily on the print medium for storage, retrieval, and dissemination of information. The Medical Literature Retrieval and Analysis System (MEDLARS) was developed by the National Library of Medicine in the early 1960s.[6] While it provided a computerized form of searching, requests for searches were submitted by mail and results returned by mail. The ability to transmit such information over telephone lines (online technology) was not available until 1971 when MEDLINE® was introduced and was limited to libraries. During this time, the drug information specialist was viewed as a person who could bridge the gap and effectively communicate drug information.[7]

In describing the training required for a drug information specialist, the following areas were identified to either need strengthening or addition to pharmacy school curricula: biochemistry, anatomy, physiology, pathology, and biostatistics and experimental design (with some histology, embryology, and endocrinology incorporated into other courses).[8] Such topics were either not incorporated or emphasized in curricula of the 1960s. In today's pharmacy curricula, most of these topics receive considerable emphasis. Pharmacists today use knowledge and skills to make clinical decisions about medication use in specific patients or a group of patients in conjunction with other health professionals. Pharmacists may be principal investigators or coinvestigators in research involving a variety of therapeutic topics including medication use, optimal dose, drug interactions, or adverse effects of new or existing medications. Likewise, publications in the area of therapeutic guidelines or other drug policy initiatives are frequently authored by a pharmacist, sometimes with support of the pharmacy professional organizations.

The development of drug information centers and drug information specialists was the beginning of the clinical pharmacy concept. It laid the groundwork for pharmacists to demonstrate the ability to assume more responsibility in providing input on patient drug therapy. Pharmacists were provided the opportunity to extend their patient care contribution by taking a more active role in the clinical aspects of the decision-making process as it related to medication therapy. By using their extensive drug knowledge and expanding their background in certain areas, pharmacists could offer their expertise as consultants on medication therapy. The tool the pharmacist would use to function in this capacity was the clinical drug literature. This role of consultant has expanded for all pharmacists and is discussed in more detail later.

The Evolution

It is useful to look at the evolution of drug information practice from the perspective of drug information centers and of practicing pharmacists. One report describes the decline in number of drug information centers nationally with the number of drug information pharmacists and other personnel being the lowest in 30 years.[9,10] A total of 81 drug information centers were identified in this survey, although there are some existing centers missing from this list and there has been some controversy at meetings of drug information practitioners regarding some centers being excluded because of the definition of drug information centers that is used. Another source of drug information center locations, the *2004 Red Book,* lists a total of 112 drug information centers nationally.[11] Determining the accurate number is difficult. The centers are identified for these two sources through various listings that have developed over the years, but no agency or organization is responsible for maintaining a list. Well-defined criteria are not established for using the titles of drug information center/service. Some centers have specialized in a particular area of drug information and their name may reflect that specific function (e.g., Center of Drug Policy). Likewise, these lists only address drug information centers listed in the United States or Puerto Rico, and not those that have been created internationally. They also exclude centers/services provided by the pharmaceutical industry. Therefore, depending on how one would define a drug information center, the number may actually be higher.

A recent survey (2003)[10] describes the current status of drug information centers compared to past years. For several years, funding for drug information centers has been provided primarily by hospitals or medical centers (73% in 2003, 82% in 1992, and 88% in 1986), or colleges or universities (37% in 2003, 35% in 1992, and 32% in 1986). However, there was a statistically significant decrease in the percentage of drug information centers funded by hospitals between 1986 and 2003. This decrease could be attributed to the economic constraints faced by the health care system in the last several years.

Drug information pharmacists working in centers appear to be better trained than those in the past and a larger percentage have a doctor of pharmacy degree (71% in 2003, and 42% in 1986 and 1992).[10] The number of individuals who have completed a drug information residency, fellowship, or MS degree program has also increased in recent years (29% in 2003 and 11% in 1992).

In addition to the responsibility of answering questions, the most commonly reported services in 2003 were preparation of newsletters (80%) and participation in pharmacy and therapeutics committee activities (79%).[10] Education appears to be a growing area of responsibility. Forty-one percent of respondents considered education to be their primary goal. There was an increase in the percentage of drug information centers that participated in any type of residency program training (83% in 2003) compared to 1976, 1980, 1986, and 1992, in which the number of centers that participated in any residency program ranged from 54 to 66%. There was also a larger number of drug information centers used for experiential training as part of a doctor of pharmacy program (95% in 2003 compared to 59% in 1992). Table 1–1 outlines several services that are typically provided by drug information centers.

There have been a few studies that have described the economic benefit of maintaining a drug information center or related activity in an academic institution or hospital. One such study examined the economic impact of drug information services responding to patient-specific requests. The resultant benefit/cost ratio was found to be 2.9:1 to 13.2:1. Most of the cost savings resulted from decreased need for monitoring (e.g., laboratory tests) or decreased need for additional treatment related to an adverse effect.[12] Another study examined the drug cost avoidance and revenue associated with the provision of investigational drug services, which are many times a responsibility of a drug information center. The annualized drug cost avoidance plus revenue was $2.6 million.[13] Although the cost avoidance varied with the type of study and disease category involved, overall, the investigational drug service accounted for substantial drug cost avoidance. These types of studies are becoming increasingly important in an era of cost containment.

DRUG INFORMATION—FROM CENTERS TO PRACTITIONERS

The responsibilities of individual pharmacists regarding the provision of medication information have changed substantially over the years. Impetus for this change was provided not only by the development of drug information centers and the clinical pharmacy concept, but also by the Study Commission on Pharmacy.[14] This external group was established to review the state of the practice and education of pharmacists and report its findings. One of the findings and recommendations stated that:

> …among deficiencies in the health care system, one is the unavailability of adequate information for those who consume, prescribe, dispense and administer drugs. This deficiency has

resulted in inappropriate drug use and an unacceptable frequency of drug-induced disease. Pharmacists are seen as health professionals who could make an important contribution to the health care system of the future by providing information about drugs to consumers and health professionals. Education and training of pharmacists now and in the future must be developed to meet these important responsibilities.

The report of the Commission was issued in 1975 and since that time drug information practice has changed both for drug information centers and individual pharmacists. The development of clinical pharmacy has helped move pharmacy forward in recognizing its capabilities to contribute to the care of patients. Clinical pharmacy was primarily thought of as an institutional patient care process and did not gain widespread acceptance outside of hospitals. Over time, the activity of the pharmacist as a medication expert for patients has gained acceptance in a variety of practice settings including community pharmacies, nursing homes, and primary and specialty practices in medicine. Pharmacists who provide patient-specific information with a goal of improving patient outcomes use the medical literature to support their choices.[15,16]

Pharmacists involved in patient care areas (e.g., hospitals, clinics, long-term care, and home health care) now frequently answer drug information questions, participate in evaluating a patient's drug therapy, and conduct medication usage evaluation activities. The provision of medication information may be on a one-on-one basis or may occur using a more structured approach, such as a presentation to a class of diabetic patients or a group of nurses in the practice facility. In either case, the pharmacist educates those who are the beneficiaries of the medication information. Pharmacists may also participate in precepting students in patient care or pharmacy environments. In any of these roles, the pharmacist must use appropriate information retrieval and evaluation skills to ensure that the most current and accurate information is provided to make decisions about medication use for those they are serving. There is a well-described systematic approach to answering drug information questions (Chaps. 2 and 3). It is important to obtain the important background information including pertinent patient factors, disease factors, and medication-related factors to determine the true question. Good problem-solving skills are required to fully assess the situation, develop a search strategy, evaluate the information, and formulate a response. It is equally important for the pharmacist to develop good communication skills to respond in a clear and concise manner, using terminology that is consistent with the patients', caregivers', or health professionals' level of understanding. Table 1–2 lists the medication information skills a pharmacist needs.

Opportunities continue to grow for the participation of the pharmacist in home health care and long-term care that require a solid therapeutic knowledge base, an understanding of the medical literature, and the ability to communicate the information through either verbal or written consultation. Pharmacists in community settings counsel patients, answer medication

TABLE 1–2. MEDICATION INFORMATION SKILLS

Assess available information and gather situational data needed to characterize question or issue
Formulate appropriate question(s)
Use a systematic approach to find needed information
Evaluate information critically for validity and applicability
Develop, organize, and summarize response for question or issue
Communicate clearly when speaking or writing, considering the audience level
Anticipate other information needs

information questions, review patient medication regimens for potential problems, and participate in helping patients manage chronic diseases.

Opportunities for pharmacists are also available in the area of veterinary pharmaceutics.
Information is needed by both the animal owner and the veterinarian. A pharmacist may need
to practically apply information from veterinary resources (e.g., *Veterinary Drug Handbook,
Textbook of Veterinary Internal Medicine*, and *National Animal Poison Control Center*) for the
benefit of an animal.

FACTORS INFLUENCING THE EVOLUTION OF THE PHARMACIST'S ROLE AS A MEDICATION INFORMATION PROVIDER

In addition to the changing philosophy of practice, several other factors are influential in the evolution of the pharmacist's role as a medication information provider. These include the prevention of adverse drug events (ADEs), growth of information technology, changes in the health
care environment with a focus on evidence-based medicine and the evaluation of outcomes, the
sophistication of medication therapy, and a more knowledgeable patient.

Adverse Drug Events

The 1999 IOM report *To Err is Human: Building a Safer Health Care System*[17] has generated
a great deal of discussion in the medical community and legislature because of the impact of
ADEs on patient health and well-being, and because of economic implications. IOM analysts
estimate that prescription medications are responsible for up to 7000 American deaths per
year, with the cost of drug-related morbidity and mortality being nearly U.S. $77 billion per
year.[17] Their definition of ADEs includes both medication errors and adverse drug reactions
(ADRs). Accurate statistics of the frequency of ADRs are difficult to assess for a particular
drug since phase I–III of clinical research includes too small a sample size and frequently medications are taken for a short duration. For instance, rofecoxib (Vioxx) was a drug approved in
1999 as a safer alternative to first-generation nonsteroidal anti-inflammatory agents for elderly
patients with pain. The drug was recalled on October 1, 2004 in the largest prescription drug
withdrawal in history.[18] The withdrawal was prompted after a new study examining the drug's
impact on bowel cancer found that the drug caused an almost twofold increase in heart attacks
and strokes. Although the Adenomatous Polyp Prevention on Vioxx® (APPROVe) trial began

enrollment in 2000 and was being monitored by an independent data safety monitoring board, it was not stopped earlier because the results for the first 18 months of the trial did not show any increased risk of confirmed cardiovascular events with Vioxx®. The actual number of ADRs nationally reported is probably underestimated because the full range of patients likely to use the medications postmarketing are not included in premarketing studies. Frequently, these studies include patients with only one disease and exclude children, pregnant women, and the elderly. If a report is identified by a health professional or consumer, the Food and Drug Administration (FDA) has a voluntary reporting program to help identify and address these issues once the medication has become commercially available. However, it is estimated that the spontaneous reporting system captures only 1 to 10% of all adverse events.[19,20] Therefore, this can be used only as a flag to stimulate further research in postmarketing surveillance studies. Communication and coordination among patients, physicians, pharmacists, and other health care professionals can help avoid these dangerous incidents.[21,22] Pharmacists should cautiously recommend newly approved therapy by weighing the risk versus benefit, with an understanding that all information regarding adverse effects may not be available yet on a newly approved product. When a product is newly approved with claims of decreased frequency of side effects, these claims need to be tempered with the understanding that the depth of information that is available regarding these products is not as good as products that have been available for many years.

There may also be ADR implications when selecting medications for a formulary. When a new medication becomes commercially available, clinicians supporting a proactive formulary system will review and decide if that medication will be available for routine use for patients immediately. Because information regarding new medications is frequently limited, it may be wise to collect data on patients in a clinical setting and compare this use against a standard of how the drug should be used once the product becomes available in an institution. This can be accomplished through a medication use evaluation (MUE) program. Because the product is new, physicians and other health professionals need to know how to prescribe (select appropriate patient population and dose), administer, and monitor the drug to avoid ADEs and provide effective therapy. Many times, adverse effects of newly approved medications do not appear until a medication is used in a group of patients with multiple medical problems who are taking several other medications. Data acquired from this MUE will verify that the medication is indeed being used as recommended, and that it has been used safely.

Adverse events associated with dietary supplements provide an additional concern, because the manufacturers do not need to submit safety or efficacy data to the FDA prior to availability.[23] Consumers and health practitioners have limited information to help them make decisions on safety. Large-scale studies that frequently include several thousand patients are required for a drug to be approved, but are not available with these products. Therefore, it is necessary to rely on reporting to the FDA *after* the supplement has become available to determine if there are safety concerns. In addition to having limited information on adverse effects, information is also limited in other areas such as appropriate dose, efficacy, and pharmacokinetics. Adverse effects that are reported to the FDA may be evaluated, and action may be taken. For instance, in 2004, the FDA prohibited sale of dietary supplements containing ephedrine alkaloids (ephedra) because of the limited data available on efficacy, and because of the risk of adverse health outcomes including myocardial infarction and stroke.[24] In other cases, a communication to health care professionals may alert them to a particular side effect. For instance, recently the FDA issued a warning citing 25 reports of hepatotoxicity worldwide with kava, a dietary supplement used for several indications including insomnia.[25] This product is still available in the United States. Because of these and other issues, most hospitals have policies regarding herbal product use.[26]

Information on ADRs in patients receiving either medications or dietary supplements is frequently coordinated through an ADR program in a hospital. The ADR program for an institution has many components including identification of suspected side effects, assessment of probability, dissemination of information (documentation in the medical record and submission to a larger database of information), and monitoring of outcomes.[22] In health care systems (e.g., hospitals), this initiative is performed by pharmacists, physicians, and other health professionals in a coordinated fashion. The ADR program is most often coordinated by the pharmacy department, and specifically, the drug information center, if available. Both medications as well as dietary supplements used for medicinal purposes are submitted to the coordinating group and evaluated in an ADR program. More information on ADEs can be found in Chap. 17.

Despite efforts to decrease the frequency of medical errors after the 1999 IOM report *To Err is Human: Building a Safer Health System*, many consumers are still dissatisfied with the quality of health care in the United States. In a recent survey,[27] 40% of respondents believed that the quality of health care has gotten worse in the past 5 years, while only 17% said that it has improved. Thirty-four percent of respondents said that they or a family member had experienced a medical error at some point in their life. Efforts are ongoing to lobby for additional funding for initiatives to decrease the risk of medical errors in the United States. Because of the pharmacists' role in helping to identify and prevent ADEs in patients, this could have future implications.

Integration of New Technologies

Computer technology has changed drastically, but positively, the ability to store and access information. Even though the amount of literature is much larger today than earlier, it is more manageable. The Internet has grown into a vast network of computers that millions of users can access in most countries. The World Wide Web (WWW), a method of sharing information over the Internet, allows the user to easily access the scientific literature, government publications, items in the news, and many other things. The information may be purely in textual form, or include graphics (e.g., GIF, JPEG), video (e.g., MPEG), or sound (e.g., WAV, MP3). Patients and health care practitioners can find information on nearly every disease and treatment, and virtual health communities and forums provide a mutually supportive environment for patients, family, and friends. A pharmacist in a local community pharmacy or rural hospital can communicate with health care professionals or their patients locally or can obtain information about a medication found only in another country. Although drug information centers have ready access to the Internet, and specialists use information from this resource on a daily basis, businesses have yet to take full advantage of this technology.[28] This is likely to change in the near future. Local area networks are frequently used to interconnect computers within a drug information center, building, or neighboring areas. The use of wide area networks will grow as institutions merge and interconnect data management functions.[29]

There is an increasing need by health professionals, as well as consumers, to get more information about medications sooner. Information is needed quickly when a new medication becomes commercially available because of the potential for health and cost implications, when a product is withdrawn from the market for safety reasons, or when data from a new study are released that could have an impact on how common ailments are treated. The lag time that occurs with the print format may not be acceptable for many direct patient care issues. The Internet allows medical information to be available sooner to both health care professionals and the public. Online repositories for articles, such as BioMed Central (<<www.biomedcentral.com>>) and PubMed® (<<www.pubmedcentral.nih.gov>>) have allowed individuals to access millions of articles quickly, easily, and free of charge. The site freemedicaljournals.com provides a comprehensive list of medical journals that are free of charge. The availability of e-journals has helped speed up the publication process to allow articles to be available electronically sooner than the print version. Hypertext links between reference lists from an article in one online journal to the original article eliminate the need to travel to a library. When the journals e-mail a table of contents (TOC) or provide an automatic alert about articles on a particular topic, this results in a more effective method of keeping up to date. E-textbooks are also available on the World Wide Web; however, the majority of printed medical textbooks with an online version require a subscription. For instance, *Harrison's Principles of Internal Medicine* (<<www.harrisonsonline.com>>) is a continually updated and expanded version of the printed text. Other textbooks are available for purchase as a CD-ROM.

Registries of ongoing clinical trials, such as ClinicalTrials.gov, provide information on the purpose and criteria for participation in these trials. This has allowed pharmacists to anticipate new therapies, and perhaps help their patients receive medications not yet FDA approved through enrollment in a clinical trial.

There are a variety of websites sponsored by different companies and individuals. In a recent survey, 85% of physician respondents had experienced a patient bringing Internet information to a visit.[30] Ninety percent of respondents perceived that the majority of these patients had brought them information because they wanted to ask their opinion. Wide availability of this information should be tempered with the need to evaluate the validity of information obtained, especially for the public. Information is many times incomplete or inaccurate.[31] Because misinformation may result in harmful behavior (e.g., discontinuing medication, increasing the doses), the availability of quality information is important. There is currently no valid instrument available to assess the quality of a website, although there are many proposed methods. However, there are some common sense criteria that can be used to examine the quality of information (accurate, up to date, authoritative authorship) on a website.[32] One site that may be helpful in providing patients with information on a range of medical conditions and management is <<http:/www.healthfinder.gov>>. However, if misinformation or inaccurate information is shared, organizations exist to monitor fraud on the World Wide Web (e.g., <<www. quackwatch.com>>).

Mailing lists, newsgroups, bulletin boards, web forums, and chat rooms have simplified the way in which peers can exchange news and share opinions. E-mail has been an effective method to keep up to date with a journal's e-mailed table of contents (eTOC), which are often sent before print publication. Several professional organizations (e.g., American Society of Health-System Pharmacists, <<http:/www.ashp.org>>) have websites that offer e-mail alert services to maintain awareness of important news affecting pharmacy, drug shortages, and awareness of their meetings.

Drug information centers have created their own sites to post information about their center and services, provide links to related sites considered to be of acceptable quality, and as a convenient means of receiving and answering drug information questions.[33] The advantage of having a request form for answering drug information questions on the web is that physicians, pharmacists, or other health professionals can access computers at their practice site. Many times, this is accessible only through an institution's Intranet. An Intranet is a network that belongs to an organization and is designed to be accessible only by the organization's members, employees, or others with authorization. The website looks and acts just like other sites, but has a firewall surrounding it, and therefore the center can provide easy access to their primary patrons without receiving extraneous questions from people outside their defined clientele.[34-36]

Likewise, the use of personal digital assistants (PDAs) has grown. A PDA offers the convenience of collecting and accessing information from a unit that can be carried in a user's pocket. There are several examples of the use of PDAs in pharmacy practice.[37-47] In certain situations, these systems can be used more conveniently than a desktop computer for online searching, to provide medication profiles, to set appointments, as a time-management tool, and to search drug information databases (e.g., general drug information text and drug interaction resources). The PDA can provide access to the formulary, order entry and verification, medication error and ADR reporting, and medication use guidelines. One area where several institutions have found PDAs to be a valuable tool in their facility is in the documentation of clinical interventions by pharmacists. One study compared the efficiency of using a PDA for documentation of clinical interventions compared to paper. The number of new interventions performed by pharmacists was divided by the number of new orders written during a 6-month period. When the PDA was used to document interventions, there was consistently more complete information and more interventions documented than when data were collected on paper (7.43% [697 PDA-documented interventions/15,979 new orders written] vs. 4.36% [919 paper-documented interventions/13,184 new orders; P < 0.001]).[44] An additional advantage of using a PDA for documentation of clinical interventions is that it decreases the time needed to aggregate the data into a database, rather than retrospectively entering data into the database. This may have some advantages in documenting reimbursement for services. In another study,[39] authors calculated their potential claims using their Medicaid reimbursement rate for pharmacists' cognitive services documented with PDAs. The amount was more than $1 million in 6 months, assuming a 100% reimbursement rate. This cost reflects total reimbursement and was not compared to paper documentation. There are some limitations to PDAs. In general, they are not considered to be secure at this time and, therefore, may not protect proprietary or confidential information. Also, the unit may compromise usability by trying to present too much information on a small screen. The advantage, however, is that this system offers a convenient and, in many cases easily updated, information tool at the bedside. Frequently, in a clinical setting, the use of a mix of desktop, laptop, or hand-held devices is optimal based on the particular clinical scenario.

Although technology affords remote-site access to medication information sources, it is critical that pharmacists have the skills to perceive, assess, and evaluate the information, and apply the information to the situation. One of the most rapidly changing technologies in health care is information technology. It is important that pharmacists not only keep up with medication use concepts, but that they also stay abreast of developments in the area of information technology in an effort to integrate new and valuable systems in a timely and efficient manner. The need for this type of training is emphasized in a recent IOM report.[5]

Future technology developments are likely to further enhance access and use of information. The medical record, including administrative information, laboratory data, and pharmaceutical information are becoming more commonly accessible in patient care areas. A properly configured medical record provides decision support, facilitates workflow, and enables the routine collection of data for performance feedback.[48] This offers opportunities for pharmacists, and in particular medication information specialists, to take a leadership role in planning and implementing computerized intervention programs that automatically educate at the point of prescribing. The use of computer-based clinical support systems that provide patient information with recommendations based on the best evidence has shown to be valuable in the patient care setting, including a reported decrease in length of hospital stay.[49-50] In one study that examined the value of using a decision support program to assist physicians in using anti-infective agents, the length of hospital stay of patients who used the recommendations was compared with a group of patients who did not always use the recommendations, and compared against a group of patients who were admitted to the unit 2 years before the intervention program. The length of hospital stay was statistically different with an average of 10, 16.7, and 12.9 days, respectively.[49]

Although the Internet has been used to transfer information instantaneously to clinicians and researchers, its value as a patient care resource and professional education tool is only starting to be tested. One of the concerns in using the Internet for transfer of patient information is patient confidentiality.[51-53] Virtual private networks (VPNs) are used to eliminate many of the technical issues surrounding security of information. Confidentiality has been addressed with new legislation referred to as the Health Insurance Portability and Accountability Act (HIPAA) to make sure that covered entities (e.g., health plans, health care providers, and health care clearing houses) limit disclosure of an individual's protected health information.[53] Once the legislation has been implemented for several years, the implications of this legislation will be more clear.

Focus on Evidence-Based Medicine and Drug Policy Development

The pharmacist's ability to apply medication information skills to drug policy decisions will be of growing importance in this changing health care environment. This can be done by identifying trends of inappropriate medication use in a group of patients and providing supporting scientific evidence to help change behavior. Continued growth in national health expenditures has raised the concern of government, insurance agencies, health care providers, and the public in identifying strategies to control spending while maintaining access to quality health care. With $216 billion spent on pharmaceuticals in 2003 (increased from $194 billion in 2002), inevitably, questions arise about the value of services received.[54-55] These increases in pharmaceutical costs are of particular concern especially in light of the recent approval of the Medicare drug benefit. The Medicare Prescription Drug Improvement and Modernization Act has several provisions that will affect pharmacy practice including one that requires participating in health plans to create medication therapy management programs to ensure that the covered medications are used appropriately by high-risk patients.[56] Likewise, the IOM recently completed a 3-year study of the uninsured with a recommendation that universal health insurance coverage be available in the United States by 2010. In 2001, uninsured Americans received $35 billion in uncompensated medical care; $30 billion was ultimately paid for with tax dollars.[57] Although a list of insurance benefits has not been defined, they will be created based on evidence of improved patient care.

In recent years, there has been a shift from a fee-for-service, inpatient focus, to a capitated, managed care, ambulatory focus.[58] Managed care—a process seeking to manage the delivery of high-quality health care in order to improve cost effectiveness—is consuming an ever-increasing portion of health care delivery. Today, providers are relying less on impressions of what *may* be happening in a practice setting and more on data that are actually being collected in that same group of patients (e.g., number of patients receiving appropriate dose of drugs). Goals are set for a particular group of patients (e.g., all patients receive beta-blocker therapy after a myocardial infarction) based on evidence found in the scientific literature. This connection of applying the scientific information to the patient care setting is made through evidence-based medicine. Evidence-based medicine is an approach to practice and teaching that integrates current clinical research evidence with pathophysiologic rationale, professional expertise, and patient preferences to make decisions for a population.[59] This has strengthened the need for pharmacists to have a solid understanding of medication information concepts and skills. Pharmacists need to be able to evaluate the medication use issues for a group of patients; search, retrieve, and critically evaluate the scientific literature; and apply the information to the targeted group of patients. Evidence-based medicine techniques are used in health care organizations in the development and implementation of a variety of quality assurance tools (e.g., therapeutic guidelines, clinical pathways, MUEs, and disease state management) in an effort to improve patient outcomes and decrease costs. All of these situations require pharmacists to use medication information skills and to have various kinds of medication information support at the practice site or easily accessible at a remote site. The process of evidence-based medicine requires that systems be developed to measure and report processes and outcomes that can be used to drive quality improvement efforts. Data can be collected and analyzed by a medication information specialist using scientific methods to support the decision-making process in a managed care organization. Outcomes research can be used to identify the effectiveness of pharmaceutical products and services in achieving desired health outcomes. Likewise, the branch of outcomes research, pharmacoeconomics, provides tools to assess cost, consequences, and efficiency.[60] This will be discussed more fully in Chap. 8.

Sophistication of Medication Therapy

The sophisticated level of medication therapy that occurs today provides pharmacists much more opportunity to lend their expertise in assessing medication information needs of professionals, patients, or family members, and providing literature to help choose the best medication to use within a class, to convey the appropriate information to help patients correctly and safely use the more potent medications, and to address administration and delivery problems. It is increasingly difficult for physicians and other health professionals to keep up with all of the developments in medication therapy, as well as keep abreast of the other information required for their practice. It is estimated that over 1600 compounds are in various stages of drug development.[61] Several of these drugs could have a substantial impact on clinical practice and drug expenditures once they are commercially available. For instance, it is anticipated that at least 560 of these medications are anticancer agents, which could have an impact on life expectancy, quality of life, and the related expenses associated with the potential need for increased ancillary care, additional physician office visits, or hospitalization.[55] It is important that drugs in the pipeline be monitored by pharmacists to provide adequate time to identify the patient population that will most benefit from the new drug and to help anticipate the cost of treating these patients compared to traditional therapy.[55,61]

There is also a trend toward individualization of health care using DNA profiling to determine potential drug effectiveness.[62] Patients may be tested for genomic patterns and their drug therapy will be altered accordingly. There are several potential benefits of using this pharmacogenomic technique: new effective treatments for a variety of medical conditions could be identified faster and in smaller samples, computer modeling can help eliminate the medications that do not work, and because this technique can help identify the best candidates for a particular drug, it can help patients become more productive sooner.[63]

The Self-Care Movement

Finally, consumers have a continually growing desire for information about their medications. The growth of the self-care movement, the increase in focus on health care costs, and the improved accessibility of health information are some of the factors that have influenced patients to participate more fully in health care decisions, including the selection and use of medications. Based on these needs, direct-to-consumer advertising (DTCA) campaigns have appeared in virtually all media including magazines, television ads, and radio reports. In 1996, for the first time ever, the amount spent on DTCA exceeded the amount spent on direct advertising to physicians.[64] In 1997, the pharmaceutical industry spent over $1 billion on DTCA, which is up 61% from 1996.[65] Today, it is estimated that pharmaceutical companies spend about $3 billion per year.[66] This increase in spending for DTCA may be in response to the increase in sales for these drugs.[67]

Likewise, there is a growing use of e-mail and the web by the public. A recent survey found that approximately 25% of individuals with home access to the Internet searched medical websites prior to arrival at a neurology clinic.[68] Unfortunately, 60% of the information was considered to be inappropriate. Because a single individual is able to serve as author, editor, and publisher of information on the Internet, there is no safeguard on the quality of information provided. The end result is a potentially misinformed consumer.[69-70] When patients find information about medications that they are either considering to start taking or are currently taking, from the Internet, through the lay press, or by DTCA, a pharmacist can help consumers critically assess the medication information and add to the information based on specific patient-related needs.

The need to critically assess information regarding complementary and alternative medicine has become increasingly important, with an estimated one of three Americans choosing to use this option.[60] The use of dietary supplements continues to grow in popularity.[71-74] This area presents a challenging situation for pharmacists because of the lack of relevant outcomes data from well-designed clinical trials. Consumers are increasingly interested in finding reliable information regarding these products; pharmacists are in an excellent position to help provide such information. One drug information center describes its experience with a devoted telephone line to provide information regarding herbal supplements.[75,76] There was an increased demand for the service over time based on a higher call volume. This is consistent with the growing use of complementary and alternative medicine nationally. They also described the challenges and limitations of finding reliable information on herbal products. Several resources are available that have information on herbal products. It is just as important that the pharmacist provides information from reliable sources, as well as identify information that is lacking, in regard to a particular product.

Groups like the National Council on Patient Information and Education (NCPIE) encourage patients to seek information when they have questions. The experience with some medication information hotlines that have been established for public access has indicated public desire and need for information.[77] Such hotlines, often established by pharmacists, are intended to enhance the relationships between pharmacists, physicians, and patients.

The changing environment affords the pharmacist many opportunities to use the full spectrum of medication information skills. Factors such as the integration of new technologies, the focus on evidence-based medicine and drug policy development, the sophistication of medication therapy, and the advent of consumerism require that all pharmacists have a strong foundation in medication information concepts.

EDUCATING FOR THE NEED

The education of pharmacists continues to evolve in scope and depth. Many areas identified as needed by the drug (medication) information specialist are now incorporated into pharmacy curricula and taught to all pharmacists. In 1991, a consensus conference in New Mexico was held to define a set of objectives for didactic and experiential training in drug information for the year 2000.[78] Twenty-three educators and practitioners participated in the conference. There were several key concepts that were developed including (1) drug information should be a required component of the pharmacy curriculum and include both didactic and competency-based experiential components (2) drug information concepts and skills should be spread throughout the curriculum, beginning the day students enter pharmacy school and (3) problem solving should be a major technique in drug information education, with the goal of developing self-directed learners. Developing these skills should provide the foundation for the pharmacist to be a lifelong learner and problem solver. Based on the work of this conference, as well as changes in the health care system, and the movement toward outcome-based education, colleges of pharmacy are redesigning their curricula to provide a more comprehensive and integrated approach to teaching medication information concepts and skills.[79–80] Communication skills are taught formally to facilitate the pharmacist's ability to transmit information to both health professionals and patients. Medication information and policy development are integrated throughout the three goal areas addressed in the pharmacy practice residency standards. Specialty practice residencies in medication information are also available in a variety of practice sites at (www.ashp.org/ directories/ residency/).

Opportunities in Specialty Practice

As the role of the practicing pharmacist changed regarding medication information activities, so has the role of the specialist. The role of the medication information specialist has changed from an individual who specifically answers questions to one who focuses on the development of medication policies and provides information on complex medication information questions. A specialist in medication information can provide leadership in a contract drug information center, medical informatics, health maintenance organizations (HMOs) and pharmacy benefit management organizations (PBMs), managed care organizations, scientific writing and medical communications, poison control, pharmaceutical industry, and academia. In a recent survey that examined the career paths of pharmacists who completed a drug information specialty residency in 2000 and 2001, the types of careers were diverse. However, the most common positions were in industry (32%), academia (21%), medical writing (12%), and as a specialist in an institution (9%).[81] A specialist in medication information can be involved in multiple activities in establishments listed in the following section.

CONTRACT DRUG INFORMATION CENTER (FEE-FOR-SERVICE)

The need for accurate information pertaining to drug therapy is more acute today than ever before in the history of health care. One estimate suggests that prescription drug expenditures will increase at an average rate of 11.1% between 2002 and 2012.[55] Within the next decade health care costs will increase at an alarming rate, with total expenditures reaching the $2.1 trillion mark. A majority of these costs will be shouldered by the private sector with a significant increase in prescription drug costs. Drug information practitioners are in an enviable position to provide a service that will improve patient outcomes and decrease health care costs through the provision of unbiased information that supports rational, cost-effective, patient- and disease-specific drug therapy. One of the best ways to deliver such information is by contracting with a drug information service with formally trained health care professionals. Potential clients include managed care groups, contract pharmacy services, pharmacy benefits managers, buying groups, small rural hospitals, chain pharmacies, and independent pharmacies. Several different fee structures have been used. A client may be charged a simple fee per question, or may be offered a detailed menu of services (written medication evaluations, continuing education programs, guideline development for particular diseases) with the final cost dependent on the number and types of services chosen by the contracting party.

Services provided within these contracts may include providing answers to drug information requests, preparation of new drug evaluation monographs, formulary drug class reviews, development of MUE criteria, providing journal reprints, pharmacoeconomics evaluations, writing a pharmacotherapy newsletter, and providing continuing education programming. Additional services the center may make available are access to online resources, access to in-house question files for sharing information on commonly asked questions, and direct access to the center's Internet home page for review of medical use evaluations, formulary reviews, and newsletters.[82] One center reports providing information on drug shortages to the American Society of Health-System Pharmacists through a grant.[83] Frequently, the contracting drug information center also has responsibilities for pharmacy services (drug information, drug policy) as part of an entire health system.

MEDICAL INFORMATICS IN A HEALTH SYSTEM

With the growth and development of new technologies (e.g., information systems), there are tremendous opportunities for an informatics specialist—an individual who has advanced medication information skills with a keen understanding of computer and information technology. This individual can help support the concepts of pharmaceutical care by improving the efficiency of workflow and increasing access to patient-specific information and the medical literature through technology by remote-site availability. This individual may also be involved in the area of institutional drug policy management. As more information is computerized (e.g., medical records), data that were accessible only through a paper record will be available for those professionals who understand the type of data that are needed for quality improvement efforts, and are able to get information efficiently out of the system.[84] As database designs evolve and become user friendly and computer systems become more sophisticated, there are increasing opportunities for applying computer technology using clinical decision support systems to enhance many aspects of the medication use process. Clinical decision support systems can integrate patient-specific information, perform complex evaluations, and present this information to a clinician in a timely manner. These systems can be used to support initiatives with ADR reporting and analysis programs, formulary management, and continuous quality improvement efforts.

HEALTH MAINTENANCE ORGANIZATIONS (HMOS)/PHARMACY BENEFIT MANAGEMENT ORGANIZATIONS (PBMS)/MANAGED CARE ORGANIZATIONS (MCOS)

A key opportunity identified in a strategic planning meeting in 1994 by the Consortium for the Advancement of Medication Information, Policy and Research (CAMIPR) was the growing role for medication information specialists in the area of medication policy development/research and technology.[85] Since pharmaceuticals account for approximately 10% of health care dollars, which is up from 7% 5 years earlier, this offers tremendous opportunities for the medication information specialist to provide leadership in the development and implementation of mechanisms to support the cost-effective selection and use of medications in HMOs, PBMs, and managed care organizations.[86] The specialist may coordinate activities relating to formulary development and implementation, ADE reporting and analysis, and therapeutic guideline development. Medical and pharmaceutical outcomes research has been an increasing interest among health care providers, payers, and regulatory agencies. With appropriate training (e.g., specialized residency in medication information practice or managed care experience) and expertise, opportunities are growing for the medication information specialist in the insurance industry, HMOs, managed care organizations, pharmacy benefits management companies, state and national government agencies (e.g., Medicaid and Medicare), as well as other groups interested in the cost-efficient use of medications.

A pharmacist in any of these organizations has the opportunity to evaluate new information for medications on the market and assess its true value in a target group of patients. Prior to approval by the FDA, drugs undergo testing in a limited number of patients. Once approved, experience in patients escalates and previously unrecognized, rare adverse events may be identified. The drug may also be found to be useful for conditions not described in the labeling. Perhaps one of the most important functions of postmarketing surveillance is in the area of ADR reporting. This type of analysis can answer questions about drug interactions, identify potential new indications for the product, and study patients in a broader population. Organizations with a relatively large patient population offer opportunities to study these issues under the leadership of a medication information specialist.

Opportunities also exist to establish guidelines for selected disease states (e.g., management of patients with diabetes mellitus) or classes of drugs (e.g., selection of appropriate antibiotic for surgical prophylaxis). Practice guidelines are becoming an increasingly important part of the biomedical literature. These clinical guidelines are systematically developed to assist practitioners and patients with decisions about health care in an effort to improve the quality and consistency of health care while minimizing costs and liability.[87] Evidence-based practice guidelines are developed through systematic reviews of the literature appropriately adapted to local circumstances and values. Key questions to consider when reviewing a practice guideline have been proposed.[88] These questions primarily rely on how accurately the guideline reflects the research used to produce it. More information on therapeutic guidelines can be found in Chap. 9.

POISON CONTROL

Poison information is a specialized area of medication information with the practitioner typically practicing in an accredited poison information center or an emergency room. Similar to the mission of traditional drug information centers, poison information centers exist to provide accurate and timely information to enhance the quality of care of patients. There are, however, several differences between a traditional drug information center and poison control center. Health professionals generate most consultations received in drug information centers, whereas, in a poison control center, most are generated from the public. Poison information centers must be prepared to provide information on the management of any poison situation, including household products, poisonous plants and animals, medications, and other chemicals. Because of the type of information that the specialist provides, nearly all requests for information to a poison control center are urgent, with an average response time of 5-minutes, compared to anywhere from 30 minutes to days for drug information centers depending on the urgency of the call and complexity of information required. A specialist in poison information therefore requires expertise in clinical toxicology, as well as an ability to obtain a complete history that correctly assesses the potential severity of exposure, an understanding of where to search for this type of information, and the ability to communicate the information and plan in a comprehensive, concise, and accurate manner to consumers with varied levels of education. Because of the unique expertise of this type of specialist, a national certification examination is offered through the American Association of Poison Control Centers (AAPCC, <<http://www.aapcc.org/>>). In addition to a poison control center providing information regarding individual patients, centers in the United States also contribute data to a larger program through the Toxic Exposure Surveillance System (TESS), which is coordinated by the AAPCC. These data can be used to compare safety profiles for similar products, to develop risk assessment guidelines for specific substances, to target national prevention programs, and to conduct postmarketing surveillance on products (e.g., chemicals).

Despite the impact that regional poison control centers have on reducing morbidity and mortality with poison exposures, they are also facing increasing emphasis on economic justification. One study used decision analysis to compare the cost-effectiveness of treatment of poison exposures with the services of a regional poison control center to treatment without access to any poison control center.[89] The average cost per patient treated with the services of a poison control center was almost half of that achieved without services of a poison control center. These results were consistent regardless of exposure type, average inpatient and emergency department costs, and clinical outcome probabilities.

PHARMACEUTICAL INDUSTRY

The pharmaceutical industry provides many career opportunities for pharmacists in a variety of areas including drug discovery, product development, information technology, training and development, scientific communications, health outcomes research, regulatory affairs, professional affairs, medical information services, and clinical research.[90–91] Within the area of medical information services, the pharmacist participates in typical types of activities such as answering drug information questions, reporting and monitoring ADRs, and providing information support to other departments. Other positions in medication information services include disease specialist, health outcomes associate, labeling associate, and medical or scientific writer. Pharmacists providing medication information in the pharmaceutical industry may also provide support for individuals responsible for drug formularies or participate in quality improvement efforts with the medication use process. In addition to providing written information on the drug product produced by the manufacturer, there are opportunities to provide additional information at pharmacy and therapeutics committees or state drug use review (DUR) boards. Pharmaceutical companies have extensive scientific data on their products; some of which are not available through other published sources or may require a formal FOI (freedom of information) request. Medication information specialists may also serve as reviewers for journal articles, evidence-based guidelines, and published drug monographs. Medication information specialists may interact with sales and marketing, participate with regulatory affairs issues, and handle product complaints.

Pharmacists with specialized training can take a leadership role in evaluating current research, helping to manage ongoing research, or designing studies to help answer questions about new indications for future use of the product. The impact of new medications on the health care environment is also felt within the pharmaceutical industry. The area of health outcomes research is fairly new and growing and offers tremendous opportunity for pharmacists to share their knowledge of the health care environment, research design, technology, and economics from the perspective of the pharmaceutical industry. As the sophistication of drug products and information management (e.g., electronic new drug applications [NDAs]) has increased, so have the opportunities for pharmacists to practice in the pharmaceutical industry and focus on using the skills of a medication information specialist.

ACADEMIA

The medication information specialist has the opportunity to provide leadership in the pharmacy curriculum, including both didactic and experiential training. In addition to teaching medication information skills that are required across practice sites, the specialist also serves as a collaborator with other faculty on cases and activity designed to reinforce drug information skills for students. Approximately one-third of drug information centers are funded by a college of pharmacy. This environment allows the student to be prepared to efficiently and accurately provide information to the appropriate audience, while emphasizing both didactic and competency-based experiential training.

SCIENTIFIC WRITING AND MEDICAL COMMUNICATION

Medical education and communications companies may provide educational programming to meet continuing education needs (e.g., symposia, workshops, and monographs) or nonaccredited or promotional activities (e.g., sales training, publication planning, and journal articles).

Over 180 companies were providing this service in 2001.[92] In addition to having good writing skills, the pharmacist also needs to have scientific expertise and literature evaluation skills.[93] More than 77% of medical education and communication companies employ at least one licensed health care professional. These professionals may have several positions including director and scientific writer. Pharmacists in this capacity would probably work closely with editors, graphic designers, meeting planners, and computer programmers. This type of information may be communicated in a variety of ways including orally, in print format, and electronically on the web (e.g., e-Medicine).

Summary and Direction for the Future

All pharmacists must be effective medication information providers regardless of their practice. As defined by the New Mexico Conference, an effective provider perceives, assesses, and evaluates medication information needs and retrieves, evaluates, communicates, and applies data from the published literature and other sources as an integral component of patient care. If the profession is to be successful in accepting patient care responsibilities, all pharmacists must have a certain minimum level of skill to survive in the changing practice environment. Developing the skills of an effective medication information provider is the foundation for the pharmacist to be a lifelong learner and problem solver. The literature is a valuable component of both of these processes and will allow the individual pharmacist to adapt to the needs of a continually changing health care system.

Opportunities abound for pharmacists to use medication information skills in all practice settings either as a generalist or a specialist practitioner. There is still the need for the practitioner to have support from drug information centers to meet special information needs, to serve as a resource on effective medication use, and to assist pharmacy practitioners as well as others in solving medication therapy situations. Individuals with special training as medication information specialists will still be needed to operate the centers and to provide leadership in the area of drug informatics, institutional drug policy, poison control, pharmaceutical industry, and in academia.

REFERENCES

1. Parker PF. The University of Kentucky drug information center. Am J Hosp Pharm. 1965;22:42–7.
2. Amerson AB, Wallingford DM. Twenty years' experience with drug information centers. J Hosp Pharm. 1983;40:1172–8.
3. Walton CA. The problem of communicating clinical drug information. J Hosp Pharm. 1965;22:458–63.

4. Lowe HJ, Barnett GO. Understanding and using the medical subject headings (MESH) vocabulary to perform literature searches. JAMA. 1994;271:1103–18.
5. Institute of Medicine. Health professions education: a bridge to quality. Washington, DC: National Academy Press; 2003.
6. Mehnert RB. A world of knowledge for the nation's health: The U.S. National Library of Medicine. J Hosp Pharm. 1986;43:2991–7.
7. Walton CA. Education and training of the drug information specialist. Drug Intell. 1967;1:133–7.
8. Francke DE. The role of the pharmacist as a drug information specialist. J Hosp Pharm. 1966;23:49.
9. Koumis T, Cicero LA, Nathan JP, Rosenberg JM. Directory of pharmacist-operated drug information centers in the United States—2003. J Health Syst Pharm. 2004;61:2033–42.
10. Rosenberg JM, Koumis T, Nathan JP, Cicero LA, McGuire H. Current status of pharmacist-operated drug information centers in the United States. J Health Syst Pharm. 2004;61:2023–32.
11. Drug topics red book. Montvale(NJ). Medical Economics; 2004.
12. Kinky DE, Erush SC, Laskin MS, Gibson GA. Economic impact of a drug information service. Ann Pharmacother. 1999;33:11–6.
13. LaFleur J, Tyler LS, Sharma RR. Economic benefits of investigational drug services at an academic institution. Am J Health Syst Pharm. 2004;61:27–32.
14. Study Commission on Pharmacy. Pharmacists for the future. Ann Arbor (MI): Health Administration Press; 1975. p. 139.
15. Hepler CD, Strand LM. Opportunities and responsibilities in pharmaceutical care. Am J Hosp Pharm. 1990;47:533–50.
16. American Society of Health-System Pharmacists. ASHP guidelines on the provision of medication information by pharmacists. Am J Health Syst Pharm. 1996;53:1843–5.
17. Kohn LT, Corrigan JM, Donaldson MS. To err is human: building a safer health care system. Washington, DC: National Academy Press; 1999.
18. Vioxx (rofecoxib) information [monograph on the Internet]. Washington: Food and Drug Administration; 2005 [accessed 2005 Oct 5]. Available from: http://www.fda.gov/cder/drug/infopage/vioxx/default.htm
19. Stricker BH, Psaty BM. Detection, verification, and quantification of adverse drug reactions. BMJ. 2004;329:44–7.
20. Landis NT. ADE rate uncertain, reporting systems inadequate, GAO tells legislators. Am J Health Syst Pharm. 2000;57:515–9.
21. Grissinger M. Adverse drug reactions: documentation is important, but communication is critical. P&T. 2004;29:5.
22. ASHP guidelines on adverse drug reaction monitoring and reporting. Am J Health Syst Pharm. 1995;52:417–9.
23. Fink JL, Vivian JC, Keller RK, editors. Pharmacy law digest. St Louis (MO): Facts and Comparisons; 1999.
24. FDA issues regulation prohibiting sale of dietary supplements containing ephedrine alkaloids and reiterates its advice that consumers stop using these products [monograph on the Internet]. Washington: Food and Drug Administration; 2004 Feb 6 [accessed 2005 Oct 5]. Available from: http://www.fda.gov/bbs/topics/NEWS/2004/NEW01021.html

25. FDA letter warning health care professionals about kava. Available from: http://www.fda.gov/medwatch/safety/2001/kava.htm

26. Ansani NT, Ciliberto NC, Freedy T. Hospital policies regarding herbal medicines. Am J Health Syst Pharm. 2003;60:367-70.

27. Wachter RM. The end of the beginning: patient safety five years after "To Err Is Human." Health Aff [serial on the Internet]. 2004 Nov 30 [accessed 2005 Oct 5]: [about 9 p.]. Available from: http://content.healthaffairs.org/cgi/content/full/hlthaff. w4.534/DC1

28. Johnson ST, Wordell CJ. Internet utilization among medical information specialists in the pharmaceutical industry and academia. Drug Inf J. 1998;32:547-54.

29. Malone PM, Young WW, Malesker MA. Wide area network connecting a hospital drug informatics center with a university. Am J Health Syst Pharm. 1998;55:1146-50.

30. Berland GK, Elliott MN, Morales LS, Algazy JL, Kravitz RL. Health information on the Internet: accessibility, quality, and readability in English and Spanish. JAMA. 2001;285:2612-21.

31. Kim P, Eng TR, Deering MJ, Maxfield A. Published criteria for evaluating health related websites: review. BMJ. 1999;318:647-9.

32. Murray E, Pollack L, Donelan K, Catania J, Lee K. The impact of health information on the Internet on health care and the physician-patient relationship: national U.S. survey among 1050 U.S. physicians. J Med Internet Res. 2003;5:e17.

33. Belgado BS. Drug information centers on the Internet. J Am Pharm Assoc. 2001;41:631-2.

34. Dugas M, Weinzierl S, Pecar A, Hasford J. Am J Health Syst Pharm. 2001;58:799-802.

35. Ruppelt SC, Vann R. Marketing a hospital-based drug information center. 2001;58;1040.

36. Erbele SM, Heck AM, Blankenship CS. Survey of computerized documentation system use in drug information centers. Am J Health Syst Pharm. 2001;58:695-7.

37. McCreadie SR, Stevenson JG, Sweet BV, Kramer M. Using personal digital assistants to access drug information. Am J Health Syst Pharm. 2002;59:1340-3.

38. Brody JA, Camamo JM, Maloney ME. Implementing a personal digital assistant to document clinical interventions by pharmacy residents. Am J Health Syst Pharm. 2001;58:1520-2.

39. Barrons R. Evaluation of personal digital assistant software for drug interactions. Am J Health Syst Pharm. 2004;61:380-5.

40. Silva MA, Tataronis GR, Maas B. Using personal digital assistants to document pharmacist cognitive services and estimate potential reimbursement. Am J Health Syst Pharm. 2003;60:911-5.

41. Reilly JC, Wallace M, Campbell MM. Tracking pharmacist interventions with a hand-held computer. Am J Health Syst Pharm. 2001;58:158-61.

42. Lau A, Balen RM, Lam R, Malyuk DL. Using a personal digital assistant to document clinical pharmacy services in an intensive care unit. Am J Health Syst Pharm. 2001;58:1229-32.

43. Lynx DH, Brockmiller HR, Connelly RT, Crawford SY. Use of PDA-based pharmacist intervention system. Am J Health Syst Pharm. 2003;60:2341-4.

44. Grasso BC, Genest R, Yung K, Arnold C. Reducing errors in discharge medication lists by using personal digital assistants. Psychiatr Serv. 2002;53:1325-6.

45. Clark JS, Klauck JA. Recording pharmacists' interventions with a personal digital assistant. Am J Health Syst Pharm. 2003;60:1772-4.

46. Clauson KA, Seamon MJ, Clauson AS, Van TB. Evaluation of drug information databases for personal digital assistants. Am J Health Syst Pharm. 2004;61:1015-24.

47. Lowry CM, Kkostka-Rokosz MD, McCloskey WW. Evaluation of personal digital assistant drug information databases for the managed care pharmacist. J Manag Care Pharm. 2003;9:441–8.

48. Elson RB, Connelly DP. Computerized medical records in primary care and their role in mediating guideline-driven physician behavior change. Arch Fam Med. 1995;4:698–705.

49. Evans RS, Pestotnik SL, Classen DC, Clemmer TP, Weaver LK, Orme JF, Jr. et al. A computer-assisted management program for antibiotics and other anti-infective agents. N Engl J Med. 1998;338:232–8.

50. Hunt DL, Haynes RB, Hanna SE, Smith K. Effects of computer-based clinical support systems on physician performance and patient outcomes: a systematic review. JAMA. 1998;280:1339–46.

51. Rind DM, Kohane IS, Szolovits P, et al. Maintaining the confidentiality of medical records shared over the Internet and world wide web. Ann Intern Med. 1997;127:138–44.

52. Frisse ME. What is the Internet learning about you while you are learning about the Internet? Acad Med. 1996;71:1064–107.

53. Giacalone RP, Cacciatore GG. HIPAA and its impact on pharmacy practice. Am J Health Syst Pharm. 2003;60:433–45.

54. Blank C. Spending on pharmaceuticals will pass $180 billion by 2008. Hosp Pharma Rep. 1998;12:54.

55. Hoffman JM, Shah ND, Vermeulen LC, Hunkler RJ, Hontz KM. Projecting future expenditures—2005. Am J Health Syst Pharm. 2005;62:149–67.

56. Altman DE. The new medicare prescription drug legislation. N Engl J Med. 350:1:9–10.

57. Institute of Medicine. Insuring America's health: principles and recommendations. Washington, DC; 2004.

58. Opportunities for the community pharmacist in managed care. Special Report. Washington, DC: American Pharmaceutical Association; 1994.

59. Ellrodt G, Cook DJ, Lee J, Cho M, Hunt D, Weingarten S. Evidence-based disease management. JAMA. 1997;278:1687–92.

60. Vermeulen LC, Beis SJ, Cano SB. Applying outcomes research in improving the medication-use process. Am J Health Syst Pharm. 2000;57:2277–82.

61. Top 10 areas of research: report on the most popular fields of drug development. Med Ad News. 2003;137:22:S22.

62. Emilien G, Ponchon M, Caldas C, et al. Impact of genomics on drug discovery and clinical medicine. Q J Med. 2000;93:391–423.

63. Epler GR, Laskaris LL. Individualization health care and the pharmaceutical industry. Am J Health Syst Pharm. 2001;58:1042.

64. Special feature: direct-to-consumer advertising. Med Mark Media. 1996;15:8.

65. Piturro M. D-T-C thrives. Managed Health Care News. 1998;14:1.

66. Young D. FDA examines direct-to-consumer advertising data. Am J Health Syst Pharm. 2003;60:2420–1.

67. Basara LR. The impact of a direct-to-consumer prescription medication advertising campaign on new prescription volume. Drug Inf J. 1996;30:715–29

68. Larner AJ. Use of Internet medical websites and of NHS direct by neurology outpatients before consultation [abstract]. J Neurol Neurosurg Psychiatry. 2002;72:140.

69. Silberg W, Lundberg GD, Musacchio RA. Assessing, controlling, and assuring the quality of medical information on the Internet. JAMA. 1997;277:1244–5.

70. Wyatt J. Measuring quality and impact on the world wide web. BMJ. 1997;314:1879–81.
71. Practice and Policy Guidelines Panel, National Institutes of Health Office of Alternative Medicine. Clinical practice guidelines in complementary and alternative medicine an analysis of opportunities and obstacles. Arch Fam Med. 1997;6:149–54.
72. McQueen CE, Shields KM, Generali JA. Motivations for dietary supplement use. Am J Health Syst Pharm. 2003;60:655.
73. Pal S. Herbal sales reach mainstream market. US Pharm. 1999;24:12.
74. Eisenberg DM, Davis RB, Ettner SL, et al. Trends in alternative medicine use in the United States, 1990–1997: results of a national survey. JAMA. 1998:280:1569–75.
75. Shields KM, McQueen CE, Bryant PJ. National survey of dietary supplement resources at drug information centers. J Am Pharm Assoc. 2004;44:36–40.
76. West PM, Lodolce AE, Johnston AK. Telephone service for providing consumers with information on herbal supplements. Am J Health Syst Pharm. 2001;58:1842–6.
77. Meade V. Patient medication information hotlines multiply. Am Pharm. 1991;NS31:569–71.
78. Troutman WG. Consensus-derived objectives for drug information education. Drug Inf J. 1994;28:791–6.
79. Ferrill MJ, Norton LL. Drug information to biomedical informatics: a three tier approach to building a university system for the twenty-first century. Am J Pharm Edu. 1997;61:81–6.
80. Gora-Harper ML, Brandt B. An educational design to teach drug information across the curriculum. Am J Pharm Educ. 1997;61:296–302.
81. Miller S, Clarke A. Impact of postdoctoral specialty residencies in drug information on graduates' career paths. Am J Health Syst Pharm. 2002;59:961–3.
82. Forrester LP, Scoggin JA, Valle RD. Pharmacy management company-negotiated contract for drug information services. Am J Health Syst Pharm. 1995;52:1074–7.
83. Fox ER, Tyler LS. Managing drug shortages: seven years' experience at one health-system. Am J Health Syst Pharm. 2003;60:245–53.
84. Woodruff AE, Hunt CA. Involvement in medical informatics may enable pharmacists to expand their consultation potential and improve the quality of health care. Ann Pharmacother. 1992;26:100–4.
85. Vanscoy GJ, Gajewski LK, Tyler LS, Gora-Harper ML, Grant KL, May JR. The future of medication information practices: a consensus. Ann Pharmacother. 1996;30:876–81.
86. Warren PN. Pharmacists to the fore. Managed Health Care News. 1997;13:20H–20I.
87. Zinberg S. Practice guidelines—a continuing debate. Clin Obstet Gynecol. 1998;41:343–7.
88. Field JM, Lohr KN, editors. Guidelines for clinical practice: from development to use. Washington, DC: National Academy Press; 1992.
89. Harrison MAJ, Draugalis JR, Slack MK, Langley PC. Cost-effectiveness of regional poison control centers. Arch Intern Med. 1996;156:2601–8.
90. Gong SD, Millares M, VanRiper KB. Drug information pharmacists at health-care facilities, universities, and pharmaceutical companies. Am J Hosp Pharm. 1992;49:1121–30.
91. Riggins JL. Pharmaceutical industry as a career choice. Am J Health Syst Pharm. 2002;59:2097–8.
92. Overstreet KM. Medical education and communication companies: career options for pharmacists. Am J Health Syst Pharm. 2003;60:1896–7.
93. Moghadam RG. Scientific writing: a career for pharmacists. Am J Health Syst Pharm. 2003;60:1899–1900.

2

Chapter Two

Modified Systematic Approach to Answering Questions

Craig F. Kirkwood • Karen L. Kier

Objectives

After completing this chapter, the reader will be able to

- When presented with a drug information question and given requestor demographics, determine pertinent background information.
- On determining and soliciting the most important background information, categorize the ultimate question and develop an efficient search strategy.
- On evaluating the drug information and literature obtained from a search, formulate a response appropriate for the sophistication of the requestor.
- List the categories of drug information questions that are appropriate for follow-up.
- Given three different practice settings, identify one potential question that would benefit from using the modified systematic approach and describe the advantages of the approach for each potential question identified.

An essential component within pharmacy practice is the ability to effectively answer questions posed by health care professionals and the lay public. In 1975, Watanabe et al.[1] presented a systematic approach for responding to drug information requests. The systematic approach comprised of five steps, as outlined in Table 2–1, and was developed to provide instructions for pharmacy students. These concepts were expanded and embellished to produce a textbook on the subject of drug information services.[2] For several years the original article and subsequent textbook served as the core for training pharmacy students and practitioners about

TABLE 2–1. SYSTEMATIC APPROACH (1975)

Step I.	Classification of the request
Step II.	Obtaining background information
Step III.	Systematic search
Step IV.	Response
Step V.	Reclassification

SOURCES: From Watanabe et al.[1]

responding to drug information requests.[3] The systematic approach principles were utilized in assuring quality for drug information service responses, training in drug information skills, and developing and enhancing programs[4-6] (see Appendix 2–1). New technologies have facilitated the labor-intensive teaching of the systematic approach to students and practitioners, either in a modified version as the subject of a computer program[7] or as a module of a more complete drug information computer program.[8] The modified systematic approach has been adapted by others and used for the combined purposes of quality assurance and student evaluation in drug information clerkships.[9]

Modified Systematic Approach

Drug information services may use the systematic approach, or an adaptation of it, as the basis for responding to drug information inquiries (see Appendix 2–2); however, the utility of this approach is not limited to the confines of a drug information center. These approaches can be applied in any area while practicing pharmacy, including community pharmacy, pharmaceutical industry, institutional pharmacy management, as well as general application in any type of professional consultation. The steps to the modified systematic approach, as described in Table 2–2, will be reviewed in this chapter.

TABLE 2–2. MODIFIED SYSTEMATIC APPROACH (1987)

Step I.	Secure demographics of requestor
Step II.	Obtain background information
Step III.	Determine and categorize ultimate question
Step IV.	Develop strategy and conduct search
Step V.	Perform evaluation, analysis, and synthesis
Step VI.	Formulate and provide response
Step VII.	Conduct follow-up and documentation

SOURCES: From Host and Kirkwood.[7]

REQUESTOR DEMOGRAPHICS

The first step in the modified systematic approach is to accept the initial question and secure requestor demographics. Although the presentation of the initial question provides insight to the requestor's sophistication and knowledge regarding the subject matter, it is important to more directly determine the requestor's position, training, and anticipated knowledge. For example, an elderly patient and cardiovascular specialist may each inquire about the availability of an investigational medication; however, each brings a different frame of reference to the request, and the approach and final response to the request will differ for each requestor. In addition to information regarding the requestor's background, it is imperative to secure a mechanism for delivery of the response, regardless of the medium (e.g., verbal, written, and e-mail). Therefore, telephone number(s), fax number, pager number, and/or address (mail or e-mail) or location, and so forth, are important facts to obtain regarding the requestor.

BACKGROUND QUESTIONS

The ability to obtain background information to develop a more complete picture of the question is essential for effectively using the modified systematic approach. Historically, this step is the most difficult for both students and practicing pharmacists. If an individual can truly answer the question "Why is the requestor asking for this information?" then adequate background information has been obtained. To answer this question, the background information must be sufficiently comprehensive.

The background questions, therefore, must be appropriate for the circumstances. Some general information should always be obtained—for example, whether the request is concerning a specific patient's condition or is truly academic. Other background questions should be specific for the nature of the request. Examples of general background questions are provided in Table 2–3; examples of specific background questions are provided in Appendix 2–3. Background question inquiry and reply, when performed optimally, should be a dialogue. During this dialogue, the sequence and exact wording of each background

TABLE 2–3. GENERAL QUESTIONS FOR OBTAINING BACKGROUND INFORMATION

The requestor's name
The requestor's location and/or pager number
The requestor's affiliation (institution or practice) if a health care professional
The requestor's frame of reference (i.e., title, profession or occupation, and rank)
The resources that the requestor already consulted
Whether the request is patient specific or academic
The patient's diagnosis, other medications, and pertinent medical information
The urgency of the request (i.e., negotiate the time response)

SOURCE: Standard Questions for Obtaining Background Information from Requestors. *Drug Information Service, Department of Pharmacy Services, Medical College of Virginia Hospitals, ca. 1990.*

question must be dependent on the flow of the verbal interaction. Rarely will one obtain adequate background information by forcibly demanding such information.

Though often neglected, it is commonly useful to ascertain which resource(s) the requestor has checked or used. This information is useful to avoid duplication of effort; however, often individuals do not know how to effectively use the resource(s) available to them. The responder may need to double-check the used resources to verify the information present or better appreciate the requestor's understanding of the subject. Knowledge of resources used is also helpful in determining the baseline sophistication of the requestor. For example, one would consider the user of the primary literature to be more sophisticated than the requestor who only used a general reference.

Requestors who are intermediaries in the transfer of information present a special challenge for obtaining background. Intermediaries may include medical students, nurses, pharmacists, and administrators' assistants—generally anyone involved in the process that is not truly the end user of the response. In some situations, the intermediary may not have sufficient information to satisfy background questions. In other cases, the intermediary may put an incomplete "twist" on the background information according to the frame of reference. When dealing with intermediaries, one must decide to work with them (i.e., educate them concerning the information needed and why it is needed) or bypass them (i.e., interact with the end user of the information directly). Each option has its strengths and weaknesses and the decision must be made on a case-by-case basis. One should not allow an intermediary with incomplete or inaccurate background information to drive the consultative process.

With practice, the process of obtaining background information can become an admirable skill. When background questions are utilized appropriately, the response to information requests or inquiries is very efficient. Like other skills, however, obtaining background information requires practice to maintain the competence.

ULTIMATE QUESTION/CATEGORIZATION OF QUESTION

After a precursor of the modified systematic approach was instituted, a survey of drug information questions answered by the Drug Information Service at the Medical College of Virginia Hospitals over a 6-month period was performed. In 85% of the questions, the subject researched (termed the ultimate question) was significantly different than the original question—such that provision of the final response would not have agreed with the initial question. For these questions (i.e., disagreement between original question and response provided), the requestor was satisfied with the response provided (i.e., the answer to the ultimate question). This disparity demonstrates that refocusing the requestor's question was useful for most of the drug information requests in the survey.

The determination of the ultimate question is important for effective use of the modified systematic approach. If background information is obtained in an open, productive exchange, the ultimate question is easily unveiled; if adequate background information is not obtained, the determination of the ultimate question may not be possible. The ultimate question may essentially be the same as the original question, particularly if the question is truly not patient specific. An example of the difference between an original question and the ultimate question (which was researched) is provided in Appendix 2–4. In this case, responding to the original question possibly would have precluded two therapeutic options—one because the original drug may not have been readily available for the specific patient's disease, and the other because an equally effective, unrestricted alternative may not have been fully considered. More information on this can be found in Chap. 3. Occasionally, the pursuit of the ultimate question provides an opportunity for injection of another professional's perspective, and this process alone may lead to consideration of other useful therapeutic approaches.

It is imperative that the requestor confirms the ultimate question prior to categorization and the development of a search strategy. To avoid having the requestor interpret the response to a different (the ultimate) question as condescending, the discussion must be tactful and oriented toward the attainment of the common goal of both the requestor and responder.

Once the ultimate question has been decided and acknowledged, the question is categorized. The categorization is useful not only for the initial development of the search strategy, but also for the determination of resources and staff training to be maintained. Categorization schemes vary among drug information services; the best scheme is the one that is closest to meeting the service needs. An example of a categorization scheme, with the selection of a category for an ultimate question, is shown in Appendix 2–2. Once an ultimate question is categorized, the development of a search strategy is initiated.

SEARCH STRATEGY

The categorization of the ultimate question prompts the resource selection process. For example, the categorization of a question as "adverse effect" suggests the use of adverse effect oriented resources. Once resources have been selected, they are prioritized based on the probability of their containing the information or data desired. Without prioritization, resources may be utilized based on ease of access or degree of comfort instead of probable efficiency. Further information on search strategy is found in Chap. 3 and the drug information resources have been thoroughly characterized in Chap. 4.

DATA EVALUATION, ANALYSIS, AND SYNTHESIS

At this step in the modified systematic approach, the information retrieved must be objectively critiqued. The techniques and skills for literature evaluation and clinical application of statistical analysis, as discussed in detail in Chaps. 6 and 7, are applied at this juncture. Application of these skills at this step is one of the opportunities to differentiate the professional from the technician through using the modified systematic approach. The analysis and synthesis must be performed with consideration of the background information, obtained previously, for the response to be pertinent and useful to the requestor.

FORMULATION AND PROVISION OF RESPONSE

Although one cannot absolutely know how another individual will use the information provided, a responder should think about how the soon-to-be-provided information may be used. This thought process should reference the background information received when formulating the search question. While it would be unethical to misrepresent results of the analysis and synthesis of the literature evaluated, one may formulate a response that discourages a reaction that the responder believes is not supported by the interpretation of the literature. As a consultant, one has a professional responsibility to clearly inform the requestor when one course of action is clearly more desirable than an alternate action. This consideration is not an issue when the analysis and synthesis of literature or information leads to an equivocal conclusion concerning two mutually exclusive courses of action.

If the literature includes conflicting data that must be presented to the requestor, one may need to use a logical argument. Should only one side of the conflict be presented, the requestor may not benefit from the complete picture or may mistrust the responder on later learning that another aspect of the conflict was not represented. The steps to follow in this scenario, after restatement of the ultimate question, are presented in Table 2–4. Despite the setting or circumstances, the formulated response must be succinct yet adequately comprehensive.

The provision of a response is essential in the modified systematic approach. If the response is not provided in a timely manner or is delivered at an inappropriate level of sophistication, conceivably the effort expended would be wasted. The subject of written communications will be considered in Chap. 11, and will not be discussed here. Verbal communications, however, are more frequently used within most practice settings. The utilization of good verbal communication skills, from confident delivery to correct pronunciation of all terms, is imperative for ideal response provision. Often the delivery of a complete response is analogous to the delivery of a presentation or lecture—one must be prepared for additional questions and, therefore, the information presented is only part of the responder's total knowledge and preparation on the subject. The remnants from the process of preparing a succinct response are typically the material used for addressing additional minor questions.

TABLE 2–4. FORMAT FOR LOGICAL ARGUMENT IN RESPONSE FORMULATION

Step I.	Present the competing viewpoints or considerations
Step II.	State the assessment of the literature or information reviewed and claim the superior viewpoint
Step III.	Succinctly refute the major strengths and present weaknesses of the inferior viewpoint
Step IV.	Defend the major weaknesses and promote the strengths of the superior viewpoint
Step V.	Reiterate the final assessment in support of the superior viewpoint.

FOLLOW-UP, FOLLOW-THROUGH, AND DOCUMENTATION

Follow-up is the process of verifying the appropriateness, correctness, and completeness of a response following the communication. Not only is follow-up "good business," it presents a professional approach to consultative assistance. Certain circumstances command follow-up. Patient-specific requests, especially if judgmental (i.e., therapeutic assistance or dosing recommendations), are outstanding opportunities for follow-up. Any situation in which a therapeutic decision was dependent on assumptions or "soft" data is also a candidate for follow-up. Pharmacy services and practices, in addition to patients and health care providers, may benefit substantially through the provision of follow-up assistance. Providing follow-up assistance for responses that subsequently led to dependent administrative decisions can enhance the perception of service delivery and the quality of the complete response.

Follow-through is the process of readdressing a request based on the availability of new data or a change in the situation or circumstances that were decisive factors in the synthesis of a response. For example, the basis of a decision to use a novel therapy in a patient may be confirmed or refuted according to a new article. In the same scenario, the development of renal failure (as a comorbidity) in this patient may prompt an update of the original response. In most circumstances, the provision of follow-through may also be perceived as good practice. Providing an update when new information becomes available supports the responder's expertise and command of the literature. The update of current information would be particularly useful in chronic patient or administrative problems.

Thorough documentation is essential for reducing liability and potentially promoting the development of a continual service. The method of documentation may be a simple form or an extensive review and summation of all processes completed. At a minimum, the ultimate question (as verified by the requestor), the materials searched (with pertinent findings noted), the response, and follow-up (or follow-through, if applicable) should be documented. For reimbursement of services and credit of service delivery, it may be necessary to record the achievement of the objectives in service provision. Regarding professional liability concerns, an attorney familiar with the requirements of the specific locality may be consulted. The documentation of improved patient outcomes subsequent to a response for information would be an optimal method for justification of practices.[10]

Conclusion

More than 30 years ago, Watanabe et al. presented a systematic approach for responding to drug information requests. The systematic approach, which consisted of five steps as outlined in Table 2–1, was developed to provide instruction for pharmacy students. Modifications of the systematic approach (an example is outlined in Table 2–2) have been utilized by others in service provision, practice quality assurance, and student evaluation. The enhancements relative to the original systematic approach are reasonable when one considers the explosion of drug information in the last 30 years; the expansion, sophistication, and patient orientation of pharmacy services today; and the growth and advancement of drug information resources over the past three decades.

Study Questions

1. A caller requests information regarding the use of aspirin for the prevention of preeclampsia.
   a. List the steps involved in the modified systematic approach to answering questions. What is the importance of each of these steps?
   b. What specifics regarding caller demographics should be secured?
   c. What questions should be asked to obtain background information from the caller? Consider different questions that could be asked depending on the focus of the request (e.g., general information, dosage, method of administration, drug interactions, drug of choice, adverse effects, and teratogenicity).
   d. Depending on its focus, the request could be categorized in several ways. Considering the possible focuses listed in part c, categorize the question and develop possible search strategies.
   e. Considering the possible focuses listed in part c and various caller backgrounds (e.g., consumer, pharmacist, and physician), evaluate, analyze, and synthesize data to be used for answering the request.
   f. For the possible scenarios listed in part e, formulate oral and written responses to the request.
   g. For the possible scenarios listed in part e, consider follow-up questions that should be asked of the caller.

2. Considering three different practice settings (i.e., hospital, community pharmacy, pharmaceutical manufacturer, ambulatory clinic, and insurance company), identify potential questions that would benefit by using the modified systematic approach in formulating a response in each of those settings and describe the advantages of the approach for each potential question identified.

REFERENCES

1. Watanabe AS, McCart G, Shimomura S, Kayser S. Systematic approach to drug information requests. Am J Hosp Pharm. 1975;32(12):1282–5.
2. Watanabe AS, Conner CS. Principles of drug information services: a syllabus of systematic concepts. Hamilton (IL): Drug Intelligence Publications; 1978.

3. Limon L, Kirkwood CF, Moore AO, Mullins PM. Evaluating drug information performance of staff pharmacists [abstract]. Paper presented at the 22nd Annual ASHP Midyear Clinical Meeting; December 1987; Atlanta, GA.

4. Kirkwood CF, Jackson D. Effect of implementation of a quality assurance program on performance of a drug information service [abstract]. Paper presented at the 20th Annual ASHP Midyear Clinical Meeting; December 1985; New Orleans, LA.

5. Kirkwood CF. Quality assurance in drug information at the Medical College of Virginia Hospitals [abstract]. Paper presented at the 22nd Annual ASHP Midyear Clinical Meeting; December 1987; Atlanta, GA.

6. Kirkwood CF, Kessler JM. Influencing physician use of a drug information service [abstract]. Paper presented at the 19th Annual ASHP Midyear Clinical Meeting; December 1984; Dallas, TX.

7. Host TR, Kirkwood CF. Computer-assisted instruction for responding to drug information requests [abstract]. Paper presented at the 22nd Annual ASHP Midyear Clinical Meeting; December 1987; Atlanta, GA.

8. Tunget CL, Smith GH, Lipsy RJ, Schumacher RJ. Evaluation of DILearn: an interactive computer-assisted learning program for drug information. Am J Pharm Educ. 1993;57(4):340-3.

9. Restino MSR, Knodel LC. Drug information quality assurance program used to appraise students' performance. Am J Hosp Pharm. 1992;49(6):1425-9.

10. Hermes ER, Kirkwood CF, Mullins PM, Pugh MC, Memmott HL. Evaluation of impact of drug information responses on patient care [abstract]. Paper presented at the 27th Annual ASHP Midyear Clinical Meeting; December 1992; Orlando, FL.

3

Chapter Three

Formulating Effective Responses and Recommendations: A Structured Approach

Karim Anton Calis • Amy Heck Sheehan

Objectives

After completing this chapter, the reader will be able to

- Develop strategies to overcome the impediments that prevent pharmacists from providing effective responses and recommendations.
- Outline the steps that are necessary to identify the true drug information needs of the requestor.
- List and describe the four critical factors that should be considered and systematically evaluated when formulating a response.
- Define analysis and synthesis and explain how they are employed in the process of formulating responses and recommendations.
- List the elements and characteristics of effective responses to medication-related queries.

Pharmacists are asked to provide responses to a variety of drug information questions every day. While the type of requestor, query, and setting can vary, the process of formulating responses remains constant. This chapter elaborates on the basic concepts and principles presented in other chapters, and introduces an organized, structured approach for formulating effective responses and recommendations.

As the medical literature expands, access to drug information resources by health care professionals and the public continues to grow. Yet many professionals and consumers lack the necessary skills to use this information effectively. This presents an opportunity and a challenge for pharmacists who wish to become bonafide drug therapy experts and assume a broader role in health care.

Regardless of specialty or practice site, pharmacists must strive to become pharmacotherapy specialists. Whether in a community pharmacy, outpatient clinic, or at the hospital bedside, pharmacists can apply their knowledge to the care of patients. Pharmacists should not be relegated to the role of information dispenser or gatekeeper. Pharmacists must extend their knowledge of drugs and therapeutics to the clinical management of individual patients or the care of large populations. Moreover, they must promote rational pharmacotherapy by ensuring that drug information is appropriately interpreted and correctly applied.

Accepting Responsibility and Eliminating Barriers

Pharmacists should recognize that their responsibility extends beyond simply providing an answer to a question. Rather, it is to assist in resolving therapeutic dilemmas or managing patients' medication regimens. Knowledge of pharmacotherapy alone does not ensure success. Moreover, isolated data or information do not provide answers to questions or ensure proper patient management. In fact, it is uncommon to find comprehensive answers in the literature that completely and effectively address specific situations or circumstances that clinicians face in their daily practices. Responses and recommendations must often be thoughtfully synthesized using information and knowledge gathered from a number of diverse sources. To effectively manage the care of patients and resolve complex situations, pharmacists also need added skills and competence in problem solving and direct patient care.

For pharmacists to provide meaningful responses and effective recommendations to drug information questions, real or perceived impediments must first be overcome. One such impediment is the false perception that most drug information questions do not pertain to specific patients. Another is the perception that the seemingly casual interactions with requestors and the lack of formal, written consultation somehow preclude the need for in-depth analysis and extensive involvement in patient management. Pharmacists sometimes oversimplify their interactions with requestors and fail to identify the context of the question or recognize its significance. Absence of sufficient background information and pertinent patient data greatly diminish the ability of pharmacists to provide effective responses.

Identifying the Genuine Need

Most queries that pharmacists receive are not purely academic or general in nature. They often involve specific patients and unique circumstances. For example, a physician who asks about the association of lovastatin and liver toxicity is probably not asking this question whimsically or out of curiosity. He or she most likely has a patient who has developed hepatic impairment that may be associated with the use of this medication. Of course, other reasonable scenarios, albeit less likely, also could have prompted such a question. Even questions that are not related to patient care must be viewed in their proper context. Requestors of information are typically vague in verbalizing their needs and provide specific information only when asked. Although these requestors may seem confident about their perceived needs, they may be less certain after further probing by the pharmacist. Requestors, regardless of background, are often uncertain about what the pharmacist needs to know to assist them optimally. Therefore, critical information that defines the problem and elucidates the context of the question is not readily volunteered, but must be expertly elicited by the pharmacist using questioning strategies (asking logical questions in a logical sequence) and other means. Such information may be essential for formulating informed responses. Failure of the requestor to disclose critical information or clarify the question does not obviate the need for such information or relieve the pharmacist of the duty to collect it. Although it is easy to assign the blame on the requestor for failing to provide needed information, pharmacists must understand that it is their responsibility to obtain it completely and efficiently. Good communication skills (both listening and questioning) are essential for enabling the pharmacist to gather relevant information and understand the "real" question and the genuine needs of the requestor. Providing responses and offering recommendations without knowledge of pertinent patient information, the context of the request, or how the information will be applied is irresponsible and potentially dangerous.

Before attempting to formulate responses, pharmacists must consider several important questions to ensure that they understand the context of the query and the scope of the issue or problem (Table 3–1). Without this information, pharmacists risk providing general responses that do not address the needs of the requestor. More concerning, however, is that the information provided can be misinterpreted or misapplied. This not only compromises the pharmacist's credibility but also can jeopardize patient care.

TABLE 3–1. QUESTIONS TO CONSIDER BEFORE FORMULATING A RESPONSE

Do I know the requestor's name, profession, and affiliation?

Does the question pertain to a specific patient?

Do I have a clear understanding of the question or problem?

Do I know if the correct question is being asked?

Do I know why the question is being asked?

Do I understand the requestor's expectations?

Do I know pertinent patient history and background information?

Do I know about the unique circumstances that generated the question?

Do I know what information is really needed?

Do I know when the information is needed and in what format?

Do I have insight about how the information I provide will actually be used?

Do I know how the problem or situation has been managed to date?

Do I know about alternative explanations or management options that have been considered or should be further explored?

Pharmacists must recognize the value and potential benefits of their contributions as members of the health care team. Lack of confidence in communicating with requestors can be a limiting factor. Because a telephone call or visit from a physician may not be perceived as a formal request for a consult, the significance of such apparently informal daily interactions easily can be overlooked. Pharmacists should understand that interactions with physicians and other clinicians present valuable opportunities for direct involvement in patient care. The lesson often missed is that there is a fine line between a simple, seemingly general drug information question and a meaningful pharmacotherapy consult. Knowing the context of the question, obtaining the pertinent patient data and background information, and understanding the true needs of the requestor often can be the difference.

Some pharmacists are quick to attempt to answer questions without adequately understanding the context or unique circumstances from which they evolved. They focus exclusively on the answer and ignore or fail to the obtain key information needed to establish the framework of the question. For example, in a question about the dose of an antibiotic, an incorrect response can be formulated and inappropriate recommendations made if one fails to consider such factors as the patient's age, sex/gender, condition being treated, end-organ function, weight and body composition, concomitant diseases (e.g., cystic fibrosis), possible drug interactions, site of infection, spectrum of activity of the antimicrobial, resistance patterns, or other factors such as pregnancy, dialysis, and other extracorporeal procedures.

In the absence of information that provides the proper context, a question about the half-life of a medication appears rather simple. However, if the question were posed for the purpose of assisting the requestor in determining a sufficient washout period for a crossover study, one would be remiss if factors other than the half-life of the parent compound were not considered. Proper determination of a washout period would mandate consideration of such factors as the activity and half-lives of known metabolites; the presence of potentially interacting medications; the effects of age, illness, or end-organ dysfunction; the persistence of pharmacodynamic effects of the medication beyond its detection in the plasma (e.g., omeprazole); and the effect of administration route on the apparent half-life (e.g., transdermally administered fentanyl).

It is very important to look beyond the initial question and recognize that the requestor's needs often go well beyond a superficial answer to the primary question. Pharmacists should always anticipate additional questions or concerns, including those that are not directly asked or addressed by the requestor. These questions nonetheless must be considered if a clinical situation is to be managed optimally. In Case Study 3–4, a question is posed about ranitidine as a possible cause of thrombocytopenia. Although the requestor may neglect to pose additional questions, the pharmacist must anticipate and consider related issues and questions (Table 3–2). Failure to address these concerns will undoubtedly result in an incorrect or inadequate response.

Finally, pharmacists must learn to rely on their patient care skills, problem solving skills, insight, and common sense. Computer databases and other specialized information sources

TABLE 3–2. IMPORTANT QUESTIONS NOT POSED BY THE REQUESTOR

Initial query posed by requestor: Can ranitidine cause thrombocytopenia?

What is the incidence of ranitidine-induced thrombocytopenia?

Are there any known predisposing factors?

Is the pathogenesis of this adverse effect understood?

How does the thrombocytopenia typically present?

Are there any characteristic subjective or objective findings?

Does thrombocytopenia due to ranitidine differ from that caused by other histamine-2 (H_2) receptor antagonists, other medications, or other etiologies?

Is the thrombocytopenia dose related?

How severe can it become?

How soon after discontinuing the drug does it reverse?

How is it usually managed?

What is the likelihood of cross-reactivity with other histamine-2 receptor antagonists?

How risky is rechallenge with ranitidine?

Are there treatments available that can be used in place of ranitidine?

Are there alternative explanations for the thrombocytopenia in this patient (including other medications, medication combinations, or underlying medical conditions)?

What complications, if any, can be expected?

---

can assist the pharmacist in identifying critical data, but over reliance on such resources without careful attention to pertinent background information and patient data can mislead even the most experienced clinician.

Formulating the Response

BUILDING A DATABASE AND ASSESSING CRITICAL FACTORS

Formulating a response involves a series of steps that must be performed completely, objectively, and in a logical sequence. This mandates the use of a structured, organized approach whereby critical factors are systematically considered and thoroughly evaluated. The steps in this process include assembling and organizing a patient database, gathering information about relevant disease states, collecting medication information, obtaining pertinent background information, and identifying other relevant factors and special circumstances. Table 3–3 outlines in detail the specific types of information that should be considered for each factor. It should be noted that only some of this information might be pertinent for a given query or case scenario.

For patient-related questions, development of a patient-specific database is one of the first steps in preparing a response. This requires collection of pertinent information from the patient, caregivers, health care providers, medical chart, and other patient records. A comprehensive medication history obtained by a pharmacist also is essential. This database invariably includes

TABLE 3–3. FACTORS TO BE CONSIDERED WHEN FORMULATING A RESPONSE

Patient Factors

Demographics (e.g., name, age, height, weight, gender, race/ethnic group, and setting)

Primary diagnosis and medical problem list

Allergies/intolerances

End-organ function, immune function, nutritional status

Chief complaint

History of present illness

Past medical history (including surgeries, radiation exposure, immunizations, psychiatric illnesses, and so forth)

Family history and genetic makeup

Social history (e.g., alcohol intake, smoking, substance abuse, exposure to environmental or occupational toxins, employment, income, education, religion, travel, diet, physical activity, stress, risky behavior, and compliance with treatment regimen)

Review of body systems

Medications (prescribed, over-the-counter, and complementary/alternative)

Physical examination

Laboratory tests

Diagnostic studies or procedures

Disease Factors

Definition

Epidemiology (including incidence and prevalence)

Etiology

Pathophysiology (for infectious diseases, consider site of infection, organism susceptibility, resistance patterns, and so forth)

Clinical findings (signs and symptoms, laboratory tests, diagnostic studies)*

Diagnosis

Treatment (medical, surgical, radiation, biologic and gene therapies, other)

Prevention and control

Risk factors

Complications

Prognosis

Medication Factors

Name of medication or substance (proprietary, nonproprietary, other)

Status and availability (investigational, over-the-counter, prescription, orphan, foreign, complementary/alternative)

Physicochemical properties

Pharmacology and pharmacodynamics

Pharmacokinetics (liberation, absorption, distribution, metabolism, and elimination)

Pharmacogenetics

Uses (Food and Drug Administration [FDA] approved and unlabeled)

Adverse effects

Allergy

Cross-allergenicity or cross-reactivity

continued

TABLE 3–3. FACTORS TO BE CONSIDERED WHEN FORMULATING A RESPONSE (*Continued*)

Medication Factors

Contraindications and precautions

Effects of age, organ system function, disease, pregnancy, extracorporeal circulation, or other conditions or environments

Mutagenicity and carcinogenicity

Effect on fertility, pregnancy, and lactation

Acute or chronic toxicity

Drug interactions (drug-drug or drug-food)

Laboratory test interference (analytical or physiologic effects)

Administration (routes, methods)

Dosage and schedule

Dosage forms, formulations, preservatives, excipients, product appearance, delivery systems

Monitoring parameters (therapeutic or toxic)

Product preparation (procedures, methods)

Compatibility and stability

Pertinent Background Information, Special Circumstances, and Other Factors

Setting

Context

Sequence and timeframe of events

Rationale for the question

Event(s) prompting the question

Unusual or special circumstances (including medical errors)

Acuity and time constraints

Scope of question

Desired detail or depth of response

Limitations of available information or resources

Completeness, sufficiency, and quality of the information

Applicability and generalizability of the information

*Factors such as disease or symptom onset, duration, frequency, severity, and so forth must always be carefully assessed.

information common to the medical and nursing databases. Because physicians, nurses, patients, and others often lack a clear understanding of the type of information needed for effective pharmacotherapy consultations, pharmacists must be able to identify and efficiently extract pivotal patient information from diverse sources.

Once these data are collected and carefully assembled, they must be critically analyzed and evaluated in the proper context before final responses and recommendations are synthesized. Background reading on topics related to the query (e.g., diseases, medications, and laboratory tests) is often essential. To effectively perform the steps outlined previously, one must begin with a broad perspective (i.e., see the "big picture") to avoid losing sight of important information. Approaching the problem haphazardly or with tunnel vision, and prematurely focusing on isolated details, can misdirect even the most skilled pharmacist.

ANALYSIS AND SYNTHESIS

Analysis and synthesis of information are the most critical steps in formulating responses and recommendations. Together they assist in forming opinions, arriving at judgments, and ultimately drawing conclusions. Analysis is the critical assessment of the nature, merit, and significance of individual elements, ideas, or factors. Functionally, it involves separating the information into its isolated parts so that each can be critically assessed. Analysis requires thoughtful review and evaluation of the weight of available evidence. While this process requires consideration of all relevant positive findings, pertinent negative finidings should not be overlooked.

Once the information has been carefully analyzed, synthesis can begin. Synthesis is the careful, systematic, and orderly process of combining or blending varied and diverse elements, ideas, or factors into a coherent response through the use of logic and deductive reasoning. This process relies not only on the type and quality of the data gathered, but also on how they are organized, viewed, and evaluated. Synthesis, as it relates to pharmacotherapy, involves the careful integration of critical information about the patient, disease, and medication along with pertinent background information to arrive at a judgment or conclusion. Synthesis can give existing information new meaning and, in effect, create new knowledge. Use of analysis and synthesis to formulate a response is much like assembling a jigsaw puzzle. If the pieces are identified and then grouped, organized, and assembled correctly, the picture will be comprehensible. However, if too many of the pieces are missing or are not arranged logically, discerning a clear image may be altogether impossible.

RESPONSES AND RECOMMENDATIONS

An effective response obviously must answer the question. Other characteristics of effective responses and recommendations are outlined in Table 3–4. The response to a question

TABLE 3–4. DESIRED CHARACTERISTICS OF A RESPONSE

Timely
Current
Accurate
Complete
Concise
Well referenced
Clear and logical
Objective and balanced
Free of bias or flaws
Applicable and appropriate for specific circumstances
Answers important related questions
Addresses specific management of patients or situations

must include a restatement of the request and clear identification of the problems, issues, and circumstances. The response should begin with an introduction to the topic and systematically present the specific findings. Pertinent background information and patient data should be succinctly addressed. Conclusions and recommendations are also included in the response along with pertinent reference citations from the literature. The format of responses (verbal or written) is discussed in Chap. 11. In formulating responses, pharmacists should disclose all available information that is relevant to the question. They should also present all reasonable options and explanations along with an evaluation of each. Specific recommendations must be scientifically sound and clearly justified.

FOLLOW-UP

When recommendations are made, follow-up always should be provided in a timely manner. Follow-up allows pharmacists to know if their recommendations are accepted and promptly implemented. Also, it is a hallmark of a true professional and demonstrates the pharmacist's commitment to patient care. Furthermore, follow-up is required for outcomes assessment and, when necessary, to reevaluate the recommendations and make appropriate modifications. Finally, follow-up allows pharmacists to receive valuable feedback from other clinicians and to learn from the experience.

Case Study 3–1

■ INITIAL QUESTION

What is the molecular weight of enalapril?

■ POTENTIAL RESPONSE IN THE ABSENCE OF RELEVANT BACKGROUND INFORMATION

Enalapril is an oral angiotensin converting enzyme (ACE) inhibitor that is indicated for the management of hypertension, symptomatic congestive heart failure, and asymptomatic left ventricular dysfunction.[1,2] The molecular weight of enalapril is 376.45.[3]

■ PERTINENT BACKGROUND INFORMATION

The requestor is a basic scientist who is conducting an *in vitro* experiment to evaluate the pharmacologic effects of enalapril. She would like to know the molecular weight of enalapril so that she can perform appropriate calculations specified for this experiment.

■ PERTINENT PATIENT FACTORS

N/A

■ PERTINENT DISEASE FACTORS

N/A

■ PERTINENT MEDICATION FACTORS

Enalapril is a prodrug that is converted *in vivo* to the pharmacologically active form, enalaprilat.[1,2] Both enalapril and enalaprilat are commercially available for use in the United States.

■ ANALYSIS AND SYNTHESIS

Considering that enalapril is a prodrug that must be converted to a pharmacologically active compound *in vivo*, and given that this researcher wishes to conduct an *in vitro* study, the researcher should use the active form of the drug in her experiment. Therefore, she should have requested the molecular weight of enalaprilat.

■ RESPONSE AND RECOMMENDATIONS

Enalapril is an oral angiotensin-converting enzyme inhibitor that is indicated for the management of hypertension, symptomatic congestive heart failure, and asymptomatic left ventricular dysfunction. Because enalapril is a prodrug that requires conversion to the active form, the requestor was advised to consider using enalaprilat in the experiment. The molecular weight of enalaprilat is 384.43.[3]

■ CASE MESSAGE

This example illustrates the importance of collecting pertinent background information, even for seemingly uncomplicated questions. Failure to understand exactly how the information that you provide will be used could result in an inaccurate or misleading response. In this case, providing the molecular weight without alerting the requestor that *in vitro* enalapril is pharmacologically inactive, would have resulted in wasted time and money, and the results of the experiment would likely have been invalid.

■ INITIAL QUESTION

What is the maximum dose of oprelvekin (Neumega®)?

■ POTENTIAL RESPONSE IN THE ABSENCE OF RELEVANT BACKGROUND INFORMATION

The recommended dose of oprelvekin in adult patients is 50 µg/kg given once daily.[4] Larger doses of oprelvekin (75 to 100 µg/kg/day) have been studied in patients with breast cancer.[5] Constitutional symptoms associated with oprelvekin therapy, such as myalgias, arthralgias, and fatigue, were noted to increase in a dose-dependent fashion. One patient who received 100 µg/kg/day of oprelvekin experienced a cerebrovascular event after the third dose. Dose escalation greater than 75 µg/kg/day was discontinued in this study, and the maximum tolerated dose of oprelvekin was determined to be 75 µg/kg/day.[5]

■ PERTINENT BACKGROUND INFORMATION

The requestor is a physician who is managing a patient with human T-cell leukemia/lymphoma virus Type I (HTLV-1)-associated adult T-cell leukemia. The patient received myelosuppressive chemotherapy and subsequently developed prolonged and severe thrombocytopenia. Oprelvekin was prescribed in an attempt to improve the patient's platelet count and allow continuation of therapy. After 4 days of oprelvekin therapy at a dose of 50 µg/kg/day, the patient's platelet count did not increase substantially. The physician would like to know if doses greater than 50 µg/kg/day of oprelvekin have been studied. She is planning to increase the patient's dose to achieve a better response.

■ PERTINENT PATIENT FACTORS

R.R. is a 44-year-old man with HTLV-1-associated adult T-cell leukemia who has been treated with zidovudine plus interferon alpha-2b and four cycles of cyclophosphamide, hydroxydaunomycin (Doxorubicin), vincristine (Oncovin®), and prednisone, the combination of which is referred to as CHOP. After these treatments, R.R. developed severe and protracted thrombocytopenia, which has prevented further treatment.

Past Medical History

- HTLV-1 adult T-cell leukemia
- Cardiomegaly (ejection fraction 0.28) secondary to azidothymidine (Zidovudine) (AZT) and interferon alpha-2b treatment

- Peptic ulcer disease
- Thrombocytopenia

Social History

- Ø alcohol
- Ø tobacco

Current Medications

- Oprelvekin 50 µg/kg/day subcutaneously
- Pantoprazole 40 mg orally daily
- Dexamethasone 40 mg orally daily
- Loperamide 4 mg orally as needed for diarrhea
- Acetaminophen 325 mg orally as needed for headache
- Ø complementary/alternative or other over-the-counter (OTC) medications

Allergies/Intolerances

No known drug allergies.

Laboratory Results

Sodium 135 mmol/L, potassium 4.9 mmol/L, chloride 103 mmol/L, CO_2 22 mmol/L, creatinine 0.6 mg/dL, glucose 91 mg/dL, blood urea nitrogen (BUN) 15 mg/dL, albumin 3 g/dL, calcium (total) 2.49 mmol/L, magnesium 0.75 mmol/L, phosphorus 3.4 mg/dL, liver function tests (LFTs) within normal limits, white blood cell (WBC) 28.3×10^9/L, Hgb 10.1 g/dL, hematocrit (Hct) 28.1%.

Date	Platelet count (per mm^3)
7/13	25,000
7/14[†]	21,000
7/15	26,000
7/16	29,000
7/17	28,000

[†]Day 1 of oprelvekin therapy.

■ PERTINENT DISEASE FACTORS

It is not known whether patients with adult T-cell leukemia respond differently to oprelvekin than those with other types of nonmyeloid malignancies.

■ PERTINENT MEDICATION FACTORS

Oprelvekin, or recombinant interleukin-11, is indicated for the prevention of severe thrombocytopenia following myelosuppressive chemotherapy in adult patients. The FDA-approved dose of oprelvekin is 50 µg/kg once daily for up to 21 days.[4] Larger doses of oprelvekin (75 to 100 µg/kg/day) have been studied in patients with breast cancer.[5] Constitutional symptoms associated with oprelvekin therapy, such as myalgias, arthralgias, and fatigue, were noted to increase in a dose-dependent fashion. One patient who received 100 µg/kg/day of oprelvekin experienced a cerebrovascular event after the third dose. Dose escalation greater than 75 µg/kg/day was discontinued in this study, and the maximum tolerated dose of oprelvekin was determined to be 75 µg/kg/day.[5] However, the manufacturer warns that doses greater than 50 µg/kg/day may be associated with an increased incidence of fluid retention and cardiovascular events in adult patients.[4] After initiation of therapy, platelet counts usually begin to increase between 5 and 9 days, with peak counts occurring after about 14 to 19 days of therapy.[5]

■ ANALYSIS AND SYNTHESIS

Because R.R. has only received 4 days of oprelvekin treatment and platelet counts are expected to increase between 5 and 9 days after the initiation of therapy, adequate time for an optimal response to oprelvekin therapy has not been reached. In addition, oprelvekin doses higher than 75 µg/kg/day have been associated with serious adverse effects in adult patients. Therefore, increasing the dose of oprelvekin in this patient is probably not necessary, and may increase the risk of serious adverse effects without providing additional therapeutic benefits.

■ RESPONSE AND RECOMMENDATIONS

Oprelvekin or recombinant human interleukin-11, is a thrombopoietic growth factor that stimulates the proliferation of hematopoietic stem cells and megakaryocyte progenitor cells, resulting in increased platelet production. Oprelvekin is indicated for the prevention of severe thrombocytopenia in patients with nonmyeloid malignancies who are at high risk for severe thrombocytopenia following chemotherapy.[4] Platelet counts usually begin to increase between 5 and 9 days after initiation of oprelvekin, with peak platelet counts occurring after 14 to 19 days of therapy.[4,5] R.R. has only received 4 days of oprelvekin treatment, which is insufficient for an optimal response. In addition, the adverse effects of oprelvekin therapy (e.g., myalgias, arthralgias, fatigue, fluid retention, and cardiovascular events) are dose dependent.[4,5] Therefore, increasing the oprelvekin dose at this time is not warranted. In fact, doing so may predispose the patient to an increased risk of adverse effects without the prospect of added therapeutic benefit.

■ CASE MESSAGE

This example demonstrates the importance of understanding the proper context of the question. In this case, the physician is asking the wrong question. The pharmacist must collect critical background information to determine the actual drug information needed. Had the pharmacist failed to collect pertinent patient information, the physician may have increased the dose of the medication after being told that doses of 75 µg/kg/day of oprelvekin have been used. This would have been inappropriate, given that this patient had not received the medication for a sufficient duration to achieve optimal response. Moreover, larger doses of this medication are associated with a higher incidence of adverse effects.

Case Study 3–3

■ INITIAL QUESTION

Are there any drug interactions between labetalol, clonidine, amlodipine, lorazepam, and minoxidil?

■ POTENTIAL RESPONSE IN THE ABSENCE OF RELEVANT BACKGROUND INFORMATION

An extensive search of tertiary[1,6–9] and secondary (MEDLINE®, EMBASE, and so forth) literature sources did not reveal any significant drug-drug interactions between labetalol, clonidine, amlodipine, lorazepam, and minoxidil. However, concomitant therapy with a beta-adrenergic antagonist, an alpha-adrenergic antagonist, a calcium-channel antagonist, and a periperal vasodilator may increase the potential for additive hypotension.

■ PERTINENT BACKGROUND INFORMATION

The requestor is a physician who is caring for a patient with severe hypertension. The physician plans to add minoxidil to the antihypertensive regimen because the patient's morning blood pressure is not optimally controlled. He would like to make sure that there are no drug interactions between minoxidil and the patient's other medications.

PERTINENT PATIENT FACTORS

S.L. is a 40-year-old Human immuno defficiency virus HIV-infected man with severe hypertension and renal dysfunction.

Past Medical History

- HIV infection (2003)
- Hepatitis C (2001)
- Hypertension × 4 years
- Renal dysfunction

Social History

- 1 to 2 pints of vodka daily × 12 years
- 1 pack per day (PPD) of cigarettes × 25 years
- History of intravenous drug abuse

Current Medications

- Labetalol 400 mg orally qd (@9 AM)
- Clonidine transdermal patch 0.3 mg/day
- Amlodipine 10 mg orally daily (@9 AM)
- Lorazepam 1 mg orally as needed for anxiety
- Multiple vitamin tablet orally daily
- Ø complementary/alternative or other OTC medications

Allergies/Intolerances

- Lisinopril (angioedema)

Laboratory Results

- Sodium 136 mmol/L, potassium 4.7 mmol/L, chloride 102 mmol/L, CO_2 24 mmol/L, creatinine 2.9 mg/dL, glucose 98 mg/dL, BUN 14 mg/dL
- Viral DNA < 100 copies/mL
- Cluster designation 4 (CD4) count 900 cells/mm^3

Blood Pressure Measurements (mmHg)

4/15		4/16		4/17	
@ 6 AM	172/116	@ 6 AM	168/110	@ 6 AM	178/114
@ noon	121/81	@ noon	116/86	@ noon	119/84
@ 8 PM	158/100	@ 8 PM	150/104	@ 8 PM	166/100

■ PERTINENT DISEASE FACTORS

It is not known whether patients with HIV infection respond differently to antihypertensive medications.

■ PERTINENT MEDICATION FACTORS

There are no primary or tertiary literature reports describing drug interactions between minoxidil and any of S.L.'s current medications.[1,6-9] A review of the patient's current antihypertensive medications suggests that the dose of each agent is appropriate for achieving adequate blood pressure control in the face of significant renal compromise.[10] However, the duration of action of labetalol is 8 to 12 hours, and this agent is typically dosed twice daily. S.L. is receiving 400 mg of labetalol daily at 9 AM.

■ ANALYSIS AND SYNTHESIS

S.L.'s blood pressure appears to be highest in the morning, just before the daily doses of labetalol and amlodipine are administered. He is receiving 400 mg of labetalol daily at 9 AM. Because the duration of action of labetalol is 8 to 12 hours, and the usual maintenance dose is 200 to 400 mg twice daily, the increase in blood pressure observed in the morning could be due, at least in part, to inappropriate dosing of labetalol. This medication should generally be administered twice daily to achieve maximal benefit. Adjustment of the labetalol dose should precede the addition of other antihypertensive agents to this patient's medication regimen. Although long-term cigarette smoking can increase the cardiovascular risk associated with hypertension, there is no indication that smoking or alcohol ingestion are contributing to this patient's present problem.

■ RESPONSE AND RECOMMENDATIONS

There do not appear to be any significant drug interactions between any of S.L.'s current medications and minoxidil.[1,6-9] Additionally, after considering the pharmacokinetics, pharmacodynamics, adverse effect profiles, and pharmaceutical properties of the patient's medications, the potential for a clinically significant drug interaction appears low. However, a review of the patient's current antihypertensive regimen suggests that the dosing of labetalol is inappropriate. The duration of action of labetalol is 8 to 12 hours, and the usual maintenance dose is 200 to 400 mg twice daily. Because S.L. is receiving 400 mg of labetalol once daily at 9 AM, the increase in blood pressure observed in the morning could be due to inappropriate labetalol dosing. The physician was directed to optimize labetalol therapy before the addition of another antihypertensive agent. If the patient's blood pressure is not controlled with proper dosing of labetalol and minoxidil therapy is required, the physician should be advised that minoxidil is usually administered with a diuretic to prevent fluid retention.

■ CASE MESSAGE

This is another example emphasizing the importance of the proper context of the question. In this case, the pharmacist was able to recommend appropriate drug therapy management, even though the initial question posed by the physician was not related to dosage and administration of labetalol.

Case Study 3–4

■ INITIAL QUESTION

Can ranitidine cause thrombocytopenia?

■ POTENTIAL RESPONSE IN THE ABSENCE OF RELEVANT BACKGROUND INFORMATION

Ranitidine has been infrequently associated with thrombocytopenia.[1,11-13] This is a relatively rare but readily reversible complication of H_2-antagonist therapy.

■ PERTINENT BACKGROUND INFORMATION

The requestor is a physician who is evaluating a patient for suspected Cushing's disease. The patient has been hospitalized for 8 days and has undergone extensive diagnostic tests, including serial blood sampling to establish the diagnosis. Over the last 4 days, the patient has experienced a rapid decline in her platelet count. The physician is aware that cimetidine can cause thrombocytopenia. Her patient is taking ranitidine, and she would like to know if the thrombocytopenia could be induced by this medication.

■ PERTINENT PATIENT FACTORS

L.B. is a 38-year-old obese woman with Type II diabetes who is being evaluated for Cushing's disease.

Past Medical History

- Gastroesophageal reflux disease (GERD) × 6 years
- Type II diabetes × 1 year

Social History

- Ø alcohol
- Ø tobacco
- no occupational or environmental exposures

Current Medications

- Ranitidine 150 mg orally twice a day (intermittently for 6 years)
- Metformin 500 mg orally three times a day (for about 8 months)
- Heparin 100 USP units/mL (as needed for flushing heparin lock)
- Ø complementary/alternative or OTC medications

Allergies/Intolerances

- Penicillin (rash)

Laboratory Results

Sodium 137 mmol/L, potassium 4.9 mmol/L, chloride 102 mmol/L, CO_2 24 mmol/L, creatinine 0.9 mg/dL, glucose 133 mg/dL, BUN 12 mg/dL, albumin 3.4 g/dL, calcium 2.35 mmol/L, magnesium 0.81 mmol/L, phosphorus 3.8 mg/dL, liver function tests within normal limits, WBC 5.6×10^9/L.

Date	Platelet count (per mm^3)
1/17	241,000
4/20[†]	230,000
4/24	212,000
4/25	159,000
4/26	114,000
4/27	97,000
4/28	81,000

[†]Day of admission.

■ PERTINENT DISEASE FACTORS

L.B.'s thrombocytopenia is of new onset and is characterized by a rapid decline in the platelet counts over a few days. This patient does not appear to have a readily identifiable medical condition as a likely cause of the thrombocytopenia. Furthermore, she does not have any clinical evidence of bleeding or thrombosis.

■ PERTINENT MEDICATION FACTORS

A review of secondary (MEDLINE®, EMBASE) and tertiary[1,14] literature sources indicates that metformin has not been reported as a cause of thrombocytopenia. Ranitidine, however, has been infrequently associated with thrombocytopenia.[1,11-13] This is a relatively rare but readily reversible complication of ranitidine therapy. Ranitidine-induced thrombocytopenia usually develops within the first 30 days of therapy, but its pathogenesis remains unclear. Most hematologic toxicities reported with the H_2-receptor antagonists appear to occur in patients with serious concomitant diseases or in those receiving other treatments more commonly associated with hematologic adverse effects.[11-13] Thrombocytopenia has been reported in about 5% of patients treated with porcine heparin.[1] Heparin-induced thrombocytopenia does not appear to be dose dependent and has been reported in patients receiving less than 500 units of heparin/day. This condition typically develops within 5 to 9 days after initiation of therapy and reverses readily after discontinuation of the drug.

■ ANALYSIS AND SYNTHESIS

Although both ranitidine and heparin have been reported to cause thrombocytopenia, heparin appears to be the most likely cause in this case. L.B. has been taking ranitidine intermittently for nearly 6 years. Thrombocytopenia induced by ranitidine usually develops within the first 30 days of therapy. Moreover, heparin-induced thrombocytopenia is a more common adverse effect and has been reported in patients receiving very small daily doses of heparin (including heparin lock flush solution). It usually develops within 5 to 9 days after initiation of therapy. Based on the presentation and temporal sequence of events, heparin-induced thrombocytopenia is the most likely explanation for L.B.'s acute drop in platelet count. Assessment of causality using the Naranjo algorithm (see Chap. 17 for more information on this algorithm) implicates heparin as a "probable" cause of thrombocytopenia in this case, with ranitidine and metformin as "possible" and "unlikely" causes, respectively.[15]

■ RESPONSE AND RECOMMENDATIONS

A review of L.B.'s current medications reveals two agents, ranitidine and heparin, that have been reported to cause thrombocytopenia.[1,6,11] Ranitidine-induced thrombocytopenia is most likely to occur within the first 30 days of therapy.[11-13] Because L.B. has been taking ranitidine intermittently for GERD for approximately 6 years, it is unlikely that ranitidine is responsible for the acute decrement in platelet count. Ranitidine, however, cannot be immediately ruled out as a possible cause. Heparin-induced thrombocytopenia is a more common adverse effect that has been reported even with very small daily doses of heparin (e.g., heparin lock flush solution).[1] The thrombocytopenia is acute and usually develops within 5 to 9 days after initiation of therapy. Based on the presentation and temporal relationship, heparin appears to be the most likely cause of thrombocytopenia in this patient. The physician was advised to discontinue the heparin lock flush solution, closely monitor the patient's platelet count, and test for heparin antibodies in order to establish the diagnosis and guide future therapy. If the platelet counts do not begin to normalize after discontinuation of heparin, other potential causes of thrombocytopenia should be considered.

■ CASE MESSAGE

This question highlights the importance of skillful problem solving. As always, collecting appropriate background information and patient data is critical. Analyzing this information before synthesizing a logical response is paramount for effective patient management. In this case, failure to recognize that the patient was receiving heparin lock flush solution could incorrectly have excluded heparin as a possible cause of the thrombocytopenia.

Conclusion

Formulating effective responses and recommendations requires use of a structured, organized approach whereby critical factors are systematically considered and thoroughly evaluated. The steps in this process include organizing a patient database, gathering information about relevant disease states, collecting medication information, obtaining pertinent background information, and identifying other relevant factors or special circumstances. Once these data are collected and carefully assembled, they must be critically analyzed and evaluated in the proper context. Responses and recommendations are synthesized by integrating data from these diverse sources through the use of logic and deductive reasoning.

Study Questions

1. Why is it necessary to gather background information and patient data? Why do pharmacists often fail to obtain this information?

2. What factors should be considered in making a recommendation regarding dosage and administration of an antibiotic? Provide a justification for each factor you select.

3. Given the question "Can naproxen cause nephrotoxicity?," list at least five related questions that also should be considered.

4. List three patient-related factors that should be considered for a question pertaining to potential drug interactions.

BIBLIOGRAPHY

Galt KA, Calis KA, Turcasso NM. Clinical Skills Program: Module 3 Drug Information. Bethesda, MD: American Society of Health-System Pharmacists Inc; 1995.

Watanabe AS, Conner CS. Principles of Drug Information Services. Hamilton, IL: Drug Intelligence Publications Inc; 1978.

REFERENCES

1. McEvoy GK, editor. AHFS drug information 2004. Bethesda (MD): American Society of Health-System Pharmacists; 2004.
2. Vasotec [package insert]. Morrisville (NC): Biovail Pharmaceuticals; 2002.
3. O'Neil MJ, Smith A, Heckelman PE, Obenchain JR, Jr., editors. The Merck Index: an encyclopedia of chemicals, drugs, and biologicals. 13th ed. Whitehouse Station (NJ): Merck & Co.; 2001.
4. Neumega® [package insert]. Philadelphia (PA): Wyeth Pharmaceuticals; 2004.
5. Gordon MS, McCaskill-Stevens WJ, Battiato LA, Loewy J, Loesch D, Breeden E, et al. A phase I trial of recombinant human interleukin-11 (Neumega® rhIL-11 growth factor) in women with breast cancer receiving chemotherapy. Blood. 1996;87(9):3615–24.
6. Klasco RK, editor. DRUG-REAX® system. Greenwood Village (CO): Thomson MICROMEDEX.
7. Hansten PD, Horne JR. Drug interactions: analysis and managment. St. Louis (MO): Facts & Comparisons; 2004.
8. Tatro DS, editor. Drug interaction facts. Philadelphia (PA): Lippincott Williams & Wilkins; 2004.
9. Zucchero FJ, Hogan MJ, Sommer CD, editors. Evaluation of drug interactions. St. Louis (MO): First Databank; 2004.
10. Bennett WM, Aronoff GR, Golper TA, Morrison G, Brater DC, Singer I, editors. Drug prescribing in renal failure. 4th ed. Philadelphia (PA): American College of Physicians; 1999.
11. Dukes MNG, editor. Meyler's side effects of drugs. 14th ed. Amsterdam (The Netherlands): Elsevier Science; 2000.
12. Yin JM, Frazier JL. Ranitidine and thrombocytopenia. J Pharm Technol. 1995;11:263–6.
13. Wade EE, Rebuck JA, Healey MA, Rogers FB. H_2 antagonist-induced thrombocytopenia: is this a real phenomenon? Intensive Care Med. 2002;28(4):459–65.
14. Glucophage [package insert]. Princeton (NJ): Bristol-Myers Squibb; 2004.
15. Naranjo CA, Busto U, Sellers EM, Sandor P, Ruiz I, Roberts EA, et al. A method for estimating the probability of adverse drug reactions. Clin Pharmacol Ther. 1981;30:239–45.

4

Chapter Four

Drug Information Resources

Kelly M. Shields • Elaine Lust

Objectives

After completing this chapter, the reader will be able to

- Differentiate between primary, secondary, and tertiary sources of information.
- Select resources relevant to different pharmacy practice areas.
- Identify the most appropriate resource for a specific drug information request.
- Describe the role of Internet and personal digital assistant (PDA) resources in the provision of drug information.
- Critique tertiary resources to determine appropriateness of information.
- Describe appropriate search strategy for use with computerized secondary databases.
- Recognize alternative resources for provision of drug information.

Introduction

The quantity of medical information and medical literature available is growing at an astounding rate. The technology by which this information can be accessed is also improving exponentially. The introduction of PDAs and Internet resources has to some extent changed the methods by which information is accessed, but not the process of providing drug information.

Pharmacists are being asked daily to provide responses to numerous drug information requests for a variety of people. It is tempting just to select the easiest, most familiar resources to find information; however, by doing that there is the possibility of missing new resources or limiting the comprehensiveness of the information found. It is for these reasons that the systematic approach discussed in Chap. 2 is helpful in order to streamline the search process.

Generally, the best method to find information includes a stepwise approach moving first through tertiary (e.g., textbooks, full-text databases, and review articles), then secondary (e.g., indexing or abstracting service), and finally primary (e.g., clinical studies) literature. The tertiary sources will provide the practitioner with general information needed to familiarize the reader with the topic. If this information is not recent or comprehensive enough, a secondary database may be employed to direct the reader to review primary literature articles that might provide more insight on the topic. Primary literature often provides the most recent and in-depth information about a topic, and allows the reader to analyze and critique the study methodology to determine if the conclusions are valid (see Chaps. 6 and 7 for more information on critiquing the primary literature).

Sometimes it may be necessary to consult news reports or other Internet sites to get background information before beginning the searching process for a request. Also, other resources, including experts or specialists in particular areas of practice, may need to be consulted. More information will be provided about these resources later in the chapter.

Often, a search for information will not employ all of these steps or require the use of all three types of resources. For example, a question regarding commercial availability of a product formulation or mechanism of action can be found quickly in a tertiary resource. The information found there may be sufficient to conclude the search and provide a response. However, a question regarding the clinical trials supporting off-label use in a specific population may require a search of primary literature.

The type of requestor may also substantially influence the resources used to respond to a question. Generally, a request from a consumer or patient could be answered more appropriately from available tertiary resources rather than a stack of clinical trials. However, if the requestor is a prescriber requesting detailed information about the management of a specific disease state and role of investigational therapies, provision of primary literature may be appropriate.

The provision of drug information is continually expanding into new areas, which may impact selection of appropriate resources. For example, increased patient use of dietary supplements and alternative therapies has caused medical professionals to seek information on these topics. Pharmacists are often expected to respond to questions about these topics and provide recommendations as to management of patients using these therapies. Also, increasing interest in the practice of veterinary pharmacy underscores the need for pharmacists to be able to practically apply drug information resources for the benefit of animal patients, animal owners, and veterinary professionals.

Tertiary Resources

Tertiary resources consist of textbooks, compendia, review articles in journals, and other general information, such as may be found on the Internet. These references may often serve as an initial place to identify information due to the fact that they provide a fairly complete and concise overview of information available on a specific topic. These resources are convenient, easy to use, and familiar to most practitioners. Most of the information needed by a practitioner can be found in these sources, making these excellent first-line resources when dealing with a drug information question.

The major drawback to tertiary resources, however, is the lag time associated with publication, resulting in less current information. Medical information changes so rapidly that it is possible that information may be out of date before it is even published. It is also possible that information in a tertiary text may be incomplete due either to space limitations of the book or incomplete literature searches by the author. Other problems that can be seen with tertiary information include errors in transcription, human bias, incorrect interpretation of information, or a lack of expertise by authors. For these reasons readers must judge the quality of tertiary references. Some questions that should be considered when evaluating tertiary literature are listed in Table 4–1.

It is impossible to compile a comprehensive list of tertiary resources that are useful in all areas of pharmacy practice. Differences in practice setting, available funding, patients seen, and types of information most commonly needed, all have an impact on which tertiary resources should be available at a specific practice site. Legal requirements for information sources available at a practice setting vary from state to state, but rarely will the minimally required texts be sufficient to meet all information needs in a practice.

Another important factor in the selection of appropriate tertiary resources includes selecting a resource focused on the type of information needed for a specific request or situation. For example, a very well-written and comprehensive therapeutics text may have very limited use in providing information regarding pharmacokinetics of a specific drug. For this reason, it is important to consider the categories of requests received in a particular practice setting to ensure that appropriate tertiary texts are available. Table 4–2 lists resources that may be useful for specific categories of drug information requests.

A brief summary of selected tertiary resources is listed to provide examples of some resources that may be useful in the practice of pharmacy. This list is not comprehensive and reflects only a limited number of resources that reflect recommendations of organizations[1] or resources commonly used in drug information settings.[2] Other suggested references may be found in *Doody's Core Titles in the Health Sciences*[1] or in the listing of core resources provided by the American Association of Colleges of Pharmacy.[3]

TABLE 4–1. EVALUATION OF TERTIARY LITERATURE

Does the author have appropriate experience/expertise to publish in this area?
Is the information likely to be timely based on publication date?
Is the information supported by appropriate citations?
Does the resource contain relevant information?
Does the resource appear free from bias or blatant errors?

TABLE 4-2. USEFUL RESOURCES FOR COMMON CATEGORIES OF DRUG INFORMATION

Type of Request	Useful Tertiary Sources	Secondary Resources
General product information	Major compendia,* Handbook of Clinical Drug Data,[4] Handbook of Nonprescription Drugs,[5] Clinical Pharmacology[6]	MEDLINE®, EMBASE, International Pharmaceutical Abstracts (IPA), Iowa Drug Information Service (IDIS)
Adverse effects	Meyler's Side Effects of Drugs,[7] Drug Therapy Monitoring System,[8] major compendia*	Reactions Weekly, MEDLINE®, EMBASE, IPA, IDIS
Availability of dosage forms	Red Book,[9] American Drug Index,[10] major compendia*	—
Compounding	Remington: The Science and Practice of Pharmacy,[11] Merck Index,[12] A Practical Guide to Contemporary Pharmacy Practice,[13] USP/NF,[14] Allen's Compounded Formulations,[15] Martindale: The Complete Drug Reference,[16] Extemporaneous Formulations,[17] Ansel's Pharmaceutical Dosage Forms and Drug Delivery Systems,[18] The Art, Science and Technology of Pharmaceutical Compounding[19]	IPA, IDIS, EMBASE, MEDLINE®
Dietary supplement	Natural Medicine Comprehensive Database,[20] Review of Natural Products,[21] Professional's Handbook of Complementary and Alternative Medicine,[22] Herbal Medicine: Expanded Commission E Monographs,[23] PDR for Herbal Medicine,[24] Herbal Medicines: A Guide for Health Care Professionals,[25] Herb Contraindications and Drug Interactions,[26] AltMedDex[27]	EMBASE, MEDLINE®, IPA, IDIS
Dosage recommendations (general and organ impairment)	Major compendia,* Drug Prescribing in Renal Failure[28]	MEDLINE®, InPharma, IPA, IDIS, EMBASE
Drug interactions	Hansten and Horn's Drug Interaction Analysis and Management,[29] Drug Interaction Facts,[30] Stockley's Drug Interactions,[31] DRUG-REAX,[32] major compendia*	Reactions, IPA
Drug-laboratory interference	Basic Skills in Interpreting Laboratory Data,[33] Laboratory Test Handbook,[34] Clinical Guide to Laboratory Tests,[35] Laboratory Tests and Diagnostic Procedures[36]	—
Drugs in pregnancy and in lactation	Drugs in Pregnancy and Lactation,[37] Drugs During Pregnancy and Lactation,[38] Drugs for Pregnant and Lactating Women,[39] Medications and Mothers' Milk: A Manual of Lactational Pharmacology,[40] REPRORISK,[41] major compendia*	Reactions, EMBASE, MEDLINE®, IDIS, IPA
Foreign drug identification	Martindale: The Complete Drug Reference,[16] Index Nominum,[42] DRUGDEX®,[43] European Drug Index,[44] Internet search engines, specific country resources	—
Geriatric dosage recommendations	Geriatric Dosage Handbook,[45] The Merck Manual of Geriatrics,[46] major compendia*	MEDLINE®, InPharma, IPA, IDIS, EMBASE

Category	Key references	Databases
Identification of product by description of dosage form	IDENTIDEX®,[47] Clinical Pharmacology,[6] Ident-a-Drug,[48] Clinical Reference Library,[49] electronic Facts and Comparisons	—
Investigational drug information	FDA website,[50] Clinicaltrials.gov,[51] MedlinePlus,[52] manufacturer websites	InPharma, Current Contents, EMBASE, MEDLINE®, LexisNexis, IPA, IDIS
Incompatibility/stability	Handbook of Injectable Drugs,[53] King Guide to Parenteral Admixtures,[54] Trissel's Stability of Compounded Formulations,[55] Extended Stability for Parenteral Drugs,[56] Remington: The Science and Practice of Pharmacy[11]	IPA, IDIS, EMBASE, MEDLINE®
Method/rate of administration	Major compendia*	
Pediatric dosage recommendations	The Harriet Lane Handbook,[57] Pediatric Dosage Handbook,[58] Neofax,[59] major compendia*	MEDLINE®, InPharma, IPA, IDIS, EMBASE
Pharmacokinetics	Clinical Pharmacokinetics,[60] Applied Pharmacokinetics and Pharmacodynamics: Principles of Therapeutic Drug Monitoring,[61] Basic Clinical Pharmacokinetics,[62] major compendia*	IPA, EMBASE, MEDLINE®, IDIS
Pharmacology	Goodman & Gilman's: The Pharmacological Basis of Therapeutics,[63] Basic & Clinical Pharmacology,[64] Principles of Pharmacology[65]	IDIS, IPA, EMBASE, MEDLINE®
Pharmacy law	Pharmacy Practice and the Law,[66] Guide to Federal Pharmacy Law,[67] State Board of Pharmacy web pages	LexisNexis
Price	Price-Chek PC, Drug Topics Red Book[9]	
Serum or urine therapeutic levels	Pharmacokinetic texts above and major compendia*	IPA, EMBASE, MEDLINE®, IDIS
Therapy evaluation/recommendations	Pharmacotherapy: A Pathophysiologic Approach,[68] Applied Therapeutics,[69] The Merck Manual,[70] Harrison's Principles of Internal Medicine,[71] Cecil's Textbook of Medicine,[72] Textbook of Therapeutics,[73] Conn's Current Therapy[74]	MEDLINE®, EMBASE, IDIS, InPharma, IPA
Toxicology information	POISINDEX®,[75] Goldfrank's Toxicologic Emergencies,[76] Casarett & Doull's Toxicology: The Basic Science of Poisons,[77] Ellenhorn's Medical Toxicology: Diagnosis and Treatment of Human Poisoning,[78] Poisoning & Toxicology Handbook,[79] Clinical Management of Drug Overdose,[80] TOXNET[81]	Reactions, EMBASE, MEDLINE®, IPA, IDIS, BIOSIS
Veterinary medicine	Veterinary Drug Handbook,[82] Textbook of Veterinary Internal Medicine,[83] Compendia of Veterinary Products,[84] FDA Center for Veterinary Medicine,[85] 5-Minute Veterinary Consult: Canine and Feline[86]	BIOSIS, EMBASE, MEDLINE®

*Major compendia referred to in this table include Facts and Comparisons,[87] AHFS Drug Information,[88] Physicians' Desk Reference,[89] DRUGDEX®,[43] Drug Information Handbook,[90] and USP DI Volume I.[91]

General Product Information

AHFS DRUG INFORMATION

American Society of Health-System Pharmacists, <<www.ashp.org>>. This drug information resource is organized by monographs containing information on both Food and Drug Administration (FDA) approved and off-label uses of medications. Information about dosing in specific populations is also included, as is a wide variety of general information about medications. Some information is also available about compatibility and stability of injectable formulations. American Hospital Formulary Services (AHFS) is available in paper text (updated annually), an intranet resource (AHFSFirstWeb), and a PDA version.

CLINICAL PHARMACOLOGY

Gold Standard, <<http://cp.gsm.com/>>. This electronic database has monographs of prescription and nonprescription products as well as some dietary supplements. The database can also screen for drug interactions, create comparison tables for prescription drugs, determine intravenous (IV) compatibility, and search for tablets by description or imprint codes. There is a patient education section also. It is available via the Internet, CD-ROM, through an organization's Intranet, or for PDAs.

DRUGDEX® SYSTEM

Thompson MICROMEDEX, <<www.thomsonhc.com>>. This electronic resource is a database within the MICROMEDEX system. It contains information about FDA-approved indications, off-label uses, pharmacokinetic data, safety information, and pharmacology. Information is also provided regarding common questions for some medications (e.g., cross-sensitivity between penicillin and cephalosporin). This resource is available via CD-ROM, PDA, and the Internet.

DRUG FACTS AND COMPARISONS

WolterKluwer Health, Inc., <<www.factsandcomparisons.com>>. This reference contains information organized by drug class. Information is provided about specific agents, including inactive ingredients in commercial preparations. There are comparative monographs of drug classes to help discern differences between agents of the same class. This resource is available via CD-ROM and online. The electronic version of this resource allows for an integrated search across a variety of Facts and Comparison publications (depending on subscription purchased).

DRUG INFORMATION HANDBOOK

Lexi-Comp, <<www.lexi.com>>. This handbook is organized in brief product monographs, where information is presented regarding clinical use, safety, and monitoring for a variety of drugs. Data are presented about FDA-approved as well as off-label use of medications. There is a limited tablet identification section as part of the electronic format. The resource also has several helpful appendices providing treatment options and comparing agents in the same class. This resource is available via CD-ROM, PDA, and online. The electronic versions allow for integrated searches of various Lexi-Comp products (depending on subscription purchased) through the online Clinical Reference Library (<<www.crlonline.com>>). The online resource also includes pricing information provided by drugstore.com.

HANDBOOK OF CLINICAL DRUG DATA

McGraw-Hill, <<www.mcgraw-hill.com>>. This information resource is organized into monographs and comparative charts. Data are provided regarding dosing, including adjustments for special populations, adverse events, pharmacology, and pharmacokinetic data. This resource serves as a quick reference rather than an in-depth review.

HANDBOOK OF NONPRESCRIPTION DRUGS: AN INTERACTIVE APPROACH TO SELF-CARE

American Pharmacists Association, <<www.aphanet.org>>. This text is organized by body system, focusing on those disease states for which self-care may be appropriate. Information is provided about comparative efficacy of various over-the-counter (OTC) agents, as well as contraindications for self-treatment, drug interactions, and other safety information. Use of treatment algorithms and patient care cases make this resource especially helpful for students and new practitioners.

PHYSICIANS' DESK REFERENCE

Thomson Healthcare, <<www.thomsonhc.com>>. This resource is a compilation of product package inserts. Additional information includes contact information for manufacturers, a list of poison control centers, and some limited tablet identification. Information from the *Physicians' Desk Reference* (PDR) is also available in an electronic online package from Thomson and via

MICROMEDEX, as well as in a PDA format. In addition to the original PDR, there are a variety of specialty texts, including the *PDR for Herbal Medicines, PDR for Nutritional Supplements, PDR for Ophthalmic Medicines,* and *PDR for Nonprescription Drugs and Dietary Supplements.*

USP DI VOLUMES I, II, AND III

Thomson Healthcare, <<www.thomsonhc.com>>. Information from the United States Pharmacopeia (USP) Drug Information (DI) resources is also included in the MICROMEDEX Healthcare Series.

Volume I contains information for the health care professional, organized into monographs based on nonproprietary names. Information that is included is similar to that in other monographs: indications, pharmacology, pharmacokinetics, safety issues, and patient counseling points.

Volume II contains advice for the lay person and includes material intended to supplement counseling by a health care professional.

Volume III includes information about therapeutic equivalence and USP/National Formulary (NF) requirements for labeling, storing, and packaging drugs. There is also information about regulations and statutes impacting pharmacy. The first portion of this volume of the resource is commonly known as the *Orange Book,* and contains the same information that is available through the FDA via <<www.fda.gov/cder/ob/default.htm>>.

USP DICTIONARY OF USAN AND INTERNATIONAL DRUG NAMES

U.S. Pharmacopeia, <<www.usp.org>>. This is the official resource for determining generic and chemical names of drugs, as well as the international nonproprietary name. Additionally, useful information such as chemical structure, molecular weight, Chemical Abstracts Services (CAS) registry number and a pronunciation guide are provided. This resource is also available in an online format (<<www.uspusan.com>>) that is updated annually at the printing of the new edition of the text.

Adverse Effects

MEYLER'S SIDE EFFECTS OF DRUGS

Elsevier Publishing, <www.elsevier.com>>. This reference, published every 4 years with annual updates, provides a critical review of international literature in the area of adverse events. Chapters are organized by drug classification; adverse events are organized by drug name and then by organ system within each drug.

Availability of Dosage Forms

AMERICAN DRUG INDEX

Facts and Comparisons, <<www.factsandcomparisons.com>>. Contains brief entries, indexed by product and generic name, with information about product use, available dosage forms and sizes, and manufacturer information. Several helpful charts are also available, including look-alike/sound-alike medications, pregnancy categories, normal laboratory values, as well as common pharmacy calculations. This print resource is updated annually and is also included in the CliniSphere CD-ROM resource.

RED BOOK

Thomson Healthcare, <<www.thomsonhc.com>>. This resource primarily contains data regarding prescription and OTC product availability and pricing. There are also a number of tables listing information such as sugar-free, lactose-free, or alcohol-free preparations. Additionally, information such as normalized device coordinates (NDC) numbers, routes of administration, dosage form, size, and strength are included.

Compounding

ALLEN'S COMPOUNDED FORMULATIONS

American Pharmacists Association, <<www.aphanet.org>>. This resource is a collection of *U.S. Pharmacist* columns that have been printed as a text. Each recipe provides method of preparation, stability, and discussion of utility of the dosage form.

EXTEMPORANEOUS FORMULATIONS

American Society of Health-System Pharmacists, <<www.ashp.org>>. This resource is a compilation of published recipes with stability data. Most products are oral formulations to reflect the unique needs of some pediatric patients. Information is also provided about legal and technical issues in compounding practices.

MERCK INDEX

Merck & Co., <<www.merck.com>>. This resource provides descriptions of the chemical and pharmacologic information about a variety of products. Data include CAS number, chemical structure, molecular weight, and physical data, including solubility, which may be especially useful in compounding. This reference is available in print, online, and on CD-ROM.

REMINGTON: THE SCIENCE AND PRACTICE OF PHARMACY

Lippincott Williams & Wilkins, <<www.lww.com>>. This classic text contains information about all aspects of pharmacy practice. There is discussion of social issues impacting pharmacy as well as information about the basics of pharmaceutics, manufacturing, pharmacodynamics, and medicinal chemistry. Information is provided regarding common compounding techniques and ingredients.

A PRACTICAL GUIDE TO CONTEMPORARY PHARMACY PRACTICE

Lippincott Williams & Wilkins, <<www.lww.com>> This text resource with CD-ROM is organized in an outline format to easily find information. Discussion of compounding techniques and explanations of additives used in compounding are very useful. Students and young practitioners may find the sample cases especially helpful.

USP/NF

United States Pharmacopeial Convention, <<www.usp.org>> This resource, available in both text and CD-ROM format, contains the official substance and product standards. Also, official preparation instructions are given for a limited number of commonly compounded products.

Some journals are especially useful for compounding "recipes", for example, the *International Journal of Pharmacy Compounding, U.S. Pharmacist,* or *American Druggist.*

Dietary Supplements

NATURAL MEDICINE COMPREHENSIVE DATABASE

Therapeutic Research Faculty, <<www.naturaldatabase.com>>. This resource is available in a text form as well as online. It provides a summary of the information available for various dietary supplements and rates the relative safety and efficacy of those products. Searches can be performed by the brand name of the supplement or by a variety of common names. The electronic version includes an interaction checker and disease state/condition search. This resource is also available for PDA.

NATURAL THERAPEUTICS POCKET GUIDE

Lexi-Comp, <<www.lexi.com>>. This resource contains information sorted by both product and disease state. Each disease state has a summary of the disease, a decision tree, a list of natural products to consider, and a listing of special considerations about these products. This product does not have the same in-depth focus on clinical trials as other resources, but instead provides a bottom line summary of the author's interpretation of the available evidence. The last section of the reference contains a variety of helpful tables summarizing commonly used herbs, herb-drug interactions, and drug-induced nutrient depletion, as well as unsafe herbs.

REVIEW OF NATURAL PRODUCTS

Facts and Comparisons, <<www.factsandcomparisons.com>>. This resource provides information about the chemistry, pharmacology, and toxicology of a number of natural products based on references to primary literature. A summary of relevant clinical trials is also available. There is also limited patient counseling information, but the strength of this resource is in the chemistry and pharmacology information. Recent revisions have dramatically increased the amount of information included in patient counseling sections. This is available in loose-leaf, bound paper, CD-ROM, and Internet-based formats.

THE COMPLETE GERMAN COMMISSION E-MONOGRAPHS

American Botanical Counsel, <<www.herbalgram.org>>. This resource was one of the first scientific-based publications available to address the therapeutic uses of herbal products. It consists of translations of German monographs prepared through the 1980s and 1990s and addresses only herbal products. Some of this information may be considered dated and other resources may contain more clinically relevant information. A follow-up publication *Herbal Medicine: Expanded Commission E Monographs* was released in 2000 and was designed to provide additional clinical information that was not present in the original work. The expanded edition provides greater number of references and more detailed descriptions of product use, but still is not the most comprehensive resource available.

PDR FOR HERBAL MEDICINES

Thomson Healthcare, <<www.thomsonhc.com>>. Products are indexed by common name and information is provided regarding action, usage, dosage, and other clinically useful information. Citations to the primary literature are also provided at the conclusion of each monograph. The focus on strictly herbal products, rather than nonbotanical dietary supplements, may limit utility in some settings.

PROFESSIONAL'S HANDBOOK OF COMPLEMENTARY AND ALTERNATIVE MEDICINE

Lippincott Williams & Wilkins, <<www.lww.com>>. This resource contains short monographs of commonly used dietary supplements, focused on the information needed for patient counseling. For some of the most common products summaries of clinical trials are also provided.

Dosage Recommendations

DRUG PRESCRIBING IN RENAL FAILURE

American College of Physicians, <<www.acponline.com>>. This resource addresses the changes in pharmacokinetics that occur as a result of renal impairment, and provides specific recommendations for dosing adjustment for medications. Information is provided in a variety of tables. Tables also include recommendations for dosage modifications for patients undergoing hemodialysis, chronic ambulatory peritoneal dialysis, and continuous renal replacement therapy. Citations to the primary literature are also provided.

Drug Interactions

HANSTEN AND HORN'S DRUG INTERACTION ANALYSIS AND MANAGEMENT

WolterKluwer Health, Inc., <<www.factsandcomparisons.com>>. This resource provides summaries of, mechanism of, and management options for reported drug interactions. The authors also provide information regarding severity of interaction and any risk factors that might predispose patients to this event. This loose-leaf reference, which is updated quarterly, provides rapid information regarding severity and likelihood of an interaction and actions needed to minimize this risk based on the case studies and primary literature available.

DRUG INTERACTION FACTS

Facts and Comparisons, <<www.factsandcomparisons.com>>. This resource provides information about drug-drug or drug-food interactions. Discussions of significance of the interaction as well as suggestions for management are included. This resource is available in both bound and loose-leaf texts. It is available electronically via CD-ROM and as part of an online subscription.

DRUG-REAX

Thompson MICROMEDEX, <<www.thomsonhc.com>>. This electronic resource is a database within the MICROMEDEX system. Information is provided about drug-drug, drug-food, and drug-supplement interactions. Discussion is provided regarding severity, management, and literature about the interaction. Available formats include CD-ROM, PDA, and the Internet.

EVALUATIONS OF DRUG INTERACTIONS

First DataBank, <<www.firstdatabank.com>>. This loose-leaf reference contains information, organized by drug class, about the management of various drug interactions. Information is provided regarding mechanism of drug interaction, recommendations for management, and clinical significance. This information is also available in the format of an electronic database.

DRUG THERAPY MONITORING SYSTEM

Medi-Span, <<www.medi-span.com>>. This CD-ROM resource offers information about drug-drug, drug-food, and drug-alcohol interactions. Discussions regarding onset of interaction, severity, mechanism, and management are provided. Summaries of primary literature are also provided.

STOCKLEY'S DRUG INTERACTIONS

Pharmaceutical Press, <<www.pharmpress.com>>. This resource, available in CD-ROM, Internet, and print formats, contains concise summaries of drug interactions with supporting primary reference citations. The text uses both British (British Approved Name [BAN]) and American (United States Adopted Name [USAN]) drug names.

Foreign Drug Identification

EUROPEAN DRUG INDEX

European Society of Clinical Pharmacy, <<www.escpweb.org>>. This resource offers information about the identification of European medications. Information is provided about dosage form, strength, and name of principle ingredients. A dictionary translating dosage form terms is also included in this reference.

INDEX NOMINUM: INTERNATIONAL DRUG DIRECTORY

Medpharm Publishers, <<www.medpharm.de>>. This drug information source contains information on drugs available in over 140 countries. Information is included regarding structure, therapeutic class, and proprietary names for single-entity medications. A CD-ROM is included containing contact information for pharmaceutical manufacturers worldwide. The information from this resource is also included in the MICROMEDEX Healthcare Series.

MARTINDALE: THE COMPLETE DRUG REFERENCE

Pharmaceutical Press, <<www.pharmpress.com>>. This resource includes information on a variety of domestic and international drugs. Proprietary names and manufacturer contact information are available for a variety of countries. Some information is provided about common herbal products as well as diagnostic agents, radioactive pharmaceuticals, and some veterinary products. This information is available in hardcopy, CD-ROM, via online subscription, and is also included in some MICROMEDEX Healthcare Series packages.

Additional resources are available that are specific to individual countries including *Diccionario de Especialidases Farmaceuticas* (Mexico), *British Pharmacopoeia* (United Kingdom), *Rote Liste* (Germany), *Dictionary Vidal* (France), *Compendium of Pharmaceuticals and Specialties* (Canada), and *Repertorio Farmaceutico Italiano* (Italy).

Geriatric Dosage Recommendations

GERIATRIC DOSAGE HANDBOOK

Lexi-Comp, <<www.lexi.com>>. The monographs in this resource contain traditional sections of drug information, but focus on dosing recommendations for geriatric patients. There is a special section of each monograph addressing concerns specific to the geriatric population. Limited references to primary literature are provided. This reference is also available online, on CD-ROM, and in PDA format.

THE MERCK MANUAL OF GERIATRICS

Merck & Co., <<www.merck.com>>. This resource, available in print and online focuses primarily on management of diseases and conditions common in geriatric patients. There is some discussion of appropriate dosing of medications in this population.

Identification of Product

IDENT-A-DRUG

Therapeutic Research Faculty, <www.indentadrug.com>>. This resource is organized by imprint codes and provides identification of drugs based on those codes. Descriptions of medications, as well as NDC numbers, are provided. Electronic and text versions of this reference are available.

IDENTIDEX®

Thompson MICROMEDEX, <<www.thomsonhc.com>>. This electronic resource is a database within the MICROMEDEX Healthcare Series. It has the ability to identify tablets and pills based on the imprint code selected. There is also limited ability to search by description of dosage form (i.e., color). Descriptions, NDC numbers, and a listing of active and inactive ingredients is provided.

Other resources, discussed elsewhere, also have some tablet identification features including *Clinical Pharmacology*, Lexi-Comp Online, *PDR*, *Redbook*, and eFacts (Facts and Comparisons online).

Incompatibility and Stability

HANDBOOK ON INJECTABLE DRUGS

American Society of Health-System Pharmacists, <<www.ashp.org>>. This resource, commonly called Trissel's, includes information regarding the compatibility and stability of various parenteral medications. Information is primarily provided in the form of charts and tables, making finding information relatively quick. This resource also provides information about routes of administration and commercially available strengths. A pocket-sized handbook and a CD-ROM version are also available.

KING GUIDE TO PARENTERAL ADMIXTURES

King Guide Publications, <<www.kingguide.com>>. Over 400 IV drug monographs are provided, focused on compatibility information. Also limited information about stability is available. This resource is available in loose-leaf, bound copy, CD-ROM, as an Internet resource, and for PDAs.

TRISSEL'S STABILITY OF COMPOUNDED FORMULATIONS

American Pharmacists Association, <www.aphanet.org>>. Information is provided on nearly 300 compounded oral, enteral, ophthalmic, and topical formulations, organized by drug name. Extensive citations of the stability and formulation studies are provided. There is also limited discussion of compatibility with other drug products.

TRISSEL'S 2 CLINICAL PHARMACEUTICS DATABASE

TriPharma, <www.trissels.info>>. This electronic resource compiles data from other Trissel publications. Information about parenteral admixtures, compounded formulations, physical compatibility, and chemotherapy formulations is included. This resource is available for an intranet, as well as via CD-ROM and the Internet.

Pediatric Dosage Recommendations

THE HARRIET LANE HANDBOOK

Mosby, <<www.mosby.com>>. This resource, assembled by medical residents, contains a succinct discussion of common diseases and conditions of newborn to adolescent patients. A significant portion of the book is dedicated to medication dosing, specifically pediatrics. This section also contains information about common side effects and dosage forms available.

NEOFAX

Acorn Publishing Inc., <<www.neofax.com>>. This reference, available in print, PDA, and online forms, contains brief drug monographs specific to neonates arranged by drug therapeutic class. Each monograph has information about dose, monitoring, adverse reactions, preparation of drug, and limited references to primary literature.

PEDIATRIC DOSAGE HANDBOOK

Lexi-Comp, <<www.lexi.com>>. The monographs in this resource contain traditional sections of drug information, but focus on detailed dosing recommendations for pediatrics. There is also information about common extemporaneous preparations. Limited references to primary literature are provided. This reference is also available online, on CD-ROM, and in PDA format.

Pharmacokinetics

APPLIED PHARMACOKINETICS AND PHARMACODYNAMICS: PRINCIPLES OF THERAPEUTIC DRUG MONITORING

Lippincott Williams & Wilkins, <<www.lww.com>>. The first section of this text includes general information about pharmacokinetics and pharmacodynamics as well as how these parameters may differ in specified patient populations. This text also addresses pharmacokinetics of specific drugs and drug classes.

BASIC CLINICAL PHARMACOKINETICS

Lippincott Williams & Wilkins, <<www.lww.com>>. This text discusses the basic principles of pharmacokinetics especially interpretation and implications of plasma concentrations. The second section of the book provides monographs and discussions focused on drugs most commonly assessed by blood concentration levels.

CLINICAL PHARMACOKINETICS: CONCEPTS AND APPLICATIONS

Lippincott Williams & Wilkins, <<www.lww.com>>. This text covers pharmacokinetic information focused on clinical applications and usages. The information is geared toward people with little or no knowledge in this area and so is best used as a learning resource rather than a quick reference.

Pharmacology

GOODMAN & GILMAN'S: THE PHARMACOLOGICAL BASIS OF THERAPEUTICS

McGraw-Hill, <<www.mcgraw-hill.com>>. This classic pharmacology text also provides information about pharmacokinetics and pharmacodynamics of a number of drugs. The focus of the resource is to provide a correlation between principles of pharmacology and contemporary clinical practice.

BASIC & CLINICAL PHARMACOLOGY

Lange, <<www.mcgraw-hill.com>>. This text, organized by therapeutic class of agents, provides general discussion of pharmacology principles as well as a more detailed discussion of specific agents. Figures and tables are used frequently to illustrate difficult material.

PRINCIPLES OF PHARMACOLOGY

Lippincott Williams & Wilkins, <<www.lww.com>>. This text is designed for medical students and offers a good discussion of pharmacology in the context of a variety of biologic processes. The use of cases with accompanying study questions makes clinical application of these principles easy.

Pharmacy Law

GUIDE TO FEDERAL PHARMACY LAW

Apothecary Press, <<www.apothecarypress.com>>. This text is geared toward students preparing to take the pharmacy licensure examination. Discussion is provided about major legislation and the impact of these laws on pharmacy practice.

PHARMACY PRACTICE AND THE LAW

Jones and Bartlett Publishers, <<www.jbpub.com>>. This resource contains information about federal laws and regulations impacting pharmacy practice. Additional implications for pharmacy practice are provided for some legislation. Information is provided about federal and state regulation of product development, dispensing, and development. Various summaries of case law are provided. Additionally, information regarding Internet pharmacies and electronic transmission of prescriptions has been added.

Information about individual state pharmacy law, as opposed to federal law, is best obtained through the individual state boards of pharmacy. A listing of state board website URLs is available at <<http://www.nabp.net/ftpfiles/NABP01/ROSTER.pdf>>. Often the board will have this information available in PDF format on the web page. The Code of Federal Regulations containing many aspects of federal law is available at <<http://www.gpoaccess.gov/cfr/index.html>>.

Teratogenicity/Lactation

DRUGS IN PREGNANCY AND LACTATION

Lippincott Williams & Wilkins, <<www.lww.com>>. As the title implies, this text (often referred to as Brigg's) focuses exclusively on information available about the use of medications in pregnant or lactating women. Summaries of the literature available regarding fetal exposure *in utero* or exposure through breast milk are provided. Animal literature is provided in cases where human literature is lacking. Additional information about recommendations by organizations such as the American Academy of Pediatrics is provided.

MEDICATIONS AND MOTHER'S MILK: A MANUAL OF LACTATIONAL PHARMACOLOGY

Pharmasoft Publishing, <<www.ibreastfeeding.com>>. Provides information on lactation and safe use of medication. Numerous case reports are cited and discussed, also some basic pharmacokinetic data of interest are provided. The text is organized by drug monograph, and for relevant sections alternative treatment options are provided.

REPRORISK

Thompson MICROMEDEX, <<www.thomsonhc.com>>. This electronic resource is a database within the MICROMEDEX Healthcare Series providing information about both teratogenicity and lactation, based on human and animal data. Descriptions of clinical experiences and references to the primary literature are provided.

Therapy Evaluation/Drug of Choice

APPLIED THERAPEUTICS: THE CLINICAL USE OF DRUGS

Lippincott Williams & Wilkins, <www.lww.com>>. This text includes information about disease states and treatment options. Information is presented in the form of cases with follow-up discussion. Its focus is on clinical case-based presentation of information. There is also a pocket-sized handbook designed to accompany the text. This print resource is updated every 3 to 4 years and comes with a CD-ROM. A version is also available for use on a PDA.

CECIL TEXTBOOK OF MEDICINE

Saunders, <<www.us.elsevierhealth.com>>. This text is available in print, CD-ROM, PDA, and Internet (<<www.cecilmedicine.com>>) formats. Information is organized by disease state and color-coded to speed usage. Information about etiology, manifestations, diagnosis, treatment, and prognosis are provided.

HARRISON'S PRINCIPLES OF INTERNAL MEDICINE

McGraw-Hill, <<www.mcgraw-hill.com>>. This text serves as a fairly comprehensive introduction to clinical medicine. It is available in text, PDA, and electronic formats. Comprehensive information is presented including pathophysiology, differential diagnosis, and disease management.

THE MERCK MANUAL OF DIAGNOSIS AND THERAPY

Merck & Co., <<www.merck.com>>. This source provides a quick summary of disease state information, including pathology, symptoms, diagnosis, and treatment. This resource is also available online as a free resource at <<http://www.merck.com/mrkshared/mmanual/home.jsp>>, and as a CD-ROM and a PDA version.

PHARMACOTHERAPY: A PATHOPHYSIOLOGIC APPROACH

McGraw-Hill, <<www.mcgraw-hill.com>>. This text focuses on the management of a variety of disease states. Information provided about disorders includes epidemiology, etiology, presentation of disease, treatment, and treatment outcomes. A CD-ROM is also available. This resource also has accompanying texts: *Pharmacotherapy Casebook: A Patient-Focused Approach* and *Pharmacotherapy Handbook*.

TEXTBOOK OF THERAPEUTICS

Lippincott Williams & Wilkins, <<www.lww.com>>. PDA, CD-ROM, and text versions of this resource are available. While the resource focuses on treatment of disease states and development of a therapeutic plan, sections regarding pathophysiology and clinical presentation are also provided.

Toxicology

CASARETT & DOULL'S TOXICOLOGY: THE BASIC SCIENCE OF POISONS

McGraw-Hill Medical Publishing, <<www.mcgraw-hill.com>>. This resource is designed to serve as a textbook rather than a quick resource for toxicology information. Extensive information is provided regarding organ- and non-organ-directed toxicity.

ELLENHORN'S MEDICAL TOXICOLOGY: DIAGNOSIS AND TREATMENT OF HUMAN POISONING

Lippincott Williams & Wilkins, <<www.lww.com>>. This resource provides toxicology and management information for a variety of drugs, household products, natural toxins, and other chemicals. Some information is presented in the form of tables, making information easier to find than some other toxicology texts.

GOLDFRANK'S TOXICOLOGIC EMERGENCIES

McGraw-Hill Medical Publishing, <<www.mcgraw-hill.com>>. This text is designed to offer a case study approach to toxicology. Initial basic toxicology data are provided but the majority of this text focuses on the management of toxicologic emergencies with a variety of common drugs, botanicals, pesticides, and other occupational or environmental hazards.

POISINDEX®

Thompson MICROMEDEX, <<www.thomsonhc.com>>. This electronic resource is a database within the MICROMEDEX Healthcare Series, providing information about presentation and treatment of many toxicology situations. The information presented is based on human case reports and animal data and is extensively referenced.

Veterinary Medicine

Practice settings that handle a large number of veterinary information questions may benefit from having access to some of the following resources. Information about additional useful resources can be found in Appendix 4–1.

COMPENDIUM OF VETERINARY PRODUCTS (CVP)

North American Compendiums, <<www.prodvm.com>>. This textbook is similar to the human *PDR* in terms of information provided and format. The resource contains the product monographs for over 4800 pharmaceutical, biologic, diagnostic, feed additive, and pesticide products that are currently available. The reference contains indicies of manufacturers and distributors, brand names/ingredients, and product categories.

FOOD AND DRUG ADMINISTRATION/CENTER FOR VETERINARY MEDICINE HOME PAGE

Food and Drug Administration (FDA) <<http://www.fda.gov/cvm/default.html>>. This website provides information for pharmacists about the legal or regulatory issues that affect the practice of veterinary pharmacy or veterinary medicine. It is useful for regulatory issues pertaining to animal health. The compliance policy guide (CPG 608.400) *Compounding of Drugs for Use in Animals* and the Animal Medicinal Drug Use Clarification Act (AMDUCA) can be found at this site, these documents are considered essential reading for any pharmacist who practices veterinary pharmacy. CVM updates are available that detail the prohibited use of drugs in certain animal populations. Updates on the judicious use of antibiotics in food-producing animals are posted at this site. A listing of all FDA-approved animal drug products, also known as the *Green Book*, is available and searchable at this site. Patent information, manufacturer lists, indications, approval numbers, general drug information, code of regulations, and trade/generic names are just a few pieces of information that can be gathered from this website.

THE 5-MINUTE VETERINARY CONSULTANT: CANINE AND FELINE

Lippincott Williams & Wilkins, <<www.lww.com>>. This is a quick reference textbook on internal medicine in canine and feline health. The resource focuses on signs and symptoms, drug indications, and laboratory interpretations. Good appendices are provided on conversion tables, lab values, drug formularies, and toxicology.

TEXTBOOK OF VETERINARY INTERNAL MEDICINE: DISEASES OF THE DOG AND CAT

W.B. Saunders Company, <<www.us.elsevierhealth.com/Veterinary>>. This is a practical, useful, and informative two-volume resource, focusing on internal medicine topics in canines and felines. The text provides extensive coverage of pathophysiology, diagnosis, and treatment of diseases affecting dogs and cats.

VETERINARY DRUG HANDBOOK

Blackwell Publishing, <<www.blackwellprofessional.com>>. This textbook is written by a pharmacist and is considered one of the most useful references for off-label drug dosages, indications, and specific drug information on human- and veterinary-labeled pharmaceuticals. Monographs are listed in alphabetical order, and categorize drugs chemistry, pharmacology, indications, dosages, contraindications, and interactions into an easily identifiable format. A client information booklet is also available.

Pharmacists should also be aware that more resources are becoming available in a variety of formats. Many resources that have been traditionally only available in a paper text are now accessible via CD-ROM, the Internet, or via PDA. Selection of the appropriate format (e.g., hardcopy, computer, and PDA) is now another factor that pharmacists should consider when selecting resources for a practice site. Electronic resources are often preferred because they may be easier to use, allow quicker access to information, allow multiple searches to be performed simultaneously, and often contain the most recent information available regarding a topic. Additionally, many electronic networked resources allow use of the same resource at more than one location. This lets many practitioners access information from a variety of physical locations rather than being restricted to only medical libraries or drug information centers.

References for PDA

The incorporation of PDAs into clinical practice settings has lead to an increase in the number of databases that provide sources of drug information. Several databases have been created by companies currently producing a variety of other well-known drug information resources, e.g., Lexi-Comp, Thompson Healthcare, and The American Society of Health-System Pharmacists. The databases available differ in terms of material covered as well as quality of coverage. A limited number of critical evaluations of these databases has been performed to aid in the selection of the highest quality databases. [92-94] Based on the limited data available, Lexi-Comp, ePocrates, and Clinical Pharmacology OnHand appear to be among the best quality PDA drug information databases available at this time. One additional study[95] evaluating the efficacy of PDA databases specifically for addressing drug interaction information found slightly different results than previous studies but did find Lexi-Interact to be one of the top performers, in addition to iFacts (<<www.skyscape.com>>).

Secondary Literature

Secondary literature refers to references that either index or abstract the primary literature with the goal of directing the user to the primary literature. The two terms, indexing and abstracting, differ slightly. Indexing consists of providing bibliographic citation information (e.g., title, author, and citation of the article), while abstracting also includes a brief description (or abstract) of the information provided by the article or resource cited. Various systems will index or abstract literature from different journals, meetings, or publications, therefore, in order to perform a comprehensive search different databases must be used.

The vast majority of secondary resources are utilized primarily in an electronic format, although some may still have a print form. Occasionally a paper resource may be used because it is less costly than an electronic database. Using a paper resource will often require more time than the electronic formats, due to the need to look at multiple editions and indexes (possibly an annual or quarterly listing). There is an additional disadvantage in that the printed sources can be searched by only one user at a time. An advantage to printed resources is their use for browsing for new information.

Electronic databases offer some advantages over print listings. Notably, for online listings, the more frequent updating of listings and information is very important. In searching most electronic databases, a user will follow a similar search strategy, with small changes to reflect differences in database systems. There are several challenges in searching secondary database systems. Systems do not index all terms in the same manner therefore it is necessary to determine what terms a database is using to conduct a successful search. For example, databases through the National Library of Medicine index terms by their Medical Subject Heading (MeSH term), while the Iowa Drug Information Service (IDIS) uses the United States Adopted Name and the International Classification of Diseases. Most computerized databases also include a free-text search option, which is very useful when the defined index terms are not identifying relevant data. This option may also be helpful when only limited data have been published or are available, perhaps before an official index term is defined.

The need to utilize a variety of terms for search strategy is illustrated in the following sample question "Is clonidine effective in the treatment of attention deficit hyperactivity disorder (ADHD) in adolescents?" It is first important to identify the key terms. These terms might include clonidine, ADHD, and adolescents. However, some databases may not recognize the term adolescent and instead may require use of the term pediatric or child. Additionally, the use of the term pediatric may just refer to the medical specialty in some resources, rather than the pediatric patient population. Therefore, it is important to recognize that different databases may require different search terms to be used. Also, the name of the disease state, attention deficit hyperactivity disorder, has changed over time and so it may be necessary to use other terms, such as attention deficit disorder.

Searches generally use Boolean operators, often AND, OR, and NOT (see Figure 4–1). The operator AND will combine two terms, returning only citations containing both of those concepts or terms. The operator OR will have an equal or greater number of returns since it will include any citation where either term is used. Use of the term NOT will always decrease the number of responses, since it eliminates any references having the term that follows that operator; therefore it should be used with caution, since it may eliminate articles that may be appropriate, simply because the term being eliminated happens to appear somewhere in the article.

For example, in the earlier clonidine for ADHD question, the appropriate search terms (*clonidine* AND *attention deficit hyperactivity disorder*) may be used with the AND operator. However, if the requestor wanted information regarding use of either clonidine or guanfacine

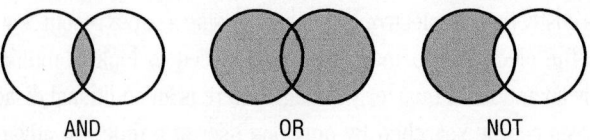

Figure 4–1. Boolean operators.

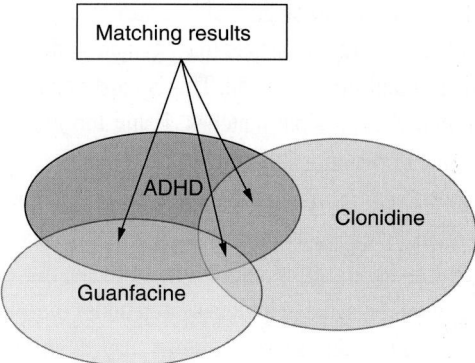

Figure 4–2. ADHD AND (clonidine OR guanfacine).

in this disease state, then the term OR might be used. See Figure 4–2 for a graphic presentation of this search. A search using OR will return a number of results equal to or greater than a search using the term AND. The term OR might also be useful when searching for a term with synonyms, for example, attention deficit disorder OR ADHD. The operator NOT would be helpful if a user wants to exclude certain topics, for example, a specific disease state. In this case, a search might be performed for ADHD NOT Tourette's disorder (see Figure 4–3). Since the use of the term NOT will exclude any article mentioning Tourette's disease, an article focused on treatment of ADHD with a small section about Tourette's disease would also be excluded. Parentheses can also be used to further streamline a search. In this example, a search may be performed for *clonidine* AND *(attention deficit disorder* OR *ADHD)*, this would retrieve articles that contain the drug of interest as well as either of the two disease states of interest. An additional example of search strategy is provided in Appendix 4–2.

Some databases will also use the terms WITH or NEAR. These operators are similar to AND, however, they require the terms to be within a certain number of words of each other. These terms may be useful when other searches are identifying a large number of articles where both terms are mentioned, but not in conjunction with each other.

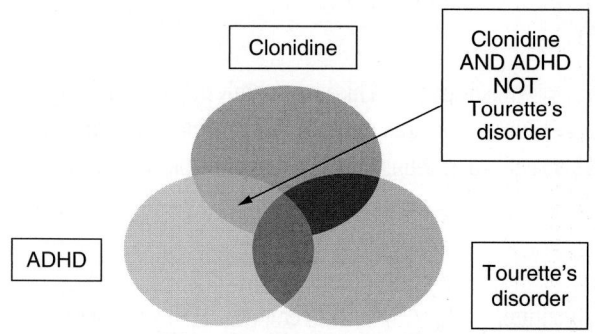

Figure 4–3. Clonidine and ADHD NOT Tourette's disorder.

Some databases allow searches to be limited by a variety of factors, including language of publication, year of publication, type of article (e.g., human study, review, and case report), or by type of journal where publication is found. This is most helpful when the initial search terms return a large number of possible matches. Using too many limits with the initial search may eliminate articles or citations that would be helpful.

One additional point to bear in mind when performing electronic searches is that the same search phrase could be indexed under a variety of search terms, and in order to provide a comprehensive search it is important to address all of those. For example, if looking for information regarding ginkgo it may be helpful to search under the common name as well as a common misspelling. So a possible search strategy may be to use the terms "ginkgo", "ginkgo biloba", the Latin name "Ginkgoaceae", as well as the misspelled word "gingko". This same principle holds true when considering disease states whose names may have changed over time.

Included below are some examples of secondary databases and types of requests they are helpful in addressing.

ANTI-INFECTIVES TODAY

Adis International, <<www.adis.com>>. This monthly service indexes important new research, adverse reactions, and pharmacoeconomic data in the area of therapies for infectious disease. Paper as well as electronic formats are available.

BIOLOGIC ABSTRACTS/BIOSIS PREVIEWS

Thompson Medical, <<www.biosis.org>>. This is a comprehensive database of biologic information, covering biologic and biomedical information. BIOSIS also covers abstracts from conferences relating to basic sciences. This is most helpful when seeking basic science information. Both print and electronic formats are available and are updated semimonthly.

CANCER TODAY

Adis International, <<www.adis.com>>. This is a monthly indexing and abstracting service summarizing current literature in the area of cancer management. Information from recent trials, case reports, and international meetings is provided. Available in print and also electronically.

CANCERLIT

National Cancer Institute, <<http://www.cancer.gov/>>. This database is maintained by the National Cancer Institute and indexes literature from a variety of sources specific to cancer literature. This resource is most useful when looking for information about oncology therapies or quality-of-life issues. This resource is updated monthly and is available electronically at <<http://www.cancer.gov/search/cancer_literature/>>.

CINAHL

CINAHL Information Systems, <<www.cinahl.com>>. This is an indexing service that covers literature primarily in the fields of nursing and allied health. This database is useful when seeking information about patient care from the perspective of allied health professionals. It is updated monthly.

THE COCHRANE DATABASE OF SYSTEMATIC REVIEWS

Cochrane Library, <<www.cochrane.org>>. This database, published quarterly, indexes Cochrane reviews about a variety of medical treatments, conditions, and alternative therapies. These evidence-based medicine reviews are based on extensive analysis of current literature and provide treatment recommendations (see Chap. 9).

CURRENT CONTENTS

Thompson Medical, <<www.isinet.com>>. This electronic service offers an overview of very recently published literature as it relates to scientific information. The clinical medicine and life science subgroups are useful for information about recent drug research or developments.

EMBASE

Elsevier, <<www.embase.com>>. EMBASE is a comprehensive abstracting service covering biomedical literature worldwide. This database covers material similar to that covered by MEDLINE®, but with greater coverage of international publications. Additionally, there is less lag time between publication and inclusion in the database. This database is useful when seeking information about dietary supplements or medications that may be available in other countries.

GOOGLE SCHOLAR

Google, <<scholar.google.com>>. An Internet search engine that is designed to target scholarly materials available online in a variety of professional areas including health care. Information from a variety of scholarly journals and publications is able to be searched, however, in some cases, the searcher may not be able to access full-text versions of articles or works due to password restrictions.

INPHARMA WEEKLY

Adis International, <<www.adis.com>>. An abstracting service that provides current literature related to pharmacotherapy. It also provides information regarding drugs in development. This resource is useful when seeking information about experimental drugs or ongoing research. While this resource is not comprehensive, it does offer a very short lag time and offers a way for users to quickly scan the literature and keep abreast of recent changes and developments.

INTERNATIONAL PHARMACEUTICAL ABSTRACTS (IPA)

American Society of Health-System Pharmacists, <<www.ashp.org>>. Coverage includes drug-related information, including drug use and development. This database also abstracts a variety of meeting presentations. The main focus of this database is pharmacy information, including pharmacy administration and clinical services, making it the most comprehensive database for pharmacy-specific information.

IOWA DRUG INFORMATION SERVICE

Division of Drug Information Service, University of Iowa, <<http://itsnt14.its.uiowa.edu/>>. This is an indexing service that allows retrieval of complete articles from a variety of biomedical publications. Indexing is done by database-specific terms, which at times makes searching challenging. This database is useful for information about standard medications. It is unique in that it provides full articles, in either PDF form or, for older articles, microfiche. There are a limited number of journals covered and not all information from a specific journal issue is covered (i.e., some articles may not be included if the editorial staff did not feel that they had sufficient focus on relevant drug or disease state information).

JOURNAL WATCH

Massachusetts Medical Society, <<www.jwatch.org>>. Journal Watch is an abstracting service including recent information, summarized by physicians, from a variety of medical literature. A general newsletter covering major medical stories of interest to generalists is published along with additional newsletters in specific specialty areas. This is most helpful when monitoring for new clinical trials involving specific medications.

LEXISNEXIS

LexisNexis Academic & Library Solutions, <<www.lexisnexis.com>>. This indexing and abstracting service covers a variety of information, including medical, legal, and business news. Some publications are available full text through this service. This resource is helpful when attempting to locate information about recent medical news or research.

MEDLINE®

National Library of Medicine, <<www.nlm.nih.gov>>. Coverage includes basic and clinical sciences as well as nursing, dentistry, veterinary medicine, and many other health care disciplines. Information comes from more than 3900 journals in 40 different languages. This database is available through a variety of services including PubMed®. A sample search is provided in Appendix 4–2.

PAEDIATRICS TODAY

Adis International, <<www.adis.com>>. This monthly indexing and abstracting service covers recent literature regarding the use of drugs in pediatrics from both biomedical literature and recent clinical meetings. Requestors seeking information about pediatric uses of medications may find this resource helpful.

PHARMACOECONOMICS AND OUTCOMES NEWS WEEKLY

Adis International, <<www.adis.com>>. This biweekly publication covers recent publications regarding economic use of health care resources, as well as information on prescribing trends, recent health care news, and regulatory updates. The focus of this publication is the economic impact of disease states and medical interventions.

REACTIONS WEEKLY

Adis International, <<www.adis.com>>. A weekly indexing/abstracting service summarizing literature involving adverse events, drug interactions, drug dependence, and toxicology data. This resource is especially useful when seeking case reports of adverse reactions or other information on drug safety.

Primary Literature

Primary literature consists of clinical research studies and reports, both published and unpublished. Not all literature published in a journal is classified as primary literature, for example, review articles or editorials are not primary literature. There are several types of publications considered primary, including controlled trials, cohort studies, case series, and case reports. Additional information about study designs commonly found in medical literature and how to evaluate them is found in Chaps. 6 and 7.

Advantages of the use of primary literature include access to detailed information about a topic and the ability to personally assess the utility and validity of study results. Additionally, primary literature tends to be more recent than tertiary or secondary literature. However, there are several disadvantages of using primary literature alone. These disadvantages include misleading conclusions based on only one trial without the context of other researches, the need to have good skills in medial literature evaluation, and the time needed to evaluate the large volume of literature available.

Due to the rapidly increasing number of specialty journals being published, it is difficult to determine which journals are essential in a pharmacy practice setting. Appendix 4–3 provides a listing of core holdings for a college of pharmacy assembled by the American Association of Colleges of Pharmacy.[96] While this list may be more extensive than what is required in many practice settings, it does provide a core listing of journals. Each practice setting will require slightly different primary literature based on the specific areas that are of greatest importance to that facility.

Obtaining the Primary Literature

Once the literature has been identified in a secondary searching system, then the actual articles can be obtained in various ways. Often a local library may carry the journal needed, or may be affiliated with other facilities that can provide that article. Some publisher websites also have access to some full-text articles. If neither of these options are available then the Loansome Doc ordering system might be used. This system is available through the National Library of Medicine and offered for a fee to any user. Articles identified in PubMed® can be easily ordered from that database through this system. Additional information about this program is available at <<http://www.nlm.nih.gov/pubs/factsheets/loansome_doc.html>>.

Internet Resources

Another method to identify relevant resources might be a general Internet search for information. This can be especially helpful to serve as a starting point for questions about unusual diseases or about marketed over-the-counter products and combination dietary supplements. For example, if a requestor asked about the use of a dietary supplement product called

GABA Plus in ADHD, it would be difficult to search for information, unless the requestor was able to provide a list of ingredients contained in the product. Often requestors may not have that information and therefore it may be necessary to search for a manufacturer's website to identify the specific individual ingredients and then look for information on the individual components. This is also helpful in identifying information or specific product claims provided by the manufacturer. Additionally, Internet searches may be useful for topics that have recently been in the news, where information is changing more rapidly than standard paper resources can be updated.

It is important to remember that different search engines use different techniques to identify web pages, and that no search engines will identify all websites. Some search engines are geared toward scholarly content (Google Scholar, <<scholar.google.com>>) or toward scientific research (Scirus, <<www.scirus.com>>), rather than general information. These might be more useful for identifying recent research about a disease or disorder, rather than the ingredients in *GABA Plus*. In order to efficiently perform a search, it is important to consider which search engine would most likely index the desired materials. Additional discussion of search engines is found in Chap. 5.

There are, however, several caveats to finding information on the Internet. The first is to carefully evaluate the quality of all information provided. There are literally millions of websites and there are no true quality assurance measures in place to evaluate the reliability of information available. There are some general tenets to keep in mind when evaluating this type of literature. Generally, sites maintained by educational institutions, not-for-profit medical organizations, or a division of the U.S. government are likely to contain high quality information, whereas information maintained by a company selling or promoting a specific product may be more questionable.

In order to assess the quality of online information, several standards and programs now exist. These include organizations such as the Health on the Net (HON code, <<www.hon.ch>>),[97] which clearly define rules to evaluate the quality of information available via a website. Many websites do not apply to organizations to be evaluated, so the lack of an organization's quality seal does not necessarily indicate that the information is of low quality.

The following criteria should be used when determining quality of online material.

- Is the source credible, without a vested interest in promoting one particular treatment or product?
- Is the information accurate and current?
- Does the site link to other nonaffiliated sites that provide good information consistently?
- Is the information appropriately detailed and referenced?
- Is it possible to identify the author of the site to contact with additional questions or comments?

Further information on evaluating websites is discussed in Chap. 5.

Alternative Information Sources

Occasionally, sufficient information cannot be obtained from standard resources, requiring instead the use of some alternative sources of information. If a question involves, for example, a recent news story reporting a removal of a medication from the market, a logical first place to find initial information would be to identify the original news story. This can be done by searching various newswire services like PR Newswire or even major news network websites such as CNN. LexisNexis, <www.lexisnexis.com>>, indexes a variety of newswire stories as well as transcripts of news reports. While this news story may not provide all the information needed, it might at least serve as a point from which to search for additional information (Table 4–3).

In some cases, there may be so little information available that it would be wise to seek out an expert in the field, for example, the use of heparin in a troche dosage form. It may be prudent to contact persons performing research in this area or practitioners who are currently using that therapy to identify information that might have been missed in an initial search. Some experts may be identified via medical organizations focusing on specific disease states, leadership of medical societies, or persons who have authored numerous papers on a specific medication or medical condition.

When looking for recent recommendations regarding treatment of a specific disease state, it may be helpful to identify an organization affiliated with that disease state. For example, when looking for treatment recommendations to manage irritable bowel syndrome it might be appropriate to contact the International Foundation for Functional Gastrointestinal Disorders (<<http://www.iffgd.org/>>) to obtain information about current practice standards as well as possible emerging therapies.

Additionally, when seeking information about a specific drug therapy, it may be helpful to contact product manufacturers via their medical information department to identify information that may be available in-house. This resource could be especially helpful for obtaining the literature that is difficult to access if a product is newly approved or identifying a possible rare adverse drug reaction.

TABLE 4–3. MAJOR NEWS SOURCES ONLINE

News Source	URL
ABC	www.abcnews.go.com
AP (Associated Press)	www.ap.org
CBS	www.cbsnews.com
CNN	www.cnn.com
FDC Reports	www.healthnewsdaily.com/FDC/Daily/hnd/TOC.htm
MSNBC	www.msnbc.msn.com
Reuters Health News	www.reutershealth.com/en/index.html
PR Newswire	www.prnewswire.com

Consumer Health Information

As consumers become more active and educated in their health care and disease management, the need for health information sources geared at consumers has increased. Currently there are a variety of sources where consumers obtain their health information. A recent survey indicated that the most common source of information about prescription medication, behind physicians and pharmacists, is the Internet.[98] Since many consumers find at least some of their information online, pharmacists should be prepared to help consumers evaluate the quality of information found online as well as recommend sites where information might be found. Table 4–4 contains a listing of just a few of the sources that may be useful for consumers.

TABLE 4–4. ONLINE CONSUMER INFORMATION SOURCES

Website URL	Maintained By	Information
www.medlineplus.gov	National Library of Medicine	Contains information about various medications as well as disease states and conditions
www.fda.gov/cder	Food and Drug Administration	Contains information about new drugs as well as dietary supplements. Also contains information about recalls of drug or food
www.gettingwell.com	Thomson Health care	Contains information about a variety of prescription drugs
www.merckhomeedition.com	Merck	This is a consumer-based version of the *Merck Manual*. It includes a variety of interactive features
www.healthfinder.gov	Department of Health and Human Services	This site contains information about a variety of common medical conditions and diseases
www.4women.gov	National Women's Health Information Center	This site contains information about the conditions and diseases of special interest to women
www.cdc.gov	Centers for Disease Control and Prevention	This site has information about the treatment and prevention of infectious diseases. It also contains a listing of public health hoaxes
dirline.nlm.nih.gov	National Library of Medicine and National Institute of Health	This contains a directory of health care organizations online
ods.od.nih.gov	National Institute of Health	This site compiles some of the scientific information available about the efficacy and safety of dietary supplements
nccam.nih.gov	National Center for Complementary and Alternative Medicine	This site is a government maintained resource describing ongoing research in the area of dietary supplements, as well as detailing efficacy information currently available

Consumers may also benefit from some text resources available at a local library. Some resources, like *The PDR Family Guide to Prescription Drugs*,[99] are published by organizations that produce references for health care professionals, while others are published by lay press companies. There is great variation in the quality of information provided from resource to resource. Some of the most popular resources may not be written at an appropriate level for a consumer to understand or may not provide helpful information for the patient. For this reason, it is important to discuss with patients what other resources they are using to find additional drug and medical information. Opening a dialogue with patients about this topic is fairly simple and can consist of open-ended questions such as "Where else have you found information on your disease state?" or "What other material have you read about your medication?"

Often, one can confidently recommend health care organizations or disease societies, both of which usually provide helpful, high quality disease-specific information geared for the average consumer. Some drug companies offer web pages with helpful disease or disease management information.

In addition to the resources aimed at consumers, there are consumer-specific sections of many tertiary resources discussed earlier. Electronic resources such as MICROMEDEX or Clinical Pharmacology have subsections dedicated to consumer-level information. Additionally text references such as *USP DI* have information written at an appropriate level for consumers.

Conclusion

Given the rapid rate at which medical information is increasing and the amount of available technology to organize and locate this information, it is easy to become overwhelmed by the volume of data available. However, as pharmacists develop a better understanding of where to access information, provision of drug information will occur more quickly. As technological advances continue, which may change the face of physical pharmacy dispensing and compounding, the need for information retrieval and interpretation will continue to grow. Pharmacists must not, however, be satisfied with merely identifying sources for drug information. Understanding where to access information is only the first step in the provision of quality drug information. Information must be interpreted and evaluated to become knowledge, as is described in other chapters. It is this unique knowledge that will enable practitioners to optimize patient care.

The information in this chapter helps provide guidance as to where specific types of drug information might be found and how to begin a search for drug information. The next several chapters will provide additional guidance on how to interpret and apply the information that is gathered.

Study Questions

1. A physician is seeking information about the use of chondroitin in the management of osteoarthritis. He sees a large number of patients in his practice and is seeking information about efficacy, safety, and appropriate dosing of this product.
   a. What are the advantages and disadvantages of tertiary resources in responding to this request?
   b. What are the advantages and disadvantages of primary literature in this scenario?
   c. What might be the appropriate key words to use to identify relevant information in a secondary database?
   d. Might information on the Internet be helpful in responding to this question?

2. A 15-year-old patient has recently been started on atomoxetine for treatment of attention deficit/hyperactivity disorder. He is taking no other medications. He has noted recently that his hair is thinning and wants to know if this might be drug related.
   a. What are the appropriate tertiary resources to consult for a response to this request?
   b. Is it necessary to consult tertiary, secondary, and primary resources for this response?
   c. If no information is found in any tertiary resources or in a search of secondary databases, where might additional information be located?

3. Consider which tertiary, secondary, and primary resources might be appropriate for the following drug information requests.
   a. A physician requests information about the use of sildenafil for treatment of female sexual arousal disorder. She also requests information about the use of any of the other phosphodiesterase 5 inhibitors.
   b. A patient has mixed all his medications together in a pill box and needs a capsule to be identified. The capsule is purple and gray and has the imprint code 224 3850.
   c. A pharmacist wants to know what current investigational drugs are being used to treat Huntington's disease.
   d. A prescriber needs to give diazepam to a 7-year-old child who is not able to swallow pills or capsules. By what other routes can this drug be given and what dose is appropriate for this patient?
   e. A patient who is visiting the United States from Sweden contacts the pharmacist asking for advice. He has had problems with acid reflux and took Artonil® at home, which relieved his symptoms well, and would like to know what would be an equivalent medication available here in the United States.
   f. A pharmacist received a prescription for dexamethasone to help reduce a tumor. The pharmacist wants to know what dose is appropriate for this use.

g. A nurse requests information about long-term use of prednisone therapy. He recalls that there are serious long-term adverse events and is curious what these events are and how they might be managed.

h. A pharmacy student is working on a presentation involving illicit drugs. She knows that there have been recent news stories about adolescents using Coricidin products for recreational use, and she is curious at what doses these products are toxic.

i. A patient is given a prescription for promethazine 25 mg orally every 6 hours to treat nausea and vomiting. The patient is currently taking sertraline 50 mg daily and Ortho Tri Cyclen Lo®. Are there any interactions between the patient's medications?

j. A 5-year-old female has a history of acid reflux; the patient was well controlled on a cisapride product with no problems. Since cisapride has been removed from the market what might an appropriate treatment option for this patient be?

k. A patient is receiving amiodarone in a bag of normal saline. The nurse wants to know if the amiodarone therapy is compatible with metronidazole.

l. A consumer contacts the pharmacy requesting information about drug screening tests. She has a drug screen scheduled 3 days from today and last night she used cocaine. She wants to know if the cocaine will be out of her system before the drug screen test.

m. A prescriber wants to know the role of cytochrome P450 3A4 in the metabolism of carvedilol.

n. A new mother has been breastfeeding her child for 3 months. The mother has recently been prescribed levofloxacin for treatment of an infection. Is it safe for her to continue breastfeeding during this therapy?

4. Consider which tertiary resource would be useful in answering the following veterinary drug information questions:

a. A woman calls you stating that her 8-month-old Great Dane puppy jumped onto her bathroom counter top and ate the entire contents of a prescription bottle containing Darvocet-N 100 #60 tables and a bar of scented hand soap.

b. A fellow pharmacist has received a request to compound injectable ivermectin 1% for beef cattle. What is this drug, its indication, and is it legal to compound this drug for food animals?

c. A newly licensed veterinarian calls and inquires about the human selective serotonin reuptake inhibitor (SSRI) class of drugs and wants to know how many have an off-label dosage for dogs?

d. A long-time client in your diabetes management clinic states that her cat was recently diagnosed with diabetes by a veterinarian. The woman is asking for information on diabetes in cats and how it is similar to different human diabetes.

e. A customer asks you about the use of herbals and nutraceuticals in dogs. What website provides this type of information for animal owners?

f. A customer approaches you and hands you a piece of paper. On the paper is written "Kaopectate for dog diarrhea." The customer states that the veterinarian directed her to get some Kaopectate® over-the-counter for her dog that has loose stools. What resources would be helpful in determining if this is an acceptable therapy and a proper dose?

REFERENCES

1. Doody's Core Titles in the Health Sciences, 2005 ed. Chicago (IL): Doody Enterprises, Inc., 2005.
2. Rosenberg JM, Koumis T, Nathan JP, Cicero LA, McGuire H. Current status of pharmacist-operated drug information centers in the United States. Am J Health Syst Pharm. 2004;61:2023–32.
3. Alphabetic listing of 2001 AACP Basic Resources for Pharmaceutical Education. American Association of Colleges of Pharmacy; 2002 Feb [cited 2004 March 1]: [41 screens]. Available from: http://www.aacp.org/site/tertiary.asp?TRACKID=&VID=2&CID=381&DID=3499
4. Anderson PO, Knoben JE, Troutman WG, editors. Handbook of clinical drug data. 10th ed. New York: McGraw-Hill; 2002.
5. Berardi RR, Popovich NG, editors. Handbook of nonprescription drugs. 13th ed. Washington, DC: American Pharmaceutical Association; 2000.
6. Clinical Pharmacology [database on the Internet]. Tampa (FL): Gold Standard Multimedia; c2004. [updated 2004 Feb 28; cited 2004 Mar 1]. Available from : http://www.cp.gsm.com
7. Dukes MNG, editor. Meyler's side effects of drugs. 14th ed. Amsterdam, The Netherlands: Elsevier; 2000.
8. Drug Therapy Monitoring System [database on the Internet]. St. Louis (MO): Wolters Kluwer Health; c2005. Cited 2005 February 10. Available from: htp://www.medi-span.com
9. Red book. 2002 edition. Montvale (NJ): Thomson Medical Economics; 2002.
10. Billups NF, Billups SM, editors. American drug index. 48th ed. St. Louis (MO): Facts and Comparisons; 2003.
11. Gennaro AR, Popovich NG, DerMarderosian AH, editors. Remington: the science and practice of pharmacy. 20th ed. Philadelphia (PA): Lippincott Williams & Wilkins; 2000.
12. The Merck index. 13th ed. Whitehouse Station (NJ): Merck & Co.; 2001.
13. Thompson JE. A practical guide to contemporary pharmacy practice. Philadelphia (PA): Lippincott Williams & Wilkins; 2004.
14. USP/NF: the official compendia of standards. Rockville (MD): United States Pharmacopeial Convention; 2004.
15. Allen LV. Allen's compounded formulations. Washington, DC: American Pharmaceutical Association; 1999.
16. Sweetman SC, editor. Martindale: the complete drug reference. 33rd ed. London: Pharmaceutical Press; 2002.
17. Jew RK, Mullen RJ, Soo-Hoo W. Extemporaneous formulations. Bethesda (MD): American Society of Health-System Pharmacists; 2003.
18. Allen LV, Popovich NG, Ansel HC, editors. Ansel's pharmaceutical dosage forms and drug delivery systems. 8th ed. Philadelphia (PA): Lippincott Williams & Wilkins; 2005.

19. Allen LV, editor. The art, science, and technology of pharmaceutical compounding. Washington, DC: American Pharmaceutical Association; 2002.

20. Jellin JM, Gregory PJ, Batz F, Hitchens K, editors. Natural medicine comprehensive database. 7th ed. Stockton (CA): Therapeutic Research Faculty; 2005.

21. DerMarderosian A, Beutler JA, editors. The review of natural products. 2004 ed. St. Louis (MO): Facts & Comparisons; 2004.

22. Fetrow CW, Avila JR, editors. Professional's handbook of complementary and alternative medicine. 3rd ed. Philadelphia (PA): Lippincott Williams & Wilkins; 2004.

23. Blumethal M, Goldberg A, Brinckmann J, editors. Herbal medicine: expanded commission E monographs. Austin (TX): American Botanical Council; 2000.

24. PDR for herbal medicines. 2nd ed. Montvale (NJ): Thomson Medical Economics; 2000.

25. Barnes J, Anderson LA, Phillipson JD, editors. Herbal medicine: a guide for health care professionals. 2nd ed. London: Pharmaceutical Press; 2002.

26. Brinker F. Herb contraindications and drug interactions. 3rd ed. Sandy (OR): Eclectic Medical Publishing; 2001.

27. Klasco RK, editor. AltMedDex [database on CD-ROM]. Vol 120. Englewood (CO): Thompson Micromedex; 2004.

28. Aronoff GR, Berns JS, Brier ME, Golpher TA, Morrison G, Singer I, et al. Drug prescribing in renal failure. 4th ed. Philadelphia (PA): American College of Physicians; 1999.

29. Hansten PD, Horn JR, editors. Hansten and Horn's drug interactions analysis and management. Vancouver: Applied Therapeutics; 2002.

30. Tatro DS, editor. Drug interaction facts. 2003 ed. St. Louis (MO): Facts and Comparisons; 2003.

31. Stockley IA, editor. Stockley's drug interactions. 6th ed. London: Pharmaceutical Press; 2002.

32. Klasco RK, editor. Drug-REAX [database on CD-ROM]. Vol 120. Englewood (CO): Thompson Micromedex; 2004.

33. Traub SL, editor. Basic skills in interpreting laboratory data. 2nd ed. Bethesda (MD): American Society of Health-System Pharmacists; 1996.

34. Jacobs DS, Oxley DK, editors. Jacobs & DeMott laboratory test handbook. 5th ed. Hudson (OH): Lexi-Comp; 2001.

35. Tietz NW, editor. Clinical guide to laboratory tests. 3rd ed. Philadelphia (PA): W.B. Saunders; 1995.

36. Chernecky CC, Berger BJ, editors. Laboratory tests and diagnostic procedures. 3rd ed. Philadelphia (PA): W.B. Saunders; 2001.

37. Briggs GG, Freeman RK, Yaffe SJ. Drugs in pregnancy and lactation. 6th ed. Philadelphia (PA): Lippincott Williams & Wilkins; 2002.

38. Schaefer C, editor. Drugs during pregnancy and lactation. Amsterdam (The Netherlands): Elsevier; 2001.

39. Weiner CP, editor. Drugs for pregnant and lactating women. New York: Churchill Livingstone; 2004.

40. Hale TW. Medications and mother's milk. 11th ed. Amarillo (TX): Pharmasoft Medical Pub; 2004.

41. Klasco RK, editor. REPRORISK [database on CD-ROM]. Vol 120. Englewood (CO): Thompson Micromedex; 2004.

42. Swiss Pharmaceutical Society. Index nominum: international drug directory. 18th ed. Germany: Medpharm; 2004.

43. DRUGDEX® [database on CD-ROM]. Vol. 120. Englewood (CO): Thompson Micromedex Health care Series; 2004.

44. Muler NF, Dessing RP, editors. European drug index. 4th ed. Stuttgart: Deutscher Aptheker Verlag; 1997.

45. Selma TP, editor. Geriatric dosage handbook. 9th ed. Hudson (OH): Lexi-Comp; 2003.

46. Beers MH, Berkow R, editors. The Merck manual of geriatrics. 3rd ed. Whitehouse Station (NJ): Merck Research Laboratories; 2000.

47. IDENTIDEX® [database on CD-ROM]. Vol 120. Englewood (CO): Thompson Micromedex; 2004.

48. Jellin JM, editor. Ident-a-drug reference. 2002 ed. Stockton: Therapeutic Research Faculty; 2002.

49. Clinical Reference Library online [database on the Internet]. Hudson (OH): Lexi-Comp; c2004 [updated 2004 Mar 1; cited 2004 Mar 3]. Available from: http://www.crlonline.com

50. U.S. food and drug administration center for drug evaluation and research [home page on the Internet]. Rockville (MD): Food and Drug Administration [updated 2004 Feb 3; cited 2004 March 1]. Available from: http://www.fda.gov/cder/.

51. ClinicialTrials.gov [home page on the Internet]. Bethesda (MD): National Institutes of Health [updated 2004 Feb 27; cited 2004 March 1]. Available from: http://www.clinicaltrials.gov

52. MEDLINE® Plus [home page on the Internet]. Bethesda (MD): National Library of Medicine and National Institute of Health [updated 2004 Mar 4; cited 2004 March 4]. Available from: http://www.nlm.nih.gov/ medlineplus/healthtopics.html

53. Trissel LA, editor. Handbook of injectable drugs. 11th ed. Bethesda (MD): American Society of Health-System Pharmacists; 2001.

54. King JC, Catannia PN. King guide to parenteral admixtures [database on the Internet]. Napa (CA): King Guide Publications; c2003 [updated 2003 Dec 31; cited 2004 Mar 1]. Available from: http://www.crlonline.com

55. Trissel LA, editor. Trissel's stability of compounded formulations. 2nd ed. Washington, DC: American Pharmaceutical Association; 2000.

56. Bing CM, editor. Extended stability for parenteral drugs. 2nd ed. Bethesda (MD): American Society of Health-System Pharmacists; 2003.

57. Gunn VL, Christian N, Barone MA, editors. The Harriet Lane handbook: a manual for pediatric house officers. 16th ed. St. Louis (MO): Mosby; 2002.

58. Taketomo CK, Hodding JH, Kraus DM. Pediatric dosage handbook. 10th ed. Hudson (OH): Lexi-Comp; 2003.

59. Young TE, Mangum B, editors. Neofax. 15th ed. Raleigh (NC): Acorn Publishing: 2002.

60. Murphy JE. Clinical pharmacokinetics. 2nd ed. Bethesda (MD): American Society of Health-System Pharmacists; 2001.

61. Burton ME, Shaw CM, Evans WE, Schentag JJ, editors. Applied pharmacokinetics and pharmacody-namics: principles of therapeutic drug monitoring. 4th ed. Philadelphia (PA): Lippincott Williams & Wilkins; 2005.

62. Winter ME. Basic clinical pharmacokinetics. 4th ed. Philadelphia (PA): Lippincott Williams & Wilkins; 2004.

63. Hardman JG, Limbird LE, editors. Goodman & Gilman's the pharmacological basis of therapeutics. 10th ed. New York: McGraw-Hill; 2001.

64. Katzung BG. Basic & clinical pharmacology. 9th ed. New York: Lange Medical Books; 2004.

65. Golan DE, editor. Principles of pharmacology. Philadelphia (PA): Lippincott Williams & Wilkins; 2005.

66. Abood RR. Pharmacy practice and the law. 4th ed. Boston (MA): Jones and Bartlett Publishers; 2005.

67. Reiss BS, Hall GD. Guide to federal pharmacy Law. 4th ed. Delmar (NY): Apothecary Press; 2005.

68. DiPiro JT, Talbert FL, Yee GC, Matzke GR, Wells BG, Posey LM, editors. Pharmacotherapy: a pathophysiologic approach. 6th ed. New York: McGraw-Hill; 2005.

69. Koda-Kimble MA, Young LY, editors. Applied therapeutics: the clinical use of drugs. 7th ed. Philadelphia (PA): Lippincott Williams & Wilkins; 2001.

70. Beers MH, Berkow R, editors. The Merck manual of diagnosis and therapy. 17th ed. Whitehouse Station (NJ): Merck Research Laboratories; 1999.

71. Kasper DL, Braunwald E, Fauci AS, Hauser SL, Longo DL, Jameson JL, editors. Harrison's principles of internal medicine. 16th ed. New York: Mc-Graw Hill; 2005.

72. Goldman L, Bennett JC, editors. Cecil textbook of medicine. 21st ed. Philadelphia (PA): W.B. Saunders; 2000.

73. Herfindal ET, Gourley DR, editors. Textbook of therapeutics. Philadelphia (PA): Lippincott Williams & Wilkins; 2000.

74. Rakel RE, Bope ET, editors. Conn's current therapy 2004. Philadelphia (PA): W.B. Saunders; 2004.

75. Klasco RK, editor. POISINDEX® [database on CD-ROM]. Vol 120. Englewood (CO): Thompson Micromedex; 2004.

76. Goldfrank LR, Howland MA, Flomenbaum NE, Hoffman RS, Lewin NA, Nelson LS, editors. Goldfrank's toxicologic emergencies. 7th ed. New York: McGraw-Hill; 1998.

77. Klasseen CD, editor. Casarett & Doull's toxicology: the basic science of poisons. 6th ed. New York: McGraw-Hill; 2001.

78. Ellenhorn MJ, Schonwald S, Ordog G, Wasserberger J, editors. Ellenhorn's medical toxicology: diagnosis and treatment of human poisoning. 2nd ed. Baltimore (MD): Williams & Wilkins; 1997.

79. Leikin JB, Paloucek FP, editors. Poisoning & toxicology handbook. 3rd ed. Hudson (OH): Lexi-Comp; 2002.

80. Haddad LM, Shannon MW, Winchester JF, editors. Clinical management of poisoning and drug overdose. 3rd ed. Philadelphia (PA): W.B. Saunders; 1998.

81. TOXNET [database on the Internet]. Bethesda (MD): National Library of Medicine [updated 2004 Jan 22; cited 2004 Mar 1]. Available from: http://toxnet.nlm.nih.gov

82. Plumb DC, editor. Veterinary drug handbook. 4th ed. White Bear Lake (MN): PharmaVet Publishing; 2002.

83. Ettinger SJ, Feldman EL, editors. Textbook of veterinary internal medicine. 5th ed. Philadelphia (PA): W.B. Saunders; 2000.

84. Dechert AA, editor. Compendium of veterinary products. 6th ed. Port Huron (MI): North American Compendiums; 2001.

85. U.S. Food and Drug Administration Center for Veterinary Medicine [home page on the Internet]. Rockville (MD): Food and Drug Administration [updated 2004 Feb 25; cited 2004 Mar 4]. Available from: http://www.fda.gov/cvm

86. Tilley LP, editor. The 5-minute veterinary consultant: canine and feline. 2nd ed. Philadelphia (PA): Lippincott Williams and Wilkins; 2000.

87. Facts and comparisons. 58th ed. St. Louis (MO): Facts & Comparisons; 2004.

88. McEvoy GK, editor. AHFS drug information. 2004 ed. Bethesda (MD): American Society of Health-System Pharmacists; 2004.

89. Physicians' desk reference. 58th ed. Montvale (NJ): Thompson PDR; 2004.

90. Lacy CF, Armstrong LL, Goldman MP, et al., eds. Drug Information Handbook. 13th ed. Hudson, OH: Lexi-Comp; 2005.

91. Drug information for the health care professional. 25th ed. Greenwood Village (CO): Thomson MICROMEDEX; 2005.

92. Clauson KA, Seamon MJ, Clauson AS, Van TB. Evaluation of core and supplemental drug information databases for the Palm OS and Pocket PC. Am J Health Syst Pharm. 2004;61:1015–24.

93. Enders SJ, Enders JM, Holstad SG. Drug-information software for palm operating system personal digital assistants: breadth, clinical dependability and ease of use. Pharmacotherapy. 2002;22:1036–40.

94. Gulbis BE, Kier KL. Comparison of drug information databases for palm OS handheld personal digital assistants. ASHP Midyear Clinical Meeting. 2002;37:P-236-E.

95. Barrons R. Evaluation of personal digital assistant software for drug interactions. Am J Health Syst Pharm. 2004;61:380–5.

96. Fuller N, Allison A, Beattie M, Bowman L, Iwanowicz S, Jackson E, et al. AACP core list of journals for libraries that serve schools and colleges of pharmacy 2003. Am Assoc Coll Pharm [online], July 2003 [cited 2004 March 1]: [6 screens]. Available from: http://www.aacp.org/site/page.asp?TRACKID=&VID=1&CID=380&DID=3619.

97. Health on the Net [home page on the Internet]. Geneva, Switzerland: Health on the Net; c2003 [updated 2004 Feb 2; cited 2004 March 1]. Available from: http://www.hon.ch/.

98. Stergachis A, Maine LL, Brown L. The 2001 national pharmacy consumer survey. J Am Pharm Assoc. 2002;42:568–76.

99. The PDR family guide to prescription drugs. 9th ed. Montvale (NJ): Medical Economics; 2002.

5

Chapter Five

Electronic Information Management

Patrick M. Malone

Links referred to in this chapter are available at www.MaloneDruginfo.com.

Objectives

After completing this chapter, the reader will be able to

- Explain how to integrate the following into his or her personal practice:
  - Searching the Internet for information necessary for pharmacy practice.
  - Providing pharmacy and drug information to others over the Internet.
  - Gathering input from health care practitioners and patients via websites.
  - Use of electronic mail (e-mail), including personal distribution lists and listservers.
  - Online discussion groups.
  - Internet collaboration.
  - Push technology.
  - How to ensure long-term data viability.
- Evaluate the credibility of Internet resources.
- Efficiently manage personal e-mail, both outgoing and incoming.

Introduction

In 1981 drug information was revolutionized when it suddenly became possible for nonlibrarians to access MEDLINE® directly. Those who first had access were required to participate in a week-long training class given in only three locations in the country and then could only access the information via dumb terminals using a 300 bits per second (bps) modem. Little did practitioners realize that they were starting down a technologic road that would quickly accelerate. A few years later some of the first pharmacy uses of what was to become the Internet were seen. At that time, some users of the Iowa Drug Information Service (IDIS) could e-mail search requests, via ARPANET (a predecessor of the Internet), to the University of Iowa, and would receive a reply with citations to the IDIS microfiche. Although the sender's computer might indicate the message was received in seconds, in reality it could take several days to make its way across the country. It would then take additional time for the reply. Certainly, this was a vast improvement over the very first MEDLINE® searches that were requested and sent via the postal system, but still was not close to what practitioners take for granted today.

Today, pharmacists can access vast amounts of data locally or from computer systems around the world in seconds, using a powerful microcomputer system that costs less than $1000, at speeds of up to 1 billion bps or more! These data can even be obtained at home at great speeds across cable TV lines or satellites. In addition to increases in amounts of data and speed, the ways data can be communicated have improved greatly and include graphics, sounds, and video. These capabilities are seen around the world to some extent or another, with an estimated 317,646,084 host computers attached to the Internet as of January 2005, up from 19,540,000 in July 1997.[1] Computer speeds are up to 360 teraflops (a teraflop is a trillion operations per second).[2] The amount of information available in computerized format has increased tremendously and is expected to increase more with the digitalization of major libraries by Google.[3,4]

The overwhelming amount of information, and its hazards, has been recognized by pharmacy organizations as an area that needs to be addressed.[5] Also, the lack of training and lack of use of resources, particularly electronic, by health care practitioners must be recognized[6] and is now being addressed in some schools of pharmacy.[7] The Institute of Medicine has also stated that health science schools need to provide further training in informatics in a report available at <<http://www.nap.edu/catalog/10681.html>>.

Initially a way to communicate data, the Internet has become a way to simply communicate. E-mail and instant messaging are widely used in business and as a means of personal communication, but may be replaced by real-time video conversations. Use of the Internet to provide telepresence may become one of its most important uses.

This chapter will describe how pharmacists can access the Internet, the methods of communicating information over the Internet, some particularly good sources of data, and how pharmacists can integrate these resources and the new information management and communication methods into their practices.

Technology—The First Step

Any microcomputer capable of running a current operating system (e.g., the current version of Windows) and web browser (e.g., Microsoft Internet Explorer, Netscape, Firefox, and Opera) is an appropriate choice for connecting to the Internet. Notebook computers are practical for the clinician moving from place to place, however, that often makes connection to the Internet more difficult. Wireless computers, along with other wireless devices, have not been used as much in health care because of concerns about security[8] and also because of potential for interference with other devices,[9] although both are becoming less of an issue. That connection to the local area network in the institution, clinic, or pharmacy, along with connection to the Internet, is vital. Pharmacists' computers must be set up to give the easiest, most transparent, access to information. It should be no more difficult to switch from a local copy of MEDLINE® to the Centers for Disease Control and Prevention (CDC) website than it is to switch from a word processing program to a spreadsheet program.

A possible replacement for personal computers, at least in some settings, is a personal digital assistant (PDA), which contains a subset of the functions, programs, and data available on a normal desktop machine.[10] It has been noted that physicians already use such equipment to perform searches of MEDLINE® or other databases,[11] retrieve patient information,[12] and set appointments, or other activities.[13] Many digital cellular phones also have web browsing functions available,[14,15] but they do not yet seem practical for most practitioners, if for no other reason than the extremely small screen. These phones may also be combined with a PDA.

The connection to the network should not be a concern to the practitioner because of security, however, some institutions are reluctant to provide practitioners easy connection from a personal computer to the Internet, or sometimes even to the hospital's network. There are a variety of methods for an institution to strike an appropriate balance between security and access. Cheryl Currid, the former head of computing at Coca-Cola®, stated a number of years ago, "PCs go on networks, period. Stand-alone computing is worthless to an organization. Demand a LAN."[16] That advice should be taken a step further today—demand quality access to the Internet![17]

In cases where the worry of an institution or clinic is the cost of an Internet connection, it should be pointed out that the Telecommunications Act of 1996 or later funding might help to offset costs.[18] Another reason that Internet connections may be absent is the concern about abuse of web surfing by the employees. This is also a valid fear, but should be addressed by clear, well-known web surfing policies that are enforced, rather than preventing Internet use altogether.[19]

Once the computer is connected to the network, appropriate software is required. Typically, the newer operating systems provide simple telnet and FTP (file transfer protocol) programs. Telnet essentially turns a computer into a dumb terminal to access mainframe-like programs. FTP allows transfer of files to or from another computer. The functions provided by these programs are relatively limited to text material or very simple functions, and are now almost always superceded by web browsers.

Popular web browsers include Microsoft Internet Explorer (<<http://www.microsoft.com>>), Netscape (<<http://www.netscape.com>>), Firefox (<<http://www.firefox.com>>), and Opera (<<http://www.opera.com>>). All have strengths and weaknesses, particularly in regard to the increasingly important topic of security, but they are likely to serve most needs of the average user. Web browsers can also provide other functions, such as e-mail, USENET News Reader, live collaboration tools, live software updates, and web page authoring tools. In addition, other programs can work in conjunction with the web browser. For example, if a word processing file is downloaded with the web browser, the browser may start the copy of Word for Windows residing on the computer and display the document in the browser window. Also, there are a variety of free reader programs that are available on the Internet to display data that are downloaded, whether or not the full version of the program has been purchased. For example, Adobe Acrobat Reader can be downloaded (<<http://www.adobe.com>>) to allow review of copies of *Morbidity and Mortality Weekly Report* (*MMWR*) from the CDC. Often, websites will alert a user to the need for these extra "plug-in" programs and will give directions for obtaining them, or provide an automatic method for installation.

Before ending this section, it is important to note that any personal computer should have antiviral protection that is updated regularly[20] along with at least one, if not several, antispyware programs (e.g., Microsoft Antispyware, Lavasoft's Ad-Aware, Spybot—Search and Destroy, and Spyware Blaster). It may also be desirable to have other forms of software protection for web browsers, e-mail, and so forth, which can be separately investigated. Protection provided by each of these programs is becoming better and updating is often automatic. Finally, any organization with networked computers must make efforts to protect data integrity and confidential information through the use of protection procedures such as firewalls, cryptography, and file server security software. Even for home use, a router switch that isolates the home network from the Internet is very useful. While there have not been any cases specific to drug information, there have been documented cases where patient record information has been altered as a prank, causing needless patient suffering—there is potential for much greater harm in the future.[21]

Information via the Internet

Information can be communicated over the Internet in many ways. This section will describe the most likely methods, provide examples of the information obtained and some likely sources of information, and provide information on how pharmacists can incorporate these capabilities into their actual practice.

THE PRESENT

It is nearly impossible to live in the United States these days without having heard of the world wide web (www). It is a very popular source of information, including health information. It has been proposed that there should be universal access to the Internet for health-related information, to help improve the information reaching underserved populations.[22]

The quality and presentation of information retrieved from the Internet has progressed from simple text-based information to multimedia extravaganzas that can be accessed through web browsers. Much of the information currently available consists of text and simple graphics, but more sophisticated presentation of information is rapidly appearing. Reasons for the simpler material include lack of more advanced information in computer format and a concern about the time that it takes to access material. Retrieval speed is particularly important to those individuals who access the Internet via modem, but such slow connections can rarely be justified anymore with the wide access to high-speed connections that are inexpensively available to most people.

In order to best address the current situation, the various features available in the current web browsers will be covered.

Incorporating Web Browsing into the Systematic Search Process

The most common use for a web browser is its original purpose—to present information from WWW servers. However, before using a browser, the first step is to recognize the need to access the Internet and the value of the information it makes available. After all, to use the Internet, a pharmacist does need special equipment and some knowledge about how to use it. Often a simple look at a common textbook (e.g., *Drug Facts and Comparisons, AHFS Drug Information*) may answer a question simply and efficiently. The key is to create an efficient search strategy. A full discussion of a systematic approach to answering a drug information question and preparing a search strategy is presented in other chapters of this book. However, a few general rules can be restated. First, if a pharmacist is familiar with references that are likely to contain the information necessary to answer a question, those references should be consulted first. For example, to check for drug interactions, a drug interaction reference would be a logical choice. Second, there is no one "right" way to search.[23] Sometimes a person will know precisely where a piece of information is located from experience, even if it is obscure. In other cases, the searcher will realize that it is so unusual a topic that an immediate jump to Internet metasearch engines is warranted. Generally, Internet WWW browsing is likely to be farther down the list after books or other resources—perhaps even after MEDLINE® searching, except in certain circumstances, such as the following:

- When a reference to the Internet is found (e.g., advertisement and citation).
- Situations where company-specific information is necessary (e.g., product package inserts).
- Items currently in the news (e.g., check sites listed in Appendix 5–13).* As a side issue, this is becoming a much more important step that needs to be pursued in any situation where the origin of the question is vague (e.g., a patient heard about something and asked a physician, who then asked the pharmacist).
- When U.S. government information is required (e.g., Food and Drug Administration [FDA]- or CDC-specific subjects—including clinical information and new drug

---

*The appendix can be found at www.MaloneDrugInfo.com.

approvals). The U.S. government has been very active in putting a great deal of information on the web (see Appendix 5–9).*

- When the information is not likely to be contained in other available sources of information (e.g., alternative medicine [see Appendix 5–1]* and tropical diseases).
- When computer-related information or software updates are needed.

Why is there so much emphasis on web browsing versus some other form of obtaining information? Quite likely the reason is that web protocols allow easy access of various types of information on disparate computer systems—they are very flexible and powerful.[24] That is why there is such emphasis on it in this book. Also, it should be pointed out that many periodicals and textbooks have become web based due to the ease of availability and use.[25] Most indexing or abstracting services are also available in network forms. Also, patient information is increasingly available through web interfaces due to the ease of use, security, and the ability to transparently tie together information residing on separate, somewhat incompatible, computer systems.[26]

Web Addresses

Once the decision to search the web is made, the pharmacist needs to log onto a computer attached to Internet and run the web browser. To obtain information, the user simply needs to put the address (referred to as a URL [uniform resource locator]) of that information in the browser, which will then find it automatically. An example of an address is <<http://druginfo.creighton.edu>>, which was the address of the author's main website. The first term in an address, which will be followed by a //, indicates the type of information provided at that site. In this case, http stands for hypertext transfer protocol, which is the technical term for the information generally contained by a site accessed with a web browser. Common types of information are as follows[27]:

- http: hypertext transfer protocol—normal web information
- https: a secure form of http, used for confidential information (e.g., credit card numbers)
- telnet: a site that requires your computer to act like a dumb terminal
- ftp: file transfer protocol—allows you to transfer software or a file of information in various formats
- news: USENET News group
- mailto: Internet e-mail address

The second term in the address (*druginfo*) is often the name of the web server that you are accessing. Typically, the main web server for a particular organization will have an address name of "www." In actuality, one computer can host multiple addresses through a process called multihoming. For example, <<http://druginfo. creighton.edu>> on the same

---

*The appendices can be found at www.MaloneDrugInfo.com.

computer as <<http://pharmacy.creighton.edu>> and several other websites. The next item in this address is the organization's general address name. These servers are at Creighton University. Finally, you will notice a three-letter extension at the end of the URL. In this case, it is .edu, which indicates that the address is that of an educational institution. Common three-letter extensions seen in the United States include:

- .biz: business
- .com: commercial (e.g., <<http://www.microsoft.com or <<http://www.netscape. com>>)
- .edu: education
- .gov: government (e.g., <<http://www.cdc.gov>> for the CDC)
- .info: information
- .mil: military
- .org: organization (e.g., <<http://www.ashp.org>> for American Society of Health-System Pharmacists)
- .net: network (network provider)

In foreign countries, addresses tend to end in a two-letter code that indicates the country (e.g., .fr = France). The country code for the United States is .us, but it is seldom used.

In addition, there can be a slash (/) followed by one or more names added onto the end of the address. These indicate the file name, including the server subdirectory. For example, <<http://druginfo.creighton.edu/links/governmt.htm>> indicates that you are accessing a file called governmt.htm in the links subdirectory (note long file names are permitted). The .htm indicates that the file is in hypertext markup language format (also sometimes abbreviated as .html). This format is standard for much of the information available on the web, however, other file formats are occasionally used. For example, the .ppt in the address <<http://druginfo.creighton.edu/PHA458/NewsletterLec/Newsletter%20Lecture.ppt>> indicates that the file is actually in Microsoft PowerPoint format. A somewhat common extension that pharmacists may run across is .pdf, which stands for portable data file. This is the format used by the Adobe Acrobat Reader (<<http://www.adobe.com>>). A variety of information, such as *MMWR* from the CDC's website, is available in this format. Other commonly seen extensions[27] are .gif (graphic image), .jpeg or .jpg (graphic image), .mov (movie/animation), .avi (movie/animation), .au (sound), .wav (sound), and .wmv (movie).

Links to Internet Sites

In many cases, the URL of a company or an organization's website may be known; after all, such addresses seem to be printed on everything now. If the URL is unknown, often a correct guess may be made. For example, the American Society of Health-System Pharmacists is commonly known as ASHP and it is an organization. Therefore, <<http://www.ashp.org>> would be a logical guess of its web address, which happens to be correct.

A second easy way to find sites is to find cross references from similar sites or sites that would have an interest in the site. For example, a logical guess of the web address for the

American Pharmaceutical Association would be <<http://www.apha.org>>, but this produces the website for the American Public Health Association. However, by going to the ASHP website, it is possible to easily find a link to the APhA website at <<http://www. aphanet.org>>. Links are in the form of text or graphics on a web page that, when clicked on with a mouse or other pointing device, will take the user to another web page. That page may simply be another page on the same website, but it could also be located on another computer halfway around the world; that is one of the major advantages to web browsing—the ease with which a user can connect from one piece of information to another without having to worry about where that information is actually located. It is also possible to find links to a variety of other useful websites at either the ASHP or APhA websites. Lists of other useful websites for pharmacists are presented in the appendices* of this chapter. It is important to note that links on websites are often shown in different colors than surrounding text or may be "boxed" by a different color. Usually, the mouse pointer will change into a different shape when passed over a link (e.g., a hand with the forefinger extended, as if to push a button), which also allows for easy identification of a link.

Using Search Engines

In many cases, the URL of a likely source of information is not known and a method of searching for the information is necessary. Fortunately, a variety of search engines have been developed for this purpose; some are general and some are specific to medically related topics, even medical specialties. Once the decision is made to use one of these search engines, it is then up to the user to decide which is most appropriate for his or her needs. Unfortunately, there does not seem to be a truly excellent search engine specific to pharmacy.

When a pharmacist needs general medical information, there are a variety of medical search engines listed in Appendix 5–23.* Even these search engines are not all encompassing, and it may be necessary to search several of them to find any information.

Each search engine uses different methods for conducting Internet searches. An in-depth explanation of the ways to use each individual service is not possible in a chapter; however, some general information can be provided. The first step is to pick the search engine that seems most likely to produce information. If a specific legitimate medical subject is to be searched, one of the medical search engines would probably be good. Also, Google Scholar (<<http://scholar.google.com>>) is a good way to access professional information, including that of medicine and pharmacy, whereas, if the need is for information that might not be supported by the medical literature (e.g., finding what is being claimed by alternate medicine marketers and finding "street information" about illegal medications), it might be better to go to one of the general search engines listed in Appendix 5–23.*

Those general search engines attempt to index as much of the WWW as possible. Some are referred to as web crawlers, since they use intelligent software agents (termed *spiders*) to crawl

---

*The appendices can be found at www.MaloneDrugInfo.com.

through sites across the Internet by exploring links on other websites.[28] Since it is virtually impossible to do this and keep entirely up to date, the various web crawlers have a specific logic as to how often a site is "crawled." More important or common sites (e.g., CNN and Microsoft) and those known to change frequently are "crawled" more often. However, by indexing everything, a search on these general engines may produce too many "hits." It is not unusual for a vague or general search on a common term to produce thousands of "hits." Needless to say, that is unmanageable and means that the search needs to be narrowed.

Even though the general search engines index a great number of websites, they are not all inclusive. A study found that no single search engine indexes more than about one-third of the Internet web pages.[29] Another publication was even less optimistic, showing that the best search engine only indexed approximately 16% of the web.[30] Also, the frequency of adding new pages and deleting "dead links" should be at least once a month,[31] with some engines being rather dated. Other web technology, such as dynamically prepared pages and frames (screens on a web browser may consist of several frames), may not be appropriately indexed by search engines. This material and other things are even referred to as the hidden Internet,[32] which is estimated to be 500 times bigger than the normally searchable web.[33] Some search engines, such as OAIster at the University of Michigan (<<http://oaister.umdl.umich.edu/o/oaister/>>), Find Articles (<<http://www.findarticles.com/>>), Library Spot (<<http://www.libraryspot.com/>>), First-Gov.gov (<<http://firstgov.gov/>>), infoplease (<<http://www.infoplease.com/>>), Director of Open Access Journals (<<http://www.doaj.org/>>), Scirus for Scientific Information Only (<<http://www.scirus.com/srsapp/>>), and Combined Health Information Database (<<http://chid.nih.gov/>>), can be useful for the pharmacist trying to access material on this hidden Internet.

Techniques to narrow a search are discussed in Chap. 4, under the secondary literature section. These techniques may include the use of logical operators (i.e., AND, OR, and NOT) or other methods (e.g., putting a phrase in quotations). Unfortunately, the various search engines implement these search methods differently. For example, in some you might put in the word "and," in others it will need to be "AND" ("and" is just treated as a text word), and in some you might have to use "+" or "&." Also, features such as truncation, phrase searching, field searching (e.g., date, URL, and language),[34] case sensitivity (e.g., finding AIDS instead of aids),[35] and additional logical operators (e.g., "NEAR," "WITH," and "BEFORE") may be available. On some search engines it is possible to search for nontextual information, such as graphic images or sounds (see Appendix 5–25).*[36]

Many search engines may restrict certain words or short words from searches (e.g., vitamin B will not be found because the "B" is too short). Because of these problems, the next rule of searching is to read the directions for using a search engine before performing anything but a very simple search on an unusual topic (i.e., one that is not likely to produce many "hits").

---

*The appendix can be found at www.MaloneDrugInfo.com.

The differences in search commands and capabilities can drastically change the quality of the search results, making more traditional secondary search programs (e.g., MEDLINE® and International Pharmaceutical Abstracts) more likely to produce useful results with a number of searches.[37] Perhaps the easiest procedure for pharmacists is to become familiar with a couple of medical and general search engines and understand the directions. If those "favorites" do not produce an answer, the searcher can then pick others to try and read their help file while preparing a search strategy.

If the search covers a topic that is very unusual and it is expected that several general search engines will need to be consulted, it may be appropriate to use a multiple web search engine, also referred to as a metasearch engine (i.e., software that allows the searching of multiple databases using a single uniform interface[38]), which will search multiple search engines concurrently. Several of these are found in Appendix 5–23.* It may be tempting to hop directly to these multiple-web search engines, but two major problems are possible, information overload and slow speeds. So it might be best to save them until other search strategies have failed. Also, depending on the specific multiple-web search engine used, there are several other possible problems. These include the inability to use all logical operators (e.g., NEAR), a limit on the number of hits to be reported from the other search engines, and possible incompatibilities between the multiple-web search engine and the general search engine (i.e., the general search engine may have changed its format and the multiple-web search engine might have not yet noted and adjusted for that change).[39]

A related, but perhaps better, alternative to metasearch engines are programs residing on a users computer that perform many of the same functions. For example, Copernic (<<http://www.copernic.com>>) provides a program that can search for a variety of types of information. This program gives a common interface and is automatically updated to best know how to interface with other search engines each time it is run.

One search engine is available for those who do not like to use or have difficulty using logical operators in their search. Mooter (<<http://www.mooter.com/>>) is a very interesting tool. When a person inputs a search term, it will graphically present options for the user to choose. For example, the phrase *drug informatics* was input and the main term with number of "hits" was displayed in a circle in the middle of the screen. Other related or more specific variations on the term, along with the number of hits for each, are then displayed in circles that are connected to the main term by a line. Users can then pick either the main term or one of the related terms. The user can then decide which direction would be best for the search. For example, if the person was interested in a career in drug informatics, the career button could be clicked to display results. This search engine is not specific to medicine, but can be helpful in obtaining specific leads. A similar search engine is found at <<http://vivisimo.com/>>.

Portal software provides a new means to search the Internet.[40] Portals have been previously mentioned in this chapter as a different name for some of the search engines; however, some of

---

*The appendix can be found at www.MaloneDrugInfo.com.

the new portal software acts as a universal interface to allow searching of not only the Internet, but also an institution's Intranet for documents, including databases, word processing documents, spreadsheets, slide presentations, and e-mail messages.[41,42] In addition, this software may use logic to aid in identifying material by context, filtering out irrelevant information based on the needs of the individual and his or her job description. The software may also be fault tolerant, using fuzzy logic to identify documents when search terms are misspelled, or will even actively search out information on a prospective basis in the background. In addition to institutions, professional organizations may offer portals, such as the National Community Pharmacists Association e-Link (<<http://ncpa.yellowbrix.com/pages/ncpa/ Headlines.nsp>>).

Before leaving the general topic of Internet search engines, additional information needs to be presented regarding Google. Over the years, there have been several search engines that people felt were the best and, thus, were used the most. Currently, Google is extremely popular and appears likely to remain so in the near future. In many cases, instead of saying "I searched for XXX," a person might say "I Googled XXX." In some cases, Google is overused because some individuals may use Google only instead of making it a part of a well-planned search.[43] There is no doubt that Google provides a powerful tool that should be properly used, but to use it to the exclusion of everything else is the equivalent of trying to build a home using only a wrench—the wrench may be vital for the plumbing work, but it is not good for sawing wood. That said, it is also important to point out that Google offers an ever-increasing group of features that are often not found in other search engines. In regard to search commands, see Table 5–1 for a list of possible useful ways to restrict searches on Google. Some can be of particular use to pharmacists, such as the ability to get definitions of medical terms and to perform measurement conversions. Also, Google Scholar (<<http://scholar.google.com>>) can be of use.[46] While it is not specific to health care, it does perform an admirable search of health-related material. For example, it appears to include all of the material in PubMed® and additional material as well. It also links to original articles, when possible, including pharmacy journals such as the *American Journal of Health-Systems Pharmacy*. In addition, it will do a reverse citation look-up similar to that seen with Science Citation Index, where the search results have a link to other web pages that link to the article or web page found in the search. This is a unique and valuable feature; however, since it is an important factor in how Google determines the order in which search results are displayed, it can mean that the older articles are displayed preferentially. While having an outdated or older reference does not mean that the material is wrong, most times, searchers are interested in obtaining the most recent material to make sure that information is not missed. Therefore, it can be valuable to click on the *cited by* link to try to obtain the most recent information.

Besides using the above search engines, a version of a classic database is available on the Internet. PubMed® (<<http://www.ncbi.nlm.nih.gov/entrez/query.fcgi? db=PubMed>>) is a version of MEDLINE® from the National Library of Medicine that is available at no charge on the Internet. Besides some of the well-known features of MEDLINE®, it provides natural language searching and even links to some of the articles that might be

TABLE 5–1. GOOGLE SEARCH COMMANDS[44,45]

Command	Use	Example
define:term(s)	Provides dictionary definition of term	define:neutropenia
filetype:extension	Used with other terms to limit search to only files with a particular file type extension	filetype:pdf
inurl:terms	Searches for a term in the URL of a web page	inurl:informatics
link:URL	Searches for pages that link to a specific web page	link:druginfo.creighton.edu
measurement in measurement	Provides conversion from one form of measurement to another	1 grain in mg
phonebook:data	Searches a residential phonebook to find either the phone number, if a name and place is input or the name if the phone number is input	phonebook: bush dc note: above search turns up the White House in Washington, DC – the dc above was for District of Columbia, but a state abbreviation and a city can be put after the name phonebook:(202) 456–1111
site:domain	Used with one or more other terms to limit a search to one specific domain (particularly helpful in searching a website with no built-in search function)	site:www.cdc.gov
video:term	Searches for videos about that term	video:pharmacy

NOTE: When the terms are input in conjunction with other terms in a Google search, it is possible to put a "+" sign in front to make sure the term is included in the web page or a "–" sign to make sure it is excluded. For example, in the first search, the following is input into Google: <<tuberculosis -filetype:pdf>>. This search will produce results of web pages that have the term tuberculosis on them, but will exclude web pages that are in .pdf format.

found and links to other databases.[47] Further research is also being indexed as part of a new service called PubMed® Central (<<http://www.pubmedcentral.nih.gov/>>). Electronic library card catalogs are also starting to provide such direct browser links to actual publications. While this information might make it tempting to drop subscriptions to the MEDLINE® database from other vendors to save money, pharmacists should take into account that the other vendors may provide value-added features and their products may be more easily accessible at a much faster speed.[48] Although different vendors use the same MEDLINE® database, results of querying the database may vary from one vendor's system to another because of different search engine capabilities and different rates of updating the database.[49] Be sure to evaluate the quality of MEDLINE® search engines before settling on one to make sure that it meets the users' needs.[50]

It should also be mentioned that many full-text publications are available on the Internet (see Appendix 5–19* for examples), which will increase over the years.[51] Users are charged in some way or the other for accessing many of these sites, mostly through advertising if not in a more direct manner. Similarly, forms of some other references (e.g., MICROMEDEX

---

*The appendix can be found at www.MaloneDrugInfo.com.

and STAT!-Ref) may be placed on an institution's network and be searched using web browsers—even from remote sites, as long as licensing restrictions are observed through the use of passwords, proxy servers, virtual private networks (VPNs), or other means. Also, libraries are recommending increases in open access (i.e., free) publishing on the Internet, including the use of Public Library of Science (<<http://plos.org>>).[52,53]

Other Search Software

Two other types of search software need to be mentioned at this point.

First, many search engines (e.g., Google,<<http://www.google.com>> and Yahoo, <<http://www.yahoo.com>>) offer a piece of software that integrates a toolbar on a web browser.[54] Similarly, the Copernic search engine (<<http://www.copernic.com>>) provides a similar toolbar, which will allow searching of multiple search engines concurrently.[55] These toolbars allow a person to search for a particular topic without first going to the search engine website. Instead, the user simply types the search into the box on that toolbar and presses the enter key. The program then goes to the search engine database and performs the search, displaying the results in the browser window.

In addition to toolbars, various search engines provide desktop search software. Two of the earliest to do this were Google[56,57] and Copernic.[44] These programs can be used to search the Internet but provide the extra feature of searching the user's computer, in addition, for files (e.g., word processing and spreadsheets), e-mail, instant messaging, contacts, or other things as an additional feature. Each of the programs has limitations as to what it will search, which must be understood by the user before installation. However, both provide additional capabilities that may be of use to pharmacists.

Evaluating Information on the Web

Finding the information is only part of the battle. Essentially anyone can put any information on the web, whether that information is valuable, worthless, disgusting, or even dangerous.[58-60] This has been noted as a particular problem by the National Library of Medicine.[61] It is necessary for pharmacists to use the skills discussed in Chaps. 4, 6 and 7. In particular, a web source should be evaluated for believability, the source (author), supporting evidence, logic, timeliness, and other factors.[62-64] Unfortunately, while there are many website evaluation methods available, there is no standard method; however, some guidelines can be applied as will be described in this section of the chapter.[65]

In classic literature evaluation, one of the first things that a person is taught to evaluate is the source of the information. In this case it would be the Internet website, which should disclose its name, location, and sponsorship (which can be important in determining conflicts of interest). Sometimes the user will know the site. For example, it might be supported by a pharmaceutical manufacturer (whose information is regulated by the FDA[66]), university, or pharmacy organization, all of which generally provide good, high-quality information. However, even if the searcher does not know the source of information or the website, there is a method for evaluating its overall quality. The Health on the Net Foundation has established an HONcode (<<http://www.hon.ch/HONcode/Conduct.html>>), which contains eight principles. These principles, if met, support the quality of the information provided by a particular website.[67] A webmaster for a particular site can apply to the Health on the Net Foundation to display their HONcode logo on a website. The webmaster is required to abide by the eight principles, and the Health on the Net Foundation does check to see that they do so, although there are cases where it has been felt that the Health on the Net Foundation needed to be more aggressive in their prevention of the misuse of their seal, particularly in the field of complementary and alternative medicine.[68] There are also many other site-rating services that might be noted on the Internet, however, not all of them are known to have acceptable criteria for rating websites.[69] It should also be pointed out that none of these site-rating services are considered to have a completely comprehensive method of doing so.[69]

A second way to evaluate the overall site is to use a piece of software that gives you information on how other people evaluate the site. One such program is called Alexa, a freeware program available at <<http://www.alexa.com/download>>.[70] This program provides information on a website such as the name, address, and phone number of the site's owner, the number of hits the site receives, and the number of votes received from Alexa users on whether they do or do not like the site. Actually, the information about who owns the site should be prominent on a site's home page—if not, beware.

Once at a particular site, the author of the information being evaluated should be considered. Unfortunately, there is great potential for problems here. There have been instances on the Internet of a person writing some piece of information claiming to be someone else—perhaps a well-known and respected individual. So, evaluation of the author's name and credentials should probably be coupled with evaluation of the source of the site itself—if the site is not trusted, do not trust that the supposed author really was the author.

Next, a good site is one that looks good and makes it easy to give feedback, and to obtain or retrieve information.[71] This includes not having huge graphics or other files that do not add to the quality of information while taking extended time to download. This certainly is not an absolute in either the good or bad directions, but can be used as one of the factors in evaluating a site.

It is also important to see how recent the information actually is. A good site will list on each page the date it was last updated.

It is worthwhile noting that some websites seem to be only a listing of other websites with links to those sites. If that is their purpose, that is fine, but if the purpose of the site is to supposedly provide good information to the user, the overwhelming number of links should be considered to be a mark against them.[72]

If the above criteria are met, the reader should use traditional literature evaluation skills to determine whether the information is clear and concise, easy to use, fully presented, unbiased, relevant, well organized, and appropriately referenced. Just as there is no perfect study or perfect printed article, there is no perfect web page. Any page is likely to have some deficiencies, and it is up to the user to determine whether those deficiencies are fatal to the usefulness of the information. Also, it must be understood that even absolutely terrible information can be useful to a practitioner in that it may be necessary to look at what patients are reading and believing to sometimes help them.

If a website is found that provides good and valuable information, it would be worthwhile to consider saving the URL. Web browsers allow saving such things as *bookmarks* or *favorites* to permit the user to get back to those addresses quickly.

Providing Information

Besides using the web to obtain information, pharmacists can use it to provide information.[73] Anyone with a connection to the Internet can have a personal website. The software to host a website is often available free or at little cost, at least for websites that will not be requiring specialized functions (e.g., secure financial transactions) and those with relatively light use. More powerful and capable web servers can be purchased from a variety of vendors. It is also possible for people to lease a website from a commercial provider. Just having the web address and some storage space for material may only cost a few dollars a month or be available as part of a subscription to an Internet Service Provider (ISP). Commercial vendors can also prepare and publish the web pages themselves, for a fee. A pharmacy or institution should have available commercial web services, by contract or internally, with adequate support, to allow best interchange of information, although individual pharmacists may use their own websites for small projects, committees, and so forth.

Preparing the material to be placed on the website can be accomplished using a variety of free or low cost software, which can be specific for web page development or be part of other software (e.g., word processor, web browser, and desktop publisher).

As to why someone would want to prepare a website, it has been suggested that there are four general uses for computer-based hypertext systems[74]:

- Macro literary systems—large libraries with computerized interdocument links.
- Problem exploration systems—support for early unstructured thinking on a particular problem.
- Structured browsing systems—can be used for reference or teaching; similar to macro literary systems, but easier to use.
- General hypertext systems—general systems for experimentation with a wide range of hypertext applications.

So, how can a pharmacist use these capabilities? Actually, it is possible to do a variety of things. First, a website can be used to provide information, just like any reference. For example, an institution's drug formulary, policies and procedures, intravenous (IV) guidelines, antimicrobial sensitivities, drug information, investigational drug protocols, and other institution-specific items can be placed on a website.[75] Such information should be interlinked to allow the user to access other information. For example, an entry in the drug formulary system might be linked to a policy and procedure stating who can use the medication, how it can be used, and/or where it can be used. Although there may be concern about making information available outside the institution, that is not a problem, because websites can have restricted access, by either location or login name and password. When access is limited to users within an institution, it is called an Intranet.

The use of dynamic html allows the preparation of informational web pages that are specific to the user. For example, it might be possible to set things up so that when a physician accesses information on a drug, information about indications, dosing, side effects, and interactions is first presented, whereas, a nurse might be first presented with information on how to administer the drug and monitor the patient. A pharmacist in the IV room could be first given information on how to prepare the drug. While the other information could be available to each of these individuals, the website can, through the dynamic html, try to best serve the likely needs of the user.

Pharmacists can also provide education to patients and health care professionals via the web, within or outside the institution.[76-78] This may be purely textual material, but can also include slides,[79] pictures, video,[80-82] and sound. Right now, the network bandwidth usually found on the patient's connection to the Internet, often restricts at least the quality of such material, but that is improving. There can also be an online testing service for classes or continuing education programs. This can have advantages over traditional examinations because the testing system may provide immediate feedback to the user—not just a grade, but also an explanation of what the user answered wrong on the test and why it was wrong.

A website can also be used to provide a place for on-line discussions, although sometimes the software is actually through an e-mail system or is separate. The author of this chapter has used this feature to conduct discussions among Pharm.D. students scattered all over the world for several years. The results have been quite good because students can provide their input to the discussion when it is convenient for them over a period of time, allowing them adequate time to think about what they wanted to say. This type of software could also be used in patient groups to improve patient education and communication between the pharmacist and the patient.

Overall, the benefits of making a website include the following[83]:

- Documents may be made available to anyone in the world with a computer and Internet access very quickly.
- Documents can be updated as often as necessary. For example, a few minutes' work will update the drug formulary for everyone in the institution for practically no expense.

- Paper may be saved, although computer use has been shown to actually increase paper use.
- Everyone can publish web documents.

Obtaining Information

Besides providing information, websites can also be used by the pharmacist to obtain information. For example, a website could have input forms to be used as a way for health care professionals on the floor to easily report adverse drug reactions or request the addition of drugs to the formulary. Information and prescriptions can be obtained from patients. Internationally, similar Internet data reporting systems have been used for epidemiologic research (e.g., FluNet, <<http://www.who.int/GlobalAtlas/home.asp>>).[84] These are suggestions and others will likely have other ideas, however, the main thing is that it is necessary to have an objective.[85] The objective(s) will likely grow, and regular updating and maintenance is necessary, but at least one good, useful reason for being on the web is necessary.

How a pharmacist puts together a website can be compared to how a newsletter would be prepared. The concepts and skills are much the same and are dealt with in greater detail in Chap. 11; however, specific points are made in Table 5–2 that can be of value.[86–90]

Also, it must be noted that pharmacists must be careful to make sure that other electronic means are used to provide or obtain information wherever it is needed. Information provided by hospital computer systems is believed to be necessary[91] and useful to decrease both adverse effects and medication errors[92,93] and improve patient safety.[94] These data might be used through the process of data mining, where large amounts of data in the institutional computer system are converted into information that can be used by decision makers.[95] Electronic information has also been found to be useful in providing reminders during drug shortages,[96] which are covered in more detail in Chap. 14. An increasingly popular source of information consists of references available for PDAs[97–104]; Chap. 4 covers a great number of these references and pharmacists are encouraged to carry appropriate ones in situations where other resources are not readily available (e.g., clinical rounding). After all, why tell someone that it will be necessary to get back to them later when it is possible to quickly obtain the information via a PDA at that time?

As a final thought in this section, EVERY document a pharmacist creates (with the possible exception of personal communications, confidential information, and material that will be submitted for journal publication[105]) should be considered for possible inclusion in website information or other databases within the institution—share information with others who need it; do not hoard it!

E-Mail

The ability to send brief, simple messages around the world in seconds is wonderful and efficient for both the sender and recipient. E-mail programs have proliferated and many are

TABLE 5–2. WEBSITE CREATION POINTS

Know the mission and goals of the website and regularly consider whether they are being addressed

Make sure the site has useful, timely, and preferably, original information

Make sure the website looks good—if it does not, it will be shunned

Use graphics, but only if they add something worthwhile to a page. Be sure to keep graphics small, so that downloads of pages will be quick

Keep the information to a reasonable length on each page (preferably just a screen full)

Make it easy to use and easy to move through and around the website. That includes providing a good search engine. A great deal of effort should be placed into interlinking data in order to make it more accessible and useful. Also, a consistent and clear method to present information to navigate around the website is necessary

Custom tailor information presented to each user

Use self-generating content, if appropriate. For example, information about formulary material may be in a database format that is dynamically prepared in the format requested by the web user at the time of access

Test out the website to make sure that things work. That includes trying all web browsers and all versions of web browsers likely to be used by people looking at the site. This can include access by rather nontraditional browsers, such as those now found on cellular telephones. If the site requires a specific web browser or version of a browser, make that very clear

Get rid of broken links to other pages or websites

Test out various methods of access for acceptability. For example, see whether the site is usable via modem—if not, get rid of big graphics, and so forth

Provide contact information (i.e., names, addresses, and phone numbers)

Keep material up to date. Also, each page should indicate the date it was last changed

Leave out unnecessary information. Huge biographies of each of the pharmacists might be good for their ego, but otherwise useless

Consider the technical support needed by the website users

Consider the costs involved for both you and the intended user

Consider the level of security needed. Such things as VPNs and firewalls may be needed

Register the site with search engines, if high traffic is desired (e.g., community pharmacy). Also, just advertise the site, perhaps at other Internet sites that may be consulted by patients

Remember to assess what the users think about the website—what is valuable and what needs to be improved or eliminated

Consider the disabled. Do you need to make the site accessible to the blind?

---

available at little or no cost, or as part of web browsers, computer operating systems, or office software suites. Free e-mail accounts are readily available (e.g., HotMail, Yahoo mail, and Gmail) and are often given out as part of a subscription to an ISP's services. As a side note, everyone should have their own business and personal e-mail addresses, and use them for those separate purposes for legal and ethical reasons. It is still possible to use a single e-mail program to process messages from multiple accounts concurrently, but the separate accounts should exist.

Think about it—a pharmacist working on a computer remembers to let someone know about something or requires some information about a situation. If there was a need to have a record of communicating with that other person, in the past would have written memo or a letter, which might have taken several days to be written, dictated, typed, and/or proofed. It would then be sent and might take several more days to work its way through the institution's mail system and, possibly, the postal system. Another possibility is to call and then jot down the information. Of course, calling might require an extended period of "phone tag." Voice mail may make things simpler, although it certainly does not easily leave a permanent record of the information and many people do not like using it. The caller might actually get the person on the phone, but that could lead to spending a lot of time on irrelevant subjects—which sometimes leads people to hope they get the voice mail box instead.[106] An e-mail program running in the background can be quickly brought up and the person's address is typed in. The address is often much easier to remember than a postal address and is in a similar format to web addresses. Also, the user generally puts in a subject and might indicate whether the message is of high priority. When it is necessary to send other information, a computer file may be attached to the message before it is sent. Whether the addressee is in the next office or the next country, the message may be received in seconds or minutes. The person can reply when there is an opportunity (quite often the reply may be received in minutes). Another advantage is that the recipient may be able to obtain the message from many locations, including long distances, as long as a computer is available. Overall, e-mail can greatly improve the speed and efficiency of brief communications and should be considered instead of a short memo or phone call that would have been used in the past. In fact it was shown in one study that the time for a specialist consultation in oncology was decreased from 19 to 6.8 working days by using e-mail.[107]

As a side issue, nowadays, instant messaging services are also used for the above functions when a quick question is to be asked and it is not necessary to maintain a record. Such programs allow typing quick messages to others and are available from companies like Microsoft (<<http://www.microsoft.com>>), America Online (<<http://www.aol.com>>), and Yahoo (<<http://www.yahoo.com>>). Unfortunately, these programs are often incompatible, so users may find that they will run several of the programs on their computer in order to contact various people. Fortunately, a product such as Trillian (<<http://www.trillian.com>>) can provide at least a subset of the services of several instant-messaging products, allowing the use of this one program to contact people on various instant-messaging systems.

It should also be noted that by using e-mail it is possible to send information to personal distribution lists previously set up on the e-mail system. For example, the chairman of a committee with members scattered throughout the institution may need to regularly send short messages to all of them (e.g., the next meeting is on Friday at 10 AM in Room XXX). An e-mail user can use the name of the mailing list as the address and have it sent to the whole group.

Depending on the set up of the e-mail system, automated routing of forms, documents (e.g., for comments), and other items may be possible. For example, filling out a request for vacation time may be as simple as filling out an e-mail form that is automatically routed to an employee's supervisor.

E-mail also gives the sender the option to automatically receive a message from the recipient's computer confirming that the message has been read, which can sometimes be important when establishing whether lack of action is due to lack of communication or other reasons. Please note, however, it can be possible for such automated messages to be disabled or incompatibilities between e-mail programs can occasionally result in the "return-receipt" message being sent when the computer receives the message, rather than when it is actually read. Also, please be aware that e-mail does not always reach individuals and the level of lost e-mails can reach 40% under certain circumstances.[108,109]

Using e-mail to communicate with patients may be an important tool in the future (as an alternative with similar functions, physicians have also used secure web messaging to patients[110]).[111] Guidelines for doing so have been published[112–114] and revolve around the ability to keep information confidential (encryption or informed consent may be necessary) and making a clear agreement with the patient as to what can be transmitted via e-mail and to which e-mail address (home vs. employer)—note that signed informed consent is suggested[115] and it is necessary to be compliant with the provisions of the Health Insurance Portability and Accountability Act of 1996 (HIPAA).[116] Detailed information about the effect of HIPAA and other regulations can be found in Chap. 12, but is applicable to all aspects of digital information management and may be a particular concern for the use of e-mail or PDAs.[117] For example, would it be acceptable to e-mail a refill reminder to an immunodeficiency syndrome (HIV)-positive patient for antiviral medications? A record of all e-mail communications should be kept as a part of the medical record and some method of assuring the identity of the medical professional (e.g., cyber notaries) may be necessary.[115] Encryption of e-mail may be necessary.[118] A medicolegal problem to be resolved is the provision of advice via e-mail, or other electronic means, across state lines. While it has been shown that physicians do have concerns about using e-mail with patients, it has been found that it does work[119] and that patients will follow recommended guidelines.[120,121]

While a health care practitioner cannot assume that the e-mail is read promptly or at all by the patient, the practitioner must make sure all e-mail communications receive an appropriate response quickly and that patients know how to contact them directly for more information or in an urgent situation.[112]

E-mail and other electronic means can now be used by physicians to send prescriptions to pharmacists in some places,[122] and the volume of such prescriptions is likely to increase in the future. There are even companies that have created PDA applications to allow transmission of electronic prescriptions to pharmacists (e.g., <<http://www.zixcorp.com/ehealth/>>).

E-mail is also used to automatically provide information to pharmacists.[122–126] Many journals provide services where pharmacists can sign up to receive the journal table of contents free. Also, a service called Highwire Press from Stanford University provides such a service for many journals (<<http://highwire.stanford.edu/>>).

Whether used for patient communications or other functions, e-mail is "discoverable" in court and employers may have permanent records of e-mail messages that the sender and recipient thought were deleted long ago. Therefore, be as careful with e-mail as is necessary with other written communications.[127] Jobs have been lost due to improper use of e-mail communications. Some suggestions for companies to protect against legal problems include the following[128,129]:

- Develop a written e-mail policy. Make it clear and usable, and then enforce it.
- Define who owns the contents of the e-mail system.
- Inform employees that old mail may be saved (e.g., backups) even if it was supposedly deleted.
- Teach employees e-mail-appropriate conduct, including the avoidance of discrimination, harassment, or other misconduct.

Listservers

Listservers are similar to the distribution lists mentioned previously. However, a server on the e-mail computer keeps the list, to which people can apply to be a member. Once the list is established, any messages sent to the list are automatically sent to all members of the list—making it easy to communicate within a group. To better explain the concept of listservers, an example will be used.

The Consortium for the Advancement of Medication Information Policy and Research (CAMIPR) is a group of drug information specialists originally brought together by Gordon Vanscoy, Pharm.D. at the University of Pittsburgh. To facilitate communications between members of the group, a listserver was established at Creighton University with the address <<camipr@creighton.edu>>. To become members of the group, people sent a message to <<majordomo@creighton.edu>>, which controls the listservers at the institution (note: majordomo is the usual address name for joining any listserver). The body of the message must contain the phrase "subscribe camipr <<yourname@youraddress.xxx>>" where <<yourname@youraddress.xxx>> is the prospective subscriber's own e-mail address (to leave the list at a later time, the same procedure is followed, substituting the word "unsubscribe" for "subscribe"). If this was a public listserver, the person would be automatically added to the e-mail address list and would receive both an automated message acknowledging joining the list (and usually providing directions on special functions of the list) and any future messages sent to the list. However, in this situation, CAMIPR has been a private listserver. This means that all applicants are approved for addition to the list. While the application procedure is the same as previously described, the result is an automated message to the listserver owner, who then sends a message approving the addition of the new listserver member back to <<majordomo@creighton.edu>>. Other commands are available for the users of the listserver, including one that will provide a list of the addresses of current members. Once a member of the listserver, a person can then send messages to the other members by addressing their e-mail to the listserver address, which in this case is <<camipr@creighton.edu>>. (Please note, this listserver has now been transferred to the Iowa Drug Information Service, which can be contacted to join the listserver).

Listservers act as a good conduit for discussions. For example, one member can pose a question or problem to the listserver. Others can then reply to the original message or to the other replies to the message. In addition to sending each of the messages in the discussion to the members' e-mail addresses, the listserver may keep a record of the discussion, which can later be posted on a website to allow someone to read a continuous account of how a discussion proceeded. Also, a listserver can be moderated.[130] This means that all messages are first approved by the "owner" of the list before other members receive them. That allows for censoring of inappropriate material.

Pharmacists can use listservers to facilitate discussion between groups. Besides the use mentioned, it may be of value for committees, classes, or other groups. Various pharmacy organizations and special interest groups currently use listservers. The advantage of listservers over distribution lists is that while the listserver is available to all members of the group, a distribution list may be developed by an individual for his or her own use. A listserver is dynamically changed for all members as others join or leave the group. The only major problem with them is that their content may be stopped by software dedicated to preventing spam (i.e., unsolicited e-mail). If that happens, the recipient may have to specifically make a change to the list of e-mail addresses that are approved for receiving.

Pharmacists often get information on listservers from acquaintances or publications, as previously mentioned. Of particular interest to some pharmacists is the listserver from the CDC (<<http://www.cdc.gov/subscribe.html>>), which automatically sends a table of contents for the *MMWR* publications.

Electronic Faxes

The ability to send and receive faxes via a fax/modem has been available for years. Recently, however, it has become possible to send or receive faxes via e-mail. In some cases, the e-mail program acts like it is sending traditional e-mail, but then accesses the fax/modem. One interesting twist is the ability to have a fax number where the fax itself is turned into an e-mail message automatically and is then forwarded to the user's e-mail address to be read and/or printed. Similar to the free e-mail addresses mentioned previously, individuals can also sign up for a free fax phone number, where the message is delivered to his or her e-mail address (e.g., contact <<http://www.efax.com>>).[131] These services also may offer additional services for a fee. For example, an 800 fax phone number may be available. Also, sending faxes without charge is possible.

How to Manage E-Mail

E-mail is a wonderful tool, but there is definitely something to be said about having too much of a good thing, with many people complaining that they are getting more than 100 messages a day, many of which are unsolicited or spam. While this may be worrisome, there are ways that people can handle numerous messages. The first rule is to avoid adding to everyone else's e-mail inbox. Yes, it is easy to send messages to groups, but do not do so unless it is really necessary. Related to that, keep what is sent short, perhaps providing a longer version for those who need it, and do not bother with colored fonts and clip art.[132] Next, remember that programs do have filter features that will allow certain mail to be handled automatically.[133] For example, unsolicited mail from certain addresses can be automatically deleted, or an automatic reply can be sent to those messages. More important messages can be filtered to a common location for review as soon as possible. Also, e-mail programs may display a few lines of all new messages allowing the user to scan, highlight, and delete unimportant messages within seconds. Finally, be sure to review e-mail regularly—probably several times a day. That way, it will not build up to unmanageable levels and will maintain the efficiency of e-mail as an advantage. This may seem like a big chore, but it does not have to be. Modern computer operating systems allow several programs to run concurrently. An e-mail program can be set to always be running in the background, so that a user going from one thing to another can quickly check for any e-mail. Also, it is often easy to have more than one screen running on one computer system, sometimes simply using obsolete hardware scavenged from computers that are being discarded.

Personal Information Managers

An item that can be covered with e-mail is the use of personal information management (PIM) software (e.g., Microsoft Outlook) and PDAs, since e-mail acts as a basis of many functions. This can be taken to be specific software or pocket devices, but in this section will only refer to the functions, not the equipment the software resides on.

Many individuals carry pocket calendars or one of a number of notebooks designed to improve their productivity by expanding the calendar with to-do lists, contact information, and other items. For some people, such hard copy resources will continue to function; however, most people should be using the electronic versions of these items.

Many versions of software are available to do a variety of items. In particular, it should combine e-mail, calendar, to-do lists, contact (e.g., address and phone number), and the innumerable notes that people commonly carry (e.g., budget numbers, directions, and purchase lists). If at all possible, an institution should have a common system that allows people better interaction and easy access from multiple locations. For example, a person wanting to schedule a meeting should be able to use the software to find when everyone is available, and then "penciling" the meeting in on the calendar of all the prospective attendees. Also, project software may send specific action items to appropriate individuals, and then monitor progress and due dates. In addition, having the institution's system track reporting and organizational structure allows specific messages to be automatically routed to the appropriate individuals. For example, an individual filling out a vacation or reimbursement request on his or her PIM will know that the request will automatically be sent to the appropriate people for review and approval, regardless of whether the usual person is on vacation or has left the company and someone else is covering the function.

For individuals who need to have a calendar immediately available (e.g., a clinician who is all over the institution, rather than sitting at a desk), synchronization with a handheld device is normal. That way, when at his or her desk, the person has the ease of use of the keyboard and screen, but can keep both the PDA and himself or herself up to date at all times. The PDA can also be used to carry other information, including reference manuals and books. Various health care-related references for PDAs (some free) are available (see Appendix 5–15).*

In the case of a small organization or individuals, there are web-based services on the Internet that will perform the services mentioned in this section.[134]

Discussions

There are two types of online discussions that are often used. One is within a group or organization as mentioned earlier, perhaps even using a portion of the e-mail software. This is commonly used for online discussions for distance education students. The other is USENET News.

USENET News can be considered a group of discussion areas on the Internet that resemble electronic bulletin board services, with areas for discussion of a wide variety of topics from the serious (e.g., adverse drug reactions) to the absurd (e.g., McDonald's ketchup). These newsgroups can be compared to *chat rooms* available from some services, such as America Online, however; in this case the discussions are asynchronous (i.e., the messages are available to people logging on later, perhaps for days or weeks) and may occur over an extended period of time. Chat rooms will be discussed further in the next section.

USENET News servers are available from a number of locations. To access the servers it is necessary to have the appropriate software. Microsoft Internet Explorer does provide such features, as do a variety of other programs. When the software is installed and an address of an available USENET News server is input, the user will be presented with a list of available discussion group topics. This list may contain thousands of topics. Not all news servers have all of the discussion areas because of limitations in storage or other reasons. These topics are broken down into a number of areas, such as sci (science), comp (computer-related), rec (recreation), and misc (miscellaneous). A common discussion group for pharmacists is sci.med.pharmacy.

Once in a particular discussion area, the pharmacist will be presented with a list of recent "postings." These resemble a list of e-mail messages, which in many ways they are. Users of the newsgroup have "posted" what they want to say, talk about, or ask about on the newsgroup. The user will see the subject and who posted it (often the users will use very vague names or nicknames, similar to CB radio "handles"). For example, at the time this is

---

*The appendix can be found at www.MaloneDrugInfo.com.

being written, a current message is titled "Aricept and Alzheimer's disease." It is a request for information. The person requesting information posted this message to his news server and it was then replicated to all other news servers carrying this discussion group around the world. By clicking on the listing, anybody can read it and it is possible to reply. It is also possible to follow the "thread" of replies to a particular original posting over time. Therefore, a newsgroup can be used to obtain and give information. However, caution is advised. The quality of the postings varies widely. People on a particular discussion group may be world-renowned experts or crackpots. They may even be posing as someone else. Therefore, particular caution is advised—even more than is necessary with websites. Studies have found that approximately 70% of the information given on USENET News is erroneous.[135,136] That is not to say there are not good groups or that they are not valuable. Some patient groups regularly exchange good and valuable information on their disease state (e.g., cancer, panic disorders, incontinence, impotence, alcohol and drug abuse, domestic violence, and sexually transmitted diseases) using USENET News[137] and this has been successfully used for disease research,[138] but it is necessary to be very careful.

It is also possible to create new public or private discussion groups, perhaps using Google's Group feature (<<http://groups-beta.google.com/>>).

Internet Collaboration

It is now possible for pharmacists to communicate directly over the Internet (i.e., voice and video pictures of themselves in real time) with other pharmacists, while working together on a document. Collaboration with other pharmacists over the Internet has been available for a while, but there has not really been any evidence that it has been used to any extent. Reasons for this may include that the possible use has not yet become widely known, pharmacists do not know what software to use (even though it might even already be on their computers as part of Microsoft Internet Explorer), their network connection may be too slow, or even that they have not yet figured out how to integrate the use into their practice methods.

In the past, such communication might have been through Internet Relay Chat (IRC), however, now it is more likely to be through Microsoft NetMeeting or another commercially available product. In the future, collaboration capabilities will be built into office software suites (e.g., word processors).[139]

In general, the only equipment necessary for collaboration is a video camera for the computer, and only if video is needed. Such equipment may be purchased for well under $100. The software is often free.

Simpler methods of communicating that might fall under this topic are the "instant messenger" type products, as was previously discussed.

Telepharmacy

Related to many of the above items, pharmacists are starting to use a variety of forms of communication over the Internet. For example, it is currently possible to make phone calls over the web (e.g., <<http://www.skype.com/>>). New ways of sending phone applets[140] (maybe as part of a refill reminder) might allow pharmacists to let patients contact them directly (both broadcast quality audio and visual) for some service via the Internet. This will be an expansion on televideo technology that is already being used for patient counseling.[141]

Pharmacists are also able to receive monitoring data from patients, for example, blood sugar readings from diabetics, peak flow and expiratory volume readings from asthmatics, and blood pressures and lipid profiles from cardiac patients.[142] It is expected that houses, and even devices in the house,[143] will be able to monitor their occupants in the future, even calling for help when necessary.

Expansion of these capabilities and education of pharmacists to use them is being promoted by pharmacy organizations.[144] Since many of the details of telepharmacy go beyond the scope of this book, the reader is referred to other sources on the topic.

Push Technology

Push technology involves software that actually sends information to users' desktops. In many ways, this can be thought of as a marriage of web browsing, e-mail, and a screen saver, in that the information may resemble that found on a website (e.g., text, graphics, audio, and video), but it is delivered directly to the desk and may be displayed by the screen saver. Optionally, it may be set up to "pop up" when specific news is available (users set their preferences), as is seen with MSNBC News Alert (<<http://www.msnbc.com/>>), or as a window at the bottom of the screen.[145] This was considered to be a concept with a great future in 1997, but the enthusiasm for it has died down. The great advantage was that users did not have to take much of an active role in getting information (other than perhaps setting up a list of preferences for their computer when the push technology was added). In addition to using commercial information feeds, this software also allowed companies to create their own information stream to the desktop,[146,147] perhaps to better inform employees about a variety of institution-related topics.

Very closely related to push technology is Really Simple Syndication (RSS), which uses aggregator software that is available on the Internet.[124,148,149] These are programs working in the background on a computer with Internet access that allow the computer to go out and download information from a variety of sites that are chosen by the user. For example, some publications or websites (e.g., Medscape, <<http://www.medscape.com>>; MSNBC, <<http://www.msnbc.msn.com/id/5216556/>>) provide information for such programs. Institutions can also set up their own RSS feed to provide information to employees. This allows the user to go to one program (the aggregator) and look at new information from numerous sources in one place, hopefully saving the time that would have otherwise been used to go from one source to another.

Push technology does have some possible use for pharmacists. First, it can be used to inform pharmacists, even about news events (perhaps filtering medical news from a news organization), and can be used within an institution for institution-related news (e.g., new formulary additions, new policies, and procedures—essentially what would have previously been provided in a newsletter). The problems with push technology include that the information is often only being displayed when people are not using their computers (i.e., their screensaver starts up when they leave the office), it still may require going into a program (e.g., RSS aggregators), or that people may find it annoying.[150]

On a related topic, it should also be pointed out that some software allows automatic updates and bug fixes over the Internet (e.g., antiviral programs and newer versions of Microsoft Windows). In the future, the cost of doing this might be paid for by subscription or may even be free (due to advertising embedded in the updates).

Information Storage

An often-neglected piece of electronic information management is the long-term storage and availability of that information.[151] It may be simple to think that is an easy problem and that all that needs to be done is to burn the information on a CD-ROM. However, that argument quickly breaks down when a person may realize that not many years ago the same was said about storage on a 5 $\frac{1}{4}''$ floppy disk, since it is now very difficult to find a 5 $\frac{1}{4}''$ floppy disk drive. It is now getting more difficult to find such common things as 3 $\frac{1}{2}''$ floppy disk drives and Zip drives. There are many methods of storage that are no longer easily available, if available at all. So, it is necessary to make sure that data that may be needed in the future are available in a form that will be usable in the future. In addition to the physical media, it is also necessary to remember that current software may not be able to read old data. For example, a current copy of Microsoft Excel is unlikely to be able to read a 1980s VisiCalc spreadsheet. Therefore, it is necessary to plan ahead if data are to be used at a time in the future. It may be necessary to transfer the information to new software data formats and hardware devices.

Classified Advertisements

It is worth mentioning that classified advertisements are available on the Internet. Pharmacists may be interested in them for such things as personnel placement, or may even put advertisements in their websites to obtain revenue to support the site.

THE FUTURE

In many ways, most people have seen the near future of information technology whenever they tune into their favorite science fiction program. Just as Star Trek in the mid-1960s anticipated today's sliding doors and personal communicators (i.e., cellular phones), current science fiction programs anticipate how information will be widely available in many forms.

To begin with, it can be assumed that there will be an increase in computers, greater availability of information (reference, bibliography, electronic drug product labeling,[152] clinical decision support systems and clinical information systems [standardized patient data], which will be a financial bonanza for the owners of that data[153]), and a huge increase in the speed and capabilities of computers. For example, it has been stated that a computer capable of similar processing power as the human brain will be available in the next few years. This includes a speed of 1 petaop (10^{15} operations per second) and storage of 10 terabytes (10^{13} characters). These capabilities will eventually be on a computer that the user wears![154] It may be referred to as a body area network (BAN). It will allow the storage and recall of everything a person reads, hears, and/or sees during the entire life. Furthermore, computers will be designed to calm the user rather than cause anxiety. Overall, more information will be available from nearly any location, with much better linkage of the pieces of information and organized in a much more useful way.[155] As a side issue, it will be further necessary for individuals to realize that they cannot possibly know all they need to know and that they will have to take advantage of these information capabilities in their professional practices.[156]

In the near future, limited advances are possible. It can be assumed that current software will have additional capabilities. Data will be presented in forms that make them easier to visualize and manipulate interactively, making them easier to understand.[157] Clinical decision support systems that physicians may use in diagnosis are expected to improve,[158,159] although there are problems with getting physicians to use them because of overconfidence.[160] Different health professionals will be tied together by computers to improve patient care through such things as electronic drug utilization review.[161] Software will be available to spot health threats, including bioterrorism.[162] In general, an increase in the amount of information and the way it is tied together will be seen. More specifically for pharmacists, their practice sites will be redesigned to take advantage of automation of all dispensing functions, so that pharmacists can spend more time on cognitive, business, and clinical functions—making sure patients have more information, and better treatment and monitoring.[163] Those pharmacists who want to avoid cognitive functions and the patients will soon be out of a job if all they can do is count, pour, lick and stick, since robotics is becoming increasingly common.[164]

Pharmacists will have to deal with digital identities, both of their patients and their own. There are already electronic identification cards for both patients and practitioners (<<http://www.abda.de/>>). Coming soon are implantable devices that may carry medical records. As might be expected, there may be information about pharmacists regarding such things as disciplinary action, but other items, such as the pharmacist's home address may come as a shock (e.g., <<http://www.hhs.state.ne.us/lis/lisindex.htm>>). Even further information may start appearing on the Internet.

Overall, it will be up to pharmacists to learn how to best use all of these capabilities to improve patient care and to obtain appropriate reimbursement for services. Others are selling drug information, medical books, and vitamins over the Internet to patients and the National Association of Boards of Pharmacy has a process to approve Internet-based pharmacies, called Verified Internet Pharmacy Practice Sites (VIPPS),[165] which is important as a number of less than reputable sites have been established to allow people to easily obtain prescription drugs. Other pharmacy services will have to follow for optimal economic survival of the profession. Pharmacists should try new technology and new ways to use that technology; it may seem crazy, but it may end up being a wonderful idea.[166]

To do all of this, pharmacists will have to learn how to use the technology, and they must be given continual training by their employers and through their own efforts. In addition to the technical aspects, pharmacists will also have to ensure that the quality of their information is good and work with the reengineering of pharmacy and medical information resources to be more useful.[167] Although pharmacy has long used computers for business type purposes, much of what this article discusses has not been covered in pharmacy training.[168] This will have to change. It will be up to pharmacists to embrace this powerful communication tool; to lead the way or others will trample them. It may seem like a lot of work, but the returns are vast and pharmacists might even find that it is enjoyable.

Acknowledgment

Portions of this chapter were reproduced, with permission, from Malone PM. Drug information technology and Internet resources. J Pharm Pract. 1998;XI(3):196–218.

Study Questions

1. What search strategies can a pharmacist use in finding information on the Internet?
2. How can the quality of information be assessed on items located on the Internet?
2. How can a pharmacist use e-mail in practice situations (include distribution lists and listservers)?
4. What items can belong on a website in your practice situation?
5. What Internet access does a practitioner need?
6. What are USENET News groups, how are patients using them, and what should a pharmacist know about them to discuss with the patients?

REFERENCES

1. Internet domain survey, January 2005 [cited 2005 Jun 15]: [1 screen]. Available from: http://www.isc.org/ops/ds/reports/2005-01/.
2. IBM Research Blue Gene Project page [homepage on the Internet] [cited 2005 June 16]. Available from: http://www.research.ibm.com/bluegene/.

3. Roush W. The infinite library. Tech Rev [serial on the Internet]. 2005 [cited 2005 Apr 8]: [about 6 p.]. Available from: http://www.technologyreview.com/articles/05/05/issue/feature_library.asp?p=0

4. Carlson S, Young JR. Google will digitalize and search millions of books from 5 leading research libraries. Chron High Educ [serial on the Internet]. 2004 Dec 14 [cited 2004 Dec 16]: [about 6 p.]: Available from: http://chronicle.com/prm/weekly/v51/i18/18a03701.htm

5. Klein CN. Pharmacy and the Internet. Am J Health Syst Pharm. 1995;52:2095.

6. Westberg EE, Miller RA. The basis for using the Internet to support the information needs of primary care. JAMIA. 1999;6:6–25.

7. Editors of ComputerTalk. The next generation: today's pharmacy students are wired to the future. A fascinating look at the innovative Shenandoah University School of Pharmacy. ComputerTalk. 1998;18(6):14–23.

8. Chen A. Hospital cures WLAN insecurity. eWeek. Feb 2003;3:35.

9. Young M, Fox BI. Wireless communications in health systems: is there a danger? Hosp Pharm. 2005;40:360–2.

10. Vecchione A. New data-collection tool speeds up reporting process. Hosp Pharm Rep. 1997;11(2):64.

11. Chin T. More doctors go online for drug information. AMNews [serial on the Internet]. 2003 [cited 2003 Sept 9]: [about 3 p.]. Available from: http://www.ama-assn.org/sci-pubs/amnews/pick_03/bisd0908.htm

12. Chen ES, Mendonça EA, McKnight LK, Stetson PD, Lei J, Cimino JJ. PalmCIS: wireless handheld application for satisfying clinician information needs. JAMIA. 2004;11:19–28.

13. Vine D, Corvalán E. 21st century physician's little black bag. Gratefully Yours. 1997 Sept/Oct;1–3.

14. Rupley S. Calling the web. Smart phones get smarter. PC Mag. 1999 Dec 14;18(22):32.

15. Brown M, Brown B. Web phones. PC Mag. 2000 Mar 7;19(5):32–4, 36.

16. Currid C. Currid's ten commandments puts electronic mail use on top. InfoWorld. 1992;14(Sept 28):58.

17. Van Name ML, Catchings B. Quality Internet access is a business basic. PC Week. 1999 Jan 11; 16(2):29.

18. Jones MG. Telemedicine and the National Information Infrastructure: are the realities of health care being ignored? JAMIA. 1997;4:399–412.

19. Nicefaro ME. Internet use policies. Online. 1998 Sept/Oct;23:31–3.

20. Bailes L. WinFAQ: PC viruses. Safe or sorry? Windows Mag. 1998;9(1):251–5.

21. Druffel L. Information warfare. In: Denning PJ, Metcalfe RM, editors. Beyond calculation. The next fifty years of computing. New York: Copernicus; 1997.

22. Eng TR, Maxfield A, Patrick K, Deering MJ, Ratzan SC, Gustafson DH. Access to health information and support. A public highway or a private road? JAMA. 1998;280:1371–5.

23. Ojala M. Beginning all over again: where to start a search. Online. 1998;22(3):44–6.

24. Lindberg DAB, Humphreys BL. Medical informatics. JAMA. 1997;277:1870–1.

25. Odlyzko AM. Will full online text have the last word? Medicine on the Net. 1997;3(8):5–12.

26. McDonald CJ, Overhage JM, Dexter PR, Blevins L, Meeks-Johnson J, Suico JG, et al. Canopy computing. Using the web in clinical practice. JAMA. 1998;280:1325–9.

27. Bourne DWA. Using the Internet as a pharmacokinetic resource. Clin Pharmacokinet. 1997;33(3): 153–60.

28. Morgan C. The search is on. Windows Mag. 1996;7(11):212–4, 216, 218, 220, 222, 224, 226, 230.

29. Lawrence S, Giles CL. Search the World Wide Web. Science. 1998 Apr 3;280:98–100.

30. Search engines' tiny bite. PC Mag. 1999 Sept 1;18(15):9.

31. Sullivan D. Crawling under the hood. An update on search engine technology. Online. 1998; 22(3):30–8.

32. How to access the "hidden" Internet. Max PC. 2005 July;38.

33. Boswell W. What is the Invisible Web? About [homepage on the Internet]. New York: About.com; c2005 [cited 2005 June 20]. Available from: http://websearch.about.com/od/invisibleweb/a/ invisible_web.htm.

34. Hock R. How to do field searching in web search engines. Online. 1998;22(3):18–22.

35. Hock R. Web search engines features and commands. Online. 1999 May/June;23(3):24–8.

36. Berinstein P. Turning visual: image search engines on the web. Online. 1998;22(3):37–42.

37. Pemberton JK, Garman N, Ojala M. Head to head. Online. 1998;22(3):24–8.

38. Webster P. Metasearching in an academic environment. Online. 2004 Mar/Apr;20–3.

39. Notess GR. Toward more comprehensive web searching: single searching versus megasearching. Online. 1998 Mar/Apr;73–6.

40. Lunt P. Search & retrieval—special agents find it for you. Imaging & Document Solutions. 1999 Apr;8(4):46–54.

41. Knorr E. The new enterprise portal. InfoWorld. 2004 Jan 12;(2):42–52.

42. Ericson J. Portal with a pulse. Portals Mag. 2002 Oct;32–5.

43. Lippincott JK. Net generation students & libraries. EDUCASE Rev. 2005 Mar/Apr;56–66.

44. Crispen P. Google 201: advanced googology. Fullerton (CA): California State University, Fullerton, 2004.

45. Use Google's advanced search tools. Max PC. July 2005;36.

46. Malone PM. New specialized search tools from Copernic and Google. Adv Pharm. 2005;3(2):156–66.

47. Kurkul D. Free MEDLINE® shakes up content providers: what it means for you. Medicine on the Net. 1997;3(9):8–15.

48. Southwick K. Free MEDLINE® ignites vendor wars. Medicine on the Net. 1997;3(9):16–7.

49. Sikorski R, Peters R. Medical literature made easy. Querying databases on the Internet. JAMA. 1997;277:959–60.

50. Detmer WM. MEDLINE® on the Web: ten questions to ask when evaluating a web based service. AMIA Internet Working Group Newsletter. 1997;3(1):11–3.

51. Webster P. Implications of expanded library electronic reference collections. Online. 2003 Sept/Oct;24–7.

52. Graeme D. Alternatives in academic publishing. Wwwtools for Educ [serial on the Internet]. 2004 Feb 23 [cited 2004 Feb 23]:[about 9 p.]. Available from: http://magazines.fasfind.com/wwwtools/ magazines.cfm?rid=626

53. Bethesda statement on open access publishing [homepage on the Internet]. 2003 June 20[cited 2004 Feb 23]. Available from: http://www.earlham.edu/~peters/fos/bethesda.htm

54. Calishain T. The next small thing. PC Mag. 2004 Mar 2;62.

55. Malone PM. RFID, searching, weblogs and more. Adv Pharm. 2004;2(3):304–12.

56. Seltzer L. Google moves desktop search out of beta. eWeek [serial on the Internet]. 2005 Mar 7 [cited 2005 Mar 7]:[about 2 p.]. Available from: http://www.eweek.com/print_article2/0,2533,a=147083,00.asp

57. Vaughan-Nichols SJ. Google Desktop is in a class by itself. eWeek [serial on the Internet]. 2005 Mar 7 [cited 2005 Mar 7]:[about 2 p.]. Available from http://www.eweek.com/print_article2/0,2533,a=147232,00.asp

58. Bailey WJ. Searching the Internet for drug information. Strategies for locating accurate and scientifically accepted information. [cited 1996 Jul 18]:[1 screen]. Available from: http://www.drugs.indiana.edu/pubs/newsline/searching.html

59. Talley CR. Trouble on the Internet. Am J Health Syst Pharm. 1997;54:757.

60. Rogers A. Good medicine on the web. The Internet is a powerful health resource, but watch where you surf. Newsweek. 1998 Aug 24, CXXXII(8):60–1.

61. Knoben JE, Phillips SJ, Snyder JW, Szczur MR. The National Library of Medicine and Drug Information. Part 2: an evolving future. Drug Inf J. 2004;38:171–80.

62. Bridges A, Thede LQ. Electronic education. Nursing education resources on the World Wide Web. Nurse Educ. 1996;21(5):11–5.

63. Alexander J, Tate M. The web as a research tool: evaluation techniques. [cited 1997 April 14]: [1 screen]. Available from: http://www.science.widener.edu/~withers/webeval.htm

64. Jacobson T, Cohen L. Evaluating Internet resources. [cited 1997 April 14]: [1 screen]. Available from: http://www.albany.edu/library/internet/evaluate.html

65. Bernstam EV, Shelton DM, Walji M, Meric-Bernstam F. Instruments to assess the quality of health information on the World Wide Web: what can our patients actually use? Int J Med Inform. 2005;74:13–9.

66. Pines WL. The challenge of the Internet. Drug Inf J. 1998;32:277–81.

67. Health on the Net Foundation packs a punch with more than just quality. Medicine on the Net. 1997;3(12):15–7.

68. Wanjek C. Attaching their HONor. Washington Post [serial on the Internet]. 2004 Apr 20 [cited 2004 Apr 23]:[about 3 p.]. Available from: http://www.washingtonpost.com/ac2/wp-dyn/A25556-2004Apr19?language=printer

69. Jadad AR, Gagliardi A. Rating health information on the Internet. Navigating to knowledge or to Babel? JAMA. 1998;279:611–4.

70. Notess GR. Alexa: web archive, advisor, and statistician. Online. 1998;22(3):29–30.

71. Silberg WM, Lundberg GD, Musacchio RA. Assessing, controlling, and assuring the quality of medical information on the Internet. JAMA. 1997;277:1244–5.

72. Murray PJ. Click here—and be disappointed? Evaluating websites. Comput Nurs. 1996;14(5):260–1.

73. Wu WK, Tucker T. Composing a pharmacy web page. US Pharmacist. 1999 Jan;32, 34–6, 38, 40, 42–4.

74. Lowe HJ, Lomax EC, Polonkey SE. The World Wide Web: a review of an emerging Internet-based technology for the distribution of biomedical information. JAMIA. 1996;3:1–14.

75. Dalton M, Enos M, Halvachs F. Use of a private intranet system by a pharmacy and therapeutics committee. Hosp Pharm. 1998;33:1365–71.

76. Appleton EL. New recipes for learning. Inside Technology Training. 1997;1(1):12–6, 18, 57.

77. Polyson S, Saltzberg S, Godwin-Jones R. A practical guide to teaching with the World Wide Web. Syllabus. 1996;10(2):12, 14, 16.

78. Kaplan IP, Patton LR, Hamilton RA. Adaptation of different computerized methods of distance learning to an external Pharm.D. degree program. Am J Pharm Educ. 1996;60:422–5.

79. Bell SJ. Mounting presentations on the web: presentation software, HTML or both? Online. 1998 Sept/Oct;62–70.

80. Moore J. Stream your presentations from the web. Windows Sources. 1998 Feb;108.

81. Hinman L. Streaming video: adding real multimedia to the web. Syllabus. 1999;12(5):18–21.

82. Major MJ. Next generation Internet and video: emerging applications. Syllabus. 1999;12(5):24, 26.

83. Levy L. Imaging takes publishing to new territories. Imaging Mag. 1998;7(3):16, 18, 20, 22.

84. Flahault A, Dias-Ferrao V, Chaberty P, Esteves K, Valleron A-J, Lavanchy D. FluNet as a tool for global monitoring of influenza on the web. JAMA. 1998;280:1330–2.

85. Peters R, Sikorski R. Building your own. A physician's guide to creating a website. JAMA. 1998;280:1365–6.

86. Olsen G. 9 design and production stages for creating web presentations. Presentations. 1997;11(4):31–3.

87. Schwartz M. Ways to doom your website. Software Mag. 1998;18(4):26.

88. What makes a great website? [cited 1999 May 13]:[1 screen]. Available from: http://www.webreference.com/greatsite.html

89. Giebel T. Make your site a success. PC Mag. 1999 Sept 21;18(16):36.

90. Hopp DI. Three topics integral to the use of the Internet for clinical trials: connectivity, communication, and security. Drug Inf J. 1998;32:933–9.

91. Durieux P. Electronic medical alerts—so simple, so complex. N Engl J Med. 2005;352:1034.

92. Oren E, Shaffer ER, Guglielmo BJ. Impact of emerging technologies on medication errors and adverse drug events. Am J Health Syst Pharm. 2003;60:1447–58.

93. Wilcox RA, Whitham EM. Reduction of medical error at the point-of-care using electronic clinical information delivery. Int Med J. 2003;33:537–40.

94. Wilson JW, Oyen LJ, Ou NN, McMahon MM, Thompson RL, Manahan JM, et al. Hospital rules-based system: the next generation of medical informatics for patient safety. Am J Health Syst Pharm. 2005;62;499–505.

95. Felkey BG, Liang H, Krueger KP. Data mining for the health system pharmacist. Hosp Pharm. 2003;38:845–50.

96. Bogucki B, Jacobs BR, Hingle J. Clinical Informatics Outcomes Research Group. JAMIA. 2004;11: 278–80.

97. Lowry CM, Kostka-Rokosz MD, McCloskey WW. Evaluation of personal digital assistant drug information databases for the managed care pharmacist. J Manag Care Pharm. 2003;9(5):441–8.

98. Keplar KE, Urbanski CJ. Personal digital assistant applications for the health care provider. Ann Pharmacother. 2003;37:287–96.

99. Galt KA, Rule AM, Houghton B, Young DO, Remington G. Personal digital assistant-based drug information sources: potential to improve medication safety. J Med Libr Assoc. 2005;93(2): 229–36.

100. McCreadie SR, Stevenson JG, Sweet BV, Kramer M. Using personal digital assistants to access drug information. Am J Health Syst Pharm. 2002;59:1340–3.

101. Ellington TM. Evaluation of OTC product information in three drug information databases for PDAs. J Am Pharm Assoc. 2003;43(1):118–20.

102. Barrons R. Evaluation of personal digital assistant software for drug interactions. Am J Health Syst Pharm. 2004;61:380–5.

103. Keplar KE, Urbanski CJ, Kania DS. Update on personal digital assistant applications for the health care provider. Ann Pharmacother. 2005;39:892–907.

104. Zabrek EM. Winners: editor's choice best health care software 2004. Pocket PC. 2005 Feb;8:74–7.

105. Guernsey L, Kiernan V. Journals differ on whether to publish articles that have appeared on the web. Chron High Educ. 1998 July 17. Available from: http://chronicle.com/free/v44/i45/45a02701.htm

106. Machrone B. Perfect talk, perfect sense. PC Mag. 1998;17(3):85.

107. Kedar I, Ternullo JL, Winrib CE, Kelleher KM, Brandling-Bennett H, Kvedar JC. Internet based consultations to transfer knowledge for patients requiring specialised care: retrospective case review. BMJ. 2003 Mar 21;326:696–9.

108. Langa F. Langa letter: e-mail—hideously unreliable. Information Week. 2004 Jan 12:[about 7 p]. Available from: http://www.informationweek.com/story/showArticle.jhtml?articleID=17300016.

109. Livingston B. Is one-fourth of your e-mail getting lost? [Internet]. Westport (CT): Jupitermedia; 2004 April 19 [cited 2004 Apr 26]. Available from: http://itmanagement.earthweb.com/columns/executive_tech/article.php/3341991.

110. Liederman EM, Morefield CS. Web messaging: a new tool for patient-physician communication. JAMIA. 2003;10:260–70.

111. Delbanco T, Sands DZ. Electrons in flight—e-mail between doctors and patients. N Engl J Med. 2004;350:1705–7.

112. Kane B, Sands DZ, AMIA Internet Working Group. Guidelines for the clinical use of electronic mail with patients. JAMIA. 1998;5:104–11.

113. Stevens L. Communicating with your patients. The promises and pitfalls of e-mail. Medicine on the Net. 1999 Apr;5(4):6–10.

114. Kuppersmith RB. Is e-mail an effective medium for physician-patient interactions? Arch Otolaryngol Head Neck Surg. 1999;125(4):468–70.

115. Spielberg AR. On call and online. Sociohistorical, legal, and ethical implications of e-mail for the patient-physician relationship. JAMA. 1998;280–1353–9.

116. HIPAA Insurance Reform [homepage on the Internet]. Washington: Centers for Medicare and Medicaid Services; [updated 2004 Sept 16; cited 2005 June 16]. Available from: http://www.cms.hhs.gov/hipaa/hipaa1/default.asp

117. Pancoast PE, Patrick TB, Mitchell JA. Physician PDA use and the HIPAA privacy rule. JAMIA. 2003;10:611–2.

118. Karagiannis K. Securing your e-mail. PC Mag. 2002 Dec 24;21(22):76.

119. Leong SL, Gingrich D, Lewis PR, Mauger DT, George JH. Enhancing doctor-patient communication using email: a pilot study. J Am Board Fam Pract. 2005;18:180–8.

120. Sands DZ. Help for physicians contemplating use of e-mail with patients. JAMIA. 2004;11:268–9.

121. White CB, Moyer CA, Stern DT, Katz SJ. A content analysis of e-mail communication between patients and their providers: patients get the message. JAMIA. 2004;11:260–7.

122. E-mail to eliminate drug confusion. Finger Lakes Times. 1999 Apr 28;7.

123. Balen RM. How to use email and the Internet to help you keep up with the literature: part I. J Inform Pharmacother [serial on the Internet]. 2002 April–June [cited 2005 June 16];9:[about 5 p.]. Available from: http://www.informedpharmacotherapy.com/Issue9/TIPS/Keeping%20up%20pt1.htm

124. Balen RM. How to use email and the Internet to help you keep up with the literature (part II): PubMed® and Allied Journal Club. J Inform Pharmacother [serial on the Internet]. 2002 Jul–Sept [cited 2005 June 16];9:[about 7 p.]. Available from: http://www.informedpharmacotherapy.com/Issue10/TIPS/Keeping%20up%20pt2.htm

125. Balen RM. How to use email and the Internet to help you keep up with the literature (part III): the therapeutic topic approach and a potential corporate strategy. J Inform Pharmacother [serial on the Internet]. 2002 Oct–Dec [cited 2005 June 16];9:[about 6 p.]. Available from: http://www.informed-pharmacotherapy.com/Issue11/TIPS/Keeping_up_pt3.htm

126. Malone PM. Slides, files and keeping up. Adv Pharm. 2004;2(2):175–80.

127. Fitgerald WL, Jr. Do you know where your e-mail messages are? Drug Top. 1998;142(1):66.

128. Wolfe D. Avoiding e-mail litigation. Network Magazine. 1999;14(1):25.

129. Steen M. Legal pitfalls of e-mail. Every company needs a clear policy, and IT needs to help draft it. InfoWorld. 1999 July 5;21(27):65–6.

130. Mack J. Secrets of a successful e-mail discussion group moderator. Medicine on the Net. 1999 Apr;5(4):12–3.

131. Faxless society. Newsweek. 1999 Feb 15;CXXXIII(7):15.

132. Howard B. Avoiding clueless e-mail. PC Mag. 1998 May 26;17(10):97.

133. Notess GR. Filtering the e-mail storm. Online. 1998 Nov: [cited 1999 Nov]:[1 screen]. Available from: http://www.online.inc.com/onlinemag/OL1998/net11.html

134. Brookshaw C. Web-based PIMS can help you stick to your schedule. InfoWorld. 1999 May 10;21(19):57–8, 66.

135. Carre S. How to separate the Internet wheat from the chaff. Drug Top. 1997;141(4):88, 90.

136. Seaboldt JA, Kuiper R. Comparison of information obtained from a Usenet newsgroup and from drug information centers. Am J Health Syst Pharm. 1997;54(1)1732–5.

137. Howe L. Patients on the Internet: a new force in health care community building. Medicine on the Net. 1997;3(11):8–16.

138. Engstrom P. How a scientist tapped UseNet for clues to an inexplicable disease. Medicine on the Net. 1997;3(3):1–4.

139. Trott B, Scannell E. Microsoft to open a new Office. InfoWorld. 1998;20(7):35.

140. Verity J. IP shakes up long distance. Windows Sources. 1998 Feb;58.

141. Keith MR. Televideo technology for patient counseling and education. Am J Health Syst Pharm. 1999;56(1):860–1.

142. Vecchione A. The net set. Hosp Pharm Rep. 1999 Apr;38–40.

143. Huang GT. Monitoring mom. Tech Rev. 2003;106(6):22–3.

144. Melby MJ. Board of directors report on the Council on Professional Affairs. Am J Health Syst Pharm. 1999;56:664–7.

145. Browserless news—free. PC Mag. 1999 Oct 5;18(17):66.

146. Rapoza J. The cost of free net tools. PC Week. 1998;15(3):47.

147. Shankar G. PointCast adds broadcast tools. InfoWorld. 1998;19(3):58C–58D.

148. Livingston B. Are you ready for RSS? InfoWorld. 2003 Apr 25:[about 3 p.]. Available from: http://www.infoworld.com/article/03/04/25/17winman_1.html

149. Livingston B. Ahoy, RSS Enterprise. InfoWorld. 2003 May 2:[about 3 p.]. Available : http://www.infoworld.com/article/03/05/02/18winman_1.html

150. Dvorak JC. When push comes to shove. PC Mag. 1997;16(6):87.

151. Malone PM. Topics in informatics. Adv Pharm. 2003;1(4):369–76.

152. Martin IG. Electronic labeling: a paperless future? Drug Inf J. 1998;32:917–9.

153. Collen MF. A vision of health care and informatics in 2008. JAMIA. 1999;6:1–5.

154. Schwartz E. Wearables have you dressed for success. InfoWorld. [serial on the Internet] 2004 June 4 [cited 2004 June 8]:[about 2 p.]. Available from: http://www.infoworld.com/article/04/06/04/23OPreality_1.html

155. Lindberg DAB, Humphreys BL. 2015—the future of medical libraries. N Engl J Med. 2005;352:1067–70.

156. Lee TH. Quiet in the library. N Engl J Med. 2005;352:1068.

157. Hawkins DT. Information visualization: don't tell me, show me! Online. 1999;23(1):88–90.

158. Hunt DL, Haynes RB, Hanna SE, Smith K. Effects of computer-based clinical decision support systems on physician performance and patient outcomes. A systematic review. JAMA. 1998;280:1339–46.

159. Westbrook JI, Coiera EW, Gosling AS. Do online information retrieval systems help experienced clinicians answer clinical questions? JAMIA. 2005;12:315–21.

160. Study: doc overconfidence hampers use of decision support software. iHealthBeat. 2005 Mar 30[cited 2005 Mar 30]:[about 1 p.]. Available from: http://www.ihealthbeat.org/index.cfm?Action=dspItem&itemID=109848

161. Monane M, Matthias DM, Nagle BA, Kelly MA. Improving prescribing patterns for the elderly through an online drug utilization review intervention. A system linking the physician, pharmacist, and computer. JAMA. 1998;280:1249–52.

162. Scott M. Software can spot threats to health. St. Petersburg Times [serial on the Internet] 2003 [cited 2003 Sept 11]:[about 2 p.]. Available from: http://www.sptimes.com/2003/09/11/news_pf/Northpinellas/Software_can_spot_thr.shtml

163. Slezak M. Eckerd shoots for the moon. Am Drug. 1998 Aug;38–41.

164. ScriptPro sells Rite Aid on automation. Drug Top. 1999 Apr 5;143(7):7.

165. Breu J. NABP starts process of certifying sites as accepted pharmacies. Drug Topics. 1999 Oct 4; 143(19):19, 23.

166. If it sounds crazy, try it. Information Week. 1994 Sept:32–37.

167. Hersh WR. Medical informatics. Improving health care through information. JAMA. 2002;288:1955–8.

168. Vecchione A. Pharmacy schools found wanting in their training on technology. Hospital Pharmacist Report. 1997 Sept;(Technology and Pharmacy '97 Suppl):22S–23S.

6

Chapter Six

Controlled Clinical Trial Evaluation

Michael G. Kendrach • Maisha Kelly Freeman

Objectives

After completing this chapter, the reader will be able to

- Explain the reasons why pharmacists need the skills to locate and evaluate current information for pharmaceutical care activities.
- List the advantages and limitations of the pharmacy/biomedical tertiary literature sources (e.g., textbooks and review articles) and continuing education programs.
- Describe the special characteristics of a controlled clinical trial that distinguish this research design as the prototype for clinical research.
- List the reasons as to why research results are not published.
- Identify Internet websites to register controlled clinical trials and obtain Institutional Review Board (IRB) information.
- Describe the peer-review process and significance to the literature publication process.
- Discuss methods to identify the potential bias of investigator/author conflict of interests and funding sources on the reliability of the clinical trial results and conclusions.
- Discuss the purpose of the clinical trial abstract and limitations of using only information from this source in problem-solving processes.
- Differentiate between internal and external validity.
- Identify key information presented in each section of a clinical trial.
- Differentiate between the specific types of data and measures of central tendency.
- Explain the effect of selection bias, inclusion/exclusion criteria, composite endpoints, and surrogate endpoints on applying the clinical trial results into practice.
- Discuss the importance of selecting proper intervention and control regimens, endpoints, sample size, study power, and statistical tests.
- Discuss the need for a well-defined study objective, randomization, and blinding within a clinical trial.

- Explain the purpose of a subject informed consent form and reasons clinical trials need IRB approval.
- Define intention-to-treat, subgroup, and interim analyses.
- Differentiate between Type I and Type II errors and discuss methods to reduce the possibility of either of these errors occurring.
- Calculate and interpret relative risk (RR), relative risk reduction (RRR), absolute risk reduction (ARR), and number-needed-to-treat (NNT).
- Interpret p values, 95% confidence interval (CI), standard deviation (SD), and standard error of the mean (SEM).
- Determine statistical significance, clinical difference, and clinical meaningfulness of the clinical trial results.
- Prepare a null hypothesis (H_0) based on the clinical trial objective and endpoints; discuss whether to reject or fail to reject the H_0 by using the clinical trial results.
- Address the importance of the clinical trial conclusions being consistent with the results.
- Explain the purpose and usage of editorials, letters to the editors, and secondary journals in critiquing clinical trials and in the decision-making process of applying the results into practice.

Pharmacists continuously rely on the biomedical/pharmacy literature for many day-to-day activities. The practice of medicine and pharmacy is dynamic, and drug facts acquired during formal education cannot sustain a health care provider in future practice. Changes include new medications, dosage formulations, and uses approved by the Food and Drug Administration (FDA), revised drug safety information (i.e., adverse drug effects and drug interactions), and updated disease state therapeutic guidelines. During 2004, more than 25 new molecular entities/biologic agents were approved by the FDA,[1] more than 40 drug safety alerts/notices were issued by the FDA,[2] and over 500 published articles classified as human, adult practice guidelines were added to the National Library of Medicine database.[3] Therefore, skills, such as drug literature evaluation, are necessary to prepare the health care provider for practice. Furthermore, pharmacists must employ methods to keep current with these advances in order to remain competent, trustworthy health care professionals.[4]

Multiple resources are available for pharmacists to provide answers to questions, care for patients, make decisions, and solve problems; but pharmacists need to recognize both the advantages and limitations of the information resources to meet the challenges encountered during the work day. Advantages include ready access and electronic formats. Potential disadvantages include biases, costs, and lag time (i.e., lack of current content) that hinder the usefulness of some references. In addition, misinterpretation of the information can lead to improper patient care.

Pharmacists must have skills in efficiently locating, critically analyzing, and effectively communicating drug information. Regardless of the pharmacy practice setting (e.g., community and institutional), pharmacists are called on to use these skills. Access to information for both health care professionals and laypersons has increased exponentially, because of improvements in technology over the past few decades. Not all information can be deemed accurate and pharmacists are repeatedly relied on, especially by laypersons, to clarify, explain, defend, and/or refute information.[4] Pharmacists are frequently consulted by other health care providers to assist in individual patient care regarding appropriate drug use.[5-7] Furthermore, pharmacists are in decision-making positions in which drugs are selected for use in a multitude of patients (e.g., third-party health care plans and drug formulary decisions).[8,9] All these activities require pharmacists to carefully review and critique the literature instead of accepting the authors' conclusions. Many studies have very positive conclusions but include study design errors, which limit the clinical usefulness of the results. Also, medical/pharmacy continuing education presentations may contain biases and/or inaccuracies while textbooks/review articles may contain misinterpreted and/or noncomprehensive information. Due to the important contribution pharmacists have in patient care, pharmacists need to have skills in identifying the strengths and limitations of the biomedical literature. This chapter is devoted to explaining and discussing core concepts for critiquing one essential type of biomedical literature, controlled clinical trials.

Biomedical/Pharmacy Literature

Three types of literature serve as information resources for pharmacists: tertiary, secondary, and primary (see Table 6–1).[10] Readers are referred to Chap. 4 in this text for more in-depth discussions of these three literature types.

TABLE 6–1. THREE TYPES OF LITERATURE

Literature Type	Description	Examples
Tertiary	Established knowledge	Textbooks, review articles, MD Consult, WebMD, Lexi-Comp
Secondary	Indexing/abstracting services (i.e., databases)	PubMed or MEDLINE (National Library of Medicine), EMBASE (Elsevier), International Pharmaceutical Abstracts (Thomson Corporation), CINAHL (Cumulative Index to Nursing and Allied Health), InfoTrac OneFile (Gale Group), Academic Lexis-Nexis (Reed Elsevier Inc)
Primary	Original research	Controlled clinical trials, case-control studies, crossover trials, case reports

Primary literature, specifically controlled clinical trials, serves as the foundation for clinical practice by providing the documentation for using therapy. Although vast amounts of primary literature articles are published each year, individuals can efficiently locate information specific and useful to their needs by incorporating appropriate search techniques.[11,12] Clinical trials are one particular type of primary literature that can be a reliable source of new information to change health care practices.[13–15] New information may either counter or serve as the root for altering existing practice regimens; thus, pharmacists need the skill of critiquing clinical trials. The special features of clinical trial design allow investigators to determine which therapeutic interventions should be used in practice.[16,17] In fact, the FDA requires clinical trials to be conducted and the results submitted before a new molecular entity (i.e., medication) can be marketed and/or receive new indications for use.[18] Proper interpretation of clinical trials is vital to providing appropriate health care. The next chapter in this text reviews evaluating publications using the other types of research designs.

In general, a controlled clinical trial consists of an investigational (intervention) group being directly compared to a control group (e.g., standard therapy, placebo).[16,17] The intervention under investigation may be a new medication, different medication dosing regimen, diet, surgery, behavioral process, exercise program, diagnostic procedure, or something else. The goal of the clinical trial is to assess the difference in effect between the investigational and control groups. The results then can allow decisions to be made regarding proper care for patients (i.e., to use or not use the investigational therapy).[16] Although the origins of a controlled trial date back to the eighteenth century,[19] a formalized process of conducting controlled clinical trials was implemented during the late 1940s.[20] However, poorly designed clinical trials are still published and the existence of a clinical trial may not translate into clinically useful information. Research has reported that results of well-designed clinical trials are considered to be of better quality and are usually more clinically relevant than clinical trials that are poorly designed.[21]

The published clinical trial is presented in a manner that explains the research process in an orderly format to improve the readers' comprehension of the project, results, and conclusions. Table 6–2 displays the style in which a clinical trial usually appears in printed resources.[22,23] This chapter discusses the information presented in these sections according to the CONSORT (Consolidated Standards of Reporting Trials) format. The CONSORT format was formulated to improve the quality of reporting clinical trials in the published literature, since inadequate reporting methods hinder the interpretation of results produced by clinical trials. CONSORT has been supported by an increasing number of medical and health care journals (e.g., *Journal of the American Medical Association* [*JAMA*]) and editorial groups (e.g., International Committee of Medical Journal Editors [ICMJE]).[23] Other research types (i.e., case-control study) can report the investigation using the style of reporting a controlled clinical trial. Therefore, one should not assume all publications using this format are controlled clinical trials.

TABLE 6–2. FORMAT AND CONTENT OF CONTROLLED CLINICAL TRIALS

Controlled Clinical Trial Section	Type of Information Presented
Abstract	Brief overview of the research project
Introduction	Research background
	Clinical trial objective
Methodology	Study design
	Patient inclusion and exclusion criteria
	Intervention and control groups
	Randomization
	Blinding
	Endpoints
	Follow-up procedure
	Sample size calculations/power analysis
	Statistical analysis
Results	Subject characteristics
	Subject dropouts/compliance
	Endpoints quantified
	Safety assessments
Discussion	Result interpretations
	Other study results compared
	Limitations
Acknowledgments	Other contributors
	Funding source
	Peer-review dates/manuscript acceptance date (not all trials)
References/Bibliography	Citations for information included from other resources (e.g., trials and reports)

Health care providers are known to base their practice style on evidence from clinical trials.[13,14,24,25] This study design is the most robust method to measure and quantify differences in effects between a therapy under study and the control group.[16,17] Many clinical studies are published annually, but not every study initiated is reported in the published literature.[26–28] Primary reasons for not publishing trials are lack of time, funds, or other resources.[27] In order to treat patients most appropriately, all relevant information and data, both positive and negative, are needed in the decision-making process.[27,29] Typically the positive studies, which conclude a favorable result for the therapy under study, are readily published whereas the publication of negative studies (a study that does not show favorable results from the new therapy) may not be published immediately, if at all.[26–28]

The existence of questionable data or poorly designed studies could lead to inappropriate therapy. Just as problematic is investigators not publishing negative clinical trial results. The suppression of data and/or failure to present information regarding negative study results is termed publication bias. An excellent illustration of this issue is the increased risk of suicide in children receiving selective serotonin reuptake inhibitors (SSRIs). Results from negative studies conducted in children prescribed SSRIs, particularly paroxetine, were not released to health care providers; but positive studies of the SSRIs were available and used as the basis of prescribing these agents to this patient type. Without the negative trial results, practitioners were unaware of the dangers of prescribing these medications to patients under 18 years of age.[26,28]

One remedy to publication bias proposed by the ICMJE and endorsed by the American Medical Association is for all clinical trials to be registered with a central body. Registering clinical trial information is not mandatory at the time of this writing so ICMJE has suggested a method to enforce clinical trial registration for the future: consideration to publish the trial in an ICMJE member journal will be given to only those trials that have been registered at or before subject enrollment has commenced. The registration policy applies to any clinical trial starting subject enrollment after July 1, 2005; also, trials that began prior to this date require registration before September 13, 2005.[28] Another recommendation to enforce trial registration is for IRB (the committee that approves human research projects) to review only those trials completing the registration process.[28] The purpose of clinical trial registration is to account for research that has been conducted in human subjects. Trial information would be accessible, so a comprehensive review of the efficacy and safety of a therapy can be performed. A registry exists that contains information and data regarding trials that were not completed or published. The Pharmaceutical Research and Manufacturers of America (PhRMA) member companies will voluntary post information regarding clinical trials addressing all disease states.[30] One website identified as an acceptable registry is <<www.clinicaltrials.gov>> (sponsored by the U.S. National Library of Medicine).[26,30] Another website, <<www.controlled-trials.com>>, is an international registry that is available for investigators to register clinical trials.[31]

Readers of the biomedical literature need to consider the issues of selective reporting, as described earlier. In addition, usually one clinical trial is not sufficient to adopt a therapy under investigation as the first choice to treat patients. Results of multiple trials are usually combined together to serve as the evidence for either incorporating a newly developed therapy into practice or changing the existing method of treating a disease (see Chap. 9).[26,32] Journal editors have an obligation and should publish negative studies. Results of these studies are important in formulating practice patterns based on the available evidence. Failure by investigators and journal editors to publish negative studies contributes to publication bias.[29,33,34]

As shown by the above discussions, the process of determining the therapy for a patient is complex and multifold. Results of both appropriately and poorly designed studies are published; in addition, some study results are concealed.[32] Thus, an essential skill required of health care providers is the ability to efficiently locate and critique the literature plus apply the results appropriately to patient care. Although, including clinical trial results into practice is partially dependent on the practitioner, assuming no barriers from third parties (i.e., insurance companies), some practitioners may readily include new therapies into their practice even though the evidence is weak.[35] These individuals are usually easily impressed with misleading study results or easily enticed by gifts from the pharmaceutical representatives.[36] In some cases, investigators may not even include their own research results into practice at their own institution.[37,38] Therefore, individuals skilled in analyzing clinical trials and comprehending the trial results are those who appropriately use the information for practice.

The intent of this chapter is for readers not to be misled by the literature, but to correctly critique the controlled clinical trial, then properly use the results and conclusions in health care practice settings. In addition to the discussions of critiquing clinical trials from this chapter, readers should use the principles of the evidence-based medicine in providing patient care (Chap. 9).

Approach to Evaluating Research Studies (True Experiments)

Many different research designs are published, but the most common of these are prospective studies in which an intervention is directly compared to a control and differences between these are measured. Examples of prospective studies include clinical trials (e.g., drug A vs. drug B; drug vs. exercise), stability of compounded drug formulation (e.g., suspension made from drug tablets), compatibility of intravenous (IV) drug mixtures, and drug pharmacokinetic interactions. Regardless of the study design and objective, fundamental elements should be present in all studies, including appropriate qualifications of the researchers conducting the research, valid investigational methods, proper research techniques, and appropriate analysis plus interpretation of the results. A similar process is used to evaluate prospective studies. A checklist for pertinent information to be included in a clinical trial is located in Appendix 6–1. Answering the questions contained in Appendix 6–1 can allow readers to determine the strengths and limitations of a clinical trial. The remainder of this chapter discusses the questions presented in the appendix plus techniques for critiquing a clinical trial.

Journal, Peer-Review, and Investigators

Numerous journals are published covering the professions of medicine and pharmacy. Health care practitioners need to regularly access professional journals (either print or electronic) to assist them in keeping current in their practice responsibilities.[35] One essential journal feature is the peer-review process. Simply defined, peer-reviewed articles are evaluated by someone other than the editorial staff (i.e., evaluation by one's peers).[33,39] Most journals incorporate the peer-review process in selecting articles for publication. Briefly, manuscripts submitted to the journal for publication consideration are screened by the editor; those deemed as potential publications are sent to individuals with expertise in the appropriate area. These individuals read the manuscript and comment on the strengths and limitations, plus offer a recommendation to the journal editor regarding accepting or rejecting the manuscript for publication. The peer-reviewers' comments are sent to the authors for the manuscript to be revised and, if necessary, resubmitted for publication consideration. In some cases manuscripts may be rejected as being too flawed or inappropriate for the journal.

Although the peer-review process increases the time required before publication, the goal is to reduce the publication of manuscripts that have inappropriate methods/design, are poorly written, and/or do not meet the needs of the journal's audience.[39] However, the peer-review process does not always prevent publication of articles without deficiencies. Readers are still required to assess the quality and critique each published article. Two journal sections can be checked for information addressing whether the peer-review process is used: instruction for authors and journal scope/purpose. Readers of the biomedical/pharmacy literature need to be aware of journals not incorporating a peer-review process. The primary purpose of these non-peer-reviewed publications is to generate profit (since authors may pay a per page fee for articles to be published and/or the journal has a high advertisement-to-text content ratio). Regardless of whether a clinical trial is published in a peer-review or non-peer-reviewed journal, the article needs to be evaluated closely for biases and interpreted appropriately.[35]

As readers become more familiar with the professional literature, they will also find that certain journals have a reputation for good quality publications, such as *New England Journal of Medicine* and *Annals of Internal Medicine*. This too can be considered in the evaluation of literature, although poor articles are still found in those well-respected journals and excellent articles are published in other journals.

Research results can be published in other venues besides journals. A very common publication type is meeting abstracts. Research presented during a professional organization meeting, whether as a platform or poster, requires an abstract to be available for meeting attendees to review. These abstracts usually undergo the peer-review process to be selected, but readers should be cautious of the abstract content. The peer-review process may not be as thorough and the entire study details are not available to the reader. Another common publication type for research is journal supplements. The purpose of such supplements is to publish a collection of articles related to a specific topic in a separate journal issue.[33] Many, but not all supplements, are sponsored by an outside entity (i.e., pharmaceutical company), which serves as another source of revenue for the journal. The articles may undergo peer-review, but the process may not be as rigorous. Not all articles published in journal supplements should be automatically discarded or classified as inferior information. An example of a very informative journal supplement is the American College of Chest Physicians' supplement addressing antithrombotic therapy.[40] Many of the articles in this supplement are authored by recognized leaders and researchers in their field of practice.

Other factors to evaluate are the investigators' credentials and the practice site of these individuals. Investigators need to be properly trained and have active practice experience in the area of study. The site where the clinical trial was conducted should not immediately endorse or condemn the quality of the research, other than it should be a site that has the capability to perform the study (i.e., have the resources to properly and completely perform the necessary study methods). The quality of the research must be evaluated because even prestigious institutions can conduct poor clinical trials. Also, persons involved with the study need to be ethical and responsible to protect patients enrolled in the study.[41] Persons with specialized credentials in biostatistics need to contribute with statistical analysis of the data. Furthermore, all authors listed should have made substantial contributions to the research and/or publication. The Uniform Requirements for Manuscripts Submitted to Biomedical Journals, prepared by journal editors, explicitly outlines the criteria for persons to be listed as authors for a published article. According to this publication, "An author is generally considered to be someone who has made a substantive intellectual contribution to a published study ...."[33] The topics of authorship and publishing are discussed in detail in Chap. 11.

Articles with authors who are employees of a pharmaceutical company should be more selectively analyzed, since there may be concern about potential bias. The pharmaceutical industry must conduct research for new therapies to be introduced to the marketplace and many companies are collaborating with academic researchers.[36,42] The concern regarding influence from the pharmaceutical industry on health care providers has not gone unnoticed, particularly involving practitioners conducting research for the pharmaceutical industry. In response, many journals now are requiring article authors to declare any conflict of interests with the research and outside interests.[33,41] "The potential for conflict of interest can exist whether or not an individual believes that the relationship affects his or her scientific judgment."[33] Authors need to state they have received honorariums and/or research grants or are members of the speaker's bureau for pharmaceutical companies. Readers should be informed of potential bias of the investigators. However, immediately discarding or discounting clinical trials in which investigators declare relationships with the pharmaceutical industry may be premature. Many investigators are required to obtain external funding for research projects and academic promotion. Clinical trials that have researchers with relationships with multiple pharmaceutical companies may not be considered to be overtly biased. Investigators have an ethical obligation to submit creditable research results for publication.[26,33] Biases may be present, but readers having the skills of identifying study strengths and limitations can still use the clinical trial results appropriately. Potential biases associated with pharmaceutical company funded research are discussed further later in this chapter.

Clinical Trial Title

The clinical trial title is important and should be carefully read by the reader. A title should be reflective of the work, unbiased, specific, and concise (i.e., usually ≤10 words), but not too general or detailed. Declarative sentences, which tend to overemphasize a conclusion, are not preferred for scientific articles.[43] In addition, the title should not be phrased as a question and randomized clinical trials should be identified in the title.[23] Furthermore, the title should include terms both sensitive (easing the task of locating the appropriate articles) and specific (excluding those not being searched for) that allow electronic retrieval of the article.[33]

The following is an example of a biased study title: "Improved bronchodilation with levalbuterol compared with racemic albuterol in patients with asthma."[44] The title implies levalbuterol to be better than racemic albuterol. Although the average change in lung function parameters was slightly greater with levalbuterol, no significant differences were reported.[44] Thus one could have been misled by reading only the title, to believe that levalbuterol is a superior agent. A suggested nonbiased title for this trial is "Bronchodilation from levalbuterol compared with racemic albuterol in patients with asthma: a randomized clinical trial."

Abstract

An abstract is considered to be a concise overview of the study or a synopsis of the major principles of the article. Abstracts include information addressing the article objective, methods, results, and conclusions. A primary use of abstracts is for readers to obtain an immediate overview of the article to determine if the entire article should be read.[45,46] Another use is publishing the abstract in secondary resources (e.g., PubMed® and International Pharmaceutical Abstracts [IPA]) for individuals conducting literature searches.

Although unique for each journal, authors are required to follow specific requirements while preparing an abstract. Many journals now require abstracts to be prepared in an organized format (i.e., structured abstract) and usually must contain ≤500 words. The structured abstract includes the following sections: objective, research design, clinical setting, participants, interventions, main outcome measurements, results, and conclusions.[33,45] Structured, compared to nonstructured, abstracts do have some advantages, including being more informative, easier to read, and generally preferred by readers.[47,48] However, structured abstracts usually require more journal space. Informative abstracts may entice some individuals to read the study, thus abstracts should be thorough, complete, and unbiased in wording selection.[48]

Abstracts should be consistent with the manuscript and should not present biased and/or inaccurate information.[45,46,48] For further information regarding abstracts and preparation, please refer to the Appendices of Chap. 11. Regardless of the abstract presentation style, readers should not make decisions based on abstract information only. Results of three published studies illustrate the dangers of reading only the abstract.[49–51] These studies provided evidence of omissions and discrepancies between the abstract and the manuscript in medical, psychology, and pharmacy journals.

In the first study, an analysis of 264 manuscript abstracts published in six leading medical journals (e.g., *JAMA* and *N Engl J Med*) demonstrates that 18% (95% CI; 6 to 30%) to 68% (95% CI; 54 to 82%) of the abstracts contained discrepancies.[50] Types of deficiencies included omissions (information in the abstract, but not in the manuscript) and/or inaccurate information (abstract information not exactly the same as the manuscript information). Similar results were reported after 400 random manuscript abstracts in eight journals of the American Psychological Association were evaluated.[49] Up to 18% of the abstracts evaluated were deficient (i.e., contained an inconsistency or omission between the abstract and manuscript). Furthermore, an evaluation of 243 abstracts of original research articles published in six pharmacy-specific journals contained omissions (24.7%; ranging from 19.5 to 36.3%).[51] Qualitative inaccuracies (19.3%), quantitative inaccuracies (25.1%), and instructions for authors inconsistencies (4.5%) also were contained in the abstracts of these pharmacy journals (e.g., *Ann Pharmacother, Am J Health Syst Pharm*). The results of these three studies emphasize the need for readers to read the entire manuscript, and not rely on the abstract, or the article title, for information to make a decision.

Introduction

The introduction section serves two specific purposes: discussing the study rationale and study purpose.[23,52] Usually, readers are first briefly educated on the issues that were the basis of conducting the study. The study investigators may state that the reason the research was conducted is due to the lack of data to answer a question or available data are conflicting regarding an issue. Every clinical trial is designed to answer one or more primary questions. The investigators should explain how the clinical trial will overcome the shortcomings of the prior research, if applicable. The study objective is often stated within the last paragraph, if not the last sentence, of this section. Better written studies present to the reader a clearly stated research purpose and this statement should be understood by the reader before continuing with the remaining article content. Studies with a well-written purpose statement enable the reader to better comprehend and assess the research methodology.

Once the clinical trial objective is determined, the investigators need to formulate a research and null hypothesis (H_0). A research hypothesis (also known as the alternative hypothesis) is stated as "a difference is present between the therapy under investigation and the control" while H_0 is stated as "no difference between these two groups" (see next paragraph for an example). After the study is completed, the researchers analyze the data and then the research hypothesis is either accepted (which also includes rejecting H_0) or rejected (which then means H_0 is accepted). Readers should recognize that not all clinical trials will include the specific research and null hypotheses in the introduction section.

An example to explain some of the material thus far included in this chapter is the Women's Health Initiative (WHI) trial, which assessed the risks and benefits of the estrogen/progestin combination in healthy postmenopausal women. The WHI trial compared conjugated equine estrogen plus medroxyprogesterone (CEE/MPE), a medication frequently prescribed to postmenopausal women, with placebo.[53] The investigators expressed in the introduction section that the rationale for conducting this clinical trial was the lack of human controlled clinical trials evaluating this product specifically for cardioprotective outcomes. Prior evaluations of this medication were predominately observational in design (i.e., not clinical trials) and reported reductions in adverse events (i.e., coronary heart disease [CHD] and hip fracture) and changes in clinical parameters (i.e., decreased lipid levels and increase bone mineral density). The actual WHI trial study objective was stated as "... to directly address whether estrogen plus progestin has a favorable or unfavorable effect on CHD incidence and on overall risk and benefits in predominantly healthy women."[53] The research hypothesis of the WHI trial is "there is a difference in the incidence of CHD between CEE/MPE and placebo" while H_0 is "there is no difference in the incidence of CHD between CEE/MPE and placebo." After reading the WHI trial introduction, the reader has a clear understanding of the study rationale and purpose: prior research did not conclusively answer the question whether CEE/MPE reduced cardiovascular (CV) risks and the results of this trial should provide health care providers with evidence to continue, or not, prescribing this medication.

The introduction section may not contain an extensive number of paragraphs. However, the presented information should concisely inform the reader of the research issues and purpose. As with all sections of a clinical trial, this section needs to be carefully read. Authors may "set-the-stage" by presenting only selective (i.e., not comprehensive) information and/or weak references (to be later discussed in the chapter) to support the rationale for conducting the study. Also, the information may be presented using biased wording, which predisposes the reader to believing the prior research was insignificant in providing evidence applicable to practice.

Methods

Following a well-designed plan is essential for the clinical trial results to be acceptable and useful to practitioners. The design of a study (i.e., methods) is important for the results to be valid, just as abiding by the blueprints is vital to building a house. The methods section of a clinical trial contains a large amount of information that includes the type of subjects enrolled, the comparative therapy description, outcome measures, and statistics. Flaws within the design of a clinical trial limit the application and significance of the results. Poor study design leads to reduced study internal validity, thus resulting in limited external study validity (see Table 6–3).[19,54] The methods section needs to be thorough in describing to the reader the process in which the study was conducted. In fact, a reader should devote the majority of time used to assess the trial in this section.

Clinical trials follow a pattern in presenting the information within the methods section.[23] This standardized format allows study details to be in an orderly fashion and quickly located. Readers of the biomedical literature should have an understanding of the overall design to appropriately critique clinical trials and use the study results for patient care-related activities.

STUDY DESIGN

Several study designs are available for investigators to select from when conducting research. The study questions the researchers wish to answer dictate which study design is selected to conduct the research.[55,56] For example, in a case where investigators wish to assess the interaction between azithromycin and cyclosporine, serum cyclosporine levels will be compared with patients taking and not taking azithromycin. Although a clinical trial can be used to conduct this research, the consequence of combining these two drugs can lead to either cyclosporine toxicity or organ transplantation rejection. This study is considered unethical to conduct in patients receiving this medication for therapeutic purposes. Thus other study techniques must be employed to answer this research question. Both investigators and readers of the literature need to identify the strengths and limitations of the research designs. Although many study designs are available, this chapter only discusses controlled clinical trials. For additional information on other study designs the reader is referred to Chap. 7.

A simple description of a controlled clinical trial is that it prospectively measures a difference in effect between two therapies. The groups are similar and treated identically with the exception of the therapies under study. The subjects in the study are assigned to one of the groups and monitored.[16,17,24,56] This study type, called parallel design, is the primary study design encountered in the literature.

TABLE 6–3. INTERNAL VS. EXTERNAL VALIDITY OF CLINICAL TRIALS

Term	Meaning	Application
Internal validity	Quality of the study design	Strong design should translate into reliable results
External validity	Ability to apply results into practice	Study results meaningful to practitioners and can be used for patient care

Controlled clinical trials offer investigators the most rigorous method of establishing a cause-and-effect relation between treatment and outcome.[17] Simply explained, the treatment under study is the cause and the consequence of giving the treatment is measured as the effect. The effect of the treatment under study is compared to the effect of the other group(s). Thus, investigators can use a clinical trial to claim that a treatment has some effect that may be important in curing or relieving disease symptoms. In addition, the magnitude (i.e., size) of the difference in the effect between the groups can be estimated.[17]

An example to briefly describe a controlled clinical trial measuring a cause and effect is a study that compared atorvastatin to placebo. The study objective was to compare atorvastatin (cause) to placebo and measure the reduction in average low density lipoprotein-cholesterol (LDL-C) levels (effect) between the two groups.[57] A clinical trial also quantifies the differences in the effect, such as atorvastatin compared to simvastatin in lowering LDL-C.[58] The results of these studies can be used to determine the magnitude of LDL-C lowering by atorvastatin and make the decision to use, or not use, this medication in practice.

The characteristics of a controlled clinical trial were the justification for selecting this study design for the WHI trial.[53] Researchers were unsure of whether CEE/MPE reduced or increased the incidence of CHD. No compelling evidence was available to document the cause and effect of this combination product for this use. The results of the WHI trial demonstrated that CEE/MPE actually increased the risk for CHD, which was the opposite effect as compared to previous noncontrolled clinical trials reported in this patient type.[53] Practitioners were under the impression for years that CEE/MPE lowered CHD risk and was beneficial to patients receiving this medication, when in reality the risks for CHD were increased. The WHI trial exemplifies the unique features of controlled clinical trials serving as a source of evidence to determine treatment plans for patients in clinical practice, as compared to other research study designs. However, as explained throughout this chapter, the results of all clinical trials cannot be automatically accepted. Each trial has to be critiqued for strengths and weaknesses.

PATIENT INCLUSION/EXCLUSION CRITERIA

The inclusion criteria list subject demographics that must be present to be enrolled into the trial, while exclusion criteria are characteristics that prevent enrollment into the trial or necessitate withdrawal from the study, if they are later determined to be present.[23] Diagnostic criteria for conditions under study and definitions of the inclusion/exclusion criteria must be included in an article reporting study results. For instance, if subjects with hypertension are the target group of individuals to be enrolled in a trial, hypertension needs to be defined in terms of the minimal and maximum systolic blood pressure (SBP) and diastolic blood pressure (DBP). The study participant features should reflect the disease under investigation, but the existence of complex and/or extensive comorbid conditions (e.g., terminal cancer, pregnancy, and numerous other disease states) in the study patients may not allow the researchers to accurately measure the differences in effect between the groups. The presence of these complex and/or extensive comorbid conditions can make for difficult decisions regarding including subjects representative of real patients versus excluding typical persons whose complicating conditions will make it impossible to accurately assess a new treatment. Whenever possible and appropriate, typical individuals with the condition being assessed, who in all probability will receive the therapy in real practice, should be represented in the trial. This includes ensuring a factual representation of the gender, race, and other demographics. Subjects with one or more (but not numerous) other disease states and taking a few other medications are usually entered into the clinical trial so the typical patients in which the therapy under investigation is intended are represented.

The inclusion/exclusion criteria are pertinent to the extrapolation of the study results (i.e., applying the study results into practice [external validity]).[54] Trial results are only applicable to the type of subject included in the study. The investigators of the WHI trial enrolled postmenopausal women with an intact uterus.[53] A slightly higher incidence of CHD was recorded in the patients taking CEE/MPE. However, this does not mean that all postmenopausal women (with or without an intact uterus) taking any formulation of estrogen are at an increased risk for CHD. The results of the WHI trial are pertinent only to similar women enrolled in the trial.

Researchers are careful in deciding which subjects to include and exclude in the clinical trial. Standard types of subjects disqualified are pregnant and lactating females; also, most clinical trials will not enroll subjects with severe conditions that may alter the medication pharmacokinetics and/or pharmacodynamics (e.g., renal and/or hepatic dysfunction). Generally the inclusion criteria attempts to include subjects that are homogeneous and are similar to the common type of patients in practice.[52]

During the process of the investigators selecting subjects to be included into a study, readers of clinical trials need to be conscious of the potential for a selection bias that may be present. A selection bias can occur due to various reasons, but can seriously affect the study results in a negative fashion. In general, a selection bias occurs after subjects meet the inclusion and exclusion criteria, but are not enrolled into the study.[59] The investigators may prevent a subject from being enrolled since this person may either positively or negatively alter the results.[16,24,59,60]

Although it is difficult for the reader to detect the above form of selection bias, the following paragraphs describe selection biases that can be more readily identified, but are not are present in all clinical trials.[59] One common form of a selection bias is requiring the subjects to complete a run-in phase (also called lead-in phase) before being officially enrolled in the study. This phase is usually short in duration (usually 2 to 4 weeks) in which the subjects may take a placebo or the therapy being investigated. The investigators should inform the reader of the intent of the run-in phase. Typical reasons include identifying subjects that may or may not be compliant with the therapy regimen, experience side effects from the therapy, or did not meet prespecific criteria (e.g., blood pressure less than a set value). Afterward these identified subjects are excluded from participating in the study even though they met the original inclusion criteria. The run-in phase produces a bias by selecting a group of subjects that does not completely represent the population since a selected group of the subjects meeting the study inclusion criteria are not included in the study and their run-in phase results are not included in the final analysis.[61]

The following examples explain a selection bias by a run-in phase. Subjects meeting the hypothetical trial inclusion criteria complete a 4-week run-in phase in which a new therapy under investigation is given to all these persons. Those persons experiencing side effects to the new therapy during the run-in phase are not allowed to be enrolled into the study. By excluding those persons eliminated after the run-in phase, the incidence and severity of the side effects of the therapy are not accurately measured during the actual study since subjects experiencing the side effects during the run-in phase were not enrolled in the study. A second example is that researchers may include a run-in phase in which only those persons achieving a preset goal are allowed to be included in the study. For instance, only subjects achieving at least a 25% reduction in LDL-C after a 4-week phase with a new therapy are enrolled in the 12-week study comparing the new therapy to placebo. By only including those with a favorable response, the final average reduction in LDL-C with the new therapy is falsely elevated since only selected subjects were allowed into the study. Those persons with less than a 25% reduction in LDL-C were excluded from the 12-week trial; if these individuals were included in the 12-week trial, the final average reduction in LDL-C most likely would have been significantly lower than actually measured.

The U.S. Carvedilol Heart Failure Study excluded subjects from the trial if they were unable to tolerate carvedilol treatment during a run-in phase. In addition, subjects who had worsening of heart failure (HF) during the run-in phase were not included in the study.[62] This clinical trial was criticized for including a run-in phase and excluding important data that may have changed the significance of the study. Subjects were excluded due to intolerance to the drug and/or death occurring while taking carvedilol during the run-in phase and these data were not included in the overall clinical trial results. Thus, the side effect profile and the incidence of death reduction with carvedilol was less accurately assessed via this trial.[63] Although excluding these data did not alter the results in a negative fashion after analyzing the data from the run-in phase with the clinical trial results,[64] some trials with a run-in phase can have biased results since this phase can allow the investigator to exclude subjects from entering the trial that would represent the patient type for the study results to be useful.

Trials including a run-in phase are not always considered to be a study limitation.[61] The investigators may stop a therapy previously prescribed to the subjects and give a placebo during the run-in phase. This allows the effects of the prior therapy to diminish and not interfere with the effects of the therapy under study. Furthermore, a clinical trial may be designed in which the investigators enroll a very specific type of subject, which can be considered a selection bias in the inclusion criteria. The purpose of this type of selection bias is to evaluate a therapy in a very unique group of individuals, usually those who met some predetermined criteria. For instance, a trial was designed so that only subjects who experienced a gastrointestinal (GI) bleed with aspirin alone were enrolled.[65] The investigators were specifically selecting a unique group of subjects (having a GI bleed due to aspirin). The combination of aspirin plus esomeprazole was compared to clopidogrel to determine which therapy had a lower incidence of GI rebleeding. Even though the trial results indicated that the aspirin plus esomeprazole combination had a lower GI rebleeding rate, this does not mean this drug combination should be used instead of aspirin alone in those people needing aspirin therapy. The results of this trial can only be used for selected patients, those who had a GI bleed while taking aspirin and need to continue antiplatelet therapy.

Investigators also should explain the process of recruiting subjects and define the time period of the recruitment.[23] Sponsors of clinical trials and investigators typically recruit subjects for clinical trials by four main strategies: sponsors may offer financial and other incentives to investigators to increase enrollment; investigators may target their own patients as potential subjects; investigators may seek additional subjects from other sources (e.g., physician referrals and disease registries); or sponsors and investigators may advertise and promote their studies. The most common means for advertising for recruitment to clinical trials is through newspapers, radio, the Internet, television, or as posters on public transportation and in hospitals.[66] The methods in which investigators recruit subjects may have implications on the generalizability of the research results to the population (i.e., external validity). Newspaper and Internet advertisements are common; however, there are inherent problems with this form of advertisement. Survey results indicate that the majority of persons who read the newspapers are older in age, Caucasian, wealthier, more educated, and own more upscale homes than the average American. Gender bias also can affect recruitment rates as it has been documented that female readers consider newspaper advertising to be more important than do male readers.[67]

Internet recruitment is not without similar problems. Typically minority and elderly individuals are less familiar and have less access to the Internet. A recent study described the process of registering persons with cancer for clinical trials via the Internet and telephone call center. Most of the subjects registered via the Internet compared to the telephone call center (88% vs. 12%). The majority of subjects who registered were female (73% vs. 27% male; $p < 0.001$), Caucasian (88.9%), and received colorectal cancer screening (59%); the median age was 49 years. No differences with respect to ethnicity or gender were observed for patients registering via the Internet compared to the call center; however, subjects registering via the Internet were significantly younger than those registering through the call center. Recruitment via newspapers and the Internet may offer some benefits in terms of recruitment, although, the lack of uniformity with respect to access to newspapers and the Internet for elderly and minority subjects may increase the difficulty of applying the clinical trial results to these underrepresented populations because of the lack of this subject type included in the trials.[68]

INTERVENTION AND CONTROL GROUPS

Once the subjects to be enrolled in the clinical trial have been selected, these persons will be assigned to either the intervention or control group. The intervention group consists of the new therapy under investigation (e.g., medication, procedure). The intervention is compared to a control so that the fundamental principle of a controlled clinical trial can be accomplished, measuring cause and effect. The control group can consist of no therapy (e.g., placebo), another therapy (aka active control) (e.g., drug and exercise), or compared to existing data (i.e., historical data). Both the intervention and control groups are to be the same in all respects other than the treatment received. Afterward, the investigators will measure and quantify a difference in effect between the group assigned to the intervention with those in the control group. Thus, any identified differences in the measured effect can be attributed to intervention rather than other factors.[16,69,70]

A key term in the phrase controlled clinical trial is control, indicating another therapy is serving as the measuring point for the effect of the intervention to be assessed. Reports have been published documenting placebo effects (i.e., measured change even though inert/inactive therapy was given).[71] Without a control, the effects measured by the intervention may be by chance or falsely quantified. For example, investigators of a study reported that oxandrolone caused an average increase in body weight in patients with chronic obstructive pulmonary disease (COPD).[72] However, all the subjects were treated with oxandrolone and no control group was included in the study. Although these patients gained weight, oxandrolone may not be the sole reason for this effect. Weight gain may have occurred naturally, even without the medication or by some unidentified reason. The results of this noncontrolled clinical trial may be the rationale for a clinical trial being conducted to evaluate the weight gaining effects of oxandrolone, but cannot be used as evidence that weight gain was solely attributed to this drug. The results of studies designed without a control can be useful (i.e., speculate causing an effect), but since no control group was present, readers cannot be certain that the intervention caused the effect.

Researchers can select from a few different types of controls: historical, placebo, or active. Historical controls are described as data that have been collected prior to the beginning of a clinical trial. Investigators conduct the study with only the intervention group and then compare the results to the existing data.[73] One advantage of using historical controls is that only one group is needed to be enrolled (thus less time, expense, and so forth). Another advantage is the usefulness of studying a disease with a low occurrence or a disease with high incidence of death or other serious sequelae in which some form of therapy should not be denied.[73] Disadvantages include usually overestimating the effect of the intervention[21] and no guarantee that similar subject types, therapeutic procedures, or techniques are exactly the same from one study period to the next.[73]

Historical controls are not used very often in published clinical trials, but are acceptable in selected situations. For example, investigators of a clinical trial evaluated the efficacy and safety of the direct thrombin inhibitor, argatroban, in patients with heparin-induced thrombocytopenia (HIT) or HIT with thrombosis syndrome (HITTS) and compared the results with a historical control. Historical controls consisted of patients who met the same inclusion/exclusion criteria who experienced HIT 4 years prior to the initiation of the trial. The use of a historical control was appropriate in this study because at the time of the study, no approved alternative therapy was available and a placebo control was deemed unethical.[74]

An intervention under study is compared to a placebo in many clinical trials to document and measure the pharmacologic effect of the intervention.[71] These studies are generally conducted as a requirement by the FDA to document that drug therapy is better than no therapy (placebo) for a given disease state (i.e., used to document cause and effect).[71] Those trials reporting a significant difference in effect of the intervention compared to placebo could be used to support the use of the intervention in treating patients. Simvastatin was compared to placebo to determine if the incidence of a death would be lowered in subjects with a history of angina pectoris or myocardial infarction (MI).[75] Before this study was conducted, health care providers did not have any information indicating that simvastatin would benefit or harm this subject type. At the time this trial was designed and initiated, persons with angina pectoris or history of MI were not routinely treated with a 3-hydroxy-3-methylglutaryl coenzyme A (HMG-CoA) reductase inhibitor (i.e., statin); thus placebo was selected as the control. But the place in therapy for the intervention may be difficult to determine when placebo is the control, since other drugs may be found to be better than the drug in question, on further research. For example, in this case, although simvastatin lowers LDL-C greater than placebo,[76] it is not directly known how simvastatin compares to other drugs that lower LDL-C based solely on these trial results.

Not all clinical trials will have a placebo as the control group for various valid reasons. For example, including a placebo as one of the groups in a trial may decrease the willingness of subjects to participate; some may not wish to be treated with a placebo.[77] But more importantly, denying therapy that has been documented to reduce morbidity and/or mortality to patients with selected diseases may be unethical. These studies would not include a placebo as the control, but instead may use active therapy (i.e., standard therapy).[71,78] Patients with cancer enrolled in a clinical trial are prime examples where trials will not include a placebo as the control.

Usually after the new therapy is compared to a placebo, a trial using an active therapy (e.g., another medication) as the control is used to assess the difference in effect between the groups. Readers should be aware that clinical trials with a placebo as the control, particularly those funded by the pharmaceutical industry, yield a larger treatment effect than if an active therapy was selected as the control group.[79] For instance, the LDL-C lowering effect is expected to be significantly greater with a new statin versus placebo instead of another statin or other lipid-lowering agent. Thus, the treatment effect may appear to be substantial versus placebo, but could be minimally different from another active drug that was used as the control. Also, the possibility exists that the new treatment in fact may be inferior in efficacy and/or safety compared to an active drug, even though the new treatment appears better in comparison to a placebo.

An appropriate control needs to be included in the study for the trial results to be applicable for practice. The use of historical or placebo as the control is acceptable in some clinical trials (as described earlier). Some studies may be designed with a control that may no longer be the preferred treatment after the trial results are published. The study may have been designed and initiated based on either recommendations of the FDA or before new therapy recommendations were available. In the Carvedilol or Metoprolol European Trial (COMET), carvedilol was compared to metoprolol tartrate (an immediate-release formulation) in patients with HF.[80] The study was published after a new metoprolol formulation (controlled/extended release) became available. The new controlled/extended-release formulation was documented to reduce mortality in subjects with HF versus placebo.[81,82] Since COMET trial investigators concluded that carvedilol reduces the incidence of mortality greater than metoprolol tartrate, practitioners question the selection of this formulation as the control. Also, practitioners were unsure of the proper interpretation of the trial results. Unanswered questions remain as to whether the controlled/extended-release metoprolol formulation would produce similar or different results as the COMET trial indicated.[83–87] It is important that an intervention in a clinical trial not be compared to an inappropriate comparator (e.g., incorrect dosage, frequency, and agent known to be inferior to standard of care).[79] Instead, the intervention needs to be compared to an appropriate therapy.[78] Thus, in clinical trials using an obsolete therapy or non-first-line therapy as the control, results indicating that the intervention is superior may not be easily applied into clinical practice since an appropriate comparator was not used.

Also, investigators including a medication as the control need to use the dosing regimen (i.e., dose and frequency) deemed suitable.[79] Standard references should be consulted to ensure that appropriate dosing regimens were included in the trial to reduce the chance of obtaining biased results. A trial concluding that a new analgesic relieved pain better than morphine dosed 0.05 mg IV every 24 hours postsurgery in otherwise healthy adult subjects is biased because an appropriate morphine regimen was not used. However, at times investigators may not know the equivalent dosing regimen of the intervention relative to the control. Investigators directly comparing rosuvastatin to atorvastatin, both 10 mg once daily for 12 weeks, reported a greater lowering of mean LDL-C with rosuvastatin (43% vs. 35%).[88] Other studies comparing these two medications have reported that average LDL-C levels are similar with atorvastatin doses two times that of the rosuvastatin dose.[89] Thus concluding rosuvastatin is a superior LDL-C lowering agent to atorvastatin based solely on the results of a single trial evaluating both agents dosed 10 mg once daily is incorrect. A more appropriate conclusion is that these two agents do not have an equivalent pharmacologic effect on this dose.

INSTITUTIONAL REVIEW BOARD (IRB)/SUBJECT CONSENT

Research projects that use humans as study subjects must be approved before investigators begin enrolling subjects into the trial. The IRB is the committee charged with ensuring that the subjects are protected and not exposed to unnecessary harm or unethical medical procedures. The name of the actual committee may differ from place to place (e.g., local ethics committee), although the purpose of the committee remains to protect the study subjects. This committee consists of both health care and nonhealthcare professionals. The rules and regulations of human research require the study to be assessed prior to the initiation of the project.

Another primary responsibility of the IRB is to approve the subject informed consent form. Before agreeing to participate in a trial, each subject is presented with a subject informed consent form that notifies the subjects of the study procedures, their rights and responsibilities of participating in the study, plus at least eight major points that include risks, benefits, compensation, voluntary participation, and right to withdraw from the study without any penalty. In addition to the content of the subject informed consent form, the IRB provides investigators with suggestions on how to write the form in language that laypersons can comprehend.[90] Additional information regarding clinical trial research can be obtained at <<http://cancer.gov/clinicaltrials/learning/page3>> while information for IRB members (i.e., training site) is at <<http://www.nihtraining.com/ohsrsite/IRBCBT/intro.html>>. Also, the reader may refer to Chap. 18 of this book. According to the Uniform Requirements, articles describing clinical trials using humans as research subjects are required to include a statement that the research was approved by the IRB (or other committee that protects subjects) and consent was obtained from the subject to participate in the research project.[33] Trials not including this information should be questioned.

BLINDING

Since clinical trials measure differences in effect between groups, outside influences (i.e., biases) should be minimized. This is especially important in studies measuring subjective outcomes (e.g., pain, depression scores). Blinding is a technique in which subjects and/or investigators are unaware of who is in the intervention or control group. Blinding techniques are incorporated to reduce possible bias (defined as "Differences between the true value and that actually obtained [are] due to all causes other than sampling variability").[24] Patients knowing that they are taking a placebo to reduce depression symptoms are very likely to report no change or worsening of the disease. The results are biased since subjects knowingly are taking a substance that does not reduce symptoms. Therefore, blinding techniques are important to reduce the influence of bias on measuring a difference in effect between the intervention and control. Three types of blinding techniques can be used in a clinical trial (see Table 6–4). The specific blinding type usually is dictated by the effect being measured during the trial.

Single-blinding and no blinding techniques are primarily incorporated in clinical trials that have study objectives not conducible to blinding (e.g., surgery vs. medication). Some trials may include a procedure that is difficult to blind (e.g., surgery) and it may not be ideal to include a placebo procedure. Imitation surgery is not without risks as death or infection-related complications are possible.[91] The use of placebo procedures to ensure a trial remains blinded, which may increase the risk of adverse effects or other dangers, is controversial and possibly unethical if the investigators do not thoroughly discuss the rationale for including and/or not using other methods to blind the trial.[92] A clinical trial designed to compare surgery to a medication is an example of using no blinding methods since both the investigators and subjects know which group the subjects have been assigned.

An example of single-blinding is that one group of subjects administered a medication subcutaneously once daily versus the other group which took an oral anticoagulation medication. The subjects were not blinded since the risk may outweigh the benefit of injecting a saline solution subcutaneously (i.e., bleeding complications may develop in persons taking an anticoagulant agent plus unnecessary injections). Since the investigators measure the occurrence of a blood clot, the subjects' knowledge of which therapy they were receiving minimized the influence on this outcome.

Double-blinding, where neither the investigator nor patient knows who is receiving which treatment, is considered the "gold standard" blinding technique and is most commonly used in clinical trials.[25] As a general rule and regardless whether the outcome is a subjective or objective measure, the study should be double-blinded. A clinical trial measuring an objective outcome usually assesses other study outcome measures (e.g., therapy side effect

TABLE 6–4. TYPES OF BLINDING

Type of Blinding	Definition
No blinding (open-label)	Investigators and subjects are aware of the assignment of subjects to the intervention or control group
Single	Either investigators or subjects, but not both, are aware of the assignment of subjects to the intervention or control group[25]
Double	Both investigators and subjects are not aware of the assignment of subjects to the intervention or control group[25]
Triple	In addition to both investigators and subjects not being aware of the assignment of subjects to the intervention or control group, trial personnel involved with data interpretation are not aware of subject assignment[22]

incidence and severity), which may be biased if double-blinding was not incorporated into the trial. For instance, double-blinding was used in the WHI trial to not only minimize biases in the objective measurements (incidence of CHD) but also subjective assessments (side effects) in those women assigned to CEE/MPE or placebo.[53]

In order to ensure that blinding remains intact, the therapy each group receives should be exact in frequency of administration, appearance, size, taste, and smell and other variables. Studies that compare regimens taken once daily to twice daily will require the once-daily group to take a placebo as the second dose (i.e., double-dummy).[16] Double-dummy methods are included in clinical trials when two therapies being compared are not the same (e.g., different routes of administration and different formulations). Patients receive two formulations, one active and one control, to ensure that blinding is maintained.[16] For example, investigators of a clinical trial evaluating the blood pressure lowering effects of amlodipine (a tablet) and the combination product of amlodipine plus benazepril (a capsule) should administer amlodipine tablets plus placebo capsules to those subjects randomized to amlodipine therapy and amlodipine/benazepril capsules plus placebo tablets to the other subjects. A similar situation may present in clinical trials in which the formulations being compared are administered via different routes. Investigators evaluating the efficacy of a once-daily oral contraceptive tablet to an intramuscular contraceptive agent administered every 3 months may allocate an intramuscular placebo to those patients randomized to once-daily oral contraceptive and a once-daily placebo tablet to those patients randomized to the intramuscular contraceptive. Each patient receives a formulation that represents each therapy and both subjects and investigators would be less likely to determine which formulation is active.

Sometimes it is necessary to triple blind a study. In addition to the trial investigators and subjects, other personnel involved with the trial (e.g., data collection, analysis, or monitoring; drug administration or dispensing) can have opinions regarding the outcome of the therapy being studied based on their interaction with the subjects involved in the trial or their experience with the intervention and/or control being assessed. These opinions may cause inappropriate data collection, measurement, analysis, and/or interpretation of the results by the study personnel. Also data collection personnel having a bias for or against the intervention may not be as consistent in their data collection procedures if they know which group the subjects were assigned. This may result in an inappropriate interpretation (e.g., overestimation of the treatment effects) of the study results.[16,21,25] Therefore, it is often necessary to blind these other individuals (triple-blinding).

RANDOMIZATION

Randomization is a distinguishing study attribute that separates controlled clinical trials from other study designs (e.g., case-control and cohort). A basic definition of randomization is "all study subjects have an equal chance of being 'assigned' to either the intervention or control group."[93] Research has indicated that the results obtained from randomized trials are more dependable than nonrandomized trials. An analysis of randomized versus nonrandomized trials reported that on average investigators of nonrandomized trials overestimated the treatment effects of the intervention compared to the control primarily due to bias.[21] Even though including randomization in a clinical trial is important for more reliable results, it is necessary to remember not all randomized trials are without faults.

Subjects are eligible for randomization after meeting the trial inclusion criteria.[16] They are randomized so the investigators cannot purposely assign selected persons to one group over another (i.e., sicker individuals in the control vs. less sick in the intervention group). Randomization minimizes bias by lowering the potential for an imbalance of risk factors or prognostic variations between the intervention and control groups.[24] A difference in effect measured by a clinical trial may result from many causes, and treatment may be just one of these. Disparities between the groups at baseline may cause a false result instead of measuring differences in effect between the intervention and control.[94] Therefore to be assured that the difference is truly due to the intervention, the groups need to be as equal as possible and other outside factors that may affect the overall results of the trial need to be equally distributed between the groups.[69] Besides reducing bias,[16,95] an additional reason to include randomization in a clinical trial is so that statistical tests are valid. Most statistical tests require subjects to be randomized so that similar groups are being compared and selected statistical tests can determine whether certain subject characteristics are equivalent between groups.[24]

Measuring differences in the effect between the intervention and control groups requires that the groups to be as similar in as many characteristics as possible (e.g., age, gender, and severity of illness) so that outside factors do not influence the results.[95] Baseline discrepancies between the groups do not allow the true difference in effect between the intervention and control groups to be measured and quantified. If unbalanced factors are present between the two groups, the outcome measure is biased, and the treatment effect may be either underestimated or overestimated.[94]

In general, an equal number of study subjects are randomized to the intervention and control groups. At times, investigators may enroll an unequal number of subjects to the intervention group versus the control group (i.e., 2:1 allocation). The purpose of this allocation type is to gather more data/information regarding the intervention group versus the control group. This unbalanced allocation may occur in a study comparing a new therapeutic intervention to placebo to measure the pharmacologic effects and is considered to be acceptable.

Many randomization techniques are available and range from very simple to complex processes. The nature of the study and outcomes measured influence the randomization procedure. Various methods are available that include random number tables and computer programs. The randomization procedures should be unbiased and unpredictable by not allowing the subjects or investigators to know in advance to which group the subject will be assigned.[16,95]

Specific randomization methods include simple (i.e., coin toss), blocked, and stratified (more advanced). Simple randomization is an easy technique to implement and includes assigning subjects according to some criteria (e.g., day of the week, subject birthday, or subject medical record number). But this method is not considered a proper randomization method since the number of subjects in the groups can be imbalanced due to the technique. If investigators assign all subjects with an office visit on a specific day of the week to one group (i.e., control), then these subjects did not have equal opportunity to be assigned to either group. This may lead to a reduction in the ability of the investigators to detect differences in effects between the two groups. Few trials use simple randomization techniques due to the limitations of this randomization method.[24]

Blocked randomization avoids group imbalances, but may complicate data analysis. Blocked randomization occurs when subjects have an equal probability of being assigned to a block of an even size and, with this type of randomization, the number of subjects in each group will be equal at some point in time. Investigators wanted to assure, for example, that after every fourth subject was randomized, there were an equal number of subjects in the intervention (A) and control (B) therapy. A block size of 4 would be used and the randomization order in which 2 subjects in the intervention group and 2 subjects in the control group would be assigned for every consecutive group of 4 subjects entering the trial. All the possible combinations would be computed: AABB, ABAB, BAAB, BABA, BBAA, and ABBA and one of these possible combinations is chosen at random.[24]

A more sophisticated randomization procedure, stratification, is designed to achieve similarities in both known and unknown baseline patient characteristics between the groups. Selected factors are identified (e.g., age, smoking, presence of other disease states) and used in determining which group the subjects will be assigned to, so significant imbalances of these factors are not present among the groups, while all subjects with any specific factor have an equal chance of being in each group.[96]

Persons randomizing study participants should be at a distant location so that they may not be able to obtain any information that could bias the randomization process. Unduly influencing the randomization sequence by randomizing subjects to either therapy based on some preference can occur through personal contact with the subject.[24] Thus to minimize these issues, investigators may contact a central randomization center, which randomizes the subject to either the intervention or control group. Investigators of all trials develop protocols and criteria prior to the initiation of a study to unblind treatment in case the safety and/or well-being of a subject is threatened.

ENDPOINTS

Clinical trials measure some effect caused by the intervention and control in order to compare these groups.[17,25,97] All trials specify one effect caused by the intervention and control as the primary endpoint, which can be referred to as "what did the investigators measure to achieve the study objective?" Since significant time, money, and effort are devoted to conduct a clinical trial, researchers usually measure a primary endpoint plus secondary end-points. These secondary endpoints are important, but not considered to be the primary pur-pose of the study. The selected primary endpoint should be a routine and useful measure.[25,97] For example, a trial evaluating the cholesterol lowering effect of a statin compared to placebo selected a change in average LDL-C value, an appropriate measure, as the primary endpoint to satisfy the study objective. However, measuring a change in serum creatinine between losartan and captopril to improve HF symptoms[98] is not ideal since serum creatinine is not the predom-inate parameter used in practice to monitor the progression or improvement in HF status.

Investigators may combine a group of endpoint measures into one primary endpoint, referred to as a composite endpoint. The group usually consists of clinical outcomes related to direct morbidity and mortality as opposed to a pharmacologic action (e.g., reduction in any incidence of stroke/MI/CV-related death vs. lowering cholesterol levels, respectively). The investigators select a group of endpoints that can occur during therapy that are considered clinically important. For example, after experiencing an MI, a therapy is prescribed to reduce the occurrence of multiple adverse outcome (i.e., reinfarction, death, and chest pain) and not just one clinical outcome. The rationale for measuring composite endpoints is to measure an overall effect of therapy, since one specific outcome cannot be deemed to be most important for the study subjects.[79,99,100]

The use of composite endpoints is not without debate.[79,99–103] The results of the individual components of the composite should be reported separately and analyzed.[99,100,102] Investiga-tors may claim that the investigational therapy is better than the control based on the overall result of the composite endpoint, even though the investigational therapy was shown to sig-nificantly affect only one or a few (but not all) of the composite endpoint components. Also, the most important component of the composite may not be affected by the intervention under study.

The following example explains composite endpoints and issues encountered with these. The investigators of the ESSENCE trial (Efficacy and Safety of Subcutaneous Enoxa-parin in Non-Q-Wave Coronary Events) used a composite primary endpoint, which consisted of death, MI (or reinfarction), or recurrent angina after 14 days of follow-up.[104] The incidence of the primary endpoint was lower with enoxaparin (intervention) than unfractionated he-parin (control) (16.6% vs. 19.8%, respectively; p = 0.02; see later portion of chapter for discus-sion of p values) in patients with angina at rest or non-Q-wave MI. However, only one of the three components of the composite endpoint was significantly different with enoxaparin, re-current angina (12.9% vs. 15.5%, respectively; p = 0.03).[104] As seen by the percentages, the ma-jority of the primary composite endpoint (~78%) consisted of recurrent angina, which is the least robust of the three outcomes.[105] Although lowering the incidence of this event is clini-cally important, this outcome is not as severe as death or reinfarction. The composite end-point effect of enoxaparin appears to be superior to heparin, even though the incidence of two of the three components of the composite endpoint indicates no difference between these two drugs. Enoxaparin was considered to be a useful therapy in this patient type, but further research was recommended to determine if the therapy reduces the occurrence of death and MI in these patients.[106]

The primary and other endpoint definitions, plus valid measuring techniques, need to be determined prior to the start of the clinical trial and incorporated in the study design.[16,25] By doing so, the investigators can be consistent throughout the trial in measuring the endpoints, thereby reducing study variances or biases. To illustrate, the WHI trial primary endpoint was CHD, defined as "acute MI requiring overnight hospitalization, silent MI determined from serial electrocardiograms (ECGs), or CHD death." In order to minimize the disparities in diagnosing a patient with MI, investigators used an established algorithm adapted from standardized criteria.[53] If the reader is informed of the measurement types and methods under investigation, he or she can judge whether practical methods were used to measure the endpoints and can determine if the study can be replicated by future investigators or by individuals wanting to implement the trial results into practice on actual patients. Furthermore, the internal and external validities of the clinical trial can be assessed. Endpoints involving human judgment (e.g., need for coronary revascularization) can also contribute to the complexity of analyzing and interpreting the study results if strict criteria or a blinded clinical events committee designed to produce valid recommendations are not incorporated and utilized during the trial.[99]

FOLLOW-UP SCHEDULE/DATA COLLECTION/COMPLIANCE

A few important issues are considered here. First, a study should be conducted for an appropriate duration and second, data need to be consistently collected throughout the entire trial. A magical number of weeks or months has not been established as a rule for all clinical trials, but the length of the study (i.e., follow-up time) should be an ideal representation to answer the question being researched.[25] Statins usually exert the maximum cholesterol lowering effect after approximately 6 weeks of stable dosing.[107] Thus, the results of a study directly comparing atorvastatin 10 mg once daily to simvastatin 20 mg once daily for 6 weeks to compare the LDL-C level lowering differences between these two agents would be considered acceptable.[58]

A number of trials do not have an extensive follow-up time and the reader may have difficulty in interpreting the results for clinical practice. For example, in one study the antipsychotic agent aripiprazole and placebo were administered to subjects for 4 weeks to determine the efficacy of aripiprazole in treating psychosis.[108] The investigators of the clinical trial detected a pharmacologic effect of aripiprazole during this time period, but the clinical effects and tolerability of the medication beyond this time period could not be assessed due to the short duration of the trial. Considering the actual duration of aripiprazole and other antipsychotic therapies for patients with psychosis exceeds 4 weeks,[109] the trial should have been longer so that investigators could determine the long-term clinical effects of this drug in practice.

Monitoring of the trial results at predetermined intervals is important throughout the duration of the trial. The Code of Federal Regulations and Good Clinical Practice guidelines for clinical research (www.fda.gov/oc/qcp/guidance.html) state that subject monitoring is required during the clinical investigation.[25] Larger trials may have a clinical trial investigator subgroup who serve as the data and safety monitoring board members. These individuals are blinded to the subject groupings and are responsible for reviewing the results obtained while the trial is ongoing. Interim analyses of the study results may indicate that the intervention produces either a favorable outcome or increased risk over the control before the established duration of the study has been completed. Typically, the protocol for discontinuing the clinical trial early is established prior to enrolling study subjects.[29,34]

By stopping the study early after finding that the intervention results in significant harm compared to the control, subjects randomized to the intervention would not be at a greater risk for experiencing the harmful effects if a trial was allowed to continue. Conversely, if the intervention was shown to be more beneficial than the control, investigators would be denying useful therapy to those subjects randomized to the control if the trial continued.[29] The WHI trial was discontinued after an average of 5.2 years of follow-up because the health risks exceeded the health benefits of continuing the trial.[53] When this study was discontinued prematurely, investigators informed subjects of the therapy they received, results of the study, and recommended discontinuation of the medication if they received the combination therapy where harm was identified.[110] In contrast, the U.S. Carvedilol Heart Failure Study was discontinued earlier than originally planned because the results documented that carvedilol decreased the occurrence of the primary endpoint (mortality) more than the control (placebo). The investigators concluded that continuing the study placed the subjects randomized to placebo at an increased risk of death.[62]

Prior to the start of the study, data collection methods are established. These should be reasonable, in that extensive time and/or procedures are not required. By doing so, incomplete follow-up by trial personnel and subjects at each follow-up time can be minimized. In addition, investigators should ensure trial personnel are properly trained and have sufficient resources to complete data collection.[111]

Another data collection and follow-up issue is measuring the compliance of therapy in the study participants.[25] This includes medication pill counts, serum drug levels, or regular follow-up communications (i.e., telephone conversations). Subjects not complying with the therapy regimen may cause inaccuracies and less reliable data. Insufficient and/or inappropriate data collection methods and noncompliance usually lead to biased results that may make the extrapolation of results to clinical practice difficult.[16]

SAMPLE SIZE

Sample size (denoted by the letter n) refers to the number of subjects randomized into a study and is of considerable importance to the validity of the study results. Financial and logistical limitations prevent all subjects with the specific inclusion criteria from being enrolled into the study.[25,111] For example, investigators want to evaluate a new drug to treat hypertension. It would be virtually impossible to enroll all people with hypertension into this clinical trial. In response, investigators will draw a representative group (i.e., sample) of individuals from all those with hypertension (i.e., population). Researchers do not wish to include too few or too many subjects in the trial. Obviously having only one subject each in the intervention and control groups is insufficient to determine differences in effect between groups since chance alone may be the reason for a difference found (if any) between the two groups. On the other hand, having too many subjects can be excessive and may expose some subjects to unnecessary treatment. The sample size should not be determined on the basis of convenience, arbitrarily, or by the number of easily recruited subjects.[112]

The number of subjects to enroll in a clinical trial is dependent on the expected magnitude of difference in the endpoint effect between the intervention and control. The expected magnitude of difference in effect between groups is estimated based on the results of previously conducted trials or other research results assessing the intervention. In general, an inverse relationship exists between the sample size and the effect size. A large sample size is needed to detect a small difference in effect between the intervention and control outcome while a smaller sample size is needed to detect large differences between the two groups.[20,112] A large sample size is needed to detect differences in blood pressure between two antihypertensive therapies (small difference in blood pressure reductions) while a smaller sample size is needed to measure the difference in relieving postoperative pain between morphine and placebo (large difference in pain relief).

Researchers utilize various procedures from table/charts to hand calculations in estimating the necessary sample size for a particular trial.[70,112] Regardless of the method selected to determine the appropriate sample size, it must be calculated prior to initiating the clinical trial. A study lacking a sample size calculation may be biased since the reader is not informed of the basis on which the investigators determined the number of subjects to enroll. Also another important issue is that the sample size is calculated based on the differences in the primary endpoint effect between the intervention and control groups. Investigators intending to measure differences in effect for other endpoints besides the primary endpoint need to include this in the process of calculating the sample size. Clinical trials consisting of larger sample sizes can be considered more reliable in measuring and detecting true difference in the effect (if it exists) between the intervention and control.[113] Consequences of a clinical trial not having a sufficient sample size (i.e., too small or too large) are discussed later in the Type I and Type II errors section of this chapter.

The importance of an appropriate study sample size is exemplified in the following example. Investigators conducted a small study (51 patients) to evaluate fenoldopam mesylate compared with 0.45% sodium chloride infusion in enhancing renal plasma flow in patients undergoing contrast angiography. Fewer subjects receiving fenoldopam developed a specific adverse event (radiocontrast-induced nephropathy [RCN]) at 48 hours than those treated with

0.45% sodium chloride infusion (21% vs. 41%, respectively).[114] One primary contributor to the large difference in the results was the small number of subjects enrolled; the incidence of RCN is increased by 4% for each subject developing this outcome. Thus, even though the percent difference was 20% (41% − 21%), this represents a difference of only five subjects developing RCN. After the results of this large difference in reducing RCN incidence were released, fenoldopam was frequently used in these patients.[115] However, the CONTRAST study (Evaluation of Corlopam® in Patients at Risk for Renal Failure—A Safety and Efficacy Trial) was designed to determine if fenoldopam reduces RCN in patients after receiving iodine-based dye (i.e., during cardiac angioplasty),[115] but this study had a much larger sample size (157 patients in the fenoldopam group and 158 in the placebo) compared to the previous study evaluating fenoldopam therapy. At 48 hours, RCN incidence was 19.9% vs. 15.9% with fenoldopam and placebo, respectively ($p = 0.45$, which indicates no statistical difference). At 96 hours, incidence was 33.6% versus 30.1%, respectively. Investigators recruited slightly greater than 300 subjects to accommodate potential subject discontinuations. Based on the results of this clinical trial, the incidence of RCN was actually higher with fenoldopam than placebo. By conducting a study with a larger sample size, the treatment effect of fenoldopam was more accurately measured compared to the study of only 51 subjects.

STATISTICAL ANALYSIS

Investigators of all controlled clinical trials statistically analyze the study results since the data are collected from a sample of the patient population. Many statistical tests are available and readers should be familiar with and have a basic understanding of those most commonly used in clinical trials. Some statistical analyses can be easily conducted using simple computer programs while others require specialized training and extensive skill. Typically, a biostatistician is consulted as one of the trial investigators to perform the statistical analysis of the trial results,[116,117] although study results may be biased by using incorrect statistical analysis, even with biostatisticians evaluating the data.[116]

The purpose of statistical analysis of the study data is to collect sufficient evidence to reject the null hypothesis (H_0) in favor of accepting the research hypothesis (H_1).[118,119] Prior to starting the study, appropriate tests are selected based on the type of data that will be collected and analyzed. Since the selection of statistical tests is dependent on the type of data,[93] an overview of the types of data is presented here. There are four types of data (see Table 6–5)[120]: nominal, ordinal, interval, and ratio (the latter two are usually referred collectively as continuous). Nominal data are categorical without any sense of order; these data can only be categorized into one of the possible groups (e.g., either dead or alive, but not both). Nominal data are mutually exclusive, meaning that the data can be in only one group. Ordinal data (i.e., ranking) are categorical data with an intrinsic order, but do not have equal intervals between units. Pain severity (or other type of subjective data) measured by a scale is a typical example of ordinal data.

TABLE 6–5. TYPES OF DATA

Type of Data	Definition	Examples
Nominal	Categorical data Data placed in one category, but not more than one category	Yes/no; alive/dead; colors of cars in a parking lot into five categories of either red, white, blue, black, or other
Ordinal	Ranking, ordered	Likert scale; visual analog scale
Interval	Data with measurable equal distances between points, but no absolute zero	Temperature in degrees Fahrenheit
Ratio	Data with measurable equal distances between points and an absolute zero	Temperature in degrees Kelvin; blood pressure, cholesterol levels, white blood count

A 5-point pain scale with a score of 0 indicates no pain while a score of 5 indicates severe pain. A 1-point change in pain intensity on this 5-point pain scale is not necessarily the same from 1 to 2 as from 4 to 5 on the scale. Interval and ratio data both have measurable equal intervals between data points, but interval data have no absolute zero while an absolute zero point is accountable for ratio data. Readers need to differentiate between the types of data to ensure that correct statistical tests were selected in addition to the study being designed appropriately with correct data collection methods. For instance, not only would blinding be included in a trial that measured pain reduction (subjective outcome), but a validated technique to measure and statistically analyze the change in pain scores is necessary.

The type of data collected also dictates the use of inferential or descriptive statistical methods. Inferential statistics are used to draw conclusions based on the sample for the application of the trial results on the population.[121,122] In other words, data are analyzed to make a conclusion of the study results from the sample that is then inferred to the population. Descriptive statistics describe the characteristics of the sample (e.g., average subject age, baseline endpoint values, number of subjects with another disease present) and the results in some studies (e.g., $X\%$ had an adverse effect). Descriptive data are typically presented as measures of central tendency (e.g., mean [average], median, and mode) and/or measure of variability (e.g., range, SD) (see Table 6–6).[123] Refer to Chap. 10 for further information on descriptive and inferential statistics.

Explaining the terms in Table 6–6 can be done best via an example of a trial in which the change in LDL-C was measured. A total of 200 subjects were enrolled in a clinical study designed to measure the reduction in LDL-C with a statin versus placebo. The LDL-C is measured in all subjects at the beginning of the trial. The values are then plotted using a histogram (see Figure 6–1). For each subject with a specific LDL-C value, a mark is placed on the graph for that value. As each subject with the same LDL-C value is plotted on the graph, an upward column for that LDL-C value forms. If the sample of subjects was randomly taken from the population, all the plotted LDL-C values would form a bell-shaped curve (also known

TABLE 6–6. DATA PRESENTATION METHODS

Type of Data	Mode	Median	Mean	Range	Interquartile Range	SD
Nominal	X					
Ordinal	X	X		X	X	
Interval and Ratio	X	X	X	X	X	X

NOTE: Mode: most frequently occurring data point; Median: midpoint of the data (point at which the data lie 50% above and below); Mean: average of the data points; Range: officially the difference between the smallest and largest data point in the data set, although usually described by listing the smallest and largest data points (e.g., "The range is from 5 to 9"); Interquartile range: difference between the scores at the 75th and the 25th percentile; SD: degree in which individual data points deviate from the mean value of the data set.

as a normally distributed data set). After all LDL-C values are obtained, the values for the terms in Table 6–6 can be calculated. As seen from the graph, the mode (most commonly occurring LDL-C value), median (point at which 50% of the LDL-C values lie above and below), and the mean (average) LDL-C are the same. In this data set, LDL-C of 145 mg/dL represents these three measures of central tendencies. In addition, the range for the LDL-C values can be determined by identifying the lowest and highest LDL-C value. The data also can be organized into quartiles, four groups containing 25% of the data points. The data are arranged from the lowest to highest value; afterward the data points are divided into four groups: 25th, 50th, 75th, and 100th percentile. Therefore, a LDL-C value that corresponds to the 75th percentile would be in the upper limit of this third quartile of the distribution. In addition, the upper limit of the 50th quartile would equal the median value for the data set. The interquartile range is the difference between the scores at the 75th and the 25th percentile.[123]

Since many trials measuring the endpoint as continuous data will present the results as an average (mean), a more detailed discussion of this measure of central tendency is warranted.

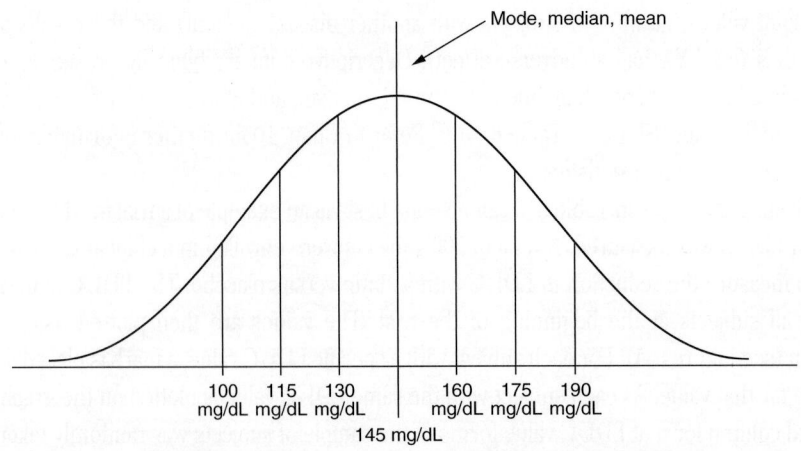

Figure 6–1. Histogram of LDL-C with standard deviation ±15 mg/dL.

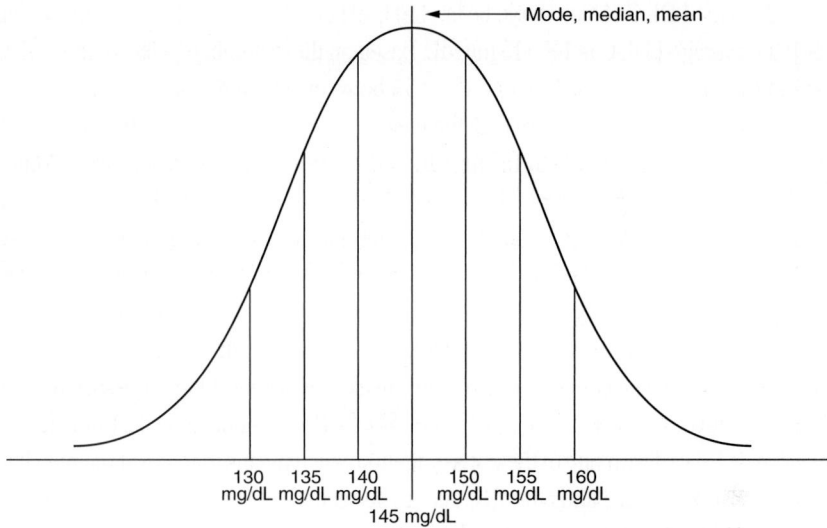

Figure 6–2. Histogram of LDL-C with standard deviation ±5 mg/dL.

Using the LDL-C example, an average LDL-C value is calculated using all the measured values. However, presenting only the average does not inform the reader of the diversity in the set of values from the sample. Thus, standard deviation (SD) is calculated using all of the LDL-C values. SD is presented with the mean value of the sample (e.g., 145 mg/dL ±15, where the former number is the mean and the latter number is the SD). The SD is important since the average LDL-C from two distinct samples may be the same, but the dispersion of the LDL-C values may be considerably different. Figure 6–2 displays another set of LDL-C values taken from a different sample of subjects. The average LDL-C value is the same as Figure 6–1, but the spread of the LDL-C values is not very diverse away from the average LDL-C value.

The presentation of the average ±SD allows the readers to calculate the percentage of LDL-C values within portions of the graph. Figure 6–3 illustrates the distribution of LDL-C within 1, 2, and 3 SD from the average in a data set that has normal distribution of the values.

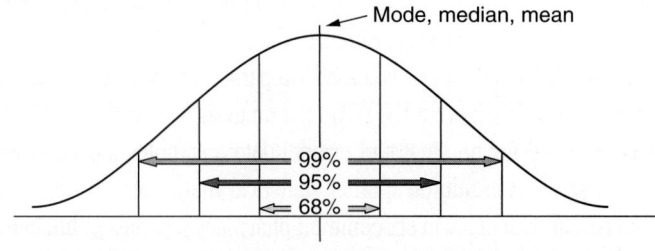

Figure 6–3. Histogram of normal distribution with standard deviations.

As a rule, ~68% of the LDL-C values would be in ±1 SD, ~95% in ±2 SD, and ~99% in ±3 SD. Using Figure 6–1, the average LDL-C is 145 ±15 mg/dL. Based on these numbers, ~68% of the LDL-C values are in the range of 130 to 160 mg/dL, ~95% between 115 and 175 mg/dL, and ~99% between 100 and 190 mg/dL. In Figure 6–2, the mean ±SD is 145 ±5 mg/dL with corresponding values of 140 to 150 mg/dL; 135 to 155 mg/dL; and 130 to 160 mg/dL, respectively. Notice that even though the average of both LDL-C data sets is the same, 95% of the LDL-C values are in the range of 115 to 175 mg/dL in Figure 6–1, but between 135 and 155 mg/dL in Figure 6–2.

Another example is presented to discuss the clinical usefulness of interpreting an average ±SD. Alpha-adrenergic antagonists were first developed to treat hypertension. However, men without hypertension receive these agents to treat benign prostatic hyperplasia (BPH).[124] Physicians may be concerned that men will experience low blood pressure if these agents are prescribed. In this example, the mean ±SD DBP was reduced by 4 ±1 mmHg in a group of subjects treated with one of these class agents, which means that 95% of the men had a reduction in DBP between 2 and 6 mmHg. As can be seen, the SD allows for the readers to assess more than just the mean for a set of data.

Although SD is commonly used, some investigators may present the standard error of the mean (SEM), which is calculated as the SD divided by the square root of the sample size $(SD/\sqrt{n})$.[122,125] As seen by this formula, the SEM is smaller than the SD, which implies a smaller dispersion of the data points away from the average. Presenting SEM instead of SD may occur when the investigators want the reader to interpret a small dispersion of the data from the mean value instead of a large variance from the mean if the SD was presented. While SD measures the deviation of the individual values from the mean of the sample, SEM measures the deviation of the individual sample means from the mean of the population.[122] The SEM identifies the variability in the population; 95% of the time, the true mean of the population lies within two SEM of the sample mean.[125] At times SEM is used appropriately (more than one clinical trial) while at most times SEM is incorrectly presented.[125] Readers should be aware of these distinctions and interpret the data accordingly.

Inferential statistics are used to determine if a statistical difference is present between the intervention and control groups. A p value is calculated based on trial results and statistical tests; afterward, the p value is compared to the alpha (α) value established prior to the beginning of the trial[121] (see section "Statistical Significance versus Clinical Difference" for further discussion, since it is necessary to discuss other issues first). The selection of the statistical test depends on the data being parametric (i.e., normal distribution) versus nonparametric. Typically, continuous data are assessed via parametric statistics; common tests are Student's t-test, analysis of variance (ANOVA), and analysis of covariance (ANCOVA). Nonparametric tests are used for nominal and ordinal data; examples are chi-square (χ^2) and Mann-Whitney U test.[93,121] A multitude of other statistical analytical procedures are available. An analysis of all research articles in six common pharmacy journals published during 2001 identified chi-square (χ^2), Student's t-test, and ANOVA as the top three most common statistical tests used.[126] Chapter 10 is devoted to a more in-depth discussion of statistical analyses.

Other statistical terms encountered while reading clinical trials are unpaired versus paired and one-tailed versus two-tailed statistical analysis. Comparing results between groups is referred to unpaired analysis, while within a group comparison is a paired analysis.[127] For example, measuring the mean change in LDL-C from baseline to 12 weeks with simvastatin would be a paired analysis. Analyzing the mean difference in the LDL-C reduction after 12 weeks between simvastatin and atorvastatin would be considered an unpaired test. Two-tailed (also known as two-sided) statistical tests are used for trials in which investigators are not sure in which direction the primary endpoint will be affected by the intervention. These tests analyze the results in both directions, for positive or negative effects in comparison to the control.[29,113] Two-tailed tests are more common because the direction of change (and the degree) is not known.[29,113] For example, a two-tailed test is used for an investigational drug compared to placebo to treat elevated LDL-C. The investigators do not know the effect of the intervention on the LDL-C levels (i.e., the levels can increase or decrease relative to the placebo). A one-tailed test is primarily used in a study in which the direction of the effect of the intervention and active control (e.g., another medication, but not placebo) are known or can go only in one direction. The intent of this study type is to measure more precisely the difference in effect between the two groups. Some investigators have used a one-tailed test to determine differences in LDL-C changes in patients receiving statins. Prior research has documented the LDL-C lowering effects of atorvastatin and simvastatin being compared to other medications or placebo. Since these research results are available, a one-tailed test could be used to increase the statistical accuracy of detecting a difference in effect between the two statins in lowering LDL-C.

TYPES I AND II ERRORS/POWER ANALYSIS

A clinical trial is conducted to test a research hypothesis that a difference in effect exists between the intervention and control treatments. Before the trial begins, investigators develop a null hypothesis (H_0; no difference between the groups) and research hypothesis (H_1; a difference is present between the groups). The trial is conducted and the investigators measure the difference in effect between the groups (if any). If a difference is present, this could actually be due to the intervention or happen by random chance.[118,119] Hypothesis testing is conducted to examine how likely any observed difference between the intervention and control would be due to chance if the H_0 were true. As the trial results diverge farther and farther from the finding of no difference, the H_0 is rejected between the intervention and control groups.[119]

Two types of errors are possible in hypothesis testing (see Table 6–7). A Type I error can occur when the H_0 is falsely rejected and the H_1 is falsely accepted. Thus, the investigators

TABLE 6–7. TYPE I AND TYPE II ERROR POSSIBILITIES

Error Type	Action/Decision	Interpretation
Type I	Statistical difference calculated, even though it is not really present Reject H_0	H_0 is really true, but was rejected, which leads to a false-positive result. The probability equals the α error rate. There is one reason for a Type I error: chance
Type II	No statistical difference calculated, even though there is one Fail-to-reject (accept) H_0	H_0 is really false, but was accepted, which leads to a false-negative result. The probability equals the β error rate. There are two reasons for a Type II error: chance or small sample size

are stating a difference in effect was measured even though there really is no difference between the intervention and control groups (also known as a false-positive finding).[95,111,113] On the other hand, a Type II error can occur when H_0 is falsely accepted and the H_1 is falsely rejected. In this case, the investigators are stating no difference in effect is present between the intervention and control even though there really is a difference between the groups (also known as a false-negative finding).[70,113,128]

Investigators attempt to control Type I and II error occurrences by setting limits on the probability of these occurring. The only reason that a Type I error can occur is by chance. Since no research is error proof, methods usually are developed to allow up to a 5% probability that chance was the reason a difference in effect was measured between the intervention and control. The process of setting the probability of a Type I error (false-positive result) to occur no greater than 5% is termed as establishing the α value.[111,113] This is also referred to setting the statistical significance to 0.05, but can also be phrased "significance level of 0.05" or setting the α rate at 0.05. Another phrase commonly used to establish the α value is "p values < 0.05 are statistically significant." This rate is the norm for most studies, but a few trials may have $\alpha = 0.01$. This latter rate indicates that the investigators are more stringent by reducing the possibility of a Type I error to 1%. However, setting $\alpha = 0.1$ is too relaxed and permits the Type I error possibility to be very high (at 10%). The α rate is a measure of how willing the researchers are to accept the chance of making a Type I error.[118] With the α rate at 0.05, this is indicating that in 1 of 20 trials, a difference in effect being measured between the groups can be due to chance.[70,111] An α rate of 0.002 indicates that in 2 out of 1000 trials, a difference in the measured effect between groups can be due to chance. Thus, the smaller the p values, the less likely chance was the reason for finding the differences. Also, the p value can be expressed as the probability of rejecting a true H_0[121] (this last statement to be explained in the "Statistical Significance versus Clinical Difference" section).

The probability of making a Type II error is referred to as beta (β).[70,113,128] Although investigators want to avoid a Type II error, appropriately designed clinical trials allow this error (false-negative) to occur no greater than 20% of the time.[70,128] Even though investigators want to avoid making both a Type I and Type II error, they are more willing to make a Type II error than

Type I error because a Type II error may be easier to determine than a Type I error.[118] Also, Type I errors are more dangerous in terms of the possible direct effects on patients (see next paragraph). Therefore, this is a reason the α rate is set lower than the β rate. Investigators, in designing the clinical trial, aim to balance the possibility of Type I and Type II errors knowing that decreasing the probability of one error may increase the probability of the other error occurring.

Making a Type I error means a difference in effect was measured by chance but really no difference in effect exists between the two groups. The danger of using a therapy no different than the control is more serious when the control is a placebo versus an active therapy. A Type II error indicates no difference was measured between the two groups. If the control group is another therapy, then the intervention is shown to be no different. If the control is a placebo, then the intervention may not be considered as a therapy to treat patients. Although the false-negative result is a concern (i.e., a useful therapy may be not used), this is less severe than a false-positive result (i.e., using a therapy that really is no different in effect than the control but was found to be so by chance).

A Type II error can occur either by chance or small sample size in which the latter is usually the reason if the error occurs.[113] The ultimate goal of each clinical trial is to ensure that the difference in effect size is properly measured between the intervention and control groups, which require a sufficient sample size.[70] One method for investigators to ensure that a sufficient number of subjects are enrolled in the trial is by conducting a power analysis. The power of a study is defined as the ability to detect a difference in the outcome between the intervention and control if a difference truly exists. Power is calculated from the β error rate (power = $1 - \beta$).[112,128] As seen from this formula, the lower the β error rate, the higher the power. Increasing the sample size then reduces the β error rate, increases study power, and reduces the chance of a false-negative result.[112] In addition, the magnitude of difference in the effect that can be detected between the intervention and control groups is related to the sample size: smaller differences in the effect between the intervention and control can be detected with larger sample sizes.[20,112]

Another factor important to ensure a clinical trial has the power to detect differences in effect is estimating the absolute difference in the effect (δ) between intervention and control groups.[24] This value is not as easily determined as the two other rates; the δ is usually based on prior preliminary research results or even consensus discussion among the researchers (i.e., educated guess).[112] For example, a study was conducted to answer the study question "is the incidence of radiocontrast-induced nephropathy (RCN) reduced with fenoldopam versus 0.45% sodium chloride infusion (placebo control)?" The incidence of RCN was estimated by the researchers to be reduced from 30% with the control to 15% with fenoldopam ($\delta = 15\%$) from the results of smaller studies evaluating fenoldopam.[115]

As seen earlier, the sample size needed is influence by the α, β, and δ values. The purpose of the sample size calculation is to provide sufficient power to be able to reject H_0 established for the clinical trial primary endpoint if it is false and should be rejected.[70] Hopefully, a clinical trial with an appropriate sample size will not lead to erroneously detecting a difference in effect when there is no real difference (Type I error), but also have a degree of certainty that the true difference in effects was not missed (Type II error).[111] A trial having an appropriate sample size increases the precision of estimating the difference in effect of the intervention compared to the control.[16] The total number of subjects completing the trial should be similar to the actual sample size calculation for the study to have appropriate power.[112] Normally, the investigators will increase the sample size by some factor above the number calculated to be necessary (i.e., 10%) to account for subject attrition and therapy noncompliance.

Results

After the methods section, the results of the clinical trial are presented. This section contains primary and secondary endpoint results and other useful information. Again this section is to be critically appraised to verify if the study objective was met, based on the data, and to evaluate the other types of outcomes that may have occurred. Normally tables, charts, figures, or other illustrative forms present many of the results, which can expedite the understanding and analysis process.

SUBJECT DEMOGRAPHICS

The first type of information provided in the results section describes the subjects actually enrolled and randomized in the clinical trial.[23] A general overview of the average subject is described, usually presented in a table of baseline information.[129] Typical information in the table includes average age, male to female ratio, disease states, and/or drug therapy among the study participants at the time of study enrollment. In addition, any complicating factors that can affect the endpoints or trial outcome may be described, such as the number of subjects who smoke, the amount of caffeine intake and so forth.

The patient baseline demographic data need to be compared between treatment groups to ensure that the groups are as similar as possible. The groups should not have any significant differences if proper randomization techniques are incorporated by the study investigators; but a few differences can still occur due to chance.[16] Significant dissimilarities between the groups that could contribute to differences in the outcome between the groups need to be closely scrutinized. If the patient baseline differences are substantial, a confounding variable is present and the study investigators must analyze the results to determine if these differences have affected the outcome of the study. Otherwise, the results may not be applicable to practice.[113]

An example of baseline subject demographics is illustrated by the selected WHI trial patient information: average age 63.3 years, 84% Caucasian, 74.1% never used hormones in the past, 36.1% were treated for hypertension, and 19.6% were taking aspirin (≥80 mg/day). Over 25 baseline subject demographics were listed in the trial and only one was significantly different between the women taking CEE/MPE versus placebo: history of coronary artery bypass graft/percutaneous transluminal coronary angioplasty (CABG/PTCA), 1.1% versus 1.5%, respectively.[53] Although a difference is present, clinical judgment suggests that the magnitude is not great and this would not significantly alter the study results in favor of one group. Although the WHI trial was randomized, a few differences in subject demographics still occurred, mostly due to chance.

SUBJECT DROPOUT AND COMPLIANCE

After the baseline subject information, data regarding the follow-up (i.e., subject dropout) and compliance should be presented. Not all subjects randomized in a clinical trial will complete the entire duration, at which time they are then termed a study dropout or stated to be lost to follow-up.[69] Reasons vary for discontinuing study participation, including lack of desire to continue, subject relocation (i.e., moving to another city), subject violating study protocol, side effects, and death. Also, not all subjects will be compliant with the therapy. Not accounting for the number of dropouts and noncompliance can have an affect on the trial results.[69,130,131] Thus, investigators need to report the number of subjects and major reasons for discontinuing the study, compliance rates, and the techniques of assessing the data for the readers to draw appropriate conclusions about the intervention understudy and subsequent trial results.

The impact of dropouts on the overall study results is dependent on the magnitude of subject discontinuations. A few subjects dropping out of the study may not cause a substantial difference in the results, whereas a sizable percentage may alter the study results significantly. No threshold of dropout rates has been established that deems the trial results to be of no clinical value. The overall effect of the dropouts on the significance of the trial results is dependent on the trial endpoints and reader interpretation. An example of dropout rates affecting trial results follows. A hypothetical clinical trial had 100 patients each in the intervention and control groups, all who had an infection. At study end, patients in the intervention group experienced greater infection cure rates (75% vs. 40%). However, 60 patients discontinued the intervention compared to only 10 patients from the control due to side effects and these data were not included in the overall study results. If all subjects were included in the analysis (counting the dropouts as therapy failures), the cure rate would be lower in the intervention than control group (30% vs. 36%). This illustrates the importance of reporting results for all subjects enrolled, not just those completing the clinical trial.

Frequently, the study results will be analyzed using data collected from all randomized subjects, regardless of whether they completed the entire study duration (i.e., results from dropouts are not discarded, but are considered to be treatment failures). This technique is referred to as the intention-to-treat (ITT) principle. Even in cases where the subject may have only taken one dose of the medication under investigation, these results are still included in the ITT analysis. The advantage of the ITT analysis is that this analysis better mimics real-life application of an intervention into practice because similar to real life, all subjects in a clinical trial may not complete therapy as prescribed.[130,131] But a concern with the ITT analysis needs to be recognized. Data from the subjects discontinuing a trial early may bias the analysis, which is of considerable importance for an endpoint measurement that worsens over time (e.g., cognitive function in subjects with dementia). The last score obtained in a subject discontinuing the trial early may suggest a better response than the last score obtained if this subject discontinued later in the trial. Analyzing data that were collected from a subject discontinuing the trial soon after it began may suggest a better outcome than if this subject discontinued later in the trial.[132]

At times, the study results are analyzed via ITT and the per-protocol (PP) procedure. The latter term refers to analyzing data only from subjects completing the trial. The advantage of this technique is for determining the effects of the intervention in subjects that followed the study protocol and completed the entire course of therapy.

An example of analyzing study data according to ITT and PP methods follows. The West of Scotland trial reported the ITT results of pravastatin lowering mean LDL-C by −15.8% compared to −26.3% via the PP analysis (from a baseline of 190 to 160 and 140 mg/dL, respectively). The change for the control group, placebo, was virtually unchanged, as expected.[133] Both the ITT and PP results can be useful to apply into practice; a subject meeting the inclusion criteria of this trial who is compliant and correctly taking pravastatin may achieve on average a LDL-C lowering of 26%, while as a whole this value would decrease by an average of 16% in the group of patients treated with this medication.

Clinical trials including only the PP results are to be scrutinized more because results from all subjects are not assessed. In certain situations, PP analysis is appropriate. PP analysis may allow estimation of accurate treatment effects for patients who have completed the study. But the reasons for the subjects still discontinuing is required in interpreting the PP analysis. Assessing the results only via PP in a trial that had the majority of subjects discontinuing due to adverse drug effects leads to overestimation of the results. If the subjects discontinued the trial due to relocating to another city, then analyzing the trial results via PP is not affected as significantly as in the prior case. Investigators not accounting for discontinuations directly caused by the therapies leads to biased results since these subjects can be counted as treatment failures but are not.

ENDPOINTS AND SAFETY

A critical component of the results section is the primary endpoint results. These results can be displayed as tables, graphs, or other illustrations. The information should be presented clearly and completely, using clear and unbiased methods. In addition, the investigators need to explain the results and present p values. Results of secondary endpoints follow and are presented in a fashion similar to the primary endpoints; however, endpoints other than the primary endpoint may not be adequately powered to detect differences in effect between the intervention and control. Therefore, if statistically significant results occur with these other endpoints, the results may be due to chance. Other endpoints should be adequately powered to draw meaningful conclusions regarding use in practice.[23]

One issue to consider in evaluating the results in some clinical trials is whether medication dosing titration is allowed in the methods. The final medication dose of one group may be maximized while the other group did not require maximum doses. The investigators may make a conclusion based on misleading information. An example is a hypothetical trial beginning with losartan 50 mg once daily. The dose is increased to 100 mg once daily and hydrochlorothiazide (HCTZ) 25 mg once daily can be added so that goal DBP of <90 mmHg is achieved. The control group received amlodipine 5 mg once daily; the dose also could be increased (to 10 mg once daily) and HCTZ 25 mg once daily could be added. Approximately 85% of patients randomized to losartan also received HCTZ while only 45% randomized to amlodipine received HCTZ. The investigators concluded that losartan was as effective as amlodipine in achieving goal DBP even though a disproportionate number of subjects received the maximum losartan dose plus HCTZ compared to amlodipine and only 15% of the losartan-treated subjects received monotherapy versus 55% of the amlodipine-treated subjects. The final losartan and amlodipine doses need to be assessed in regards to the number of subjects receiving the higher medication dose and those with HCTZ. The number of patients who received HCTZ should also be assessed to determine if clinically meaningful results can be drawn between losartan and amlodipine despite differences in doses and HCTZ therapy. Readers should be cautious in accepting the investigator conclusion that two drugs are equal in effect in a trial with methods that allow dose titrations and/or additional medications added to therapy without analyzing the final doses.

Safety assessments or tolerability of all therapies should be included in the results section.[23] Investigators need to implement valid methods of defining, collecting, and analyzing these results. As with the secondary endpoints, the study may not be powered sufficiently to definitively quantify the safety/tolerability of the intervention. In addition, the frequency and severity of these results may be dissimilar to those observed in clinical practice. Investigators are required to monitor the subjects closely and collect these data.[41] Other factors to be considered include the clinical trial duration, limited sample size, and exclusion of selected subjects from being enrolled into the trial.

Surrogate Endpoints

Investigators of some clinical trials select a primary endpoint that can be classified as a surrogate endpoint,[134] which is described as "a measure of the efficacy of a treatment can be defined as laboratory values (e.g., HDL-C/LDL-C), symptoms (e.g., pain), or clinical parameters (e.g., blood pressure), which are employed as a substitute for a clinical endpoint (e.g., morbidity, mortality). Here it is assumed that changes in the surrogate endpoint can be directly translated into changes in the definitive clinical endpoint."[135] The primary reason surrogate endpoints are selected for clinical trials is to quickly measure an effect at a lower expenditure.[135] Also, surrogate endpoints are measured instead of clinical endpoints due to a lower clinical trial financial burden and shorter time commitment. The established efficacy and other data collected from trials measuring surrogate endpoint provide the rationale for larger trials with clinical endpoints (i.e., MI, stroke, and death).[25] The following conditions should be fulfilled before a surrogate endpoint is considered as a valid substitute for a clinical endpoint: convenience (easily and readily assessable); well-established relationship between the surrogate and clinical outcomes; and determination of clinical benefit as a result of changes in the surrogate endpoint.[135]

An example of a surrogate endpoint is a reduction in mean LDL-C levels. In a study comparing atorvastatin and simvastatin, the mean change in LDL-C was measured after 6 weeks of therapy.[58] Lowering LDL-C is considered a surrogate endpoint because even though atorvastatin lowered mean LDL-C levels slightly more, this difference cannot be extrapolated to indicate that atorvastatin is better than simvastatin in reducing CV adverse events (e.g., MI and CV death). A study to document which statin to select in treating patients would require a few years, rather than 6 weeks of therapy, and many more patients than the 1300 enrolled in this study to measure LDL-C lowering differences. The use of the surrogate endpoint allows a quick comparison that may lead to longer trials that will determine the clinical benefit.

The primary limitation of surrogate endpoints is illustrated by the following example. Investigators of the WHI trial documented a reduction in mean LDL-C levels, which did not correspond with a lower incidence of adverse CV events. Change in mean LDL, total, and HDL cholesterol levels were greater (–12.7, –5.4, and +7.3%, respectively) from baseline with CEE/MPE than placebo. However, the incidence of CHD was higher with CEE/MPE (0.39% vs. 0.33%).[136] Thus, the use of surrogate endpoints to support benefit in clinical outcomes is not always guaranteed.

SUBGROUP ANALYSIS

Investigators often analyze the results of subsets of the study subjects as divided into various groups that often include gender, age, and presence of diseases or other complicating factors (i.e., diabetes vs. no diabetes).[137] Reasons to analyze the results in these subgroups vary, but usually relate to providing additional information in these specific patient types as opposed to just the overall trial results from all the randomized subjects. The WHI trial investigators conducted multiple subgroup assessments. The investigators evaluated the primary endpoint according to various demographics that included age, aspirin use, race/ethnicity, and statin use.[53]

Another example of a subgroup analysis is elderly patients (>65 years of age) enrolled in trials evaluating the reduction in the risk of adverse events (e.g., MI and stroke) with statins.

Although the investigators may be able to obtain more information from a trial by using subgroup analysis, limitations and other issues need to be recognized.[23,79,134,137,138] A few prerequisites should be present before subgroup analyses are conducted. First, the clinical trial should be well-designed with sound study methods. Subgroup analysis results from flawed studies may be of no importance. Second, the investigator may have conducted a multitude of subgroup analyses and only reported the statistically significant results. As the number of statistical evaluations increases, the likelihood of finding a statistical difference by chance alone increases. Therefore, multiple subgroup analyses should be avoided. Third, the power of the assessment is reduced, since results from a smaller number of subjects are analyzed as compared to the entire trial sample. Reduced power may lead to false-positive results.[137,138] Fourth, the primary endpoint should be statistically significant before subgroup analyses are conducted; otherwise investigators may be searching for statistically significant results.[138] Fifth, the subgroup analyses should be defined prior to the initiation of the trial and have documented justification to be conducted (e.g., past studies results suggest an effect in this group). Also, the ITT data are preferred for these evaluations since subject discontinuations may not be balanced between the two groups. Sixth, outcomes that can be influenced by either the intervention or control (i.e., compliance) should not be selected for a subgroup analysis. Lastly, the reader needs to review appropriate subgroup analysis, but keep the primary endpoint as their focus.[137]

The reader should recognize both positive and negative features of subgroup analyses. Further details of the trial results in a specific patient type are provided and may be the justification to conduct clinical trials with a larger sample with just this subject type. For instance, the PROSPER study was the first study to evaluate a statin (pravastatin) specifically in the elderly to reduce adverse events (primary endpoint measured as a combination of definite or suspected death from CHD, nonfatal MI, and fatal or nonfatal stroke). Prior clinical trials evaluating reduction of clinical events (e.g., MI, death) with a statin enrolled few elderly subjects. Analysis of the results in only the elderly subjects of these trials suggested statins were clinically useful for this patient type. Thus, investigators conducted a specific clinical trial in which elderly men and women between 70 and 82 years of age with a history of, or risk factors for, vascular disease (e.g., coronary, cerebral, or peripheral) or at risk (e.g., hypertension, diabetes, and smoking) were enrolled. The incidence of the primary endpoint was lower with pravastatin than placebo (16.2% vs. 14.1%; p = 0.014).[139] The results of this study provided the evidence to prescribe a statin (specifically pravastatin) in this patient type, instead of extrapolating this decision on subgroup analysis of previous statin studies that included elderly individuals (but not as the primary subject type).

However, subgroup analysis limitations need to be recognized. Overinterpretation of subgroup results can occur, usually because the overall study results did not demonstrate the desired difference in effect as expected by the investigators.[134] The sample size included in a clinical trial is based on the primary endpoint for all enrolled subjects. Reducing the sample size via a subgroup analysis can lead to a positive result that may have occurred by chance.[79,130,137,138] An illustration of this effect was documented by the African American Antiplatelet Stroke Prevention Study (AAASPS),[140] which was conducted in response to the subgroup analysis of Ticlopidine Aspirin Stroke Study (TASS).[141] The TASS investigators documented a lower incidence of nonfatal stroke or death from any cause in subjects with recent transient or mild persistent focal cerebral or retinal ischemia taking ticlopidine compared to aspirin (17% vs. 19%; p = 0.048). In addition to this overall study result, the investigators reported fewer cases of stroke and death with ticlopidine compared to ASA in a subgroup analysis of African Americans enrolled in this trial. The AAASPS results documented a slightly higher incidence of the composite endpoint (recurrent stroke, MI, or vascular death) in patients taking ticlopidine compared to aspirin (14.8% vs. 12.4%; p = 0.12). Although the study designs of these two studies were not identical, the AAASPS results serve as an example to the limitations of selecting therapy based on subgroup analysis. Thus, practitioners should be aware that although subgroup analysis may document greater benefits in selected individuals, the differences in effect may be due to chance or other factors.

ANCILLARY VERSUS ADJUNCTIVE THERAPIES

Clinical trials are designed to have identical groups with the only difference between the groups being the assignment to the intervention or control. At times, the study design may allow ancillary therapy to be included, in which subjects can take another therapy that can distort or interfere with the results.[69] The effect of the ancillary therapy on the study results needs to be assessed and included in the study evaluation. However, readers should not confuse ancillary therapy with adjunctive therapy. Some studies may include in the methods an adjunctive therapy, which all participants receive, while ancillary therapy is not equally distributed between the intervention and control groups. Thus, any significant difference in effect between the outcomes measured between the groups should be due to the therapies under investigation, not the adjunctive therapy. An example is a study comparing atorvastatin with simvastatin to lower LDL-C, where each patient has to follow a specified diet.[58] Although this diet can lower LDL-C, all patients are receiving the diet and any effects of the diet on the LDL-C change should be similar between the groups. However, ancillary therapy with antacids (amount not regulated, patient takes as many as they wish) in a study comparing heartburn relief between esomeprazole as needed versus lansoprazole taken everyday can lead to biased results.[142] At the end of the study, esomeprazole relieved heartburn symptoms better between the two groups, but the investigators did not report the antacid amount consumed by patients in either group (i.e., the average daily intake could have been 8.2 tablets vs. 1.2 tablets for the esomeprazole vs. lansoprazole group, respectively).

Antacids can reduce heartburn symptoms, but a significant imbalance may have been present between the two groups, which could be the reason esomeprazole was reported to relieve symptoms better.

Another type of ancillary therapy may be present in clinical trials, particularly as a rescue therapy. Rescue therapy is used to achieve a desired endpoint/outcome when the intervention under investigation fails to produce the desired outcome. This additional treatment can cause the measured outcome to be achieved, but needs to be measured separately from those subjects not receiving the rescue therapy. For instance, a medication (e.g., Headache B Gone) may be evaluated in a clinical trial to relieve migraine headache pain. Those subjects not having pain received by Headache B Gone are to take rescue therapy, (i.e., another pain reliever). Although the pain was relieved after the rescue therapy, the overall number of subjects meeting the endpoint (pain relief) from the intervention or control should not include the subjects taking rescue therapy. Those subjects achieving pain relief with the rescue therapy are to be reported separately. Otherwise, the results would be biased since the total number of subjects with pain relief is not based upon only the intervention vs. control.

Discussion/Conclusion

The primary purpose of discussion/conclusion is to evaluate and interpret the results of the clinical trial. The investigators should begin with a summary of the key findings of the study. Potential explanations of the study results should be addressed. The investigators should discuss the internal validity and external validity.[23] The investigators should also interpret the trial results in comparison with results of other similarly designed studies. Also, the trial may be discussed in comparison to other trials assessing the intervention or the disease state under investigation. Furthermore, the clinical trial limitations are identified and discussed.[23] Even though all clinical trials have limitations, these may vary from minor to those that seriously hinder the usefulness of the results. The discussion section should also address the clinical importance of the clinical trial results and how these results should be used in practice. All of this information should allow the reader to understand the application of the clinical trial results in practice. However, this section needs to be read just as carefully as the other clinical trials sections. This section can contain biased wording. In addition, only selected items may be discussed in relationship to the clinical trial.[79]

The investigators should ensure that strategies are included within the study design to minimize biases that may occur. Some of the strategies can include blinding, randomization, and appropriate inclusion/exclusion criteria. In addition, investigators should not be biased in interpreting the results of the trial. Readers should determine the degree to which the study results compare with patients encountered in practice. One of the most commonly cited criticisms of clinical trials by clinicians is the lack of external validity of the trials and this may be one explanation for the under use of reportedly favorable treatment options in clinical trials by clinicians.[143] Although some investigators may report beneficial results of an intervention under investigation, the patient population in the clinical trial may be so dissimilar to patients encountered in practice that clinicians are not convinced that the favorable results may be beneficial in their patient population. Several issues may potentially affect the external validity of the clinical trial and should be evaluated to assess the effects of the results in practice. These include the setting of the trial, selection of patients, characteristics of randomized patients, differences between the trial protocol and routine practice, outcome measures, follow-up, and adverse effects of treatment.[143] If the characteristics of the patients and setting are very different from those encountered in practice, the clinical usefulness of the reported information may be questionable.

Study strengths and limitations should be addressed in the discussion section. Potential limitations may include small sample size, short duration of the study, endpoint assessment techniques, or other factors that hinder the clinical usefulness of the study. The investigators should also address methods to circumvent trial limitations in subsequent clinical studies. Although there is no minimum or maximum limitation number that investigators should address, a thorough discussion of the limitations should be provided so that readers can determine the applicability of the trial results to their patient population.

Comparison of the current study to previous studies should be conducted. According to the results of one study, discussion sections of trial reports were lacking complete analysis of previous clinical trial results.[144] A total of 33 randomized trials were identified in 19 issues of leading medical journals (e.g., *Annals of Internal Medicine* and *JAMA*) in May 2001. The authors of four reports claimed that their study was a the first of its kind study; however, reports of similar trials were located for one of these studies. In three of the reports, systematic reviews of earlier trials were mentioned; however, no attempts to incorporate the results of the new trial with the existing results were identified in the remaining 27 reports. The results of other trials should be included to allow the reader to assess the results of the current trial in context to previous trial results. The readers can determine if the study was the first study that adds substantial information to the wealth of knowledge surrounding a topic or a me-too study that adds no new information to existing knowledge. The discussion section should also address future concerns and unanswered questions.

The conclusion section should provide an overall research recommendation to the readers. The investigators' conclusion should focus on the primary endpoint results, especially if no statistically significant differences between the intervention and control groups were observed, rather than favorable, secondary endpoint results. Conclusions should be limited to only that information discussed in previous sections of the trial; no new information should be discussed in this section. Also, the conclusions should be aligned with the results of the trial. Investigators should not make erroneous conclusions that are not supported by the results of the trial.

Clinical Trial Result Interpretation

STATISTICAL SIGNIFICANCE VERSUS CLINICAL DIFFERENCE

Once the clinical trial is completed, the investigators calculate a p value for the endpoints using the collected study results and statistical tests. The p value is an abbreviation for probability value and is compared to the α value established prior to the beginning of the clinical trial that serves as a benchmark against which p values are compared to determine if statistical significance is present. Also, since the entire population is not included, the investigators have to estimate the difference in effect from the sample.[118,119,145] Without statistical analysis, the likelihood of chance being the reason for any measured difference in effect is not known.[113] A p value for the primary endpoint that is less than the α value indicates that the H_0 is rejected and a statistically significant difference is declared between the intervention and control groups. This also indicates that chance alone was not the likely reason that a difference in effect was measured. H_0 is accepted (failed-to-be-rejected) with a p value equal to or greater than the α value and no statistically significant difference is declared.[119,145]

Statistical significance does not automatically mean a clinical difference in the effect between the intervention and control groups.[146] (See next section regarding the assessment of clinical difference.) The reader needs to make a decision to determine if the intervention is worth using instead of the control therapy, which can be dependent on the judgment and experiences of the reader. Not all statistically significant studies have clinically different results (see Figure 6–4). A p value less than the α value only represents the probability that a true H_0 has been rejected. In other words, the p value can be translated into "what is the probability of the difference in the effect between the intervention and control due to chance?"[118] Lower p values indicate a lower probability that chance could be the reason a difference in effect was measured between the intervention and control. Alternatively stated, "what is the chance of observing this difference if there really was no difference between the two groups?"[113] Recall that a Type I error is possible after rejecting the H_0; the results may be statistically significant due to chance.

Another paramount issue in understanding clinical trials is that the p value does not express the magnitude of difference in the effect between the intervention and control.[119] Statistically significant results signify that the alternative hypothesis (H_1) is accepted; H_1 states that the difference in effect is not equal between the intervention and control. H_1 only states that a difference in the effect is present between the intervention and control. The reader cannot conclude that a clinical difference is present between the intervention and control groups solely on a p value less than α.[113,121]

In addition, specific p values should be stated in the text of the article (i.e., p = 0.0012 instead of p < 0.05) to be more informative and helpful to the reader.[113,119] Also, all p values should be presented in conjunction with the endpoint results (i.e., "The clinical trial concluded that drug A lowered mean DBP more than placebo, –12 vs. –3 mmHg, respectively (p = 0.001)"

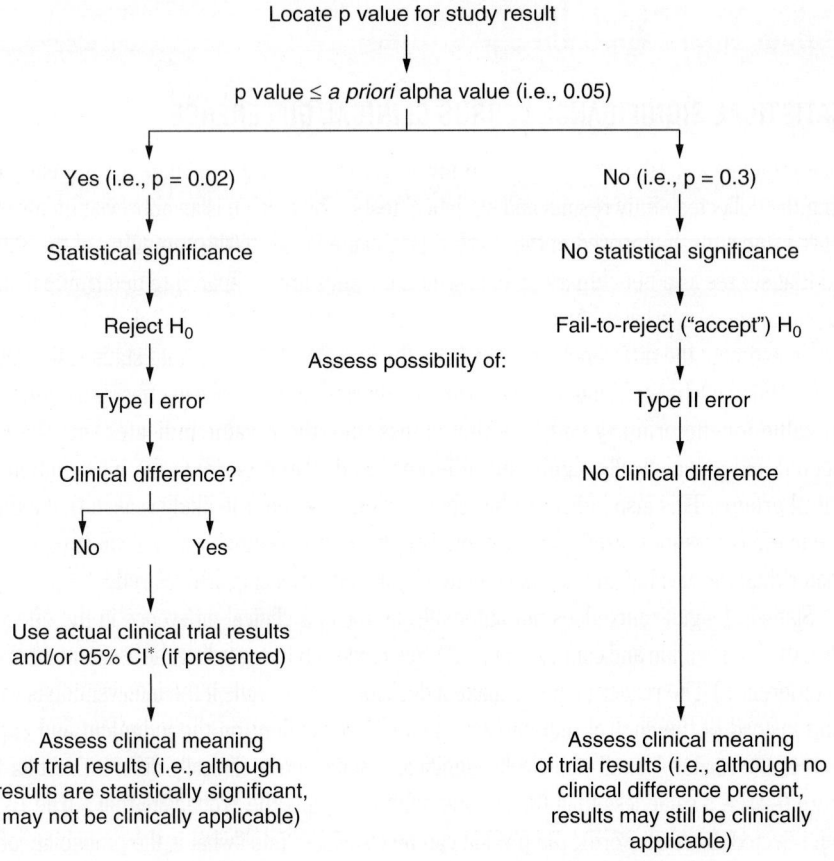

*95% Confidence interval.

Figure 6–4. Determining statistical significance, clinical difference, and clinical meaningfulness.

as opposed to "The clinical trial concluded that drug A lowered mean DBP more than placebo (p = 0.001)"). Readers encountering p values presented without the endpoint results should consider this a red flag. This situation should prompt the reader to ask "were the endpoint results not presented with the p value because the actual difference in the effect was minimal?" Without the endpoint results being presented, only statistical significance can be concluded with the p value; clinical differences in the effect cannot be assessed without the accompanying endpoint results. See the next section for further discussion of this issue.

ASSESSING CLINICAL DIFFERENCE

This step of analyzing and critiquing a clinical trial begins with p values less than the α value (see Figure 6–4). An important step in assessing clinical differences in effect between the intervention and control is to analyze the magnitude of difference between the endpoint results.[113,146] However, no magic formula is available to conclude whether clinical difference exists between the intervention and control.[119,146] The process of a reader concluding a clinical difference is usually based on clinical knowledge and experience and may be relative in the reader's opinion to whether clinical difference is present or not. For example, an antihypertensive therapy lowers mean DBP by 14 mmHg versus 3 mmHg with placebo in subjects with a mean baseline DBP of 98 mmHg. In this case, the results are clinically different due to 11 mmHg average difference and subjects are achieving goal DBP values from baseline (<85 mmHg). However, atorvastatin lowering mean LDL-C by 1.7% greater than simvastatin (37.1% vs. 35.4%; p = 0.0097[58]) can be considered not clinically different in subjects with a mean baseline LDL-C of 181 mg/dL. The mean LDL-C was reduced by <2% more with atorvastatin than simvastatin, a difference that most likely is not associated with producing clinical differences in effect. In addition, the actual mean LDL-C lowering was almost identical (66 mg/dL) and the mean LDL-C level at study end was <116 mg/dL in both groups.

Some readers may consider the trial results to be clinically different while others may not. In fact, two people may have different conclusions after reading the same clinical trial. One person may consider the difference in effect between the intervention and control to be clinically different while the other may not. This situation is very common in health care practice of interpreting clinical trials. In response, readers must justify their own conclusion regarding their decision of clinical difference. A few suggestions and examples are provided to assist in determining clinical difference.

Understanding the instrument that was used in measuring the endpoint is important in assessing clinically significant differences in trials. For example, ordinal data typically uses scales or ranking (e.g., pain and depression scales).[120] Thus the definitions of the minimum and maximum numbers of these scales need to be known. As an example, investigators of a hypothetical clinical trial concluded that glucosamine (500 mg three times a day) reduced pain greater than placebo in men with osteoarthritis (OA) of the knee. Pain intensity difference at rest was assessed by a 10-point visual analog scale (0 = no pain; 10 = severe pain). The mean (SD) scores were 3.6 (2.5) with placebo versus 3.3 (2.5) with glucosamine (p = 0.03) at the end of the trial. Although results are statistically significant between glucosamine and placebo, the mean difference in scores between these two groups is minimal, only 0.5 points on a 10-point scale. Stating a clinical difference between glucosamine and placebo would be considered incorrect.

Note that the above clinical trial example reported the average for ordinal data. According to the information presented earlier in this chapter, only the median and mode are to be used in presenting this type of data. Investigators of clinical trials commonly present the mean for ordinal data when reporting results of clinical trials, although this practice may not be appropriate. This issue has been debated, both for and against this method of summarizing the data.[151]

Another issue to consider is that clinical trials with too large of a sample size (i.e., over-powered) lead to smaller p values versus those with smaller sample sizes.[112,119] The magnitude of the p value is dependent on sample size; small differences in effect can be statistically significant with large sample size.[113] Thus, statistically significant results can occur even though a small absolute difference in effect is present. An example of this issue is a clinical trial that compared esomeprazole (n = 2624) versus lansoprazole (n = 2617). The primary endpoint, incidence of erosive esophagitis healing, was statistically significant in favor of es-omeprazole (92.6% vs. 88.8%; p = 0.0001).[147] The investigators (and marketing advertisements) conclude esomeprazole to be superior to lansoprazole, although the absolute difference in healing was only 4% between these two drugs. In addition, a significant number of subjects in each group (>88%) experienced erosive esophagitis healing. Readers can debate whether the difference in effect is clinically different.

A data assessment technique that can be misleading is converting a continuous endpoint measure into a dichotomous value. For instance, blood pressure (continuous value) is measured after an intervention (rofecoxib) and control (celecoxib) are administered. Those subjects with a blood pressure above a predefined cut-off point are classified as being hypertensive (nominal data because subject has a blood pressure value below or above this cut-off point). Significantly more subjects taking rofecoxib versus celecoxib were diagnosed with systolic hypertension (17% vs. 11%, respectively; p = 0.032). However, the mean change in SBP values was +2.6 mmHg versus –0.5 mmHg, respectively (p = 0.007).[148] These two data sets assessed together indicate that rofecoxib may not negatively affect SBP compared to celecoxib. The actual SBP in the subjects taking rofecoxib may have just exceeded the cut-off hypertensive value (increase >20 mmHg with absolute value >140 mmHg) while just below this value for the celecoxib (i.e., 141 mmHg vs. 139 mmHg, respectively). The absolute difference between these two blood pressure values is minimal (2 mmHg), but the number of subjects counted as hypertensive is different (6%). The change in SBP between these two medications does not appear to be clinically different. Even though the measured endpoints between subjects randomized to the intervention are numerically close to the control, the subjects were categorized differently based on cut-off blood pressure values. This example illustrates the potential biases of this form of data analysis and presentation.

CONFIDENCE INTERVALS

More clinical trials are including 95% CI with the study results, which can assist in assessing clinical difference between the intervention and control. CI provide data that address the size of effect (e.g., mean reduction in DBP) of the intervention under investigation in a clinical trial by presenting a range that likely covers the true but unknown value.[149,150] Although the basis of accepting or rejecting the H_0 is based on the p value, a limitation of the p value is that the magnitude of difference in effect between the intervention and control groups of a clinical trial is not known, since it is not able to be determined based on a statistical calculation.[119,146] Because of this, the use of a CI can assist in judging the clinical usefulness of the study result.[113] Clinical trials report the effect of an intervention as a point estimate, a single value that can be considered to represent the true effect (e.g., mean reduction in DBP; incidence of MI). For instance, an angiotensin converting enzyme (ACE) inhibitor lowered mean DBP by 8 mmHg; this value would be termed the point estimate. If the study was repeated, a similar, but not exact, reduction in mean DBP may occur (e.g., –10 and –12 mmHg). The presentation of the results only as a point estimate provides the reader with limited information. Clinical trials presenting 95% CI in conjunction with the point estimate enables readers to further critique the study results and determine the usefulness for practice.

CI provides an indication of the outcome within the population and is interpreted as a range of values in which the true value is included. The 95% CI for an average is calculated using the SEM from the trial sample. Recalling the formula for SEM, the SD is divided by the square root of the sample size $(SD/\sqrt{n})$. A 95% CI is equivalent to approximately 2 SEM from the sample mean, with an exact formula of: mean $\pm(1.96 *SEM)$. The SEM is used as opposed to the SD since SEM is more reflective of the population variance, while SD is indicative of the sample.[119,150] A 95% CI is not the only CI reported in the literature and readers of clinical trials need to recognize the changes in the interpretation. A 99% CI indicates more confidence the true, but unknown, endpoint value is in this range than a 95% CI. Thus, the 99% CI range is wider in value than a 95% CI, whereas a 90% CI range is more narrow (i.e., less confident).[150,151]

A 95% CI for a point estimate is a common method of data presentation. Investigators of a clinical trial reported that the mean reduction in DBP with an ACE inhibitor was –11.3 mmHg (95% CI, –8.2 to –14.4 mmHg) in subjects with a mean baseline DBP of 99 mmHg. This indicates that the investigators are 95% confident that the mean DBP reduction in the population is between –8.2 and –14.4 mmHg. An important issue to recognize in interpreting a 95% CI is that there is a lower probability for the mean reduction in DBP at the upper and lower end of the 95% CI range compared to numbers near the point estimate value.[122] The further away a value within the 95% CI range lies from the point estimate, the lower the probability that this value is the actual value for the population. A low probability exists that the ACE inhibitor lowers mean DBP in the population by only –8.2 mmHg compared to a higher probability that mean DBP reduction is closer to the point estimate of 11.3 mmHg (the same is true with the upper end of the 95% CI).

Within this trial, the ACE inhibitor was compared to HCTZ and the mean DBP reduction with HCTZ was –9.9 mmHg (95% CI, –7.5 to –13.3 mmHg). The same principles are used to interpret this 95% CI: the investigators are 95% confident that the mean reduction of DBP in the population with HCTZ is between 7.5 and 13.3 mmHg. In addition, these two 95% CI ranges can be compared to determine any difference in effect between these two agents. Since both 95% CI ranges overlap considerably, no difference in effect is concluded.[113,119,151]

However, if no overlap of the 95% CI for the two groups is present, a clinical difference can be concluded.

Another common method of data presentation is calculating a 95% CI for the difference of the point estimates between two groups. In the above trial example, the point estimate of mean DBP lowering with the ACE inhibitor was –11.3 mmHg while –9.9 mmHg for HCTZ. The difference in mean DBP between these two equals –1.4 mmHg (–11.3 – (–9.9) = –1.4). The 95% CI for the difference in the point estimates is calculated to be –3.9 to +1.1 mmHg. This is interpreted as being 95% confident that the difference in mean DBP reduction can be 1.1 mmHg greater with HCTZ (e.g., –13.1 mmHg for HCTZ vs. –12 mmHg for ACE inhibitor) or 3.9 mmHg greater with the ACE inhibitor (e.g., –16.9 mmHg for ACE inhibitor vs. –13 mmHg for HCTZ). Notice the upper end of the 95% CI of the difference in point estimates is a positive number (+1.1 mmHg). This does not indicate that the mean DBP was increased, only that the difference in mean DBP lowering was 1.1 mmHg greater with HCTZ compared to ACE inhibitor (e.g., –12 – (–13.1) mmHg for ACE inhibitor and HCTZ, respectively). Also in this 95% CI is the number 0; this indicates with 95% CI that no difference in mean DBP between these two groups (e.g., –13.2 – (–13.2) mmHg for both agents equals zero). If no zero is in the 95% CI of the difference between the two point estimates, then a clinical difference in effect between the intervention and control could be concluded. Again, the interpretation of clinical difference using 95% CI is dependent on clinical experience and appropriate assessment. A 95% CI without a zero in the range does not always indicate a clinical difference between the intervention and control. For example, a 95% CI for mean DBP lowering in a trial comparing an ACE inhibitor and HCTZ was –1.9 to –0.5 mmHg. Even though this 95% CI range does not contain a zero, a mean difference of only 0.5 to 1.9 mmHg greater DBP lowering effect with one agent would not be considered clinically different.

INTERPRETING RISKS AND NUMBERS-NEEDED-TO-TREAT

Some clinical trials are designed to determine if a reduction in an adverse event occurs with the intervention compared to the control. Examples of an adverse event are incidence of MI, stroke, hospitalization, or death. Since the endpoint is dichotomous (i.e., occurred or did not occur), the results can be set up in a table, as illustrated in Table 6–8. As seen from the table, the subjects randomized to the intervention are represented by either A (number of subjects

TABLE 6–8. PRESENTING NOMINAL DATA STUDY RESULTS

Group	Adverse Event	
	Yes	No
Intervention	A	B
Control	C	D

experiencing the adverse event) or B (those without the adverse event). Subjects assigned to the control group and experiencing the adverse event are designated by C while those without the adverse event by D.[151,152]

Afterward, the investigator (or reader) can calculate the measures of association (RR, RRR, ARR, and NNT). These four calculations provide another method to interpret the clinical difference in effect between the intervention and control of clinical trials measuring a nominal endpoint. Table 6–9 displays the formulas to calculate these four values and also provides a description of these measures.[151,152] A description of interpreting these values follows. The RR is calculated as the proportion of the intervention group experiencing the adverse event divided by the proportion of the control group with the event. The RR equaled to 1 indicates no difference between the intervention and control (i.e., the incidence of the adverse event was not increased nor decreased with the intervention compared to control). Anytime a numerator divided by a denominator calculates to 1, these two variables are equal. The RR < 1 signifies the intervention lowered the risk of the adverse event compared to the control; a lower proportion of the intervention group compared to the control experienced the adverse event. The RR > 1 indicates the intervention increased the risk of the adverse event; a greater proportion of the intervention group had the adverse event compared to control. As an example, a RR of death equal to 0.70 was reported in a clinical trial in which subjects were randomized to either simvastatin (n = 2221) or placebo (n = 2223).[75] The RR was calculated by dividing the proportion of the subjects who died taking simvastatin (n = 182) by the proportion of those who died taking placebo (n = 256). The calculation of RR for this trial: (182/2221)/(256/2223). The RR is <1, which indicates simvastatin lowered the risk of death by almost one-third of the baseline risk compared to placebo. RRR indicates the relative change in the adverse event rate between the intervention and control groups. The RRR was calculated as 30% (1 − 0.70); thus the risk of experiencing death was 30%

TABLE 6–9. MEASURES OF ASSOCIATION DESCRIPTION AND FORMULAS

Measure of Association	Description	Formula
RR	Amount of risk removed by the intervention compared to the control	$[A/(A + B)]/[C/(C + D)]$
RRR	Percentage of baseline risk removed	$1 - RR$
ARR	Percentage of subjects treated with the intervention spared the adverse outcome compared with the control	$[C/(C + D)] - [A/(A + B)]$
NNT	Number of subjects needed to be treated to prevent one adverse event. A time course is included that represents the average (or median) duration of follow-up during the trial	$1/(ARR)$

lower by treating these subjects with simvastatin instead of placebo. ARR refers to the difference in the adverse event rate between the intervention and control groups. A higher proportion of subjects taking placebo died (n = 256 of 2223 or 11.5%) compared to those taking simvastatin (182 of 2221 or 8.2%). The ARR for death associated with simvastatin in this trial equals 3.3% (ARR = 11.5% – 8.2%); thus 3.3% of the subjects receiving simvastatin were spared death compared to placebo. The NNT of this study equals 30 (NNT = 1/0.033), meaning 30 subjects need to be treated for a median of 5.4 years with simvastatin instead of placebo to prevent one case of death. The trial had a median follow-up time period of 5.4 years.

Many clinical trials present an endpoint as a relative change, which can be a misleading value. For instance, the RRR of invasive breast cancer associated with tamoxifen was 49% compared to placebo. Although this value appears very beneficial to subjects at risk for breast cancer, the absolute risk needs to be evaluated besides just the RRR value. The actual incidence of invasive breast cancer was 1.33% (89 of 6681 subjects treated with tamoxifen) versus 2.61% (175 of 6707 subjects treated with placebo), which calculates to an absolute difference of 1.28% (ARR). Even though almost 50% less subjects (a relative difference) developed invasive breast cancer with tamoxifen, this represents only a difference of 86 of almost 6700 subjects.[153]

All four measures of association can be calculated for clinical trials measuring nominal data and assessed together for the reader to determine the clinical difference in effect between the intervention and control. As seen by the simvastatin example above (plus Table 6–9), the same study result (e.g., death) can be presented using four different methods with different meanings. However, readers should not be misled by clinical trials that only present and discuss one of these values, which usually is the most appealing value (i.e., the one that seems to show the greatest difference) of these. In fact, studies have documented that practitioners are more inclined to select a therapy presented as RRR more often if the same study result was presented as all four values (ARR, RR, RRR, NNT).[154] Thus, investigators may be biased and selectively present the most appealing of these four values to mislead the reader in concluding a greater difference in effect among the intervention and control, even though the difference may be minimal.

CI also can be calculated for nominal endpoints presented as RR or hazard ratio (HR). The same formula for RR is use to calculate HR, which refers to whether the hazard of the adverse event (i.e., MI and hospitalization) is lowered or increased with the intervention compared to the control.[155] According to the formula for RR (and HR), a calculated value of 1 signifies that the incidence of the adverse event is equal between the intervention and control (i.e., numerator and denominator are equal and therefore no difference).[113,151] As previously mentioned, a RR < 1 signifies that the intervention lowered the risk and a RR > 1 is interpreted as the intervention increasing the risk of the adverse event compared to the control. Therefore investigators of a clinical trial presenting an RR (or HR) with a 95% CI that lies entirely on one side of 1 (i.e., up to 0.99 or 1.01 and upward) indicates a difference in effect between the intervention and control. The 95% CI range for death in the simvastatin study was entirely below 1 (0.58 to 0.85),[75] which is interpreted as the investigators are 95% confident that the RR of death associated with simvastatin is between 0.58 and 0.85 for the population. Also since 1 is not in this range, the investigators are 95% confident that the RR of experiencing the adverse event is reduced with simvastatin (i.e., difference in effect). Using the WHI trial as another example, the calculated HR for the primary endpoint was 1.2 with a 95% CI of 1.09 to 2.01.[53] This information indicates that the investigators are 95% confident that the risk of CHD is increased with the CEE/MPE versus placebo in the population since the HR is >1. Also, the investigators were 95% confident that this combination medication increased CHD risk in the population since the 95% CI for this endpoint did not go below 1. However, a 95% CI containing the value of 1 indicates that the intervention may have neither lowered nor increased the risk (or hazard) of the adverse event. For instance, in the WHI trial, the HR for death due to other causes was 0.92 (95% CI, 0.74 to 1.14).[53] The 95% CI range lies on both sides of 1 and indicates that the risk of death could be lowered to 0.74 or increased to 1.14 with CEE/MPE. Furthermore, the HR could equal 1, a value indicating the risk being equal (i.e., no difference between CEE/MPE and placebo). Thus, the investigator (or reader) would conclude that CEE/MPE is no different than placebo in decreasing or increasing the risk of death.

"NO DIFFERENCE" DOES NOT INDICATE "EQUIVALENCY"

Clinical studies reporting p values greater than the α value translate into no statistical significance; thus no clinical difference in effect is declared between the intervention and control groups. The H_0 is accepted (fail-to-be-rejected) and the H_1 is rejected; in response, the statement of "no difference" is accepted.[118,145] The H_0 is not written to state that the intervention and control are the same, but to state that there is no difference in the effect (i.e., endpoint measurement) between the intervention and control. Studies accepting the H_0 have the possibility of a Type II error. A difference in effect between the intervention and control groups may be present, but, either by chance or a small sample size, the difference in effect was not detected. In this latter instance, the clinical trial may not have been powered sufficiently to detect the difference. Usually (but not all of the time) clinical trials in which the H_0 is accepted have too small of a sample size.[113] In fact, some studies may even be designed with an insufficient sample size so the investigators may claim equivalence between the intervention and active control after rejecting the H_0 even though a trial with an appropriate sample size could detect a difference. But unfortunately, the trial results are incorrectly interpreted as though the intervention and control are the same. This situation can occur in articles and/or presentations that are biased. However, the correct interpretation should be "no difference" detected. As one author stated, "absence of evidence is not evidence of absence."[112]

ASSESSING THE CLINICAL MEANINGFULNESS OF THE RESULTS

All clinical trial results, whether statistically significant or not, need to be evaluated for the clinical meaningfulness (i.e., relevance).[121] In other words, "What do these results mean to practice?" Small treatment effects and/or differences may be statistically different, but really not mean much clinically.[60,79,113] For example, an antihypertensive medication lowered mean DBP by 5 mmHg versus 2 mmHg for placebo (p = 0.04). The H_0 was rejected due to statistical difference. However, mean baseline DBP was 98 mmHg and this antihypertensive medication only lowered mean DBP to 93 mmHg, which is still classified as hypertensive.[156] Thus, practitioners would not consider these results to be clinically meaningful. In other words, these results are not useful in treating patients with hypertension.

On the other hand, a small difference in effect that is statistically different may be of clinical importance, depending on the perspective of the reader. A long-term care pharmacist who specializes in geriatrics may consider a trial reporting a reduced number of incontinence episodes, on average, by two in a 24-hour period with a new anticholinergic agent compared to placebo to be clinically meaningful compared to a pharmacist who does not routinely care for elderly patients. The new drug may reduce nursing time and improve the overall quality of life in patients with incontinence.

Not all clinical trials reporting nonstatistically significant results are completely devoid of clinical importance. The overall effect of the intervention and control need to be assessed. A study compared lansoprazole (30 mg; n = 421) to omeprazole (20 mg; n = 431); each group received once-daily therapy for a duration of 8 weeks. The healing rates of erosive reflux esophagitis were 87.2% versus 87%, respectively, via ITT analysis (p = NS).[157] No clinical difference is concluded from this study, but these results would be considered to be clinically meaningful (i.e., clinically relevant) since >85% of patients were healed with either therapy.

STANDARD OF CARE

Clinical trial results of the intervention may be statistically significant and clinically different than the control, but may be not clinically practical. The clinical trial methods need to be reviewed for the ability to replicate these into everyday patient care. A clinical trial may be designed to consist of technologies and/or include personnel that may not be readily accessible in patient care areas. Another issue to consider is the demands on the actual patient. At times, investigators offer incentives (i.e., monetary compensation and free medical care) for the subjects to strictly follow the study protocol (i.e., more motivated to be compliant). But in practice, real patients may not be as eager to follow an intricate schedule. For example, bismuth subsalicylate can be taken as a prophylaxis against traveler's diarrhea.[158] Although a clinical trial reported that the suspension of subsalicylate bismuth 60 mL four times daily reduced the incidence of this unfortunate experience during travel,[159] some individuals may not be willing to adhere to this dosing schedule. Another issue to consider before applying the clinical trial results into practice is the normal care for patients with the disease/condition under study. Endpoint results of an intervention may be statistically significant and clinically different from the active control, but the control is not normally prescribed for patients with the disease/condition.[79]

Bibliography/References

References are a very important part of the manuscript. The reference or bibliography section is at the end of the manuscript and provides documentation to support the information provided in the manuscript or acknowledgement for the work of other authors.[43] Any material that the author uses in the manuscript should be appropriately cited. References included in the manuscript should be recent (e.g., outdated articles should not be used unless the results of the article are pertinent to the manuscript) and complete. Readers should scan the references listed in the bibliography to determine if the authors used material from reputable sources. In addition, authors should refrain from extensively citing only their own work.[160] References typically should be listed in a numerical order (e.g., Arabic numerals) as they appear in the manuscript; however, several referencing styles exist and are journal dependent. At a minimum, the information in the reference section should be sufficient to lead the reader to locating the same article. Some readers may wish to verify the cited information, while others search for articles in the reference section to gather additional information regarding a topic.[43]

Acknowledgments

Individuals contributing to the clinical trial, but who do not meet the requirements for authorship, can be recognized in this section (see Chap. 11 for more information). Examples of persons identified are those providing manuscript preparation, technical assistance, or donors of equipment or supplies. Medical writers or editors also may be listed if their contributions were significant. A collaboration or group may receive recognition in the acknowledgement section; however, many journals have a prespecified amount of space for the acknowledgment section that must be adhered to by authors. Authors must obtain written permission from persons acknowledged before listing in this section, so that the readers do not infer endorsements of the data and conclusions from these contributors.[33,43]

Other types of information may be included in this section. Such items are financial support (see below for more information) and an indication that the manuscript underwent peer-review, signified by a series of dates and titled received/revised/accepted. Typically, there are at least 4 to 8 weeks between these dates since it is necessary to allow time for the reviewers to comment, the authors to revise and then for another review of the manuscript. Some journals only present the manuscript acceptance date. This date allows readers to determine the lag time between the article being accepted in final form to publication. Hopefully, a minimal time period is between acceptance and the publication date, which increases the chances that the article content remains current.

Funding

Due to the enormous expense required to conduct a clinical trial, investigators seek financial assistance to conduct the research. Various funding sources are available that include pharmaceutical companies, government agencies (e.g., National Institutes of Health [NIH]), national organizations (e.g., American Cancer Society), university grants (e.g., faculty development grants), and private donations. According to an assessment of 500 randomly selected clinical trials published in five highly recognized medical journals from 1981 to 2000 (e.g., *N Engl J Med* and *JAMA*), the primary funding source (36% of the studies) was the pharmaceutical industry, either independently or jointly. In addition, a trend was observed toward a greater percentage increase of trials with pharmaceutical industry support over this time period. Furthermore, the study results documented a significant increase in the number of authors being affiliated with a pharmaceutical company.[161]

During 2003, an estimated $33 billion was spent by the pharmaceutical companies for research and development (which includes clinical drug trials); approximately 80% of this figure consisted of domestic research and development.[162] The pharmaceutical industry is responsible for a significant amount of the clinical research conducted worldwide. Thus, readers of industry-sponsored research should be cognizant of possible conflicts of interest, defined as "a set of conditions in which professional judgment concerning a primary interest (such as a patient's welfare of the validity of research) tends to be unduly influenced by a secondary interest (such as financial gain)"[163] that may result in potential bias. Conflicts of interest arise because the industry may be prompted to publish articles as a means of making their product appear better for a disease state in relation to the standard of care. This research may result in methodological bias, premature termination of trials for nonscientific/ nonethical reasons, or reporting/publication bias.[164,165]

The study design, result presentation style, data interpretations, and study conclusions should be assessed appropriately to determine if the funding source had any influences on the overall clinical trial. A clinical trial should not be automatically rejected by the reader due to the funding agency. For instance, pharmaceutical companies need to determine the clinical usefulness of newly developed medications. These companies are expecting to profit from the new medication being approved by the FDA and marketed to prescribers. Many organizations (e.g., government and nonprofit) are not prime candidates to offer funding for these studies, which leaves the pharmaceutical company to sponsor the study.

Not all investigator-pharmaceutical industry relationships have the potential to cause a conflict of interest, but readers should decide if a publication is biased. In fact, many well-designed, clinically important studies documenting a reduction in morbidity and mortality have been sponsored by the pharmaceutical industry and these have changed the standards of practice in treating patients.

However, there have been reports in the literature of selected pharmaceutical companies terminating studies for various reasons unrelated to efficacy and safety,[165, 166] employing inappropriate comparators,[167] using inappropriate study samples,[168] and suppressing the results of negative studies.[165,169] Furthermore, reports have been published that indicate a favorable conclusion of studies financially supported by the pharmaceutical industry, which can be referred to as publication bias. This type of sponsored research usually yields larger treatment effects than not-for-profit funded studies.[79,165]

Research has documented that the conclusions of some trials funded by for-profit organizations significantly were in favor of the experimental drug as the treatment of choice. But not all pharmaceutical industry-sponsored research is biased; many study results are clinically meaningful. Readers need to be aware that the pharmaceutical company has a lot at stake for an investigational drug to be approved by the FDA. In response, the pharmaceutical company attempts to design a clinical trial to meet the FDA-approval standards. However, the methods of presenting (i.e., Results section), interpreting (i.e., Introduction and/or Discussion sections), and summarizing the data and results (i.e., Conclusion) can be biased and are not governed by the regulations of the FDA. Consequently readers need to evaluate the trial data critically to assess the appropriateness and validity of the reported conclusions based on the trial results.[170]

Commentaries/Clinical Trial Critiques

All journals should provide its readership the opportunity for correspondence to exchange ideas about a topic or relay new information about articles published in the journal.[33,43] Commentaries can be essential in assisting readers interpreting and/or critiquing articles published within the journals by identifying strengths and limitations of the original research, an update to published information, or questions to the authors of the original research manuscript.

Editorials, defined as, "a written expression of opinion that may reflect the official position of the publication,"[43] are short essays from the editor or other experts in a particular field that are written to convey additional opinions about an article, typically, in the same issue of a journal. Not all editorials reflect the ideas/thoughts of the journal because these are opinions of the editorial author. Although editorials may contain some bias, this literature should always be considered when evaluating a clinical trial by providing additional insight of the results and aid in the comprehension of the clinical application of the trial results. For instance, an editorial in response to the WHI trial was published in the same journal issue. The editorial author addressed many issues regarding results of prior estrogen research, suggestions for using the WHI trial results into practice, and concluded "do not use estrogen/progestin to prevent chronic disease."[171]

Several issues should be considered during the preparation or evaluation of editorials. Quality editorials are original; those editorials with nonoriginal ideas need to include a clear justification of repeating these ideas. The editorial objective should be clearly presented and reflect a complete message. The content should be significant to merit publication. The editorial points should be timely with respect of the publication in which the author is responding. Finally, the editorial author should mention the facts clearly and the material should be applicable to the readership of the publication.[172]

Not all original research reports are accompanied by an editorial. Persons seeking an editorial associated with a clinical trial can use a few methods to locate the publication. First, the journal issue that contains the clinical trial will list the editorial title in the journal issue table of contents. Another, not always present in all clinical trials, is a notation printed on the first page of the clinical trial referring the reader to another page (i.e., "For comment, see page …"; "Commentary, page …"). The first page of the WHI trial states "For editorial comment see p. 266."[53] Readers not having access to the actual clinical trial or journal issue table of contents can locate the trial citation in PubMed® (using the Single Citation Matcher at <<http://www.pubmed.gov>>). Those clinical trials with an accompanying editorial will contain a notation of "Comment in" and an abbreviated journal citation (i.e., journal name, date, plus volume, issue, and page numbers). Another method is to search the clinical trial topic (i.e., via Medical Subject Heading term in PubMed®) and limit the search to the publication type of editorial.

Some journals/websites are published for the primary purpose of providing editorials/commentaries addressing a clinical trial. These resources are known as secondary journals and are independent of the journals that directly publish the clinical trials.[35,79,173] Secondary journals are publications that assist the busy practitioners in a few vital methods: keeping them current regarding important and relevant studies, plus presenting key study information in a concise format. Clinical trials are presented, usually in a structured abstract style, but not just "copying and pasting" the exact abstract prepared by the trial investigators. These prepared abstracts may present additional and/or more precise information. In addition, a commentary addressing the study strengths, limitations, and application into practice is authored by a leading practitioner in the field of study. Readers should use these resources while critiquing the biomedical/pharmacy literature.

Examples of secondary journal websites include <<http://www.theheart.org>>, and <<http://www.medscape.com>>. Typically these publications provide an overview of the study followed by a commentary. Medscape is particularly useful for pharmacists since pharmacy-specific topics are addressed in a section of this website. *ACP Journal Club* is an online and print resource in which biomedical literature (i.e., original research and systematic reviews) is selected based on predefined criteria and summarized by an expert in the field in the form of structured abstracts followed by a commentary. More than 100 journals are reviewed and are selected due to their potential impact on clinical practice.[174]

Another example is *Journal Watch,* a print and online resource that is published twice a month in print[175] and numerous times per week on the Internet.[176] Approximately 50 to 55 articles are summarized per month from >180 general and specialty journals by physicians and a commentary is provided to help clinicians determine the impact of the research results on their practice.[176] Several specialty editions of *Journal Watch* are available including Journal Watch Dermatology, Emergency Medicine, Gastroenterology, and Infectious Diseases.[175]

A further example of clinical trial commentaries is Patient-Oriented Evidence That Matters (POEMS), a commentary publication produced by the *Journal of Family Practice*. Each month, 10 articles are presented from 90 journals reviewed by the editorial board pertaining to the practice of primary care in an attempt to address primary care issues, present outcomes research data, and improve practice.[177]

LETTERS-TO-THE-EDITOR

Letters-to-the-editor can provide valuable insight into original research and can include various types of contributions. These may be in the form of comments, addenda, or updates from previously published articles, alerts regarding potential problems in practice, observations/comments on trends in medication use, opinions on trends or controversies in therapy or research, or original research. Authors of letters-to-the-editor must adhere to strict guidelines from the journals regarding the length, number of tables, and format of the publication.[178] The primary content of letters-to-the-editor is feedback from the journal readers regarding the published materials in the journal. Typically, these letters are published within 3 months of the original publication. The letters may disagree with the design, result interpretation, and/or conclusions of the publication. Also, the letters may ask for additional information that can be used to interpret/clarify, comprehend, and/or critique the information within the publication. Afterward, the authors of the original publication often provide a response to each letter.

Conclusion

All pharmacists need skills for efficiently locating, critically evaluating, and effectively communicating drug information, regardless of the practice setting. As the role of the pharmacist in direct patient care continues to increase, incorporating these skills on a daily basis is essential. A multitude of literature is published each year and the quality varies significantly. Readers of the literature should not immediately accept the authors' conclusions but assess the strengths and limitations of the source. The information within this chapter identifies and discusses many issues to consider while reading and analyzing the clinical literature. Although every clinical trial has limitations, those trials with appropriate design and well-presented results are still important to apply into clinical practice. Using the proper techniques in evaluating clinical trials can allow pharmacists to contribute as a problem solver and decision maker in the health care profession.

Study Questions

1. Explain the importance of pharmacists incorporating appropriate literature evaluation skills into their daily practice activities.

2. An open-labeled, controlled clinical trial was conducted to determine if linezolid is comparable to ampicillin-sulbactam to treat diabetic foot infections. Subjects were randomized to either linezolid 600 mg twice a day (n = 227) or ampicillin-sulbactam 3 g every 6 hours (n = 121) for 7 days. The primary endpoint was overall cure, defined as resolution of all clinical signs and symptoms of infection and a healing wound after ≥5 days of therapy. Results of the trial demonstrated a higher overall cure rate with linezolid than ampicillin-sulbactam: 81% (165/203) versus 77% (77/108), respectively (4% difference; 95% CI, –6 to 15%). Adverse effects included diarrhea, nausea, anemia, thrombocytopenia, vomiting, anorexia, and dyspepsia; however, no statistically significant differences in adverse effects between groups were observed (p = 0.82). The investigators concluded that linezolid is as least as effective as comparators among patients with various infections.
   a. Is a parallel design the best study design to use for this research question?
   b. Was an appropriate clinical trial objective and endpoint included in the clinical trial? Explain your response.
   c. Is IRB approval required before this clinical trial is initiated? Explain your response.
   d. Does this clinical trial design require the subjects to complete a subject informed consent form? Explain your response. Describe the purpose of this form.
   e. Define open-label; describe the advantages and disadvantages of open-labeled trials.
   f. Use the 95% CI to discuss the measured difference in effect of the primary endpoint between these two groups.

3. Prior to publishing the clinical trial described in question #2, the editor informs the investigators that peer-review is necessary.
   a. Describe the peer-review process.
   b. Discuss methods in which a reader can determine if the publication was subject to the peer-review process.
   c. List limitations to the peer-review process.

4. The investigators of the clinical trial described in question #2 disclose that Pfizer, the manufacturer of linezolid, funded the research.
   a. Discuss reasons investigators need to disclose potential conflicts of interest.
   b. Identify issues that should be considered while interpreting clinical trials funded by the manufacturer of the intervention.

5. Read the excerpt of the following clinical trial summary and answer the questions that follow.

A randomized, controlled clinical trial was conducted to assess atorvastatin as primary prevention for CV adverse events in subjects with total cholesterol (TC) levels ≤251 mg/dL. The primary endpoint was a reduction in the occurrence of nonfatal, including silent MI, and fatal CHD. Investigators also assessed the following secondary endpoints: total number of CV events and procedures, total coronary events, nonfatal MI and fatal CHD, all-cause mortality, CV mortality, fatal and nonfatal stroke, and fatal and nonfatal HF. Tertiary endpoints included occurrence of silent MI, unstable angina, chronic stable angina, peripheral arterial disease, life-threatening arrhythmias, development of diabetes mellitus, and development of renal impairment. Subjects included in the trial were diagnosed with hypertension, regardless of administration of antihypertensive medications. Also subjects had at least three CV disease risk factors: left-ventricular hypertrophy, specific abnormalities on echocardiogram, Type II diabetes mellitus, peripheral arterial disease, previous stroke or transient ischemic attack, male gender, ≥ 55 years of age, microalbuminuria or proteinuria, smoker, TC to HDL-C ratio ≥ 6, or premature family history of CHD.

Subjects were randomized to atorvastatin 10 mg once daily (n = 5168) or placebo (n = 5137). Neither investigators nor subjects knew which treatment they were receiving. A sample size of ≥18,000 was estimated for a 5-year follow-up time period to detect at least a 30% greater reduction in the primary endpoint with atorvastatin. The investigators estimated that a 10% β error was possible. All results were analyzed using the intention-to-treat analysis via chi-square. p values < 0.05 were considered statistically significant. The trial was concluded earlier (median 3.3 years) than originally planned.

The majority of the clinical trial participants were white (95%) and male (81%); the average age was 63 years. The mean number of additional CV risk factors was 3.7 per person. The mean baseline TC was 212 mg/dL and LDL-C was 131 mg/dL. Almost 99% of the randomized subjects had data at the closure of the clinical trial. The incidence of the primary endpoint in the atorvastatin group versus placebo group was 1.9 and 3%, respectively (HR = 0.64; 95% CI, 0.5 to 0.83; p = 0.0005). The mean TC and LDL-C level reductions at the clinical trial conclusion were 19% and 29%, respectively, in the atorvastatin treatment group. The nonprimary endpoints, resulting in statistically significant incident reductions in the atorvastatin treatment versus placebo were total CV events including revascularization procedures (p = 0.0005); total coronary events (3.4% vs. 4.8%; p = 0.0005); and primary endpoint, excluding silent MI (p = 0.0005). Subgroup analysis of subjects with diabetes (n = 2532) indicates no statistically significant reduction in the primary endpoint with atorvastatin. However, analysis of subjects aged >60 years (n = 6570 and fairly equally distributed between the two groups) experienced a significant reduction in the primary endpoint in the atorvastatin group versus placebo (2.2% vs. 3.4%; HR = 0.64; 95% CI, 0.47 to 0.86; p = 0.0027). The investigators concluded that CV adverse events can be lowered using atorvastatin 10 mg in nondyslipidemic, hypertensive subjects at moderate risk for CV events.

a. During a medical/pharmacy meeting, a physician submits the investigators' abstract of the above clinical trial as evidence that all patients with dyslipidemia should be treated with atorvastatin. Do you agree or disagree with this statement? Explain your response.

b. Was the primary endpoint an appropriate endpoint for the study question? Explain your response.

c. What is a composite endpoint? Should this type of endpoint be used for this clinical trial?

d. State the type of data that describes the primary endpoint.

e. State all the measure(s) of central tendency that can be used for the primary endpoint.

f. Define the type of blinding included in the article. Describe whether this clinical trial was either "strengthened" or "weakened" by the blinding type.

g. Define randomization. Describe whether this clinical trial was either strengthened or weakened by including randomization in the study design.

h. Was appropriate subject inclusion criteria included? Is a selection bias present? Explain your responses.

i. Discuss the significance of the ITT principle being included in the study design.

j. Was a power analysis conducted? If so, was the calculation and resulting percentage appropriate? Discuss the significance of including a power analysis in the study design.

k. State the H_0 (based on the primary endpoint).

l. State the p value for the primary endpoint. Was an appropriate α value included in this clinical trial? Explain your response.

m. State whether the primary endpoint was statistically significant or not. Explain your response.

n. State whether to fail-to-reject (accept) or reject the H_0. Explain your response.

o. State the type of error that can occur (based on the primary endpoint). What is/are the potential cause(s)?

p. Interpret the primary endpoint results using the 95% CI.

q. Calculate and interpret the measures of association for the primary endpoint (ARR, RRR, NNT).

r. Based on the information provided, describe whether the primary endpoint was clinically different between the intervention and control groups. Explain your response.

s. During the meeting, the physician also is very adamant that all elderly patients (>60 years) with dyslipidemia should receive atorvastatin therapy because a reduction in nonfatal, including silent MI, and fatal CHD was observed in this clinical trial. Is this appropriate? Explain your response.

   t. Total CV events including revascularization procedures between groups resulted in statistically significant differences. What other conclusions can be drawn from this result?

6. Investigators conducted a trial to compare mean change in LDL-C levels in subjects receiving a low carbohydrate (n = 35) versus a conventional diet (n = 35). The median reduction in LDL-C at 3 months for both groups was 10 mg/dL. The mean change in LDL-C levels at 3 months was –11.74 ±4.7 mg/dL and –9.74 ±1.2 mg/dL (p = 0.007), respectively.

   a. Differentiate between the mean and median values for the change in LDL-C levels.

   b. What values of change in LDL-C level at 3 months in the low carbohydrate group is represented by ±1 SD?

7. Describe other resources that are available to assist in critiquing and interpreting clinical trials.

REFERENCES

1. CDER new molecular entity (NME) drug and new biologic approvals in calendar year 2004. [accessed 2005 Jan 2]. Available from: http://www.fda.gov/cder/rdmt/NMEDY2004.HTM.
2. Safety alerts for drugs, biologics, devices, and dietary supplements. [accessed 2005 Jan 2]. Available from: http://www.fda.gov/ medwatch/SAFETY/2004/safety04.htm.
3. National Library of Medicine (PubMed®). [accessed 2005 Jan 2]. Available from: http://www.ncbi. nlm.nih.gov/entrez/ query.fcgi.
4. Levy S. Consumers say "thank you!" Drug Topics. 2004;148(6):44–6, 49, 50, 52.
5. Calis KA, Hutchison LC, Elliott ME, Ives TJ, Zillich AJ, Poirier T, et al. Healthy people 2010: challenges, opportunities, and a call to action for America's pharmacists. Pharmacotherapy. 2004;24: 1241–94.
6. Curtiss FR. Clinical pharmacist intervention in a primary care medical group reduces financial losses [editorial]. J Manag Care Pharm. 2004;10:355.
7. Hepler CD. Clinical pharmacy, pharmaceutical care, and the quality of drug therapy. Pharmacotherapy. 2004;24:1491–8.
8. ASHP Council on Professional Affairs. ASHP guidelines on the pharmacist's role in the development, implementation, and assessment of critical pathways. Am J Health Syst Pharm. 2004;61:939–45.
9. Czubak R, Tucker J, Zarowitz B. Optimizing drug prescribing in managed care populations: improving clinical and economic outcomes. Dis Manag Health Outcomes. 2004;12:147–67.
10. Wright SG, LeCroy RL, Kendrach MG. The three types of biomedical literature and systematic approach to handle a drug information request. J Pharm Pract. 1998;XI:148–62.
11. Greenhalgh T. How to read a paper. The MEDLINE® database. BMJ. 1997;315:180–3.
12. Lowe HJ, Barnett GO. Understanding and using the medical subject headings (MeSH) vocabulary to perform literature searches. JAMA. 1994;271:1103–8.
13. Rosenberg W, Donald A. Evidence based medicine: an approach to clinical problem-solving. BMJ. 1995;310:1122–6.
14. Sackett D, Richardson W, Rosenberg W, Haynes R. Evidence-based medicine: how to practice and teach EBM. London, UK: Churchill Livingstone; 1997.

15. Whitcomb ME. Why we must teach evidence-based medicine. Acad Med. 2005;80:1–2.

16. Green SB. Design of randomized trials. Epidemiol Rev. 2002;24:4–11.

17. Sibbald B, Roland M. Understanding controlled trials. Why are randomised controlled trials important? BMJ. 1998;316:201.

18. New drug application (NDA) process. [accessed 2005 Jan 2]. Available from: http://www.fda.gov/cder/regulatory/ applications/NDA.htm.

19. Gehlbach S. Interpreting the medical literature. 4th ed. New York: McGraw-Hill; 2002.

20. Doll R. Controlled trials: the 1948 watershed. BMJ. 1998;317:1217–20.

21. Kunz R, Oxman AD. The unpredictability paradox: review of empirical comparisons of randomized and nonrandomized clinical trials. BMJ. 1998;317:1185–90.

22. Kendrach MG, Anderson HG. Fundamentals of controlled clinical trials. J Pharm Pract. 1998;XI:163–80.

23. Moher D, Schulz KF, Altman D. The CONSORT statement: revised recommendations for improving the quality of reports of parallel-group randomized trials. JAMA. 2001;285:1987–91.

24. Friedman L, Furberg C, DeMets D. Fundamentals of clinical trials. 3rd ed. New York: Springer; 1998.

25. Lader EW, Cannon CP, Ohman EM, Newby LK, Sulmasy DP, Barst RJ, et al. The clinician as investigator: participating in clinical trials in the practice setting: Appendix 1: fundamentals of study design. Circulation. 2004;109:e302–e304.

26. DeAngelis CD, Drazen JM, Frizelle FA, Haug C, Hoey J, Horton R, et al. Clinical trial registration: a statement from the International Committee of Medical Journal Editors. JAMA. 2004;292:1363–4.

27. Krzyzanowska MK, Pintilie M, Tannock IF. Factors associated with failure to publish large randomized trials presented at an oncology meeting. JAMA. 2003;290:495–501.

28. Rennie D. Trial registration: a great idea switches from ignored to irresistible. JAMA. 2004;292:1359–62.

29. DeMets DL, Pocock SJ, Julian DG. The agonizing negative trend in monitoring of clinical trials. Lancet. 1999;354:1983–8.

30. Pharmaceutical companies to make more information available about clinical trials. [accessed 2005 Jan 10]. Available from: http://www.phrma.org/mediaroom/press/releases/06.01.2005.1112.cfm.

31. Grass G. Clinical trial registration. N Engl J Med. 2005;352:198–9.

32. Kaptchuk TJ. Effect of interpretive bias on research evidence. BMJ. 2003;326:1453–5.

33. Uniform requirements for manuscripts submitted to biomedical journals: writing and editing for biomedical publication. [accessed 2004 Dec 10]. Available from: http://www.icmje.org.

34. Armstrong PW, Newby LK, Granger CB, Lee KL, Simes RJ, Van de Werf F, et al. Lessons learned from a clinical trial. Circulation. 2004;110:3610–4.

35. Cook DJ, Meade MO, Fink MP. How to keep up with the critical care literature and avoid being buried alive. Crit Care Med. 1996;24:1757–68.

36. Blumenthal D. Doctors and drug companies. N Engl J Med. 2004;351:1885–90.

37. Majumdar SR, Chang WC, Armstrong PW. Do the investigative sites that take part in a positive clinical trial translate that evidence into practice? Am J Med. 2002;113:140–5.

38. Naylor CD. Putting evidence into practice. Am J Med. 2002;113:161–3.

39. Weller A. Editorial peer-review. Its strengths and weaknesses. Medford (NJ): American Society for Information Science and Technology; 2001.

40. Hirsh J, Guyatt G, Albers GW, Schunemann HJ. The seventh ACCP conference on antithrombotic and thrombolytic therapy: evidence-based guidelines. Chest. 2004;126:172S–3S.

41. Lader EW, Cannon CP, Ohman EM, Newby LK, Sulmasy DP, Barst RJ, et al. The clinician as investigator: participating in clinical trials in the practice setting. Circulation. 2004;109:2672–9.

42. Studdert DM, Mello MM, Brennan TA. Financial conflicts of interest in physicians' relationships with the pharmaceutical industry—self-regulation in the shadow of federal prosecution. N Engl J Med. 2004;351:1891–1900.

43. Iverson C, Flanagin A, Fontanarosa P, Glass R, Glitman P, Lantz J, et al., editors. American Medical Association Manual of Style. A guide for authors and editors. 9th ed. Baltimore (MD): Williams & Wilkins; 1998.

44. Nelson HS, Bensch G, Pleskow WW, DiSantostefano R, DeGraw S, Reasner DS, et al. Improved bronchodilation with levalbuterol compared with racemic albuterol in patients with asthma. J Allergy Clin Immunol. 1998;102:943–52.

45. Peat J, Elliott E, Baur L, Keena V. Scientific writing: easy when you know how. London: BMJ Books; 2002.

46. Widerquist JG. Abstract writing. Hosp Mater Manage Q. 2000;22:58–63.

47. Dupuy A, Khosrotehrani K, Lebbe C, Rybojad M, Morel P. Quality of abstracts in 3 clinical dermatology journals. Arch Dermatol. 2003;139:589–93.

48. Hartley J. Current findings from research on structured abstracts. J Med Libr Assoc. 2004;92: 368–71.

49. Harris AH, Standard S, Brunning JL, Casey SL, Goldberg JH, Oliver L, et al. The accuracy of abstracts in psychology journals. J Psychol. 2002;136:141–8.

50. Pitkin RM, Branagan MA, Burmeister LF. Accuracy of data in abstracts of published research articles. JAMA. 1999;281:1110–1.

51. Ward LG, Kendrach MG, Price SO. Accuracy of abstracts for original research articles in pharmacy journals. Ann Pharmacother. 2004;38:1173–7.

52. Cuddy PG, Elenbaas RM, Elenbaas JK. Evaluating the medical literature. Part I: abstract, introduction, methods. Ann Emerg Med. 1983;12:549–55.

53. Rossouw JE, Anderson GL, Prentice RL, LaCroix AZ, Kooperberg C, Stefanick ML, et al. Risks and benefits of estrogen plus progestin in healthy postmenopausal women: principal results from the women's health initiative randomized controlled trial. JAMA. 2002;288:321–33.

54. Motheral B. Research methodology: hypotheses, measurement, reliability, and validity. J Manag Care Pharm. 1999;4:382–8

55. Hulley SB, Cummings SR, Browner WS, Grady D, Hearst N, Newman TB. Designing Clinical Research. 2nd ed. Philadelphia (PA): Lippincott Williams & Wilkins; 2001.

56. Mednick D, Day D. Method is everything: evaluating results by study design. J Manag Care Pharm. 1997;3:66–8, 71–2, 75–6.

57. Bakker-Arkema RG, Davidson MH, Goldstein RJ, Davignon J, Isaacsohn JL, Weiss SR, et al. Efficacy and safety of a new HMG-CoA reductase inhibitor, atorvastatin, in patients with hypertriglyceridemia. JAMA. 1996;275:128–33.

58. Karalis DG, Ross AM, Vacari RM, Zarren H, Scott R. Comparison of efficacy and safety of atorvastatin and simvastatin in patients with dyslipidemia with and without coronary heart disease. Am J Cardiol. 2002;89:667–71.

59. Berger VW, Exner DV. Detecting selection bias in randomized clinical trials. Control Clin Trials. 1999;20:319–27.

60. Naylor CD, Guyatt GH. Users' guides to the medical literature. X. How to use an article reporting variations in the outcomes of health services. The Evidence-Based Medicine Working Group. JAMA. 1996;275:554–8.

61. Berger VW, Rezvani A, Makarewicz VA. Direct effect on validity of response run-in selection in clinical trials. Control Clin Trials. 2003;24:156–66.

62. Packer M, Bristow MR, Cohn JN, Colucci WS, Fowler MB, Gibert EM, et al. The effect of carvedilol on morbidity and mortality in patients with chronic heart failure. U.S. Carvedilol Heart Failure Study Group. N Engl J Med. 1996;334:1349–55.

63. von Olshausen K, Pop T, Berger J. Carvedilol in patients with chronic heart failure. N Engl J Med. 1996;335:1318–9; author reply 1319–20.

64. Packer M, Cohn JN, Colucci WS. Carvedilol in patients with chronic heart failure [response]. N Engl J Med. 1996;335:1319–20.

65. Chan FK, Ching JY, Hung LC, Wong VW, Leung VK, Kung NN, et al. Clopidogrel versus aspirin and esomeprazole to prevent recurrent ulcer bleeding. N Engl J Med. 2005;352:238–44.

66. Recruiting Human Subjects. Pressures in industry-sponsored clinical research. Department of Health and Human Services Website. [accessed 2005 Mar 24]. Available from: http://oig.hhs.gov/oei/reports/oei-01-97-00195.pdf.

67. Hebert R. Newspaper advertising could distort research results. Nicotine Tob Res. 2000;2:317–8.

68. Wei SJ, Metz JM, Coyle C, Hampshire M, Jones HA, Markowitz S, et al. Recruitment of patients into an internet-based clinical trials database: the experience of OncoLink and the National Colorectal Cancer Research Alliance. J Clin Oncol. 2004;22:4730–6.

69. Guyatt GH, Sackett DL, Cook DJ. Users' guides to the medical literature. II. How to use an article about therapy or prevention. A. Are the results of the study valid? Evidence-Based Medicine Working Group. JAMA. 1993;270:2598–601.

70. Julious SA. Sample sizes for clinical trials with normal data. Stat Med. 2004;23:1921–86.

71. Vickers AJ, de Craen AJ. Why use placebos in clinical trials? A narrative review of the methodological literature. J Clin Epidemiol. 2000;53:157–61.

72. Yeh SS, DeGuzman B, Kramer T. Reversal of COPD-associated weight loss using the anabolic agent oxandrolone. Chest. 2002;122:421–8.

73. Baker SG, Lindeman KS. Rethinking historical controls. Biostatistics. 2001;2:383–96.

74. Lewis BE, Wallis DE, Berkowitz SD, Matthai WH, Fareed J, Walenga JM, et al. Argatroban anticoagulant therapy in patients with heparin-induced thrombocytopenia. Circulation. 2001;103:1838–43.

75. Randomised trial of cholesterol lowering in 4444 patients with coronary heart disease: the Scandinavian Simvastatin Survival Study (4S). Lancet. 1994;344:1383–9.

76. Simons LA, Nestel PJ, Calvert GD, Jennings GL. Effects of MK-733 on plasma lipid and lipoprotein levels in subjects with hypercholesterolemia. Med J Aust. 1987;147:65–8.

77. Avenell A, Grant AM, McGee M, McPherson G, Campbell MK, McGee MA, et al. The effects of an open design on trial participant recruitment, compliance, and retention—a randomized controlled trial comparison with a blinded, placebo-controlled design. Clin Trials. 2004;1:490–8.

78. Tramer MR, Reynolds DJ, Moore RA, McQuay HJ. When placebo controlled trials are essential and equivalence trials are inadequate. BMJ. 1998;317:875–80.

79. Montori VM, Jaeschke R, Schunemann HJ, Bhandari M, Brozek JL, Devereaux PJ, et al. Users' guide to detecting misleading claims in clinical research reports. BMJ. 2004;329:1093–6.

80. Poole-Wilson PA, Swedberg K, Cleland JG, Di Lendra A, Hanrath P, Komajda M, et al. Comparison of carvedilol and metoprolol on clinical outcomes in patients with chronic heart failure in the carvedilol or metoprolol european trial (COMET): randomised controlled trial. Lancet. 2003;362:7–13.

81. Effect of metoprolol CR/XL in chronic heart failure: metoprolol CR/XL randomised intervention trial in congestive heart failure (MERIT-HF). Lancet. 1999;353:2001–7.

82. Hjalmarson A, Goldstein S, Fagerberg B, Wedel H, Waagstein F, Kjekshus J, et al. Effects of controlled-release metoprolol on total mortality, hospitalizations, and well-being in patients with heart failure: the metoprolol CR/XL randomized intervention trial in congestive heart failure (MERIT-HF). MERIT-HF Study Group. JAMA. 2000;283:1295–302.

83. COMET published, but arguments over metoprolol dose continue. [accessed 2004 June 23]. Available from: <http://www. theheart.org/viewEntityDispatcherAction.do?primaryKey=383844>.

84. COMET: arguments persist one year later. [accessed 2004 June 23]. Available from: http://www. theheart.org/viewEntityDispatcherAction.do?primaryKey=581450.

85. Bal SK. Does the choice of beta-blocker affect outcome in chronic heart failure? CMAJ. 2003;169:1188.

86. Furberg CD, Psaty BM. Carvedilol was more effective than metoprolol tartrate for lowering mortality in chronic heart failure. ACP J Club. 2004;140:5.

87. Wikstrand J, Fagerberg B, Goldstein S, Kjekshus J, Wedel H. COMET: a proposed mechanism of action to explain the results and concerns about dose. Lancet. 2003;362:1076–7; author reply 1077–8.

88. Davidson M, Ma P, Stein EA, Gotto AM, Jr., Raja A, Chitra R, et al. Comparison of effects on low-density lipoprotein cholesterol and high-density lipoprotein cholesterol with rosuvastatin versus atorvastatin in patients with Type IIa or IIb hypercholesterolemia. Am J Cardiol. 2002;89:268–75.

89. Kendrach MG, Kelly-Freeman M. Approximate equivalent rosuvastatin doses for temporary statin interchange programs. Ann Pharmacother. 2004;38:1286–92.

90. Mertl SL. The fundamentals of Institutional Review Board operations. J Pharm Pract. 1996;IX: 437–43.

91. Macklin R. The ethical problems with sham surgery in clinical research. N Engl J Med. 1999;341:992–6.

92. Horng S, Miller FG. Is placebo surgery unethical? N Engl J Med. 2002;347:137–9.

93. Riegelman RK. Studying a study and testing a test: how to read the medical literature. 4th ed. Philadelphia (PA): Lippincott William & Wilkins; 2000.

94. Guyatt G, Rennie D. User's guide to the medical literature. Essentials of evidence-based clinical practice. Chicago, IL: AMA Press; 2002.

95. Collins R, MacMahon S. Reliable assessment of the effects of treatment on mortality and major morbidity, I: clinical trials. Lancet. 2001;357:373–80.

96. Roberts C, Torgerson D. Randomisation methods in controlled trials. BMJ. 1998;317:1301.

97. Roland M, Torgerson D. Understanding controlled trials: what outcomes should be measured? BMJ. 1998;317:1075.

98. Pitt B, Segal R, Martinez FA, Meurers G, Cowley AJ, Thomas I, et al. Randomized trial of losartan versus captopril in patients over 65 with heart failure (Evaluation of Losartan in the Elderly Study, ELITE). Lancet. 1997;349:747–52.

99. Freemantle N, Calvert M, Wood J, Eastaugh J, Griffin C. Composite outcomes in randomized trials: greater precision but with greater uncertainty? JAMA. 2003;289:2554–9.

100. Lubsen J, Kirwan BA. Combined endpoints: can we use them? Stat Med. 2002;21:2959–70.

101. Freemantle N, Calvert M, Wood J, Eastaugh J, Griffin C. Use of composite endpoints to measure clinical events [letter]. JAMA. 2003;290:1457.

102. Lauer MS, Topol EJ. Clinical trials—multiple treatments, multiple endpoints, and multiple lessons [editorial]. JAMA. 2003;289:2575-7.

103. van Leth F, Lange JM. Use of composite endpoints to measure clinical events. JAMA. 2003;290:1456-7; author reply 1457.

104. Cohen M, Demers C, Gurfinkel EP, Turpie AG, Fromell GJ, Goodman S, et al. A comparison of low-molecular-weight heparin with unfractionated heparin for unstable coronary artery disease. Efficacy and Safety of Subcutaneous Enoxaparin in Non-Q-Wave Coronary Events Study Group. N Engl J Med. 1997;337:447-52.

105. Armstrong PW. Heparin in acute coronary disease—requiem for a heavyweight? [editorial] N Engl J Med. 1997;337:492-4.

106. Ohman EM. Enoxaparin reduced combined coronary events in unstable angina and non-Q-wave MI at 14 and 30 days [comment]. ACP J Club. 1998;128:34.

107. Expert Panel on Detection, Evaluation and Treatment of High Blood Cholesterol in Adults. Executive summary of the third report of the national cholesterol education program (NCEP) expert panel on detection, evaluation, and treatment of high blood cholesterol in adults (Adult Treatment Panel III). JAMA. 2001;285:2486-97.

108. Potkin SG, Saha AR, Kujawa MJ, Carson WH, Ali M, Stock E, et al. Aripiprazole, an antipsychotic with a novel mechanism of action, and risperidone vs placebo in patients with schizophrenia and schizoaffective disorder. Arch Gen Psychiatry. 2003;60:681-90.

109. American Psychiatric Association. Practice guidelines for the treatment of psychiatric disorders. Arlington (VA): American Psychiatric Association; 2004.

110. Frequently asked questions about the WHI estrogen plus progestin trial: issues specific to health care providers. Womens Health Initiative Participant Website. [accessed 2005 Mar 24]. Available from: http://www.whi.org/ faq/faq_eplusp_hcp.php#2.

111. Lader EW, Cannon CP, Ohman EM, Newby LK, Sulmasy DP, Barst RJ, et al. The clinician as investigator: participating in clinical trials in the practice setting: Appendix 2: statistical concepts in study design and analysis. Circulation. 2004;109:e305-7.

112. Whitley E, Ball J. Statistics review 4: sample size calculations. Crit Care. 2002;6:335-41.

113. Guller U, DeLong ER. Interpreting statistics in medical literature: a vade mecum for surgeons. J Am Coll Surg. 2004;198:441-58.

114. Tumlin JA, Wang A, Murray PT, Mathur VS. Fenoldopam mesylate blocks reductions in renal plasma flow after radiocontrast dye infusion: a pilot trial in the prevention of contrast nephropathy. Am Heart J. 2002;143:894-903.

115. Stone GW, McCullough PA, Tumlin JA, Lepor NE, Madyoon H, Murray P, et al. Fenoldopam mesylate for the prevention of contrast-induced nephropathy: a randomized controlled trial. JAMA. 2003;290:2284-91.

116. Altman DG, Goodman SN, Schroter S. How statistical expertise is used in medical research. JAMA. 2002;287:2817-20.

117. Delgado-Rodriguez M, Ruiz-Canela M, De Irala-Estevez J, Llorca J, Martinez-Gonzalez A. Participation of epidemiologists and/or biostatisticians and methodological quality of published controlled clinical trials. J Epidemiol Community Health. 2001;55:569-72.

118. Guyatt G, Jaeschke R, Heddle N, Cook D, Shannon H, Walter S. Basic statistics for clinicians: 1. Hypothesis testing. CMAJ. 1995;152:27–32.

119. Whitley E, Ball J. Statistics review 3: hypothesis testing and p values. Crit Care. 2002;6:222–5.

120. Gaddis ML, Gaddis GM. Introduction to biostatistics: Part 1, basic concepts. Ann Emerg Med. 1990;19:86–9.

121. Salkind NJ. Statistics for people who (think they) hate statistics. Thousand Oaks (CA): Sage Publications; 2000.

122. Whitley E, Ball J. Statistics review 2: samples and populations. Crit Care. 2002;6:143–8.

123. Whitley E, Ball J. Statistics review 1: presenting and summarising data. Crit Care. 2002;6:66–71.

124. AUA guideline on management of benign prostatic hyperplasia (2003). Chap. 1: Diagnosis and treatment recommendations. J Urol. 2003;170:530–47.

125. Glantz SA. Primer of biostatistics. 5th ed. New York: McGraw-Hill; 2002.

126. Lee CM, Soin HK, Einarson TR. Statistics in the pharmacy literature. Ann Pharmacother. 2004;38:1412–8.

127. Swinscow TDV. Statistics at square one. London: British Medical Association; 1983.

128. Kirby A, Gebski V, Keech AC. Determining the sample size in a clinical trial. Med J Aust. 2002;177:256–7.

129. Elenbaas JK, Cuddy PG, Elenbaas RM. Evaluating the medical literature, Part III: results and discussion. Ann Emerg Med. 1983;12:679–86.

130. DeMets DL. Statistical issues in interpreting clinical trials. J Intern Med. 2004;255:529–37.

131. Hardin JM. Principle of intention to treat analysis in clinical studies: its use and controversies. J Pharm Pract. 1998;XI:231–8.

132. Le Bars PL, Katz MM, Berman N, Itil TM, Freedman AM, Schatzberg AF. A placebo-controlled, double-blind, randomized trial of an extract of Ginkgo biloba for dementia. North American EGb Study Group. JAMA. 1997;278:1327–32.

133. Shepherd J, Cobbe SM, Ford I, Isles CG, Lorimer AR, MacFarlane PW, et al. Prevention of coronary heart disease with pravastatin in men with hypercholesterolemia. West of Scotland Coronary Prevention Study Group. N Engl J Med. 1995;333:1301–07.

134. Bucher HC, Guyatt GH, Cook DJ, Holbrook A, McAlister FA Users' guides to the medical literature: XIX. Applying clinical trial results. A. How to use an article measuring the effect of an intervention on surrogate endpoints. Evidence-Based Medicine Working Group. JAMA. 1999;282:771–8.

135. Weihrauch TR, Demol P. Value of surrogate endpoints for evaluation of therapeutic efficacy. Drug Inf J. 1998;32:737–43.

136. Manson JE, Hsia J, Johnson KC, Rossouw JE, Assaf AR, Lasser NL, et al. Estrogen plus progestin and the risk of coronary heart disease. N Engl J Med. 2003;349:523–34.

137. Cook DI, Gebski VJ, Keech AC. Subgroup analysis in clinical trials. Med J Aust. 2004;180:289–91.

138. Oxman AD, Guyatt GH. A consumer's guide to subgroup analyses. Ann Intern Med. 1992;116:78–84.

139. Shepherd J, Blauw GJ, Murphy MB, Bollen EL, Buckley BM, Cobbe SM, et al. Pravastatin in elderly individuals at risk of vascular disease (PROSPER): a randomised controlled trial. Lancet. 2002;360: 1623–30.

140. Gorelick PB, Richardson D, Kelly M, Ruland S, Hung E, Harris Y, et al. Aspirin and ticlopidine for prevention of recurrent stroke in black patients: a randomized trial. JAMA. 2003;289:2947–57.

141. Hass WK, Easton JD, Adams HP, Jr., Pryse-Phillips W, Molony BA, Anderson S, et al. A randomized trial comparing ticlopidine hydrochloride with aspirin for the prevention of stroke in high-risk patients. Ticlopidine Aspirin Stroke Study Group. N Engl J Med. 1989;321:501–7.

142. Tsai HH, Chapman R, Shepherd A, McKeith D, Anderson M, Vearer D, et al. Esomeprazole 20 mg on-demand is more acceptable to patients than continuous lansoprazole 15 mg in the long-term maintenance of endoscopy-negative gastro-oesophageal reflux patients: the COMMAND Study. Aliment Pharmacol Ther. 2004;20:657–65.

143. Rothwell PM. External validity of randomised controlled trials: "to whom do the results of this trial apply?" Lancet. 2005;365:82–93.

144. Clarke M, Alderson P, Chalmers I. Discussion sections in reports of controlled trials published in general medical journals. JAMA. 2002;287:2799–2801.

145. Anderson G, Kendrach MG, Trice S. Basic biostatistics and hypothesis testing. J Pharm Pract. 1998;XI:181–95.

146. Cook D, Sackett DL. On the clinically important difference [editorial]. ACP J Club. 1992;117:A16.

147. Castell DO, Kahrilas PJ, Richter JE, Vakil NB, Johnson DA, Zukerman S, et al. Esomeprazole (40 mg) compared with lansoprazole (30 mg) in the treatment of erosive esophagitis. Am J Gastroenterol. 2002;97:575–83.

148. Whelton A, Fort JG, Puma JA, Normandin D, Bello AE, Verburg KM, et al. Cyclooxygenase-2—specific inhibitors and cardiorenal function: a randomized, controlled trial of celecoxib and rofecoxib in older hypertensive osteoarthritis patients. Am J Ther. 2001;8:85–95.

149. Borenstein M. The case for confidence intervals in controlled clinical trials. Control Clin Trials. 1994;15:411–28.

150. Guyatt G, Jaeschke R, Heddle N, Cook D, Shannon H, Walter S, et al. Basic statistics for clinicians: 2. Interpreting study results: confidence intervals. CMAJ. 1995;152:169–73.

151. Guyatt GH, Sackett DL, Cook DJ. Users' guides to the medical literature. II. How to use an article about therapy or prevention. B. What were the results and will they help me in caring for my patients? Evidence-Based Medicine Working Group. JAMA. 1994;271:59–63.

152. Jaeschke R, Guyatt G, Shannon H, Walter S, Cook D, Heddle N. Basic statistics for clinicians: 3. Assessing the effects of treatment: measures of association. CMAJ. 1995;152:351–7.

153. Fisher B, Costantino JP, Wickerham DL, Redmond CK, Kavanah M, Cronin WM, et al. Tamoxifen for prevention of breast cancer: report of the National Surgical Adjuvant Breast and Bowel Project P-1 Study. J Natl Cancer Inst. 1998;90:1371–88.

154. Kendrach MG, Covington TR, McCarthy MW, Harris CM. Calculating risks and number-needed-to-treat: a method of data interpretation. J Manag Care Pharm. 1997;3:179–83.

155. Feinstein AR. Principles of medical statistics. Boca Raton (FL): Chapman & Hall; 2002.

156. Chobanian AV, Bakris GL, Black HR, Cushman WC, Green LA, Izzo JL, Jr., et al. The seventh report of the joint national committee on prevention, detection, evaluation, and treatment of high blood pressure: the JNC 7 report. JAMA. 2003;289:2560–72.

157. Castell DO, Richter JE, Robinson M, Sontag SJ, Haber MM. Efficacy and safety of lansoprazole in the treatment of erosive reflux esophagitis. The Lansoprazole Group. Am J Gastroenterol. 1996; 91:1749–57.

158. Advice for travelers. Treat Guidel Med Lett. 2004;2:33–40.

159. DuPont HL, Sullivan P, Evans DG, Pickering LK, Evans DJ, Jr., Vollet JJ, et al. Prevention of traveler's diarrhea (emporiatrics enteritis). Prophylactic administration of subsalicylate bismuth. JAMA. 1980;243:237–41.

160. Mosdell KW. Literature evaluation I: controlled clinical trials. In: Malone PM, Mosdell KW, Kier KL, Stanovich JE, editors. Drug information: a guide for pharmacists. 2nd ed. New York: McGraw-Hill; 2001. p. 160.

161. Buchkowsky SS, Jewesson PJ. Industry sponsorship and authorship of clinical trials over 20 years. Ann Pharmacother. 2004;38:579–85.

162. Profile Pharmaceutical Industry 2004. Focus on Innovation. New Medicine, New Hope. [accessed 2005 Jan 29]. Available from: http://www.phrma.org/publications/publications//2004-03-31.937.pdf.

163. Thompson DF. Understanding financial conflicts of interest. N Engl J Med. 1993;329:573–6.

164. Chopra SS. MS JAMA: industry funding of clinical trials: benefit or bias? JAMA. 2003;290:113–114.

165. Lexchin JR. Implications of pharmaceutical industry funding on clinical research. Ann Pharmacother. 2005;39:194–7.

166. Lievre M, Menard J, Bruckert E, Cogneau J, Delahaye F, Giral P, et al. Premature discontinuation of clinical trial for reasons not related to efficacy, safety, or feasibility. BMJ. 2001;322:603–5.

167. Gotzsche PC, Johansen HK. Meta-analysis of prophylactic or empirical antifungal treatment versus placebo or no treatment in patients with cancer complicated by neutropenia. BMJ. 1997;314: 1238–44.

168. Rochon PA, Berger PB, Gordon M. The evolution of clinical trials: inclusion and representation. CMAJ. 1998;159:1373–4.

169. Blumenthal D, Campbell EG, Anderson MS, Causino N, Louis KS. Withholding research results in academic life science. Evidence from a national survey of faculty. JAMA. 1997;277:1224–8.

170. Als-Nielsen B, Chen W, Gluud C, Kjaergard LL. Association of funding and conclusions in randomized drug trials: a reflection of treatment effect or adverse events? JAMA. 2003;290:921–8.

171. Fletcher SW, Colditz GA. Failure of estrogen plus progestin therapy for prevention [editorial]. JAMA. 2002;288:366–8.

172. Annals of Pharmacotherapy journal website. [accessed 2005 Jan 29]. Available from: http://www.hwbooks.com/annals/ guides.html#eo.

173. Devereaux PJ, Manns BJ, Ghali WA, Quan H, Guyatt GH. Reviewing the reviewers: the quality of reporting in three secondary journals. CMAJ. 2001;164:1573–6.

174. ACP Journal Club Purpose and Procedure. [accessed 2005 Jan 29]. Available from: http://www.acpjc.org/shared/purpose_ and_procedure.htm.

175. About Journal Watch. [accessed 2005 Jan 29]. Available from: http://general-medicine.jwatch.org/misc/about.shtml.

176. About Journal Watch Online. Available from: http://www.jwatch.org/misc/about.shtml. [accessed 2005 Jan 29].

177. Journal of Family Practice Website: POEMS. [accessed 2005 Jan 29]. Available from: http://www.jfponline.com/ poems/poems.asp.

178. Columns of AJHP. American Journal of Health-System Pharmacy website. [accessed 2005 Jan 29]. Available from: http:// www.ajhp.org/misc/about.dtl.

7

Chapter Seven

Literature Evaluation II:
Beyond the Basics

Karen P. Norris • Carrie J. Johnson • H. Glenn
Anderson, Jr., • Patrick J. Bryant • Elizabeth A.
Poole • Cydney E. McQueen • Linda R. Young

Objectives

After completing this chapter, the reader will be able to

- Describe study designs published in the biomedical literature.
- Describe examples of true experiments other than the controlled clinical trial.
  - Discuss the potential utility and questions to ask when evaluating an n-of-1 trial.
  - Describe limitations of data provided in case studies, case reports, and case series.
  - Compare differences between a case study and an n-of-1 trial.
  - Describe guidelines for the conduct of stability studies.
  - State the methods used in bioequivalence trials, criteria for establishing bioequivalence, and potential sources of error in bioequivalence trials.
  - Describe potential errors in the interpretation of data from postmarketing adverse event surveillance studies.
  - Discuss the use and analysis of programmatic research.
- Describe the characteristics of observational trial design.
  - Describe situations where cohort, case-control, and cross-sectional study designs are most useful and disadvantages of these designs.
  - Define relative risk as it relates to cohort studies and odds ratios as they relate to case-control studies.
  - Discuss types of potential bias within observational study designs and methods to control for potential bias.
- Describe a method for organizing and ranking quality of trials based on fundamental differentiating study design characteristics.

- Describe the scenarios regarding the impact of power (or lack of power) on interpretation of study results.
- Differentiate between three types of literature reviews: narrative review (nonsystematic review), systematic review (qualitative), and meta-analysis (quantitative).
  - List key questions to ask when evaluating a systematic review.
  - Identify potential sources of error and bias in a meta-analysis.
- Discuss use and evaluation of practice guidelines.
- Describe common quality-of-life (QOL) measures utilized in health outcomes research.
- Identify common issues encountered in dietary supplement (botanical and nonbotanical) medical literature.

Introduction

Question: Why is it important to understand principles of study design and evaluation beyond the prospective, randomized, controlled, clinical trial, and other "true experiments?"

Answer: Principles that apply to well-designed interventional trials (discussed in Chap. 6) also apply to other types of study designs; however, there are situations where other research designs are more effective in answering specific questions or are the only data available to answer the questions. For example, only a handful of small controlled trials may be available to address a particular clinical situation. This is apparent in the many small trials of gabapentin for treatment of neuropathic pain. In this case, a meta-analysis may be more effective at answering the question because data from these small trials can be pooled to achieve statistical power needed to answer the question. As another example, it may not be feasible to study the toxicity of certain agents (e.g., cardiovascular risks associated with cyclooxygenase inhibitors) in prospective controlled clinical trials; therefore, pooled data or observational epidemiologic research, such as retrospective case-control studies or cohort studies, must be employed. Thus, literature evaluation skills unique to designs discussed in this chapter must be mastered in order to critique these studies effectively.

Question: Why "reevaluate" literature that has already undergone peer-review and publication in a reputable journal?

Answer: In light of vast amounts of rapidly emerging "evidence," in conjunction with busy practitioner schedules, an understanding of inherent strengths and limitations of multiple types of medical literature gives the practicing health care professional a powerful clinical tool, most notably in cases where a peer-review process has left a lot to be desired. One may scan articles of interest for trial design and rigor within that design to determine which articles are worth precious reading time. Selected articles can then be more carefully reviewed to determine the relative validity of that article compared to previously published reports, including those which demonstrate opposing results. From this process, the clinician can draw appropriate evidence-based conclusions.

Ultimately, good literature evaluation skills allow clinicians to make the best recommendations and decisions for subsequent patient care, whether for one specific patient, or for large patient populations.

The intent of this chapter is to introduce readers to the types of literature frequently encountered beyond the interventional, prospective, randomized, controlled, clinical trial. Other true experiments encountered in the literature are discussed, including n-of-1 trials, analytical research such as stability studies, and pharmacokinetic research such as bioequivalency studies. Programmatic research is another true experiment important to pharmacy practice, and is included as well, along with survey research and postmarketing surveillance studies. The chapter will address issues related to observational study designs, such as cohort, case-control, cross-sectional, case studies, or case series and will present types of potential bias in observational trials and methods to control that potential for bias. A method for organizing studies according to fundamental differentiating characteristics of trial design (interventional vs. observational, controlled vs. uncontrolled, prospective vs. retrospective) is presented, which may be used to facilitate the process of evidence-based decision-making. Differences between nonsystematic (narrative) and systematic (qualitative and meta-analysis) reviews are addressed, as is an introduction to health outcomes, quality of life (QOL) research. Finally, utility and evaluation techniques specific to each type of literature are provided. Readers are encouraged to utilize techniques of critiquing clinical trials and to incorporate principles of evidence-based medicine (EBM) as described in this and other chapters of this text.

Experimental Study Design

The randomized, controlled, clinical trial, sometimes referred to as an interventional trial, is one form of true experimental study design. The intervention provided could be in the form of a treatment, an educational program, or a medical procedure. Students often ask why the strongest experimental designs are not used exclusively by all individuals performing research. "Doing the best with what one has" may be the best answer. Study designs are developed in an effort to reasonably achieve three key research objectives: to have equivalent sampling groups, to isolate and control the intervention, and to obtain reliable measurements of

TABLE 7–1. COMMONLY ENCOUNTERED BIOMEDICAL LITERATURE

Study Design	Study Purpose
Clinical study (true experiment)	Determine cause and effect relationships
N-of-1 study	Compare effects of drug to control during multiple observation periods in a single patient
Stability study	Evaluate stability of drugs in various preparations (e.g., ophthalmologic, intravenous, topical, and oral)
Bioequivalence study	Assess the bioequivalency of two or more products
Programmatic research	Determine the impact and/or economic value of clinical services
Cohort (follow-up) study	Determine association between various factors and disease state development
Case-control (trohoc) study	Determine association between disease states and exposure to various risk factors
Cross-sectional study	Identify prevalence of characteristics of diseases in populations
Case study, case report, or case series	Report observations in a single patient or series of patients
Survey research	Study the incidence, distribution, and relationships of sociologic and psychologic variables through use of questionnaires applied to various populations
Postmarketing surveillance study	Evaluate use and adverse effects associated with newly approved drug therapies
Narrative review	Nonsystematic, subjective summary of data from multiple studies
Systematic review	Systematic, qualitative, and objective summary of data from multiple studies
Meta-analysis	Combine, statistically evaluate, and summarize data from multiple studies
Outcomes studies (pharmacoeconomic and health related-QOL measures)	Compare outcomes (QOL) and costs (pharmacoeconomics) of drug therapies or services

ABBREVIATION: QOL = quality of life.

the response. Attainment of these objectives requires significant resource allocation, including time, materials, subjects, and money. Interventional designs require large quantities of each resource. These studies may be impractical or inefficient when investigating rare outcome incidences, when finances are limited, or when concerns arise regarding the ethical feasibility of allocating patients to potentially hazardous interventions. Table 7–1 lists commonly encountered biomedical literature.

TRUE EXPERIMENTS—BEYOND THE CONTROLLED CLINICAL TRIAL

N-of-1 Trials

Randomized, controlled trials are not feasible for many diseases and therapies. Furthermore, if results from controlled trials are available, restrictive inclusion criteria of the trial may make it difficult to apply results from the trial to individual patients routinely encountered in clinical practice.[1] N-of-1 trials attempt to apply the principles of clinical trials, such as randomization and blinding, to individual patients.[1] N-of-1 trials are useful when the beneficial effects of a particular treatment in an individual patient are in doubt. It is advantageous if the treatment has a short half-life (allowing multiple crossover periods without carryover effects) and is being used for symptomatic relief of a chronic condition.[1,2] An n-of-1 trial can be used to determine whether a drug is effective in an individual patient.[2] Taken as a whole, a group of n-of-1 trials can help to identify characteristics that differentiate responders from nonresponders.[2] Trials of multiple doses can identify the most effective dose and the clinical endpoints most influenced by the drug.[2]

An n-of-1 trial can be likened to a cross-over study conducted in a single subject in that a patient receives treatments in pairs (one period of the experimental therapy and one period of either alternative treatment or placebo) in random order.[2] As described below, the study usually consists of several treatment periods that are continued until effectiveness is proven or refuted.[2] Randomization to active drug or placebo and blinding of the physician and patient to the treatment being administered helps to reduce treatment order effects, placebo effects, and observer bias. Desired outcomes are identified prior to initiation of the study to ensure that objective criteria that are meaningful to both the physician and patient are used to assess treatment efficacy.[1]

N-of-1 trials may improve appropriate prescribing of drugs in individual patients. For example, carbamazepine may be an option for relief of pain in a patient with diabetic neuropathy, but definitive information on the efficacy of such treatment is limited. Therefore, investigators may conduct an n-of-1 trial to determine whether such therapy is useful in a particular patient. N-of-1 trials are especially useful when long-term treatment with a specific drug may result in toxicity and the physician wishes to determine whether benefits outweigh potential risks.[1]

The effectiveness of n-of-1 trials has been evaluated.[3,4] Of 57 n-of-1 trials completed, 50 (88%) provided a definite clinical or statistical answer to a clinical question leading to the conclusion by the authors that n-of-1 trials were useful and feasible in clinical practice.[3] Simply stated, the goal of an n-of-1 trial is to clarify a management decision.[3] Of 34 completed n-of-1 trials evaluated over a 2-year period, 17 (50%) were judged to provide definitive results.[4] Overall, physician confidence in the therapy was found to increase or decrease depending on the direction of trial results.[4]

When encountering a published n-of-1 trial, several considerations must be made. General requirements have been recommended for n-of-1 trials.[5] Readers should determine whether the treatment target (or measure of effectiveness) was evaluated during each treatment period.[5] This target should be a symptom or diagnostic test result, but must be directly relevant to the patient's well-being (e.g., the visual analog scale for pain in the example of carbamazepine). Two other critical characteristics of an n-of-1 study are that the symptom under investigation shows a rapid improvement when effective treatment is begun and that this improvement regresses quickly (but not permanently) when effective treatment is discontinued.[5]

Other questions to ask when evaluating n-of-1 trials include:

1. Was the treatment period long enough to include an exacerbation of the condition? (A general rule is that if an event occurs an average of once every X days, then a clinician needs to observe 3 X days to be 95% confident of observing at least one event);
2. Can a clinically relevant treatment target be measured? (It is advisable to measure symptoms or the patient's QOL directly, with patients rating each symptom at least twice during each study period); and
3. Can sensible criteria for stopping the trial be established? (Specification of the number of treatment pairs in advance strengthens the statistical analysis of the results and it has been advised that at least two pairs of treatment periods are conducted before unblinding).[2]

N-of-1 trials provide more objective information than case reports or case studies (as will be described in a later section) and are useful for providing definitive information for drug prescribing in individual patients. See Table 7–2 for a comparison of n-of-1 trials and case studies. Questions to ask when evaluating n-of-1 trials are provided in Appendix 7–1.

STABILITY STUDIES/*IN VITRO* STUDIES

Stability studies determine the stability of drugs in various preparations (e.g., ophthalmologic, intravenous, topical, and oral) under various conditions (e.g., heat, freezing, refrigeration, and room temperature). Stability studies are extremely important to the practice of pharmacy. For example, pharmacists who prepare intravenous solutions for use by patients at home often want to know how long a drug admixed in a particular solution is stable or if freezing increases the length of time an admixture is stable to determine how many intravenous admixtures may be dispensed at a time. It is also important for pharmacists involved with extemporaneous compounding to know the length of time a particular preparation is stable.

TABLE 7–2. COMPARISON OF N-OF-1 TRIALS AND CASE STUDIES

	N-of-1 Trial	Case Study
Design	Prospective	Retrospective (most often)
Predefined methods	Yes	No
Clearly defined outcome measures	Yes	No
Randomization	Yes	No
Blinding	Yes	No
Multiple treatment periods	Yes	Not usually

SOURCE: Adapted from Spilker B.[33]

Unfortunately, the quality of stability studies conducted in the past has been poor, which prompted Trissel et al. to prepare study guidelines.[6] These guidelines state that investigators conducting stability studies should provide a complete description of study methodology and test conditions. Appropriate, validated assays should be used. Samples should include a baseline time zero measurement and an appropriate number of samples to assess stability over the time period. For example, if the goal of the study is to determine the stability of an antibiotic at room temperature then taking measurements at, for example, time zero and 30 days may not be adequate. Planning the study so that testing is done at multiple time points (i.e., time zero, 6 hours, 12 hours, 18 hours, and 24 hours) would yield more information about the degradation timeline of the product. As with all studies, conclusions should be consistent with the results. Questions to ask when evaluating stability studies are provided in Appendix 7–1.

BIOEQUIVALENCE STUDIES

An ever-increasing number of generic products are becoming available in the marketplace and there is a need to establish that the quality, safety, and efficacy of these generic drugs are the same as the brand name product.[7] The health care practitioner is often placed in the position of having to select one from among several apparently equivalent products for individual patients or for use on formularies of health care organizations. The more skilled the health care practitioner is at interpreting the data, the more comfortable he or she will be in selecting the appropriate product for the specific patient or organization.

Bioequivalence trials are often conducted under standardized conditions in a small number of normal, healthy adult volunteers because of availability and lack of confounding factors in this population.[8] Data from healthy volunteers, however, may not reflect the population for whom the medication is prescribed. Single doses of the test and reference drugs are administered and blood or plasma levels of the drug are measured over time. Multidose studies are also conducted on occasion to establish bioequivalence at steady state. A two-treatment crossover study design in 24 to 36 healthy adult subjects is usually used so that the subject serves as his or her own control, thus improving precision of results.[9]

Bioequivalent products are products that are equivalent in rate and extent of absorption (by definition, based on the opinions of Food and Drug Administration ([FDA]) medical experts, the rate and extent of absorption differ by ±20% or less).[8,9] The area under the blood concentration-time curve (AUC) is used to assess the extent of absorption, and the maximum or peak drug concentration (C_{max}) is used to assess the rate of absorption, these are the primary pharmacokinetic criteria used in bioequivalence studies.

If the average blood ratios (AUC and C_{max}) of a generic product to a brand-name product of the active ingredient lie entirely within the boundaries of a 90% confidence interval of 80 to 125%, products are considered bioequivalent.[8,9] The confidence interval limits are determined by the following method where two situations are tested: (1) whether a generic (test) product is significantly less bioavailable when substituted for a brand (reference) product, and (2) whether a reference product is significantly less bioavailable when substituted for a test product.[9] Numerically expressed, the first test determines the lower acceptable limit of the confidence interval (80%) with an average test/reference ratio of 80%, while the second test determines the upper limit of the confidence interval with an average reference/test ratio of 80%, but this ratio is also expressed by convention as a test/reference ratio, thus is 125% (the reciprocal of 80%).

Similarly, for approval of a generic product, a manufacturer must show that a 90% confidence interval for the ratio of the mean response of its product compared to that of the innovator product is within the limits of 0.8 to 1.25 (80 to 125%).[8,9]

When evaluating bioequivalence studies, readers should note whether the acceptable age and weight range for the subjects is defined in the methods and clinical parameters used to characterize a normal, healthy adult (e.g., physical examination observations and hematologic evaluations) are described.[10] Subjects should be free of all drugs, including caffeine, nicotine, and other recreational drugs, for at least 2 weeks prior to testing and usually fast overnight prior to dosing.[10] Subjects are usually nonsmokers and may also have limitations placed on caffeine intake because both factors may affect blood levels of the product in question.[10] Subjects should also be free of all dietary supplements (botanical and nonbotanical), as many of these products can interact with products under bioequivalence review. Bioequivalency testing may be performed in both fasting and fed states to assess the impact of food on bioavailability; however, food intake should be closely monitored and controlled. Food can impact the rate and absorption of some products. For example, a high fat meal may affect absorption of highly lipophilic products. Additionally, methods should define sample-collection times, which should be based on the half-life of the drug, as well as collection techniques and storage methods of samples.[10]

When examining the results of bioequivalence studies, lack of statistical significance does not equate with bioequivalence.[11] The rate and extent of absorption for products must be compared. This is a commonly encountered problem. Tests for statistical significance are generally based on the premise that two products are assumed to be the same until proven otherwise. DiSanto provides the example that if the data presented are highly variable (wide range of values identified by a large standard deviation), it would be possible to show that there was no statistically significant difference between an AUC of 100 units versus an AUC of 40 units.[11] In this example, the test for statistical significance does not demonstrate that the AUCs are truly similar; it actually shows that the data were too variable from patient to patient to be able to detect a 60 unit (%) difference in areas, even if the difference existed.[11]

One of the most common errors in the use of bioavailability data is comparing two products based on data obtained from separate studies.[11] Different subject populations, study conditions, and assay methodologies are all reasons why comparisons of data from different studies are dangerous and can lead to false conclusions.[11] For example, a formulary committee may locate two generic products that have each shown equivalence to the brand product in two separate studies. A false conclusion can be made that both generic products are bioequivalent to each other. As another example, for some products, multiple assays are available for measuring serum levels. Using the same assay, results for the two drugs may demonstrate equivalence; however, if one assay type is used for the reference drug and another assay type is used for the test drug, the results may not demonstrate equivalence because the sensitivity and specificity of assays may be different.

It is very important, therefore, that a thorough investigation of the methods of the bioequivalence study is made. All subjects should receive the drug under the same conditions, and all blood levels should be taken at the same intervals. The reader must be assured that confounding factors (for example, increased weight, increased alcohol intake, and initiation of smoking) were minimized between treatment periods (crossover periods). For example, if a patient started to smoke during the crossover period, the serum levels of the drug may be affected on the next assay because smoking may alter the pharmacokinetics of the drug.

Current FDA regulations require bioequivalence between the generic product and the brand name product be demonstrated, but do not require that bioequivalence among generic copies of the same brand name drug be demonstrated. As a result, it is a common concern whether these generic drugs can be used interchangeably.

As a guide to health care practitioners in evaluating the bioequivalence of prescription drug products, the scientific and medical evaluations by the FDA are published in the USPDI: Volume III, Approved Drug Products and Legal Requirements (also known as the Orange Book) and are also available on the FDA website at <<http://www.fda.gov/cder/orange/adp.htm>>.[9] A coding system is used for efficient determination of the equivalence status of a particular product (first letter) and to provide additional information based on the FDA evaluations (second letter). This coding system is described in the initial pages of the USPDI. Products rated A are considered therapeutically equivalent to their pharmaceutical equivalents. Products rated B may have documented bioequivalence problems, or there may be a significant potential for such problems and no adequate studies demonstrating bioequivalence. A rating of B may also indicate that the quality standards are inadequate or the FDA has insufficient data to determine equivalence.

For example, multisource products having the same strength, same ingredients, same dosage form, and same route(s) of administration will usually be coded AB if there is a study submitted demonstrating bioequivalence.[9] A product coded BX is one for which the data are not sufficient to determine therapeutic equivalence and the product is assumed to be therapeutically inequivalent.

Bioequivalence studies represent an increasingly important part of the medical literature. When evaluating such trials for application in clinical practice, it is important to focus on the methods of the study. Specifically, the reader must determine if a crossover study design was used, if the assay was validated, and if consistent conditions were maintained to minimize subject variability (i.e., food intake, timing of blood levels, and nicotine use). Questions to ask when evaluating bioequivalence studies are provided in Appendix 7–1.

PROGRAMMATIC RESEARCH

Another type of true experiment important to the practice of pharmacy is research focused on the impact and economic value of programs and services provided by pharmacists in community and institutional settings. Programmatic research is particularly important because limited resources and budget constraints demand that only those services that improve patient care in a cost-effective manner be implemented. The body of evidence in support of the economic benefit of pharmacists providing clinical pharmacy services has grown over the past decade, and is diverse.[12] The evidence includes contemporary practice sites and services, and has improved in the strength of study design and methodology, and "economic, clinical and humanistic outcome assessments in many practice environments have been performed."[13,14] Pharmacists, working in interdisciplinary settings with physicians and other health care providers, have demonstrated that they can improve drug therapy effectiveness, efficiency, and safety.[15] The American College of Clinical Pharmacy has published a succession of position statements which review published literature regarding the value of clinical pharmacy services.[12-15] These position papers discuss strengths and limitations of existing literature, and include recommendations for further studies in order to facilitate continued documentation of value provided by pharmacists in progressive roles and settings, while utilizing methodology that ensures a high level of evidence-based rigor. Questions to ask when evaluating programmatic research are provided in Appendix 7–1.

Observational Study Design

The key distinguishing feature between observational and interventional design is the inclusion or omission of an investigator-initiated intervention. Observational study designs do not involve an intervention, rather, subject groups are based on presence or absence of a disease or exposure with observations being made and recorded regarding patient characteristics. The observational study design seeks to evaluate questions based on less rigidly controlled practice conditions than those used in experimental study designs. Research questions are addressed by comparing outcomes or experiences of patients arising from naturally occurring assignment to different treatments, subject characteristics, or exposures.[16,17] For instance, if an agent is particularly toxic and of no therapeutic value, it would be unethical to ask subjects to voluntarily expose themselves to the agent, thus an observational study would be used.[18] An example of this type of situation is the evaluation of risk factors for diseases such as cancer. An investigator wishing to evaluate the toxicity of environmental or industrial hazards or the teratogenicity of drugs administered during pregnancy would have to employ epidemiologic research techniques such as cohort or case-control studies to study these problems. These research techniques allow associations rather than cause and effect relationships to be determined. Thus, when evaluating overall results of any observational study (case-control, cohort, cross-sectional, or case study), it is important to remember that a correlation or an association between exposure and outcome does not prove causation.[19] The reader of such studies must consider other factors that are possibly related to both the exposure and outcome.[19]

The following discussion will present observational study designs commonly encountered within health literature: the cohort, case-control, cross-sectional designs, and case studies. Strengths and weakness of each will be discussed, along with evaluation techniques.

See Table 7–3 for differentiating factors between observation trial designs: cohort, case-control, and cross-sectional.

COHORT STUDIES

The cohort study—synonymously termed a follow-up, longitudinal, or incidence study—is the strongest observational study design. In this design, the investigator recruits a disease-free subject population and divides the population into two groups: those identified as either exposed or unexposed to a factor of interest. Subjects are then followed prospectively as development of a disease state of interest is observed during the study period.[18,20] Figure 7–1 provides a schematic of a cohort design.

The Nurses Health Study (NHS) is an example of the traditional prospective cohort design.[21] Approximately 120,000 nurses participated by answering biannual surveys beginning in 1976 and ending in 1986. The 1976 survey established baseline aspirin exposures and, for study inclusion, required absence of outcome occurrence at study inception. Subsequent follow-up surveys established incidences of fatal and nonfatal cardiovascular outcomes within the study sample.

TABLE 7–3. CHARACTERISTICS OF OBSERVATIONAL STUDY DESIGNS

Observational Study Design	Prospective Data Collection	Retrospective Data Collection	Exposure Known at Beginning of Study	Outcome Known at Beginning of Study	Study Determines Exposure Status	Study Determines Outcome Occurrence
Cohort	X		X			X
Case-control (trohoc)		X		X	X	
Cross-sectional	X				X	X

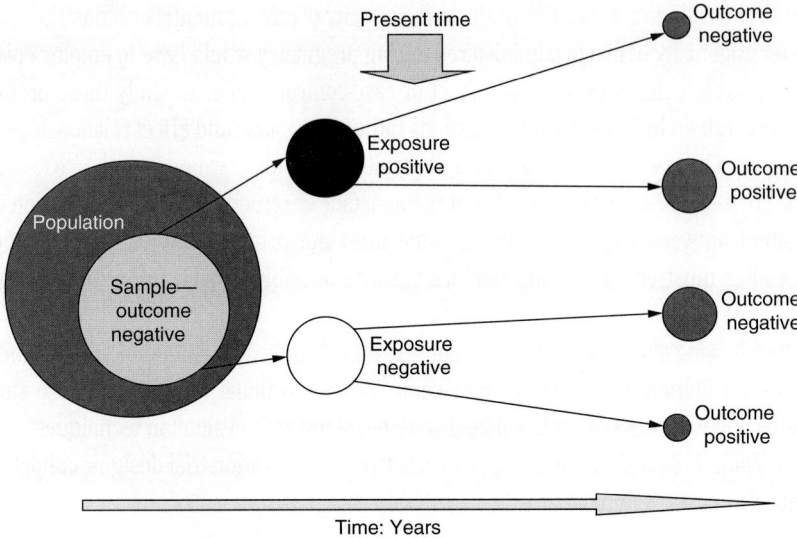

Figure 7–1. Schematic diagram of a cohort study.

When evaluating cohort studies, the research question must be stated clearly and unambiguously with relevant inclusion and exclusion criteria described in detail.[22] It is imperative that exposed and unexposed individuals are similar in terms of demographic characteristics so that susceptibility to the disease state is equal except for presence of the risk factor under investigation.[23] This is best achieved if subjects are randomized to exposure or no exposure; however, randomization is often not feasible, as in the case of toxicity questions.[23] Selection bias can occur if exposed and unexposed subjects do not have an equal chance of developing the outcome due to differential exposure to an additional important causative agent.[22] For example, a trial assessing the impact of asbestos exposure on lung cancer having more smokers as subjects in the unexposed group, results in selection bias. Furthermore, information bias can occur if the same efforts to measure outcomes are not made for both the exposed and unexposed groups.[19,22] Bias may be further introduced if follow-up rates differ for the two groups; outcome incidences will reflect follow-up rates rather than risk factor exposure rates.[22] In order to assess results of a cohort study accurately, the reader must examine study methods for evidence of these sources of bias.

Cohort designs have many advantages.[24] This design is uniquely capable of investigating outcomes from rare exposures, such as the relationship of pharmacy technicians preparing intravenous chemotherapy to subsequent development of cancer. Another advantage of a cohort design is that disease incidence rates may be determined utilizing this design; rates are not reliably ascertained with the case-control design.

Primary disadvantages of cohort studies are expense and time consumption.[24] For example, with rare outcomes, such as the occurrence of aplastic anemia with use of clozapine, a prospective investigation may require extremely large numbers of patients, require decades of data collection, and accrue large project costs to acquire answers. It takes many years for adequate assessment of disease development or to establish disease-free status.[19] Such research questions are investigated with more efficiency with the case-control design. Studies where loss to follow-up exceeds 20% in either the exposed or nonexposed cohort should be interpreted with caution.[19] Other factors to consider when evaluating cohort studies are provided in Appendix 7–1.

Relative risk is calculated from the data and provides information about the incidence of outcomes.[18] For example, consider the hypothetical situation presented in Table 7–4 in which the effects of industrial formaldehyde exposure on the development of chronic respiratory illness (i.e., chronic obstructive pulmonary disease and emphysema) were assessed. Risk for development of respiratory illness is 200/2000 (or 0.10) for those exposed to formaldehyde and 30/2000 (or 0.01) for unexposed subjects. Relative risk is equal to the ratio of these two numbers (0.10/0.01 or 10). In this case, risk of respiratory illness is 10 times greater in individuals exposed to formaldehyde. If relative risk is equal to one, the same risk exists for both exposed and unexposed subjects; if less than 1, a lower risk exists for individuals exposed to the factor and if greater than 1, a higher risk exists for those exposed.[18,23] Relative risk gives an idea of the magnitude of an effect, but does not provide information about precision or statistical significance of the result.[22] Alternatively, calculation of confidence intervals (usually at a level of 95%) are utilized for evaluation of statistical significance of results. The confidence interval provides a range in which the true value for the population lies. The wider the confidence interval, the less precise the result. Because a relative risk of 1 indicates no difference exists between groups, the confidence interval cannot include 1 and still maintain statistical significance. In the formaldehyde example described above, the relative risk is calculated as 10. If the 95% confidence interval is determined as 7 to 14, then the true risk of formaldehyde contributing to respiratory illness is contained within that interval, i.e., is at least 7 times and up to 14 times greater in individuals exposed to formaldehyde. Statistical difference is provided, since the range 7 to 14 excludes 1, the point where no difference exists between groups.

TABLE 7–4. COHORT STUDY—DETERMINATION OF RELATIVE RISK, EFFECT OF INDUSTRIAL FORMALDEHYDE EXPOSURE ON THE DEVELOPMENT OF RESPIRATORY ILLNESS

Risk Factor	Respiratory Illness	No Respiratory Illness	Total
Formaldehyde exposure	200	1800	2000
No industrial exposure to formaldehyde	30	1970	2000
Total	230	3770	4000

CASE-CONTROL STUDIES

Case-control studies—also termed case-referent, case history, or retrospective studies—are a type of observational study that offer an epidemiologic research alternative to cohort studies, which require a large number of subjects, and are often expensive and time-consuming.[18] Case-control studies seek to retrospectively identify potential risk factors of diseases or outcomes. In a case-control study, subjects (cases) with a particular characteristic or outcome of interest (e.g., disease) are recruited, matched with, and compared to a similar group of subjects (controls) who have not experienced the characteristic or outcome.[18,25,26] Data regarding exposures are collected retrospectively via patient interviews or by reviewing subject data records, and the two groups are compared to identify possible risk factors or contributors for development of the disease or outcome of interest. Of note, not only is the outcome of interest known at the beginning of the study, but also which subjects (cases) the outcome occurs in is also known. This is a key differentiating factor for case-control versus cohort study design. See Figure 7–2 for a schematic of the case-control research design.

Again because cohort studies require large subject numbers, and are often expensive and time-consuming, case-control studies are more useful when diseases occur infrequently or many years after exposure,[25] and are considered most efficient for studying rare diseases.[19] Because case-control studies are conducted in the opposite direction (i.e., retrospectively) of randomized clinical trials and follow-up studies, and are designed to determine cause rather than effect, they are sometimes called trohoc studies (i.e., cohort spelled backward).[25]

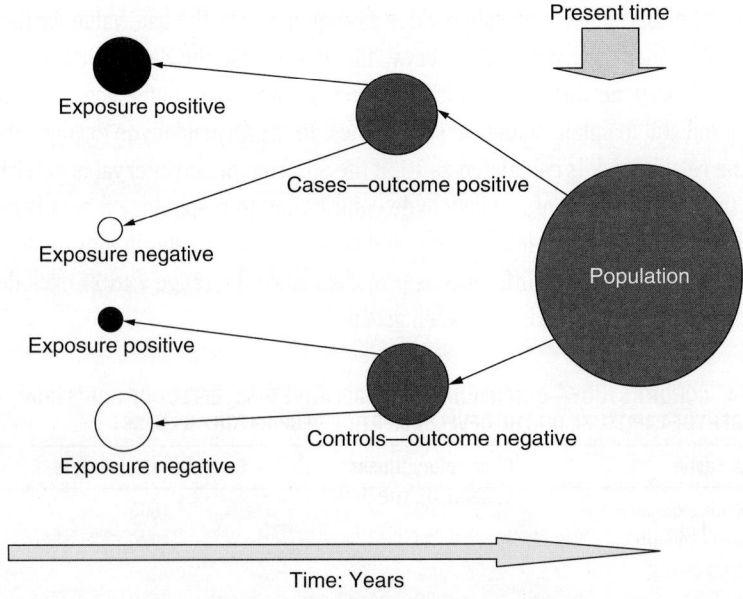

Figure 7–2. Schematic diagram of a case-control study.

Exposure of study subjects to the risk factor should reflect what occurs in the general population. If subjects with higher or lower exposure rates to the risk factor are excluded from the study, determination of possible associations between the exposure and a particular disease may be biased and inaccurate.[25] For example, case-controls often use subjects drawn from hospitalized populations, whose risk factor exposure may differ from individuals in the community; a problem termed, Berkson's bias.[25] Table 7–5 presents this and other types of bias that may be found within observational study designs, along with methods which provide control of potential biasing factors.

Predisposition to the disease of interest should be similar in both cases and controls, except for exposure to the risk factor under investigation, but it is extremely difficult to ensure that this occurs.[22,27-28] Matching is often used to assure that cases and controls are similar. With matching, each case has a comparable control in terms of demographic and exposure characteristics. Often it is difficult to determine which variables should be used to match cases to controls (e.g., sex, age, and date of admission). Such matching allows assessment of only the risk factor under investigation and no other variables that may have contributed to the disease.[25,26,29] Matching may even result in a negative impact on the interpretation of study results if cases and controls are matched for a factor that is itself related to exposure.[19]

Cases and controls should undergo the same diagnostic evaluation to determine presence or absence of the disease under investigation (e.g., endoscopy for ulcer disease), because detection of a disease is more likely to be found in individuals who undergo extensive diagnostic testing.[27] In addition, individuals administering the tests should be blinded to the presence or absence of the risk factor to eliminate "diagnostic-review bias."[25,27] A problem is that many diagnostic tests can only be performed in individuals suspected of having a particular disease state due to risks associated with their use.

Case-control study designs have both benefits and disadvantages. As mentioned earlier, case-control studies are relatively inexpensive and can be accomplished in a shorter timeframe than cohorts.[30] Both of these advantages are related to how subjects are recruited and data are acquired. When rare events are studied prospectively in a cohort design, recruitment of large samples is required due to the uncertainty of events occurring during the study period and the resulting need to assure study power. In contrast, case-control studies reduce the need for large sample sizes, as subjects are recruited based on *a priori* knowledge of occurrence of outcomes.

Most limitations inherent to case-control studies are due to the retrospective design.[26] Overall, the two major methodological issues include appropriate selection of controls and accurate determination of the level of exposure.[22] Historical data used in case-control studies may be inaccurate or incomplete.[25,26,28] When patients are interviewed regarding historical events, anamnestic equivalence may not be ensured.[27] For example, patients with the disease state may be more likely to recall events preceding development

TABLE 7–5. TYPES OF BIAS THAT MAY OCCUR WITHIN OBSERVATIONAL STUDY DESIGNS AND METHODS OF CONTROL

Category of Bias	Name of Bias	Description	Methods of Control	Cohort	Case-Control	Cross-sectional
Selection bias	Admission rate (Berkson) bias	Admission rates of exposed and unexposed cases and controls differ, resulting in a distortion of odds of exposure in hospital-based studies	A priori define inclusion and exclusion criteria All groups of subjects should have undergone identical diagnostic testing and there should be no difference in how exposure or disease status is determined		X	
	Nonresponse bias	Nonrespondents may exhibit exposures or outcomes that differ from respondents, resulting in over or under estimation of odds or risk	Match or adjust for confounding variables Use more than one control group	X	X	X
	Prevalence-incidence (Neyman) bias	Timing of exposure identification causes some cases to be missed		X	X	
	Unmasking bias	An innocent exposure causes a sign or symptom that precipitates search for a disease, but does not itself cause the disease		X	X	±
Information bias	Family history bias	Family members tend to share more information with family members who have similar diseases or exposures. Those family members without the disease or exposure may be unaware. Family historical information may vary widely depending on whether the person is a case or a control	Establish a priori explicit criteria for data collection methods on exposures and outcomes Blinded interviewer and subject to the hypotheses investigated Standardize data collection procedure, i.e., train observers, develop and refine survey questions and methods of recording answers	X	N/A	X

Bias	Description	Prevention/Control			
Recall bias	Difference in how data collection occurs exists between cases and controls, or the exposed and unexposed, resulting in an abnormally high rate of recall of exposure or outcome in one group	Maintain aggressive contact with subjects to limit attrition (cohort designs) For surveys, obtain response rates ≥80% Assess for effects of potential confounders	X	N/A	X
Exposure suspicion bias	Knowledge of a subject's disease status may influence both intensity and outcome of a search for exposure		X	N/A	±
Data analysis bias Post hoc significance bias	When decisions regarding level of significance are selected *a posteriori*, conclusion may be biased	Establish *a priori* the statistical methods to be used to evaluate data Report how missing data are handled	X	X	X
Data dredging bias	When data are reviewed for all possible associations without prior hypotheses, results are only suitable for hypothesis-forming activities	Assess associations between confounders and exposures and outcomes	X	X	X
Significance bias	Confusing statistical significance with clinical significance		X	X	X
Correlation bias	Correlations do not equate with causation; concluding that correlation equates with causation can lead to serious errors		X	X	X

Source: Adapted from Risk. In: Fletcher RH et al.[24]

230 DRUG INFORMATION: A GUIDE FOR PHARMACISTS

of the disease than patients who are healthy, since patients with disease are more likely to have contemplated factors they believe may have contributed to disease development (recall bias), so there should be some explanation in the study addressing the issue of recall bias. Investigators who collect data also may question individuals exposed to the disease more intensely than control subjects. To reduce variation in data obtained for cases and controls, data collectors should be blinded to the status of the subjects as cases or controls.[25]

Another prominent disadvantage is that information about the exposure and outcome is collected simultaneously, so it is difficult to sort out the temporal relationship between the two.[22] For instance, it is often difficult to determine if the exposure preceded the outcome, a situation termed protopathic bias, where the disease may lead to exposure to the risk factor rather than vice versa.[22,27] Consider the following illustration. Abnormal vaginal bleeding may be an early sign of uterine cancer. Vaginal bleeding, however, may lead to prescribing of hormonal therapies such as progesterone. An investigator may later erroneously conclude that use of progesterone was associated with development of uterine cancer when in fact the cancer preceded use of the progesterone in this case.[27]

Some experts have suggested use of several control groups selected on the basis of different criteria in an attempt to reduce some of the biases discussed above.[25] If results of comparing cases to the various control groups are in agreement with one another, bias in the control groups is unlikely to be present.[25]

During case-control studies, odds ratios are calculated. Odds ratio is an estimate of risk ratio.[18] Consider the situation presented in Table 7–6 where industrial exposure to formaldehyde in patients with and without respiratory illness is assessed. Odds of exposure to formaldehyde is 20/180 (0.11) in the cases with respiratory illness and 2/195 (0.01) in the controls. The odds ratio is calculated as 0.11/0.01 (11), which approximates the risk ratio determined in the cohort study example. Interpretation is the same; greater than one denotes increased risk, equal to one indicates no effect, and less than one indicates a protective effect. As with cohort studies, 95% confidence intervals should be calculated.[23]

Questions to ask when evaluating case-control studies are provided in Appendix 7–1.

TABLE 7–6. CASE-CONTROL STUDY—DETERMINATION OF ODDS RATIOS IN INDUSTRIAL FORMALDEHYDE EXPOSURE IN PATIENTS WITH RESPIRATORY ILLNESS

Risk Factor	Respiratory Illness	No Respiratory Illness	Total
Formaldehyde exposure	20	5	25
No industrial exposure to formaldehyde	180	195	375
Total	200	200	400

CROSS-SECTIONAL STUDIES

Cross-sectional studies or prevalence studies can be thought of as a "snapshot" because data are collected and evaluated at a single point in time.[14,20] This type of study design is hypothesis generating as opposed to hypothesis testing and is not suited for testing the effectiveness of interventions.[22] Typical examples of cross-sectional studies are surveys that evaluate opinions or situations at a fixed point in time and studies focused on description, diagnosis, and mechanisms of disease states.[31] For a hypothetical situation concerning rofecoxib (Vioxx™), a cross-sectional study design could be developed to look into a large insurance database and determine how many people died suddenly within 5 years of receiving rofecoxib. Cross-sectional studies are relatively quick and easy to perform and may be useful for measuring current health status or setting priorities for disease control.[22]

A study is classified as cross-sectional because measurements are taken at a single point in time, even though observations may cover a period of several months or years.[31] For example, a survey of smokers is cross-sectional when the questionnaire is administered once; however, the questions contained in the survey may focus on smoking habits over the past 10 years.

As in other observational trial designs, the research question and the relevant inclusion and exclusion criteria must be clearly and unambiguously stated.[22] Also, selection of cases must be clearly described because the starting point for the study is disease status of the subject.[19]

Problems that may occur during cross-sectional studies include errors in data collection and transient effects that may influence observations.[31] Because measurements occur at only one point in time, inaccuracies in data collection may go unnoticed because there are no prior data for comparison. In studies where multiple observations occur, outlier data, which may represent data collection errors, are more easily recognized. Transient effects are temporary occurrences that are found at the time a cross-sectional study is conducted, but are not identified if the study were repeated. A good example of transient effects is student evaluations of university professors. If a professor chooses to have students evaluate a course after a particularly grueling examination, chances are the evaluations would be poor based on students' response to the examination just taken. However, if the evaluations were administered after a curve had been applied for final grades, students may reflect on the course positively based on overall knowledge they received from the instructor, rather than a single negative experience. Transient effects are difficult to identify by a study evaluator. They may only be uncovered through retrospective evaluation of the study by the investigator. The investigator must perform a thorough assessment of all factors that may have impacted the results of the trial. Questions to ask when evaluating cross-sectional studies are provided in Appendix 7–1.

CASE STUDIES, CASE REPORTS, AND CASE SERIES

A case study—also sometimes referred to as a case report and referring to a single patient, or a case series, referring to a group of patients, has no control or comparison group, and simply reports on the clinical course of a particular patient or group of patients. In these studies observations are described that are related to a drug or technology applied to a single patient or group of patients.[32] The defining characteristic of these studies is this: cases are not compared to a control group, thus do not take into consideration other influencing factors which may also have played a role in observed outcomes. In contrast to n-of-1 trials, a case study (usually an observational study) does not apply principles of clinical trials, such as randomization and blinding, to individual patients. Usually retrospective, the case study does not involve multiple treatment periods, whereas an n-of-1 trial is prospective and includes multiple treatment periods. Comparisons of single patient clinical trials (n-of-1) and case studies are presented in Table 7–2.[33]

Interpretation of case studies can be difficult.[34] Design and methods describing conduct of a case study are not well-defined or agreed on.[34] For example, beneficial effects attributed to a drug or treatment under investigation may actually be a function of spontaneous regression of signs and symptoms of the disease, a placebo effect, and/or related to physicians' attitudes that may influence patient outcome.[32]

Case studies, however, are an integral part of the biomedical literature. They have played an important role in identifying treatments for rare disorders where large subject pools cannot be identified.[34] Case studies, reports, or series may also be useful for early recognition of drug toxicities and teratogenicity.[31] A newly recognized value of case reports is utilization for understanding potential toxicities of dietary supplement products (botanical and nonbotanical). Because the FDA does not regulate these products and adverse event reporting is scarce, often safety information is not well-defined for these products. Thus, published case reports may play a somewhat larger role for dietary supplements in suggesting potential safety problems than for traditional drug products.

When possible, results should be confirmed with randomized clinical trials. Case studies, reports, and series serve as an important initial step in the formulation of hypotheses[32]; however, only when case studies, reports, or series show a beneficial effect of a drug or treatment in diseases whose outcomes are consistently grim or when all other treatments have failed can results be applied to patients in clinical practice.[31,32] Questions to ask when evaluating case studies, case reports, or cased series are provided in Appendix 7–1.[34]

Survey Research

Survey research is used to study the incidence, distribution, and relationships of sociologic and psychologic variables.[35] It is used to collect information from a sample and generalize the findings to a larger, target population.[36] Data obtained from survey research have been used for many purposes, including helping investigators identify, assess, and compare respondents' ideas, feelings, plans, beliefs, and demographics.[36] In pharmacy practice, surveys may be used to determine how programs should be implemented by utilizing the opinions of experts with experience in a particular area, to study effectiveness of a program by questioning individuals who have used its services, or to understand attitudes and behaviors of patients or members of the profession. For example, directors of pharmacy may survey other hospitals to determine salary ranges in order to decide whether salary increases are needed to remain competitive in the job market. The ability to critically evaluate such literature has become a necessity for the practicing pharmacist due to an increased emphasis on this type of research in the medical literature.[36]

There are two basic types of surveys seen published in the biomedical literature. Descriptive surveys attempt to identify psychosocial variables such as attitudes, opinions, knowledge, and behaviors in a population, while explanatory surveys attempt to explain causal relationships between variables.[37] These dependent variables such as knowledge and behavior are often compared to independent variables such as age, sex, or education.[38]

Several types of data are collected in survey research and include incidence, attitudinal, knowledge, and behavior measurements. Incidence data try to determine the occurrence of events without drawing any relationships between variables.[38] An example of incidence data is the morbidity or mortality data reported weekly in the Centers for Disease Control and Prevention's Morbidity and Mortality Weekly Report (<<http://www.cdc.gov/mmwr>>). Manpower data are also incidence data frequently reported in pharmacy literature.[38] The number of residency-trained specialists in drug information centers is an example of data that might be collected in a nationwide manpower survey. Attitudinal data such as job satisfaction surveys often try to compare this dependent variable with independent variables such as age, education, or salary. Knowledge data attempt to document a person's knowledge or level of understanding about a specific topic. Examples include surveys asking physician's knowledge of retail prices of medications or pharmacist's knowledge of state pharmacy laws.[38] Behavior data document what a person actually does in a particular situation rather than what he or she says he does on a mail survey. Observing the number of specific points that a pharmacist addresses during patient education sessions is an example of behavior data.[38]

Data collection for surveys may involve questionnaires, examination of historical records, telephone interviews, face-to-face interviews, or panel interviews.[39] Well-conducted surveys have several important characteristics—they are objective and carefully planned, data are quantifiable, and subjects surveyed are representative of the target population.[39] In evaluating survey research, just like any other research, one must ask if the results are reliable and valid and if they can be generalized.[36]

Four sources of error have been described that can threaten the precision and accuracy (i.e., reliability) of survey results and must be evaluated by readers.[36] The first type of error, coverage error (sampling bias), occurs when there is a discrepancy between the target population and the population from which the sample was derived. This type of error can compromise the ability to generalize study results.[36] For example, people without telephones or unlisted numbers would be excluded from a sample frame of names from a telephone directory.

Sampling error (or random error) occurs when the researcher surveys only a subset (sample) of all possible subjects within the population of interest.[36] The use of random sampling procedures and larger sample sizes can be used to minimize sampling error. Sampling error is a statistical term that describes the rate of random error in sample selection. It describes variation around the true value of the population mean seen when multiple samples are pulled from the same population.[40] Sample error is reported usually as the mean ±1 standard error from the mean (SEM).

Measurement error (response bias) occurs when the collection of data is influenced by the interviewer or when the survey item itself is unclear from the respondent's point of view. When measurement error occurs, a subject's response cannot be compared to other responses.[36] The survey method used to collect the data may be one source of measurement error.[36] Face-to-face interviewers may influence the responses of the person being surveyed.[36] The survey instrument itself may be ambiguous and open to interpretation.[36] Bias can be introduced into a survey by the cover letter or sponsoring body; either may lead the respondent to one desired response rather than measuring the true reponse.[36] A fourth type of measurement error occurs when a respondent replies with a preferred or more socially acceptable answer rather than the real answer. A well-designed survey takes into account the abilities and motivation of the respondent to respond correctly (i.e., written at an appropriate educational level). Parallel forms (usually consisting of alternatively worded items placed throughout the survey) of either specific survey items or the entire survey instrument have been used to increase reliability of mail survey research. The use of such forms requires the calculation of correlation coefficients between the parallel items and survey instruments.

Accurate assessment of measurement error relies on the provision of the questionnaire or tool used to collect data so that readers may analyze wording. Unfortunately, however, many articles relating results of survey research do not include the actual questionnaire used in the survey due to space and ownership issues. Lengthy questionnaires take up valuable journal space and the publisher may decide not to include them. Some authors do not want to give away the intellectual work that they invested in developing a good questionnaire and decide not to publish it. These factors make it impossible for the reader to evaluate wording and thus objectivity of questions.

Finally, nonresponse error (nonresponse bias) occurs when a significant number of subjects in a sample do not respond to the survey when responders differ from nonresponders in a way that influences, or could influence, the results.[36] Generally, researchers strive for response rates in the 80 to 90% range so that nonresponders will not alter the author's conclusions.[38] Other authors argue that response rates of 80% for face-to-face interviews, 70% for telephone interviews, and 50% for mailed questionnaires are acceptable.[37] Additionally, evaluating responses of early versus late responders presumes that late responders are more like nonresponders, which may not hold true.

In order to accurately assess the survey's validity (i.e., robustness) and evaluate these potential sources of error and bias, the methods section, which must be explicit, should be heavily scrutinized. Foremost, a description of study methodology with enough detail to replicate the study should be provided. Additionally, the methods section should relate each type of error associated with survey research and state how investigators attempted to control those errors.[40]

Attempts to assess validity of the survey and efforts made to validate factual data should be described. For example, demographics of individual hospitals can be verified using American Hospital Association data. Asking more than one question about a concept can increase the internal validity of a survey.[36] For example, a respondent who answers yes to a positively worded statement would be expected to answer no to the same concept when worded in a negative fashion. A coefficient alpha that measures correlation between items should be calculated and reported in the article if this technique is used.[36] The coefficient alpha is interpreted in the same fashion that coefficients of reliability are interpreted, (i.e., 0 indicates no consistency between responses while 1 indicates complete consistency).

The methods section should report sample size, along with a description of how it was determined. The validity of both survey research and clinical trials relies on sample size. In order to have sufficient statistical power to demonstrate a difference between two groups, studies must have an adequate sample size. In designing survey research, the population of interest is first determined then subdivided into smaller groups around a variable of interest. For example, the population of interest may be all patients who attend a pharmacist-managed asthma clinic. This population could be subdivided into smaller groups based on the severity of asthma and then surveyed as to level of customer satisfaction. In establishing sample size for survey research, investigators must then determine the minimum number of subjects that must be sampled for the sample to be representative of the entire population.[40] This determination is made by consulting references that describe variability in sampling.[40]

Additionally, the reader should evaluate the comprehensiveness, probability of selection, and efficiency of the sample frame. A sample is comprehensive if all members of a population had a chance to be chosen and no one was systematically excluded.[40] Determining efficiency of a sample relates to how well the sample frame excluded individuals who are not the subject of the survey. For example, to survey elderly people, it is appropriate to survey all households to determine if elderly individuals live there.[40] In addition to providing information about the sampling frame, the methods section should provide a description of interviewers (age, sex, ethnicity, and so forth) and the effect interviewers may have had on the data.

Sampling strategy and response rates should also be stated. The methods section should supply the reader with enough information to assure that nonresponse error was assessed and measures were taken to control it.[36] Repeated attempts to obtain completed questionnaires from initial nonrespondents will yield higher response rates and more accurate results than if no follow-ups are performed.[41] For example, attempts at other times of the day should be made for phone surveys and a second reminder postcard should be sent for mailed surveys. Additionally, one way to minimize the problem of poor response rates is to sample (by phone) a small group of nonresponders to determine if their responses differ substantially from responders, although this may not be possible.[39] If results do not differ, the survey remains valid. Furthermore, authors should relate as much information about nonrespondents as is possible. Although survey result information has not been gathered, authors may have demographic and geographic data based on addresses and other information originally obtained.

The methods section should also describe techniques used to assess the reliability (i.e., can the results of the survey be repeated by another investigator) of the survey instrument and present the results of reliability estimates.[36] In general, the higher the reliability estimate, the more confidence the reader may place in the results published.[36] Chap. 10 provides a more complete review of reliability coefficients. Additionally, any relevant elements of the survey research administration process (i.e., whether a pretest or pilot test was used) should be described. A pretest or pilot test is an assessment of a questionnaire made before full-scale implementation to identify and correct problems such as faulty questions, flawed response options, or interviewer training deficiencies.[41] Subjects administered the pretest not only answer the survey questions, but also answer questions about the clarity, length, and ease of understanding of the actual instrument and may contribute other questions they think should be included.[37]

Of note, informed consent is generally not required in survey research as the risk is minimal and the respondent has the opportunity to withdraw from participating every time a new question is asked.[40] If the respondent does withdraw part way through the survey or interview, the data should not be included in the final analysis. In situations where sensitive information might potentially harm the subject, asking for an informed consent document to be signed allows the researchers the opportunity to reassure their commitment to confidentiality and reinforce the limits of how the data can be used.

Surveys are a commonly used research tool and are capable of providing a wealth of information on many aspects of a given target population. Ensuring validity of information gained through survey research, however, relies on critical evaluation of results through a thorough assessment of the study's internal rigor.[36] The ability to evaluate such research results is highly dependent on the amount and quality of information presented in the methods section.[36] A guide for critique of mail survey research has been published[36] and questions to ask when evaluating survey research are available in Appendix 7–1.

Postmarketing Surveillance Studies

Prior to approval by the FDA, drugs undergo testing in a limited number of patients. Once approved, experience in patients escalates and previously unrecognized, rare adverse events may be identified. The drug also may be found to be useful for conditions not described in the product labeling.

Postmarketing surveillance studies are phase IV studies that follow drug use after market approval and are sometimes referred to as pharmacoepidemiologic studies. They are useful in identifying new, potentially serious effects of drugs. A number of drugs have been removed from the market after approval following identification of such problems (e.g., fenfluramine, rofecoxib [Vioxx™], valdecoxib [Bextra®], and more recently, hydromorphone hydrochloride extended release capsules [Palladone™]). Postmarketing surveillance studies also allow assessment of drug use outside of product labeling and may identify areas for further research.

Many types of study designs are used in phase IV studies including cross-sectional, case-control, cohort, and even experimental designs (randomized-controlled clinical trials). These studies can answer questions about drug interactions, identify potential new indications for the product, and gather information about the consequences of overdose, and efficacy in a larger and broader population (patients with different disease states and demographics that may not have been fully evaluated in the original clinical trials).[42] The principles of literature evaluation described in previous sections are also applicable to these studies.

Perhaps one of the most important functions of postmarketing surveillance is in the area of adverse event reporting. Currently, most of the information on postmarketing safety of the product comes from spontaneous adverse reaction reports. Reporting of events associated with a product by the health care practitioner to a regulatory agency or the pharmaceutical company that markets the product are the primary means for gathering this information. Each pharmaceutical company is required to maintain a database of these spontaneous reports. This database is monitored for increases in frequency of certain events or the appearance of serious unexpected events. If it is determined that there is a causal relationship between the drug and the event, the product labeling may be changed to reflect either new events or events with increasing frequency.

There are several limitations to this type of data collection. The information is taken from the reporter who must make a diagnosis and assessment of causality, data may be underreported because it is a voluntary system and this may bias the estimation of incidence, reports may vary in quality and thoroughness, and the database may not be suitable for detecting adverse reactions with high background rates in the population.[42] See Chap. 17, for additional information. Questions to ask when evaluating postmarketing surveillance studies are provided in Appendix 7-1.

Pulling It all Together: Organizing and Ranking Studies _____

When reviewing published studies, it is not uncommon to become overwhelmed with a collection of papers, all seemingly pertinent to the clinical question under evaluation, and often including conclusions of two or more research reports that may be in opposition. How does one sort through the studies and efficiently determine which of those articles are of highest quality? A good place to begin is by categorizing trials based on fundamental differentiating study design characteristics. One may quickly sort articles by study design by asking a few specific questions.

One method developed and utilized at University of Missouri, Kansas City (UMKC) School of Pharmacy allows division into five broad categories of study design, and is illustrated in Tables 7–7 and 7–8.[43] Additionally, see Figure 7–3 for scenarios regarding reviewer evaluation of power status and implications for interpretability of trial results.

Subsequent analysis of strengths and limitations of individual trials within and between the five categories provides the clinician insight into varying levels of confidence for decision-making or recommendations derived from aggregate trial analysis. The clinician should make firm recommendations and decisions based on results of well-controlled interventional investigations, and make only cautious recommendations and decisions when only results of uncontrolled clinical observations exist, especially when risk to patients is involved.

TABLE 7–7. BROAD CATEGORIZATION OF TRIALS, BY STUDY DESIGN*

Controlled (Or Comparison Group Included)				Uncontrolled
Controlled vs. uncontrolled trials Rationale: Studies lacking a control or comparison group are typically not useful for broad decision-making				
Interventional		Observational		
Interventional vs. observational trials Rationale: Interventional trials can show cause and effect, while observational trials can only indicate a correlation or association. See discussion in this chapter entitled Case-Control Studies				
Powered	No power Sometimes referred to as *low power* (e.g., power not calculated or power calculated but not met)	Prospective	Retrospective or having a historical component	
Powered vs. no power Rationale: Interventional trials are most useful when powered to detect a difference if one exists.		Prospective vs. retrospective Rationale: A prospective cohort design allows for better elimination and/or control of extraneous variables, thus producing more reliable results than a retrospective look at data.		

*See also, Figure 7–3, power algorithm.
SOURCE: Adapted from Bryant PJ.[43]

TABLE 7–8. STUDY CATEGORIZATIONS

Interventional, Powered	Interventional, No Power	*Decreasing rigor* Observational, Prospective	Observational, Retrospective	Uncontrolled
Randomized, controlled trials, with power calculated and met	Randomized, controlled trials, unpowered (low power)	Cohort studies	Case-control studies (trohoc)	Case series, case reports, case studies

Other methods for categorizing and ranking studies utilized by organizations that perform evidence-based literature evaluations are discussed further in Chap. 9.

Review Articles

Once a reader understands differences between individual study designs and characteristics for evaluating strengths and weaknesses within individual studies, it will become easier to analyze differences between publications which attempt to combine results from multiple studies, generally termed review articles.

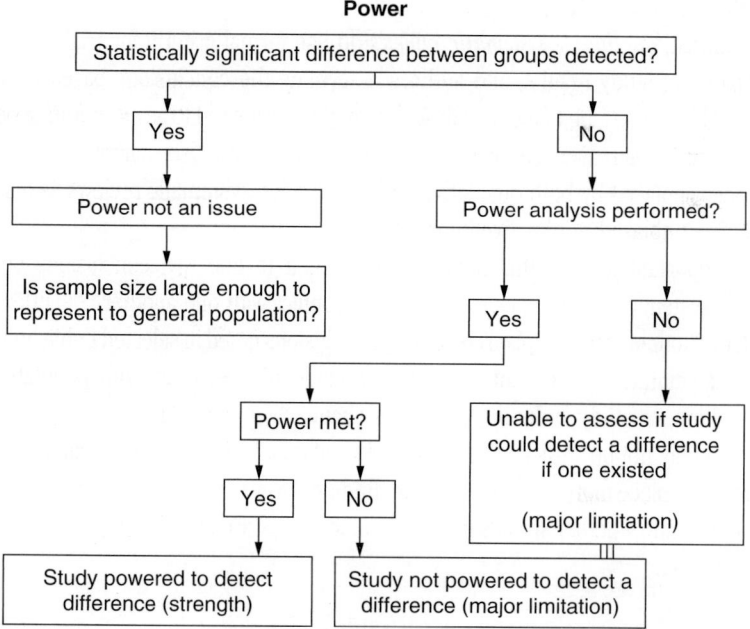

Figure 7–3. Power algorithm.
Several scenarios exist with regard to power status and subsequent interpretability of clinical trial results. This power algorithm diagrams the different power scenarios and subsequent interpretability of trial results. *(Refer to Chap. 6 for more discussion regarding the power concept.)* (Source: Developed by Richardson AD and Bryant PJ for Evidence-Based Medicine course, PHA 326, University of Missouri, Kansas City School of Pharmacy, 1999.)

Review articles, consisting of analysis and interpretation of previously conducted research studies, are classified as tertiary literature, although they are often used as secondary sources because they can lead readers to primary literature references. Review articles discussing treatment of disease states or clinical aspects of drug therapy enable pharmacists to gain insight into a topic or question of interest and may provide more current information than textbooks.

The term *review* encompasses three very different entities—the nonsystematic (narrative) review, the systematic review (qualitative review), and the meta-analysis (quantitative review). Reviews are becoming more common in the literature and are relied on as an efficient method for keeping up with the large amount of information presented to the health care professional each day.

Although the purpose of review articles is to present the "truth" found among conflicting and variable primary literature, this does not always occur. Reviews may be subject to author biases or inaccuracies or in the literature search.[44] Narrative (nonsystematic) literature reviews generally do not apply systematic methods such as formal criteria for selection of studies, and they address broad rather than focused clinical questions. They often educate readers about the author's interpretations of selected evidence, rather than using a systematic approach to evidence evaluation. Frequently, authors are experts on the topic and know the conclusions prior to conducting the review.

In contrast, *qualitative systematic reviews* do use formal criteria for trial selection and interpretation of study results, and authors determine the conclusions based on the data reviewed. This is also true of meta-analyses (sometimes referred to as *quantitative systematic reviews*). Due to increased emphasis on evidence-based practice, narrative reviews have largely been replaced by both qualitative and quantitative systematic reviews as a source of authoritative, unbiased, summative information.

It is important to note that it is not uncommon to find that conclusions of general overviews, systematic reviews, or meta-analyses conflict with one another.[45,46] Differences in research methodology may explain conflicting conclusions noted in selected published studies. Other explanations for discordant conclusions include differences in study populations, type of intervention, or study endpoint, as well as chance.[46] In some cases, the amount of high quality data may not be sufficient to come to a valid conclusion; in others, clinical judgment of authors may place more weight on certain findings over others. Readers of review articles need to determine whether studies included in the review are broad enough to apply to their clinical situation.

NARRATIVE (NONSYSTEMATIC) REVIEWS

A narrative (nonsystematic) review is a summary of research that lacks a description of systematic methods. Narrative reviews are considered tertiary literature because they provide information in much the same manner as found in textbooks, but are sometimes used like secondary references because they also contain extensive and "up-to-date" bibliographies. Narrative reviews may pertain to one specific clinical question or disease state, or to topics related to pharmacy administration (e.g., Pharmacy and Therapeutics Committees).

Techniques can be applied to evaluate the quality of narrative reviews (Appendix 7–1). Such skills are necessary, considering the poor quality of many published narrative reviews.[44] As a specific example of shortcomings of narrative reviews, Joyce and associates[47] found that citation of the literature is influenced by the review authors' discipline and nationality. For example, infectious disease specialists reviewing a disease state were more likely to cite laboratory literature than psychiatrists reviewing the same disease state while the reverse was true for neuropsychiatry literature; a review author in the United Kingdom was more likely to cite articles that originate in the United Kingdom than in other countries. This study also found that, of 89 reviews, only 3 (3.4%) described the methods used in the literature search. Legitimate differences in authors' clinical judgment can also affect results. For example, if a treatment has been shown to be effective and has a 7% incidence of a fairly severe adverse event, some authors will feel this is an acceptable risk compared to risks of the disease state, while others will deem that level of risk unacceptable.

SYSTEMATIC REVIEW—QUALITATIVE

If the purpose of nonsystematic reviews is to "find the truth," then the purpose of the systematic review is "finding the whole truth."[48] Cook and associates describe systematic reviews as scientific investigations with predefined methods and original studies as their subjects.[49] Two general types of systematic reviews exist. The term qualitative systematic review has been applied to a summary of results of primary studies where the results are not statistically combined.[49] In contrast, a quantitative systematic review, or meta-analysis, has been described as a systematic review that uses statistical methods to combine the results of two or more studies.[49] Perhaps, more appropriately, meta-analyses can be thought of as a specific methodological and statistical technique (or tool) for combining quantitative data. Table 7–9 illustrates the primary differences between qualitative and quantitative systematic reviews.[49]

Systematic overviews that summarize scientific evidence (in contrast to nonsystematic narrative reviews that mix opinions and evidence) are becoming increasingly prevalent. These overviews address questions of treatment, causation, diagnosis, or prognosis and are considered superior to nonsystematic (narrative) reviews of any given topic.[45]

Qualitative systematic reviews should concentrate on a clearly defined issue that is of importance to practice.[45,46] Specific criteria should be used to select articles from the primary literature to be included in the review.[45] For valid conclusions to be derived from qualitative systematic reviews, authors must clearly define the study population or topic of interest and include only those studies using valid research methods.[45] For example, authors would have

TABLE 7–9. COMPARISON OF NONSYSTEMATIC REVIEWS, QUALITATIVE SYSTEMATIC REVIEWS, AND QUANTITATIVE SYSTEMATIC REVIEWS (META-ANALYSIS)

Feature	Nonsystematic Review	Qualitative Systematic Review	Quantitative Systematic Review
Clinical question	Often broadly defined	Clearly defined and focused	Clearly defined and focused
Literature search	Methods of literature search usually not explicitly described	Explicit description of predefined and comprehensive search strategy	Explicit description of predefined and comprehensive search strategy
Studies included	Methods for determining which studies to include not usually described	Predefined inclusion and exclusion criteria	Predefined inclusion and exclusion criteria
Includes unpublished literature	Not usually	Possibly	Possibly
Blinding of reviewers	No	Yes	Yes
Analysis of data	Variable and subjective	Rigorous and objective	Rigorous and objective
Results statistically evaluated	No	No	Yes

SOURCE: Adapted from reference Cook DJ, et al.[49]

the choice of assessing patients who are either pre- or postmenopausal in a qualitative systematic review focused on the utility of chemotherapy in improving survival following mastectomy in breast cancer patients. Conclusions of this qualitative systematic review are likely to be very different depending on which subsets of breast cancer patients are selected. In addition, the authors' initial literature search would probably reveal a collection of studies that use a wide variety of research techniques. Only those studies meeting strict criteria for validity as discussed in Chap. 6 should be included in the review. Poorly controlled, nonrandomized, unblinded studies should be excluded to produce the most reliable results.

Authors should use a variety of resources to identify studies for the qualitative systematic review. Use of a single database is not likely to capture all relevant studies and results in reference bias. A combination of databases (such as MEDLINE® and EMBASE), study bibliographies, and experts in the field should be used to identify studies for evaluation.[45,46]

Consideration should be given to inclusion of unpublished data (e.g., data on file at the manufacturer or personal communication with investigators) in addition to published studies, because it has been determined that published studies are more often of a positive nature than unpublished studies, a situation termed publication bias.[45] The benefit of using unpublished studies is to include more data from which to draw a conclusion. A drawback is that unpublished studies have likely not undergone a peer-review and revision process; errors and unclearly stated conclusions may be present. Language bias, in which only articles published in the author's primary language are used, may also affect results. In order to reduce selection bias, review authors choosing articles should be blinded to (1) names of the study authors (to avoid political or personal issues), (2) institution of publication, and (3) results of the studies. For the initial choice of study inclusion, only the methods section should be reviewed.[50,51] In addition, because of the subjective nature of some aspects of analysis, two or more authors should critique each study under consideration and all evaluators should concur on which studies will be included in the qualitative systematic review.[45]

Data should be summarized in table format.[45] Outcomes described in the qualitative systematic review article should be meaningful, and, if the trial is a clinical trial, clinically important.[45] For example, improved survival rates is a more desirable endpoint than reduction in total cholesterol for the hydroxymethylglutaryl-CoA (HMG-CoA) reductase literature. Authors should also assess benefits versus risks associated with the therapy under review, if possible.[45]

"All reviews, narrative and systematic alike, are retrospective, observational research studies and are therefore subject to systematic and random error."[49] Just as for nonsystematic reviews, techniques can be applied to evaluate the quality of systematic reviews.[52] Questions to ask when critiquing systematic reviews are provided in Appendix 7–1.

SYSTEMATIC REVIEWS—QUANTITATIVE (META-ANALYSES)

Meta-analyses are now widely used to provide supporting evidence for clinical decision-making. Meta-analysis is a technique that has been developed to provide a quantitative and objective assessment.[53] In a meta-analysis, results of previously conducted clinical trials are combined and statistically evaluated.[50,53] Meta-analyses are designed to provide greater insight into clinical dilemmas than individual clinical trials. They are especially useful when previous studies have been inconclusive or contradictory, or in situations where sample size may have been too small to detect a statistically significant difference between treatment and control groups (i.e., low power). Sacks and colleagues[50] have described the following purposes for performing a meta-analysis: "(1) to increase the statistical power for primary endpoint and for subgroups, (2) to resolve uncertainty when reports disagree, (3) to improve estimates of size of effect, (4) to answer new questions not posed at the start of individual trials, and (5) to bring about improvements in the quality of the primary research."

Meta-analysis has been used to address important clinical questions, such as whether aspirin reduces the risk of pregnancy-induced hypertension, cholesterol lowering decreases mortality, fluoxetine increases suicidal ideations, or estrogen replacement therapy increases the risk of breast cancer.[53] Meta-analysis can be used to look at both clinical trials and epidemiologic research, such as follow-up and case-control studies, and is particularly useful when definitive trials cannot be conducted, results of available trials are inconclusive, or while awaiting the results of definitive trials.[50,51,53] For the hypothetical situation regarding drug A used for the treatment of myocardial infarction, suppose that there are a number of small clinical trials suggesting that the product increases sudden death through proarrlythmic effects. A meta-analysis could potentially be performed to statistically combine the results of these small trials and increase the power of the finding (association or lack of association of drug A with increased sudden death).

Methodological problems with meta-analyses have lead to controversy surrounding their use in clinical decision-making. When results from multiple trials are combined, biases of the individual studies are incorporated and new sources of bias arise. The quality of the meta-analysis depends on the quality of the individual studies used to develop the meta-analysis.[54] Indeed, LeLorier and coworkers have compared the results of a series of large, randomized, controlled trials with those of previously published meta-analyses examining the same questions.[54] They found that outcomes of 12 large, randomized, controlled trials studied were predicted inaccurately by previously published meta-analyses 35% of the time.[54] The randomized, controlled clinical trials corresponded to meta-analyses in terms of population studied, therapeutic intervention, and at least one outcome. In this study, 46% of divergences in results involved a positive meta-analysis being followed by a negative randomized, controlled trial while the remaining 54% of identified divergences involved a negative meta-analysis followed by a positive randomized, controlled trial. Reasons for divergences as cited by the authors included the heterogeneity of the trials included in the meta-analyses and publication bias (tendency of investigators to preferentially submit studies with positive results for publication).[54]

Several points should be considered when evaluating meta-analyses. A quality meta-analysis must clearly define the clinical question addressed by the analysis.[50,51] As with qualitative systematic reviews, details of literature searches that were conducted to locate primary research articles must be given and criteria for inclusion of studies in the meta-analysis must be determined prior to conducting the analysis.[50,51,53] Because computerized searches may not locate all of the relevant articles, other resources such as textbooks, experts in the field, and reference lists from clinical studies should also be consulted.[50] Whether to include trials from gray literature (i.e., trials that have not been published in peer-reviewed journals but are available from the author or perhaps the manufacturer of a drug, is controversial).[55] As discussed with qualitative reviews, there is the risk of using data that have not been peer-reviewed; the benefit is more data to increase the power of statistical analysis.

Trials included in and excluded from the meta-analysis should be listed, along with explanation of reasons for exclusion. Strict standards should be established prior to the initiation of the meta-analysis to ensure that criteria used for inclusion of participants, administration of the principal treatment, and measurement of outcome events are similar in all trials studied.[54] Types of patients, their diagnosis, treatments, and therapeutic endpoints used in the original clinical studies should be given. The source of financial support for the original articles should be identified; however, as with analysis of individual trials, this becomes a major source of concern only when evidence of possible bias is present (e.g., strong positive conclusions, when results are inconclusive or only weakly positive).[50,51] Interpretation of meta-analyses results are limited by what studies were (or were not) included, how homogeneous (or heterogeneous) the studies were, and the methodological quality of the studies.[19]

A major problem of meta-analyses is the issue of publication bias found by LeLorier and associates described above.[50,52,53] It has been documented that researchers are more likely to publish studies that demonstrate positive effects of drugs. Therefore, studies that show lack of efficacy are less likely to be located than those that demonstrate beneficial effects of a drug. Just as for quantitative reviews, authors of meta-analyses should be blinded and choose trials that match prespecified criteria based solely on the methods section of studies.

Authors should address the validity of articles used in the meta-analysis (see Chap. 6) such as randomization techniques, compliance, blinding, appropriate dosing and length of studies, and intent-to-treat analyses.[50,53] Some experts believe that studies should be weighted based on quality, but this practice is controversial because such assessments are subjective.[53]

The studies should be similar enough to allow pooling of data.[50,51] Statistical tests that evaluate homogeneity should be used to assess similarity of studies.[51] The more statistically significant the results of these tests, the more likely differences in study results are due to chance alone. If results of tests of homogeneity are not significant, the studies are heterogeneous and differences in study results may be due to research design, rather than chance alone. Caution should be used when pooling results of heterogeneous studies.

Appropriate statistical analyses should be undertaken (usually the Mantel-Haenszel test), probability of false-positive (e.g., Type I error) and false-negative (e.g., Type II error) results should be discussed, and 95% confidence intervals, which provide the range of values where the true value lies 95% of the time, should be calculated.[50]

Finally, sensitivity analyses should be conducted to determine how the results of the meta-analysis vary depending on use of different assumptions, tests, and criteria and the economic implications of the meta-analysis should be considered.[50,51] Use of the above criteria when conducting meta-analyses has improved in recent years.[53] However, recently the usefulness of meta-analysis have been questioned when the results of subsequent randomized, controlled trials did not support previously published meta-analyses on the same subject as described above.[54]

Overall, meta-analyses should be interpreted with caution, remembering that conclusions depend on the quality of the studies included and findings of subsequent randomized, controlled trials may differ from those of the meta-analysis.[19] Meta-analyses, on the surface, appear to be an extremely valuable tool allowing the practitioner to efficiently stay abreast of new information; however, oversimplification may lead to inappropriate conclusions.[54] Like all types of research evidence, meta-analyses require careful analysis to determine their validity and their applicability in practice.[55] Questions for readers to consider when evaluating the quality of published meta-analyses have been published and a list is provided in Appendix 7–1.[56]

Of note, an important source of systematic reviews (both qualitative and meta-analyses) is the Cochrane Handbook (published by the Cochrane Collaboration), which is available in paper, CD-ROM, and Internet format (<<http://www.cochrane.org/resources/handbook/index.htm>>). Thirty-six reviews published in the Cochrane Database of Systematic Reviews were compared to a randomly selected sample of 39 meta-analyses or systematic reviews published in journals indexed by MEDLINE® in 1995.[57] Cochrane reviews were more likely to include a description of the inclusion and exclusion criteria (35/36 vs. 18/39; p < 0.001) and an assessment of trial quality (36/36 vs. 12/39; p < 0.001). By June 1997, 18 of 36 Cochrane reviews had been updated as compared to 1 of 39 reviews listed in MEDLINE®. Overall, the authors concluded that "Cochrane reviews appeared to have greater methodological rigor and were more frequently updated than systematic reviews or meta-analyses published in paper-based journals."[57]

Practice Guidelines

Three types of practice guidelines are published at the present time: evidence-based or "explicit," formal consensus-based, and informal consensus-based. These various types are differentiated by the source of information used to develop the practice guideline as well as the rigor of the process for evaluating that information. EBM and explicit practice guidelines utilize a rigorous systematic process involving review and critical evaluation of the medical literature to develop final recommendations. Informal and formal consensus-based practice guidelines utilize experience of experts in the area to draw conclusions and develop recommendations. This is useful for those instances where the evidence is not complete or conclusive to allow the development of a final recommendation, thus experts are used to assist completion of practice guidelines using their expertise in those deficient areas. More information regarding differentiating characteristics of the development of various practice guidelines are discussed in Chap. 9.

Practice guidelines are created primarily for facilitating clinical decision-making, improving the quality of health care, providing consistent treatment across environments, decreasing costs, diminishing professional liability, and identifying individualized alternative treatment.[58,59] Key questions to be considered when evaluating a practice guideline are proposed.[60,61] These questions primarily identify the developmental process used to produce guidelines and are summarized in Appendix 7–1 and in detail in Chap. 9.

Useful guidelines provide information regarding therapeutic options and most appropriate choices for a specific disease and patient.[62] Important attributes for useful guidelines include: validity, reproducibility/reliability, clinical applicability, clinical flexibility, accessibility, clarity, multidisciplinary development process, scheduled review, and documentation.[63]

To be applicable, practice guidelines must be regularly maintained. Research has shown that within 2 years of development, a practice guideline may become outdated.[61]

Practice guidelines are becoming a common tool to use for patient population decisions. Factors are identified that influence the impact of a particular practice guideline.[64] One of the most important factors is strength of the evidence used to develop guidelines. Other factors include intensity of dissemination, follow-through of dissemination, type of problem addressed, source of guidelines, physician participation in development and adoption, form and specificity of the guideline recommendation, legal considerations, and financial/administrative issues. Additional information regarding practice guidelines is discussed in Chap. 9.

Health Outcomes Research

Health outcomes research encompasses literature pertaining to discussion of pharmacoeconomic, therapeutic, and nontherapeutic outcomes (such as number of visits to emergency room and number of hospital admissions), along with QOL outcomes. Readers are referred to Chap. 8 for information on evaluating pharmacoeconomic outcome studies. Therapeutic and nontherapeutic outcomes are covered in previous sections. This section will focus on evaluating literature that includes QOL outcome measures.

QUALITY-OF-LIFE MEASURES

Clinical trials have traditionally focused on health outcomes related to physical or laboratory measurements of response.[65] How the patient feels and functions relative to daily activities is not always captured by these measurements. A patient's perception of well-being can be the most important outcome in specific disease states. Investigators make assumptions that changes in therapy improve the patient's QOL. These assumptions require testing. For this reason, additional health outcome measurements have been developed to address a patient's QOL.

QOL is a term that has acquired several different definitions. General agreement exists that QOL is a multidimensional concept focusing on impact of a disease and treatment relative to well-being of a patient.[65] Physical and social environment affects QOL. Emotional and existential reactions to this physical and social environment also have an influence. Health-related quality of life (HR-QOL) is an accepted term used to represent the value assigned to quality and quantity of life "as modified by impairments, functional states, perceptions, and social opportunities that are influenced by disease, injury, treatment, or policy."[66] Direct measure of HR-QOL is impossible. Only inferences from patient symptoms and reported perceptions provide measurement of HR-QOL.

Two types of HR-QOL measurements exist: health status assessment and patient preference assessment.[56] Heath status assessment is a self-assessment that measures multiple aspects of a patient's perceived well-being. This assessment is primarily designed to either compare groups of patients receiving different treatments or effect of a treatment for a single group over time. Thus, health status assessments are most often used in clinical trials comparing treatment regimens. Context of questions used range from perceived impact of disease and treatments to disease frequency and severity. Examples of health status assessments include Functional Living Index-Cancer (FLIC), European Organization for Research and Treatment of Cancer (EORTC QLQ-C30), and the Functional Assessment of Cancer Therapy (FACT).[67-69] Health status assessments take approximately 5 to 10 minutes to complete.

Patient preference assessments reflect an individual's decision-making process at a time when the eventual outcome is unknown.[65] These assessments measure the patient's tradeoff between quality and quantity of life. For example, a patient with a terminal illness may be assisted with decision-making of treatment options based on a time trade-off instrument. This instrument is designed to assess a patient's preference with respect to their wishes regarding QOL versus quantity of life. Specifics of patient preference assessments are beyond the scope of this discussion because they are seldom used in clinical trials.

Two types of instruments are used to measure HR-QOL: generic and disease-specific.[70] Generic instruments assess HR-QOL in patients both with and without active disease. An example of a generic instrument is Sickness Impact Profile, a health profile instrument that attempts to measure multiple aspects of HR-QOL. Generic instruments are useful for comparing completely different groups or following groups after treatment is discontinued. Disease-specific instruments are narrower in scope, more sensitive, and focus on specific treatment or disease impact. These instruments relate to areas investigated by clinicians.

A battery of several disease-specific instruments can be used to obtain a comprehensive understanding of impact associated with different interventions. For example, a variety of disease-specific instruments, including sleep, sexual dysfunction, and physical activity, can be used to demonstrate differing effects of antihypertensive therapy on HR-QOL. HR-QOL trials should use validated HR-QOL instruments.[71] Reviewers can confirm validation of HR-QOL instruments from statements, backed by citations, indicating the questionnaires have been validated. Lack of these references or some other description of a validation process should cause concern and skepticism. Similarly, use of a combination or a series of valid HR-QOL measurements as described above should also document validity for the resultant HR-QOL battery. In practice, this integrative approach may reduce validity of HR-QOL measurements due to interactions of the various instruments on one another. Investigators must document the validity of each test used in a series as well as validity of the series as a whole. Reviewers should be aware of potential bias or problems resulting from this.

When reviewing a study containing HR-QOL measurements, the reader should consider several study characteristics,[72] and list of suggested questions to ask when reviewing these trials are provided in Appendix 7–1. Reviewers should not only identify potential biases, but then determine impact of each bias on the final results reported by investigators.

Because there is no commonly accepted method to determine clinical significance of changes in most HR-QOL measurements, interpretation of HR-QOL results from clinical trials can be difficult.[72,73] A standardized method to indicate appropriate interpretation of clinically important changes and/or differences between groups in HR-QOL measurements is needed.

Trials measuring HR-QOL should be powered to detect a statistically significant difference.[65] Adequate sample size is calculated by the investigator to meet a designated level of power with a resultant number of subjects required to detect a statistically significant difference, if a difference truly exists. For example, if a study required 400 patients in each group to meet power but only 270 patients in each group were included in the final statistical analysis, power would not have been met. This is particularly important if no difference is noted between groups, in which case a difference may actually exist, but due to inadequate sample size that difference was not detected. Inadequate enrollment to allow for attrition, large patient dropout rates, and numerous protocol violators all contribute to a reduced sample size. Often HR-QOL is designated as a secondary endpoint with study power calculated to detect differences in only primary outcome measurements. Note that if subgroups are analyzed, sample size of those subgroups must also be determined prior to analysis, and sample sizes adequate to meet power. Additional information regarding power can be found in Figure 7–3 in this chapter and in Chap. 6.

Authors should document inclusion and applicability of relevant HR-QOL measurements in the assessment instrument.[74,75] For instance, if the study is evaluating a drug for treatment of a particular disease state, rheumatoid arthritis, outcome measurements should be specific to this disease (e.g., outcome measures for rheumatoid arthritis would include mobility, hand activities, personal care, home chores, and interpersonal activities). The HR-QOL measurements represent unique personal perceptions that reflect how individual patients feel about their health status and/or nonmedical aspects of their lives. These perceptions can be difficult to capture, resulting in HR-QOL measurements that inadequately reflect patient's values and preferences.[77] The reviewer should evaluate the HR-QOL measurements to determine if individual patients are given opportunities to express opinions and reactions rather than just an assessment of disease progression. For example, the HR-QOL measurement instrument for hand activities associated with rheumatoid arthritis should capture patients' perception of how well they can move their hand, not just a determination of range of hand motion. In addition, the HR-QOL instrument should be sensitive to changes in patients' status throughout the clinical trial and should measure aspects of their lives considered important by the patients.[76,77] Benchmarking these measures with those used in similar published studies helps identify standard or accepted measurements for a specific disease state.

These can be difficult parameters to isolate and thus, many measurements of HR-QOL fall short of capturing this important concept.[77] Trials overlooking important issues related to patients' health status and/or nonmedical aspects of their lives can provide misleading results.

Timing of HR-QOL measurements should be appropriate to answer research questions.[65] This timing of test administration should be related to the anticipated timing of clinical effects. In some cases, outcomes may lag behind clinical effects and in other situations they could precede clinical effects. For instance, when evaluating a subject's perception of mood improvement following initiation of a course of antidepressant drug therapy, the measurement should not occur for several weeks to allow the medication adequate time to demonstrate efficacy. Alternatively, a HR-QOL measurement of overall QOL related to cancer therapy may include pretreatment anxiety and anticipatory nausea preceding a chemotherapy session.

HR-QOL measurements should occupy the same timing within test sequences. For example, it is recommended that HR-QOL measurements be obtained at the beginning of clinic visits, unless there are substantial reasons provided by the authors to perform these tests at a different time. This is due to cognitively demanding assessment instruments and the fact that most subjects are "fresher" at the beginning of the visit. Additionally, if several measurements are obtained for each subject throughout the course of a trial, care should be taken to ensure similar timing between subjects occurs for sequential testing.

The mode of data collection is important because self-reporting is sufficient with some types of questions, while other specific types of questions are better asked by an interviewer.[65] When a trained interviewer is used, interview location is important to obtaining unbiased answers. In a case regarding a treatment for a terminal illness, the patient may be more interested in QOL, while the family member is prioritizing quantity of life. An interview conducted in the presence of that family member could affect that patient's QOL response. Thus, HR-QOL measurements are best obtained in a private setting to reduce risk of biased responses.

Results are usually reported as a composite; however, individual patient data are often reported in smaller studies; for instance, when a rare disease limits sample size. When individual patient data are reported, the reviewer should attempt to determine if patients' answers were potentially biased due to their awareness of this public disclosure.

Assessment instrument response rates are critical since nonresponse can introduce significant bias into the results.[78] In addition, data should be reasonably complete throughout the study since missing data can suggest investigator bias.[65] The reviewer should determine if data appear to be randomly missing. If a pattern of missing data is recognized, e.g., if a specific question or group has been excluded, the omission should be explained by authors. In this situation, the reviewer should determine if missing data have the potential to counter the author's hypothesis, thus identifying one explanation for incomplete data reporting. Reviewers must determine if HR-QOL measurements in a multicenter trial were performed at all sites. If HR-QOL measurements are not performed at all sites, authors should provide the reason for this methodology deviation.

Repeated use of HR-QOL measurements can lead to a training effect on the patient and/or interviewer, resulting in misleading conclusions.[77] The reviewer should determine if this effect is present and how that effect results. Showing test subjects their prior responses to HR-QOL measurement questions in an attempt to decrease variability should generally not be done unless acceptable supportive rationale for this procedure is given by the authors.

For the HR-QOL analysis, appropriate statistical tests should be used for the type of data analyzed such as use of categorical tests such as the Mann-Whitney U test for nonparametric data. For example, data regarding attitudes regarding patient satisfaction with use of inhaled insulin may be measured by a Likert scale (ordinal data), and should be analyzed using nonparametric tests. All specific analytical features should be described at the time of trial design (e.g., *a priori*). A reviewer should look for an author explanation of which specific tests are used on QOL data and should not assume that the same statistical tests are used on the QOL data as are discussed for the other trial outcomes (i.e., efficacy or safety outcome data) if not directly discussed. Selective reporting of favorable or statistically significant results is also a problem. Both positive and negative findings, in addition to neutral or insignificant results, should be reported for completeness.

Several other items are worth consideration when evaluating trials with HR-QOL outcome measurements. Use of HR-QOL measurements for reporting of adverse drug events is not appropriate.[72] Trials should evaluate efficacy, safety, and HR-QOL separately and as distinctly different outcomes. An assumption that adverse events determine HR-QOL (or vice versa) can lead to erroneous results. For instance, consider a trial with breast cancer patients in whom surgery and chemotherapy is expected to eradicate all cancer cells. An appropriate assessment of HR-QOL outcomes for some patients may be positive despite troublesome adverse reactions such as low blood counts, decreased energy, and increased susceptibility to infection, based on perception that treatment will ultimately result in a complete cure. Alternatively, other patients HR-QOL outcomes may reflect poor QOL, even in the absence of treatment-related adverse events but instead, due to an overall situational depression. Without separate assessments of adverse events experienced and HR-QOL outcomes, linking adverse events with QOL can result in inaccurate interpretations.

Finally, culturally defined factors may impact patient's QOL and assessment of HR-QOL measurements. Validity of HR-QOL measurements across different cultures or subcultures should be considered by the reviewer. For instance, a HR-QOL instrument may effectively measure outcomes for HIV-infected men living in the United States, but may be completely inadequate for measuring outcomes in HIV-infected women living in Africa. Assessment instruments must account for and reflect the variability between outcomes perceived as important to patients, considering that perceptions may be quite diverse between cultures, must be assessed accordingly.

Dietary Supplement Medical Literature

Dietary supplement (botanical and nonbotanical) information is a growing body of medical literature that many pharmacists find themselves delving into more frequently as patients continue to use dietary supplements. As with standard drug literature, the ability to discern solid clinical evidence from weak clinical evidence is an important skill to aid pharmacists in making dietary supplement recommendations to patients and other health care professionals.

The provision of dietary supplement information is not dissimilar to that of standard drug information. Evidence may be described and ranked according to the quality of the literature supporting or refuting dietary supplement product claims. The same evidence-based criteria utilized for drug literature analysis apply to the dietary supplement literature for determining study strengths and weaknesses. Thus, large, well-designed, randomized, controlled clinical trials or well-done meta-analyses lend stronger support versus uncontrolled or retrospective data, case series or reports, and experiential testimonials. However, it is not unusual to have only poorly designed published trials supporting or refuting a dietary supplement product's claims. For some products, the only data available concerning theoretical actions, interactions, and side effects are animal and/or *in vitro* data. Often these trials use chemical extracts or single chemical agents from a natural source.

Unlike standard medications, dietary supplements are not legally required to be proven safe and effective in humans prior to marketing. In situations where the only safety and efficacy data for a product are theoretical, from case reports or flawed trials, or from animal and/or *in vitro* studies, pharmacists must weigh risks of the interaction or side effect occurring against possible benefits when counseling or recommending a product to the patient.

While many evidence-based principles are easily applied to dietary supplement literature, what follows are some issues unique to dietary supplement trials as well as the most commonly encountered methodological flaws. Chemical entity standardization, inclusion of international literature, adequate trial duration and sample size, limited high quality evidence-based literature, and quality and purity of product formulations are specifics to consider in addition to standard literature evaluation criteria.

STANDARDIZATION

One important characteristic to look for in a dietary supplement study is standardization. Plant-derived products often contain many different chemical entities that fluctuate depending on growing and harvesting conditions of the plant, the plant's age, and which part of the plant is used. There may be one or more chemical entities that are considered active constituents, which may or may not be accurately identified. Others may be marker compounds that allow scientists to estimate levels of chemicals that are less easily assayed. Standardization of one chemical entity, either an active constituent (if known) or a marker compound, is used to "calibrate" the product. Using a standardized chemical concentration allows for uniformity between study product and marketed product, as well as between various brands of one product. When evaluating dietary supplement product trials, it is important to assess standardization methods used by investigators. Investigators should discuss and document the plant or chemical substance as well as the strength or salt form utilized in the trial.

Plant parts are also important to consider. If a trial evaluated the use of an herb's root, but the product in question contains leaves and flowers, the results often cannot be extrapolated. This can also apply to non-plant-based products with different salt forms such as glucosamine. For example, glucosamine sulfate has a great deal of evidence documenting benefit in osteoarthritis patients, while other salt forms of glucosamine have little or no supportive evidence.

INTERNATIONAL TRIALS

The majority of dietary supplement trials are conducted outside the United States in Europe and Asia. Studies published in non-English language journals may be overlooked when doing a literature search. EMBASE (<<http://www.embase.com>>) is a large, commonly used database that indexes abstracts from international journals. While abstracts can be used to get an idea of the volume of potential supportive data, they do not contain enough information to properly analyze the quality of a full trial.

DURATION

As with drug clinical trials, duration of therapy is important. Inadequate duration for appropriate assessment is a common flaw in dietary supplement trials. Some dietary supplements may take several weeks to several months before patients experience benefit. Dietary supplements may appear less efficacious than they actually are if study duration is too short. And, as with drug clinical trials, shorter study periods cannot always predict outcomes or safety issues associated with long-term use.

TRIAL SIZE

Small subject population is another common flaw with dietary supplement trials. Small-sized groups may not have adequate statistical power to detect a potential difference between a dietary supplement versus placebo. Adverse reactions or drug interactions can be overlooked in smaller groups versus a larger one. In addition, a small subject population can decrease trial generalizability to broader patient populations.

LACK OF EVIDENCE

Few large, controlled, methodologically sound clinical trials exist for most dietary supplements. Many products have only animal, *in vitro*, or theoretical data to support their claims. However, more sound studies are underway as dietary supplement use becomes more prevalent and acceptable.

OTHER SPECIAL CONSIDERATIONS

Unlike prescription drugs, dietary supplements are not regulated for labeling or purity by the FDA. The bottle the consumer purchases in the health store or supermarket is not guaranteed to be labeled or dosed appropriately. Therefore, even when clinical evidence clearly supports use of a herb or supplement, the patient may not experience a benefit because the product is mislabeled, dosed subtherapeutically, or incorrectly standardized.

Dietary supplements can be adulterated with heavy metals or prescription medications. ConsumerLab (<<http://www.consumerlab.com>>) is an example of an organization that independently evaluates specific brands of dietary supplements for accurate labeling and purity. Approved or validated products receive a seal of approval companies may place on product labels. Manufacturers may also voluntarily agree to have manufacturing plants and products inspected to earn approval from agencies such as the USP-Dietary Supplement Verification Program (USP-DSVP, <<http://www.uspverified.org>>). Approved manufactures may display a seal of approval on product labels and are listed on the USP-DSVP website.

Dietary supplement use continues to be prevalent despite fluctuations in age groups and specific product popularity.[79] Pharmacists must serve as reliable and approachable information resources for dietary supplement information just as they do for other medications. Dietary supplements are often placed with over-the-counter products near the pharmacy, making the pharmacist easily accessible for consumer questions and counseling. The ability to effectively evaluate dietary supplement literature is essential to making informed recommendations and appropriately counseling patients with dietary supplement questions.

Conclusion

Many types of study designs are published in the biomedical literature. Each type of design is appropriately geared to answer specific clinical questions and each has a unique set of problems. Careful evaluation using techniques outlined in this chapter is necessary for appropriate application of the results from these studies to clinical practice.

Study Questions

1. Describe the differences between odds ratio and relative risk as they pertain to cohort and case-control studies. Why is it important to use confidence intervals when describing these parameters?
2. Compare and contrast experimental and observational study designs.
3. Compare and contrast the temporal relationship of:
   a. The cohort study design and the cross-sectional study design
   b. The cohort study design and the case-control study design
4. Describe how the validity of results obtained through survey research is assessed.
5. Describe a method for organizing and ranking trials by study design.
6. Explain the effect in a trial reporting no difference between efficacy rates for regular insulin versus inhaled insulin where a power calculation has been performed.
7. For each of the following scenarios, identify the type, advantages and disadvantages, and important points to consider when critiquing each study design.
   a. A physician designs a crossover study to prospectively evaluate the use of ibuprofen for chronic fatigue syndrome in an individual patient.
   b. Leucovorin calcium and fluorouracil often have been combined in the same solution and infused over multiple days by using a portable infusion pump. However, precipitation and clogging of the portable pump lines and catheters have been reported. A study was conducted to further evaluate the compatibility of this combination.
   c. An investigator evaluates the question of whether or not different levothyroxine products can be use interchangeably.
   d. It is hypothesized that hormone replacement therapy (HRT) in postmenopausal women may play a beneficial role in preventing osteoporosis. A group of patients receiving HRT and a group of patients not receiving HRT are followed over a 20-year period. The development of osteoporosis as assessed by bone mineral density in each group is compared and the relative risk associated with the use of HRT and the development of osteoporosis is calculated.
   e. There is a concern that the use of HRT in postmenopausal women may cause an increased risk of breast cancer. A study is conducted to test this hypothesis. A group of patients admitted to the hospital with the diagnosis of breast cancer is compared to a group of patients admitted to the hospital without breast cancer. The groups are matched by age, sex, date of admission, and other confounding factors such as alcohol use. Use of HRT in each group is assessed and compared. An odds ratio for the risk of breast cancer related to use of HRT is calculated.
   f. An investigator identifies a study sample of women aged 20 to 45 years. During a single office visit, the investigator measures bone mass in the women. He also questions them

about their past and present exercise habits. The investigator determines that women involved with rigorous exercise before the onset of menses have a greater bone mass.

g. A pharmacist notes that a patient develops erythema multiforme after administration of phenytoin. The pharmacist reports her observations regarding this patient.

h. A smoking cessation clinic has been developed and implemented at a community pharmacy. A questionnaire is mailed to all patients using the clinic within the past month to assess patient satisfaction.

i. A new antipsychotic agent is approved by the FDA. Following approval, the manufacturer of the antipsychotic agent creates a registry with several major hospitals and health maintenance organizations to monitor how the drug is used and the adverse effects associated with the use of the drug.

j. A pharmacist publishes an educational summary describing types, use, side effect profile, and cost of available oral contraceptives.

k. A pharmacist systematically gathers and analyzes the evidence for efficacy and cost-effectiveness of topical treatments of superficial fungal infections of the skin and nails of the feet. An explicit description of methods used in selecting and analyzing the data is provided. Statistical analysis is not used in combining the results of individual trials.

l. Conflicting reports exist about the effect of combining heparin with thrombolytic therapy on mortality in acute myocardial infarction. An investigator systematically identifies both published and unpublished studies in this area, combines the results, and statistically evaluates the data.

m. Guidelines for the use of thrombolytics are developed and published to aid in appropriate prescribing of these agents.

n. An investigation of the impact of intensive therapy (drug therapy, blood glucose monitoring, exercise, and diet) on the QOL for diabetic patients is conducted and published.

o. An efficacy trial for glucosamine for treatment of rheumatoid arthritis is conducted and published.

Acknowledgments

• Authors wish to gratefully acknowledge Antoine D. Richardson and Patrick J. Bryant, University of Missouri, Kansas City, School of Pharmacy, for contribution of the Power algorithm (Figure 7–3), and Rafia S. Rasu, Clinical Assistant Professor, University of Missouri, Kansas City, School of Pharmacy, for consultation regarding the Health Outcomes section.

REFERENCES

1. Larson EB, Ellsworth AJ. N-of-1 trials: increasing precision in therapeutics [editorial]. ACP J Club. 1993 July/Aug: A16–7.

2. Cook DJ. Randomized trials in single subjects: the N of 1 study. Psychopharmacol Bull. 1996;32: 363–77.

3. Guyatt GH, Keller JL, Jaeschke R, Rosenbloom D, Adachi JD, Newhouse MT. The n-of-1 randomized controlled trial: clinical usefulness. Our three year experience. Ann Intern Med. 1990; 112:293–9.

4. Larson EB, Ellsworth AJ, Oas J. Randomized clinical trials in single patients during a 2-year period. JAMA. 1993;270:2708–12.

5. Guyatt G, Sackett D, Taylor DW, Chong J, Roberts R, Puosley S. Determining optimal therapy-randomized trials in individual patients. N Engl J Med. 1986;314:889–92.

6. Trissel LA, Flora KP. Stability studies: five years later. Am J Hosp Pharm. 1988;45:1569–71.

7. Chow SC. Individual bioequivalence—a review of the FDA draft guidance. Drug Inf J. 1999;33:435–44.

8. The United States Pharmacopeial Convention, Inc. Food and Drug Administration Center for Drug Evaluation and Research approved drug products with therapeutic equivalence evaluations. USPDI, 19th ed., Vol. III: Approved drug products and legal requirements. Massachusetts; 1999:I/5–I/17.

9. The United States Pharmacopeial Convention, Inc. Food and Drug Administration Center for Drug Evaluation and Research approved drug products with therapeutic equivalence evaluations. USPDI, 25th ed., Vol. III: Approved drug products and legal requirements. Massachusetts; 2005:I/5–I/17.

10. Malinowski HJ. Bioavailability and bioequivalency testing. In: Gennaro AR, Chase GD, Marderosian AD, Hanson GR, Medwick T, Popovich NG, et al., editors. Remington: the science and practice of pharmacy, 20th ed. Philadelphia (PA): Lippincott Williams & Williams; 2000. p. 995–1004.

11. DiSanto AR. Bioavailability and bioequivalency testing. In: Gennaro AR, Chase GD, Marderostan AD, Harvey SC, Hussar DA, Medwick T, et al., editors. Remington's pharmaceutical sciences, 18th ed. Easton (PA): Mack Publishing; 1990. p. 1451–8.

12. Willett MS, Bertch KE, Rich DS, Eveshehefsky L. Prospectus on the economic value of clinical pharmacy services. A position statement of the American College of Clinical Pharmacy. Pharmacotherapy. 1989;9:45–56.

13. Economic evaluations of clinical pharmacy services: 1988–1995. Pharmacotherapy. 1996;16(6): 1188–1208.

14. Evidence of the economic benefit of clinical pharmacy services: 1996–2000. Pharmacotherapy. 2003;23(1):113–32.

15. Collaborative drug therapy management by pharmacists: 2003. Pharmacotherapy. 2003;23(9): 1210–25.

16. Mann CJ. Observational research methods. Research design II: cohort, cross sectional, and case-control studies. Emerg Med J. 2003;20:54–60.

17. Gottlieb M, Anderson G, Lepor H. Basic epidemiologic and statistical methods in clinical research. Urol Clin North Am. 1992;19:641–53.

18. Feinstein AR, Horwitz RI. Double standards, scientific methods, and epidemiologic research. N Engl J Med. 1982;307:1611–7.

19. Dolan MS. Interpretation of the literature. Clin Obstet Gynecol 1998;41:307–14.

20. Grimes DA, Schulz KF. Cohort studies: marching toward outcomes. Lancet. 2002;359:341–5.

21. Manson JE, Stampfer MJ, Colditz GA, Willett WC, Rosner B, Speizer FE, at al. A prospective study of aspirin use and primary prevention of cardiovascular disease in women. JAMA. 1991;266:521–7.

22. Peipert JF, Glennon Phipps M. Observational studies. Clin Obstet Gynecol 1998;41:235–44.

23. Hartzema AG. Guide to interpreting and evaluating the pharmacoepidemiologic literature. Ann Pharmacother 1992;26:96–98.

24. Risk. In: Fletcher RH, Fletcher SW, Wagner EH, editors. Clinical epidemiology: the essentials, 3rd ed. Baltimore (MD): Williams & Wilkins; 1996. p. 94–110.

25. Hayden GF, Kramer MS, Horwitz RI. The case-control study. A practical review for the clinician. JAMA. 1982;247:326–31.

26. Niemcryk SJ, Kraus TJ, Mallory TH. Empirical considerations in orthopaedic research design and data analysis. Part I: strategies in research design. J Arthroplasty. 1990;5:97–103.

27. Horwitz RI, Feinstein AR. Methodologic standards and contradictory results in case-control research. Am J Med. 1979;66:556–64.

28. Study design: The case-control approach. In: Gehlbach SH, editor. Interpreting the medical literature, 4th ed. New York: McGraw-Hill; 2002:31–54.

29. Gullen WH. A danger in matched-control studies. JAMA. 1980;244:2279–80.

30. Typology of observational study designs. In: Kleinbaum DG, Kupper LL, Morganstern H, editors. Epidemiologic research: principles and quantitative methods. New York: John Wiley & Sons; 1982. p. 62–95.

31. Bailar JC, Louis TA, Lavori PW, Polansky M. A classification of biomedical research reports. In: Bailar JC, Mostellar F, editors. Medical uses of statistics, 2nd ed. Boston (MA): NEJM Books; 1992. p. 141–56.

32. Jaeschke R, Sackett DL. Research methods for obtaining primary evidence. Int J Technol Assess Health Care. 1989;5:503–19.

33. Spilker B. Single patient clinical trials. Guide to clinical trials. New York: Lippincott-Raven; 1996. p. 277–82.

34. Lukoff D, Edwards D, Miller M. The case study as a scientific method for researching alternative therapies. Altern Ther Health Med. 1998;4:44–52.

35. Kerlinger FN. Foundations of behavioral research, 2nd ed. New York: Holt, Rinehart & Winston; 1973. p. 401.

36. Harrison DL, Draugalis JR. Evaluating the results of mail survey research. J Am Pharm Assoc. 1997;NS37:662–6.

37. Shi L. Health services research methods. In: Williams S, editor. Delmar series in health services administration. Albany (NY): International Thomson Publishing; 1997.

38. Manasse H, Lambert R. Types of research: a synopsis of the major categories and data collection methods. Am J Hosp Pharm. 1980;37:694–701.

39. Segal R. Designing a pharmacy survey. Top Hosp Pharm Manage. 1985:37–45.

40. Fowler F. Survey research methods. In: Bickman L, Rog D, editors. Applied social research methods series, Vol. 1. Newbury Park (CA): Sage; 1993.

41. Fairman K. Going to the source: a guide to using surveys in health care research. J Manag Care Pharm. 1999;5:150–9.

42. Spilker B. Classification and description of phase IV postmarketing study designs. Guide to clinical trials. New York: Lippincott-Raven; 1996. p. 44–58.
43. Bryant PJ. Applying evidence-based medicine to dietary supplements. Pharm Diet Suppl Alert. 2000;1(1):S1–S2.
44. Mulrow CD. The medical review article. State of the science. Ann Intern Med. 1987;106:485–8.
45. Oxman AD, Cook DJ, Guyatt GH. Users' guides to the medical literature. VI. How to use an overview. JAMA. 1994;272:1367–71.
46. Oxman AD, Guyatt GH. Guidelines for reading literature reviews. CMAJ. 1988;138:697–703.
47. Joyce J, Rabe-Hesketh S, Wessely S. Reviewing the reviews. The example of chronic fatigue syndrome. JAMA. 1998;280:264–6.
48. Mulrow CD, Cook DJ, Davidoff F. Systematic reviews: critical links in the great chain of evidence [editorial]. Ann Intern Med. 1997;126:389–91.
49. Cook DJ, Mulrow CD, Haynes RB. Systematic reviews: synthesis of best evidence for clinical decisions. Ann Intern Med. 1997;126:376–80.
50. Sacks HS, Berrier J, Reitman D, Pagano D, Chalmers TC. Meta-analyses of randomized control trials. An update of the quality and methodology. In: Bailar JC, Mosteller F, editors. Medical uses of statistics, 2nd ed. Boston (MA): NEJM Books; 1992. p. 427–42.
51. Einarson TR, Leeder JS, Koren G. A method for meta-analysis of epidemiological studies. Drug Intell Clin Pharm. 1988;22:813–24.
52. Greenhalgh T. Papers that summarize other papers (systematic reviews and meta-analyses). BMJ. 1997;315:672–5.
53. Gibaldi M. Meta-analysis. A review of its place in therapeutic decision-making. Drugs. 1993;46:805–18.
54. LeLorier J, Gregoire G, Benhaddad A, Lapierre J, Derderian F. Discrepancies between meta-analyses and subsequent large randomized, controlled trials. N Engl J Med. 1997;337:536–42.
55. Cook DJ, Guyatt GH, Ryan G, Clifton J, Buckinham L, William A, et al. Should unpublished data be included in meta-analyses? Current conviction and controversies. JAMA. 1993;269:2749–53.
56. Thacker SB, Stroup DF, Peterson HB. Meta-analysis for the practicing obstetrician-gynecologist. Clin Obstet Gynecol. 1998;41:275–81.
57. Jadad AR, Cook DJ, Jones A, Klassen TP, Tugwell P, Moher M, et al. Methodology and reports of systematic reviews and meta-analyses. JAMA. 1998;280:278–80.
58. Zinberg S. Practice guidelines—a continuing debate. Clin Obstet Gynecol. 1998;41:343–7.
59. Rush AJ, Crismon ML, Toprac MG, Trivedi MH, Rago WV. Consensus guidelines in the treatment of major depressive disorder. J Clin Psychiatry. 1998;59(Suppl 20):73–84.
60. Hayward RS, Wilson MC, Tunis SR, Bass EB, Guyatt G. Users' guide to the medical literature. VIII. How to use clinical practice guidelines. A. Are the recommendations valid? JAMA. 1995;274:570–4.
61. Shekelle PG, Ortiz E, Rhodes S, Morton SC, Eccles MP, Grimshaw JM, et al. Validity of the agency for health care research and quality clinical practice guidelines: how quickly do guidelines become outdated? JAMA. 2001;286(12):1461–7.
62. Wilson MC, Hayward RS, Tunis SR, Bass EB, Guyatt G. User's guide to the medical literature. VII. How to use clinical practice guidelines. B. What are the recommendations and will they help you in caring for your patients? JAMA. 1995;274:1630–2.

63. Field MJ, Lohr KN. Clinical practice guidelines: directions for a new program. US Institute of Medicine Committee to advise the public health service on clinical practice guidelines, US Dept. of Health and Human Services. Washington, DC: National Academy Press; 1990.

64. Katz DA. Barriers between guidelines and improved patient care: an analysis of AHCPR's unstable angina clinical practice guideline. Health Serv Res. 1999;34(1):377–89.

65. Fairclough DL. Design and analysis of quality of life studies in clinical trials. Boca Raton (FL): Chapman & Hall; 2002.

66. Patrick D, Erickson P. Health status and health policy: allocating resources to health care. New York: Oxford University Press; 1993.

67. Aaronson NK, Cull AM, Kaasa S, Spranger MAG. The European Organization for Research and Treatment of Cancer (EORTC) modular approach to quality of life assessment in oncology: an update. In: Spilker B, editor. Quality of life and pharmacoeconomics in clinical trials, 2nd ed. Philadelphia (PA): Lippincott-Raven; 1996. p. 179–89.

68. Cella DF, Bonomi AE. The functional assessment of cancer therapy (FACT) and functional assessment of HIV infection (FAHI) quality of life measurement system. In: Spilker B, editor. Quality of life and pharmacoeconomics in clinical trials, 2nd ed. Philadelphia (PA): Lippincott-Raven; 1996: p. 203–10.

69. Clinch JJ. The functional living index-cancer: ten years later. In: Spilker B, editor. Quality of life and pharmacoeconomics in clinical trials, 2nd ed. Philadelphia (PA): Lippincott-Raven; 1996. p. 215–225.

70. Guyatt GH, Jaeschke R, Feeny DH, Patrick DL. Measurements in clinical trials: choosing the right approach. In: Spilker B, editor. Quality of life and pharmacoeconomics in clinical trials, 2nd ed. Philadelphia (PA): Lippincott-Raven; 1996. p. 44–5.

71. Juniper EF, Guyatt GH, Jaeschke R. How to develop and validate a new health-related quality of life instrument. In: Spilker B, editor. Quality of life and pharmacoeconomics in clinical trials, 2nd ed. Philadelphia (PA): Lippincott-Raven; 1996. p. 49–56.

72. International Society for Pharmacoeconomics & Outcomes Research Consensus Group. ISPOR quality of life regulatory guidance issues. ISPOR Website 1999:26 screens. Available from: http://www.ispor.org/workpaper/consensus/index.asp

73. Samsa G, Edelman D, Rothman ML, Williams GR, Lipscomb J, Matchar D. Determining clinically important difference in health status measures. A general approach with illustration to the Health Utilities Index Mark II. Pharmacoeconomics. 1999;15:141–55.

74. Bowling A. Measuring health: a review of quality of life measurement scales, 2nd ed. Philadelphia (PA): Open University Press; 1997.

75. Spilker B. Quality of life trials. Guide to clinical trials. New York: Lippincott-Raven; 1996:370–8.

76. Guyatt GH, Naylor CD, Jniper E, Heyland DK, Jaeschke R, Cook DJ. User's guides to the medical literature. XII. How to use articles about health-related quality of life. JAMA. 1997;277:1232–7.

77. Gill TM, Feinstein AR. A critical appraisal of the quality of quality of life measurements. JAMA. 1994;272:619–26.

78. Sanders C, Egger M, Donovan J, Tallon D, Frankel S. Reporting on quality of life in randomized controlled trials: bibliographic study. BMJ. 1998;317:1191–4.

79. Kelly JP, Kaufman DW, Kelley K, Rosenberg L, Anderson TE, Mitchell AA. Recent trends in use of herbal and other natural products. Arch Intern Med. 2005;165:281–6.

Chapter Eight

Pharmacoeconomics

James P. Wilson • Karen L. Rascati

Objectives

After completing this chapter, the reader will be able to

- Describe the advantages and disadvantages of the different types of pharmacoeconomic analyses.
- List and explain 10 steps that should be found in a well-conducted pharmacoeconomic study.
- List the six steps in a decision analysis.
- Apply the use of pharmacoeconomic evaluation techniques to the formulary decision process, including decision analysis.
- Apply a systematic approach to the evaluation of the pharmacoeconomic literature.
- List at least four applications specific to pharmacy, where pharmacoeconomic methodology is commonly employed.

Many changes have recently taken place in health care. The continued introduction of new technologies, including many new drugs, has been among these changes. From 2000 to 2003, over 300 new drugs were approved by the Food and Drug Administration (FDA).[1] New biotechnology drugs can cost over $10,000 per course of therapy. The increase in the number of new drugs combined with the increase in costs of drugs provides a great challenge for managed care organizations (MCOs) as they struggle to deliver quality care while minimizing costs.[2]

Pharmacy and therapeutics (P&T) committees are responsible for evaluating these new drugs and determining their potential value to organizations. Evaluating drugs for formulary inclusion can often be an overwhelming task. The application of pharmacoeconomic methods to the evaluation process may help streamline formulary decisions.

This chapter presents an overview of the practical application of pharmacoeconomic principles as they apply to the formulary decision process. Students and pharmacists are often asked to gather and evaluate literature to support the decision process. For a more in-depth review of the principles and concepts of pharmacoeconomics, refer to the references at the end of the chapter.

Pharmacoeconomics—What Is It and Why Do It?

Pharmacoeconomics has been defined as the description and analysis of the costs of drug therapy to health care systems and society—it identifies, measures, and compares the costs and consequences of pharmaceutical products and services.[3] Decision-makers can use these methods to evaluate and compare the total costs of treatment options and the outcomes associated with these options. To show this graphically, think of two sides of an equation: (1) the inputs (costs) used to obtain and use the drug and (2) the health-related outcomes (Figure 8–1).

The center of the equation, the drug product, is symbolized by R_x. If only the left-hand side of the equation is measured without regard for outcomes, this is a cost analysis (or a partial economic analysis). If only the right-hand side of the equation is measured without regard to costs, this is a clinical or outcome study (not an economic analysis). In order to be a true pharmacoeconomic analysis, both sides of the equation must be considered and compared.

Relationship of Pharmacoeconomics to Outcomes Research

Outcomes research is defined as an attempt to identify, measure, and evaluate the end results of health care services. It may include not only clinical and economic consequences, but also outcomes, such as patient health status and satisfaction with their health care. Pharmacoeconomics is a type of outcomes research, but not all outcomes research is pharmacoeconomic research.[4]

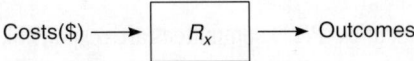

Costs($) ⟶ R_x ⟶ Outcomes

Figure 8–1. The pharmacoeconomic equation.

Models of Pharmacoeconomic Analysis

The four types of pharmacoeconomic analyses all follow the diagram shown in Figure 8–1—they measure costs or inputs in dollars and assess the outcomes associated with these costs. Pharmacoeconomic analyses are categorized by the method used to assess outcomes. If the outcomes are assumed to be equivalent, the study is called a cost-minimization analysis (CMA); if the outcomes are measured in dollars, the study is called a cost-benefit analysis (CBA); if the costs are measured in natural units (e.g., cures, years of life, blood pressure), the study is called a cost-effectiveness analysis (CEA); if the outcomes take into account patient preferences (or utilities), the study is called a cost-utility analysis (CUA) (Table 8–1). Each type of analysis includes a measurement of costs in dollars. Measurement of these costs is discussed first, followed by further examples of how outcomes are measured for these four types of studies.

Assessment of Costs

First, the assessment of costs (the left hand side of the equation) will be discussed. A discussion of the four types of costs and timing adjustments for costs follow.

TYPES OF COSTS

Costs are calculated to estimate the resources (or inputs) that are used in the production of an outcome. Pharmacoeconomic studies categorize costs into four types. Direct medical costs are the most obvious costs to measure. These are the medically related inputs used directly to provide the treatment. Examples of direct medical costs would include costs associated with pharmaceutical products, physician visits, emergency room visits, and hospitalizations.

TABLE 8–1. FOUR TYPES OF PHARMACOECONOMIC ANALYSES

Methodology	Cost Measurement Unit	Outcome Measurement Unit
Cost-minimization analysis (CMA)	Dollars	Assumed to be equivalent in comparable groups
Cost-benefit analysis (CBA)	Dollars	Dollars
Cost-effectiveness analysis (CEA)	Dollars	Natural units (life years gained, mm Hg blood pressure, mmol/L blood glucose)
Cost-utility analysis (CUA)	Dollars	Quality-adjusted life year (QALY) or other utilities

Direct nonmedical costs are costs directly associated with treatment, but are not medical in nature. Examples include the cost of traveling to and from the physician's office or hospital, babysitting for the children of a patient, and food and lodging required for the patient and their family during out-of-town treatment. Indirect costs involve costs that result from the loss of productivity due to illness or death. Please note that the accounting term indirect costs, which is used to assign overhead, is different from the economic term, which refers to a loss of productivity of the patient or the patient's family due to illness. Intangible costs include the costs of pain, suffering, anxiety, or fatigue that occur because of an illness or the treatment of an illness. It is difficult to measure or assign values to intangible costs.

Treatment of an illness may include all four types of costs. For example, the cost of surgery would include the direct medical costs of the surgery (medication, room charges, laboratory tests, and physician services), direct nonmedical costs (travel and lodging for the preoperative day), indirect costs (cost due to the patient missing work during the surgery and recuperative period), and intangible costs (due to pain and anxiety). Most studies only report the direct medical costs. This may be appropriate depending on the objective of the study or the perspective of the study. For example, if the objective is to measure the costs to the hospital for two surgical procedures that differ in direct medical costs (for example, using high-dose vs. low-dose aprotinin in cardiac bypass surgery), but that are expected to have similar nonmedical, indirect, and intangible costs, measuring all four types of costs may not be warranted.

In order to determine what costs are important to measure, the perspective of the study must be determined. *Perspective* is a pharmacoeconomic term that describes whose costs are relevant based on the purpose of the study. Economic theory suggests that the most appropriate perspective is that of society. Societal costs would include costs to the insurance company, costs to the patient, and indirect costs due to the loss of productivity. Although this may be the most appropriate perspective according to economic theory, it is rarely seen in the pharmacoeconomic literature. The most common perspectives used in pharmacoeconomic studies are the perspective of the institution or the perspective of the payer. The payer perspective may include the costs to the third-party plan, the patient, or a combination of the patient co-pay and the third-party plan costs.

TIMING ADJUSTMENTS FOR COSTS

When costs are estimated from information collected for more than a year before the study or for more than a year into the future, adjustment of costs is needed. If retrospective data are used to assess resources used over a number of years, these costs should be adjusted to the present year. For example, if the objective of the study is to estimate the difference in the costs of antibiotic A versus B in the treatment of a specific type of infection, information on the past utilization of these two antibiotics might be collected from a review of medical records. If the retrospective review of these medical records dates back for more than a year, it may be necessary to adjust the cost of both medications by calculating the number of units (doses) used per case and multiplying this number by the current unit cost for each medication.

If costs are estimated based on dollars spent or saved in future years, another type of adjustment, called discounting, is needed. There is a time value associated with money. Most people (and businesses) prefer to receive money today, rather than at a later time. Therefore, a dollar received today is worth more than a dollar received next year—the time value of money. Discount rate, a term from finance, approximates the cost of capital by taking into account the projected inflation rate and the interest rates of borrowed money and estimates the time value of money. From this parameter, the present value (PV) of future expenditures and savings can be calculated. The discount factor is equal to $1/(1 + r)^n$, where r is the discount rate and n is the year the cost or savings occur. For example, if the costs of a new pharmaceutical care program are $5000 per year for the next 3 years, and the discount rate is 5%, the PV of these costs is $14,297 [$5000 year 1 + $5000/1.05 year 2 + $5000/(1.05)^2 year 3]. The most common discount rate currently seen in the literature is 5%, the approximate cost of borrowing money today.

Assessment of Outcomes

The methods associated with measuring outcomes (the right-hand side of the equation) will be discussed in this section. As shown in Table 8–1, there are four ways to measure outcomes, and each type of outcome measurement is associated with a different type of pharmacoeconomic analysis. The advantages and disadvantages of each type of analysis will be discussed in this section.

COST-MINIMIZATION ANALYSIS

For a CMA, costs are measured in dollars, and outcomes are assumed to be equivalent. One example of a CMA is the measurement and comparison of costs for two therapeutically equivalent products, like glipizide and glyburide.[5] Another example is the measurement and comparison of using prostaglandin E_2 on an inpatient versus an outpatient basis.[6] In both cases, all the outcomes (e.g., efficacy, incidence of adverse drug interactions) are expected to be equal, but the costs are not. Some researchers contend that a CMA is not a true pharmacoeconomic study, because costs are measured but outcomes are not. Others say that the strength of a CMA depends on the evidence that the outcomes are the same. This evidence can be based on previous studies, publications, FDA data, or expert opinion. The advantage of this type of study is that it is relatively simple compared to the other types of analyses because outcomes need not be measured. The disadvantage of this type of analysis is that it can only be used where outcomes are assumed to be identical.

Examples

A hospital needs to decide if it should add a new intravenous antibiotic to the formulary, which is therapeutically equivalent to the current antibiotic used in the institution and has the same side effect profile. The advantage of the new antibiotic is that it only has to be administered once per day versus three times a day for the comparison antibiotic. Because the outcomes are expected to be nearly identical, and the objective is to assess the costs to the hospital (e.g., the hospital perspective), only direct medical costs need to be estimated and compared. The direct medical costs include the daily costs of each medication, the pharmacy personnel time used in the preparation of each dose, and the nursing personnel time used in the administration of each dose. Even if the cost of the new medication is a little higher than the cost of the current antibiotic, the lower cost of preparing and administering the new drug (once a day vs. three times per day) may offset this difference. Direct nonmedical, indirect, and intangible costs are not expected to differ between these two alternatives and they need not be included if the perspective is that of the hospital, so these costs are not included in the comparison.

Mithani and Brown[7] examined once-daily intravenous administration of an aminoglycoside versus the conventional every 8-hour administration (Table 8–2). The drug acquisition cost was $Can (Canadian dollars) 43.70 for every 8 hours dosing, and $Can 55.39 for the single dose administration. Not including laboratory drug level measurements, the costs of minibags ($Can 29.32), preparation ($Can 13.81), and administration ($Can 67.63) were $Can 110.76 for the three-times daily administration versus $Can 42.23 (minibags $Can 10.90, preparation $Can 6.20, and administration $Can 25.13) for the single daily dose. With essentially equivalent clinical outcomes, the once-daily administration of the aminoglycoside minimized hospital costs ($Can 97.62 vs. $Can 154.46).

COST-BENEFIT ANALYSIS

A CBA measures both inputs and outcomes in monetary terms. One advantage to using a CBA is that alternatives with different outcomes can be compared, because each outcome is

TABLE 8–2. EXAMPLE OF COST MINIMIZATION

Type of Cost	Every 8 Hours	Once Daily
Drug acquisition cost	$43.70	$55.39
Minibag cost	$29.32	$10.90
Preparation cost	$13.81	$6.20
Administration costs	$67.63	$25.13
Total cost	$154.46	$97.62

NOTE: Costs are presented in Canadian dollars.

converted to the same unit (dollars). For example, the costs (inputs) of providing a pharmacokinetics service versus a diabetes clinic can be compared with the cost savings (outcomes) associated with each service, even though different types of outcomes are expected for each alternative. Many CBAs are performed to determine how institutions can best spend their resources to produce monetary benefits. For example, a study conducted at Walter Reed Army Medical Center looked at costs and savings associated with the addition of a pharmacist to its medical teams.[8] Discounting of both the costs of the treatment or services and the benefits or cost savings is needed if they extend for more than a year. Comparing costs and benefits (outcomes in monetary terms) is accomplished by either of the two methods. One method divides the estimated benefits by the estimated costs to produce a benefit-to-cost ratio. If this ratio is more than 1.0, the choice is cost beneficial. The other method is to subtract the costs from the benefits to produce a net benefit calculation. If this difference is positive, the choice is cost beneficial. The example at the end of this section will use both methods for illustrative purposes.

Another more complex use of CBA consists of measuring clinical outcomes (for example, avoidance of death, reduction of blood pressure, and reduction of pain) and placing a dollar value on these clinical outcomes. This type of CBA is not seen often in the pharmacy literature, but will be discussed here briefly. This use of the method still offers the advantage that alternatives with different types of outcomes can be assessed, but a disadvantage is that it is difficult (and some argue distasteful) to put a monetary value on pain, suffering, and human life. There are two common methods that economists use to estimate a value for these types of consequences, the human capital approach and the willingness-to-pay approach. The human capital approach assumes that the values of health benefits are equal to the economic productivity that they permit. The cost of disease is the cost of the lost productivity due to the disease. A person's expected income before taxes and/or an inputted value for nonmarket activities (e.g., housework and child care) is used as an estimate of the value of any health benefits for that person. The human capital approach was used when calculating the costs and benefits of administering a meningococcal vaccine to college students. The value of the future productivity of a college student was estimated at $1 million in this study.[9] There are disadvantages to using this method. A person's earnings may not reflect their true value to society, and this method lacks a solid literature of research to back this notion. The willingness-to-pay method estimates the value of health benefits by estimating how much people would pay to reduce their chance of an adverse health outcome. For example, if a group of people is willing to pay, on average, $100 to reduce their chance of dying from 1:1000 to 1:2000, theoretically a life would be worth $200,000 [$100/(0.001 − 0.0005)]. Problems with this method include what people say they are willing to pay may not correspond to what they actually would do, and it is debatable if people can meaningfully answer questions about a 0.0005 reduction in outcomes.

TABLE 8–3. CBA EXAMPLE CALCULATIONS

	Year 1 Dollars (No Discounting in Year 1)	Year 2 Dollars (Discounted Dollars)	Year 3 Dollars (Discounted Dollars)	Total Dollars (Discounted Dollars)	Benefit-to-Cost Ratio Dollars (Discounted Dollars)	Net Benefit Dollars (Discounted Dollars)
Costs of A	$50,000 ($50,000)	$20,000 ($19,048)	$20,000 ($18,140)	$90,000 ($87,188)		
Benefits of A	$40,000 ($40,000)	$40,000 ($38,095)	$40,000 ($36,281)	$120,000 ($114,376)	$120,000/$90,000 = 1.33:1 ($114,376/$87,188 = 1.31:1)	$120,000 – $90,000 = $30,000 ($114,376 – $87,188 = $27,188)
Costs of B	$40,000 ($40,000)	$30,000 ($28,571)	$30,000 ($27,211)	$100,000 ($95,782)		
Benefits of B	$45,000 ($45,000)	$45,000 ($42,857)	$45,000 ($40,816)	$135,000 ($128,673)	$135,000/$100,000 = 1.35:1 ($128,673/$95,782 = 1.34:1)	$135,000 – $100,000 = $35,000 ($128,673 – $95,782 = $32,891)

Example

An independent pharmacy owner is considering the provision of a new clinical pharmacy service. The objective of the analysis is to estimate the costs and monetary benefits of two possible services over the next 3 years (Table 8–3). Clinical Service A would cost $50,000 in start-up and operating costs during the first year, and $20,000 in years 2 and 3. Clinical Service A would provide an added revenue of $40,000 each of the 3 years, Clinical Service B would cost $40,000 in start-up and operating costs the first year and $30,000 for years 2 and 3. Clinical Service B would provide added revenue of $45,000 for each of the 3 years. Table 8–3 illustrates the comparison of both options using the perspective of the independent pharmacy with no discounting and when a discount rate of 5% is used. Although both services are estimated to be cost beneficial, Clinical Service B has both a higher benefit-to-cost ratio and a higher net benefit when compared to Clinical Service A.

COST-EFFECTIVENESS ANALYSIS

A CEA measures costs in dollars and outcomes in natural health units such as cures, lives saved, or blood pressure. This is the most common type of pharmacoeconomic analysis found in the pharmacy literature. An advantage of using a CEA is that health units are common outcomes practitioners can readily understand and these outcomes do not need to be converted to monetary values. On the other hand, the alternatives used in the comparison must have outcomes that are measured in the same units. If more than one natural unit outcome is important when conducting the comparison, a cost-effectiveness ratio should be calculated for each type of outcome. Outcomes cannot be collapsed into one unit measure in CEAs as they can with CBAs (outcome = dollars) or CUAs (outcome = quality-adjusted life years [QALYs]). Because CEA is the most common type of pharmacoeconomic study in the pharmacy literature, many examples are available. Bloom et al.[10] compared two medical treatments for gastroesophageal reflux disease (GERD), using both healed ulcers confirmed by endoscopy and symptom-free days as the outcomes measured. Law et al.[11] assessed two antidiabetic medications by comparing the percentage of patients who achieved good glycemic control as the outcome measure.

A cost-effectiveness grid can be used to illustrate the definition of cost effectiveness. In Table 8–4, cells D, G, and H (lightly-shaded cells) are cost-effective choices, while cells B, C,

TABLE 8–4. COST-EFFECTIVENESS GRID

Cost Effectiveness	Lower Cost	Same Cost	Higher Cost
Lower effectiveness	A	B	C
Same effectiveness	D	E	F
Higher effectiveness	G	H	I

TABLE 8–5. LISTING OF COSTS AND OUTCOMES

Alternative	Costs for 12 Months of Medication	Lowering of LDL in 12 Months (mg/dL)
Current preferred medication	$1,000	25
New medication	$1,500	30

LDL: low density lipoprotein.

and F (darker-shaded cells) are not cost effective, and the remaining cells might be cost effective if the added benefits are determined to be worth the added costs. The unshaded cells A, E, and I are situations when a more subjective, complex judgment is needed.

Example

An MCO is trying to decide whether to add a new cholesterol-lowering agent to its preferred formulary. The new product has a greater effect on lowering cholesterol than the current preferred agent, but a daily dose of the new medication is also more expensive. Using the perspective of the MCO (e.g., direct medical costs of the product to the MCO), the results will be presented in three ways. Table 8–5 presents the simple listing of the costs and benefits of the two alternatives. Table 8–6 shows the cost-effectiveness ratio for each alternative. Table 8–7 shows the marginal (or incremental) cost effectiveness (the extra cost of producing one extra unit) of the new medication compared to the current medication. A marginal cost-effectiveness ratio is calculated by determining the added cost divided by the added benefit. Most economists agree that a marginal cost-effectiveness ratio is the more appropriate way to present CEA results. The costs and benefits of the medications are estimated for only 1 year; discounting is not needed.

Clinicians must then wrestle with this information—it becomes a clinical call. Many economists will argue that this uncertainty is why cost effectiveness may not be the preferred method of pharmacoeconomic analysis.

COST-UTILITY ANALYSIS

A CUA takes patient preferences, also referred to as *utilities*, into account when measuring health consequences.[12] The most common unit used in conducting CUAs is QALYs, which

TABLE 8–6. COST-EFFECTIVENESS RATIOS

Alternative	Costs for 12 Months of Medication	Lowering of LDL in 12 Months	Average Cost per Reduction in LDL
Current preferred medication	$1,000	25 mg/dL	$40 per mg/dL
New medication	$1,500	30 mg/dL	$50 per mg/dL

LDL: low density lipoprotein.

TABLE 8–7. MARGINAL COST-EFFECTIVENESS RATIO

Alternative	Costs for 12 Months of Medication	Lowering of LDL in 12 Months	Marginal Cost per Marginal Reduction in LDL
Current preferred medication	$1,000	25 mg/dL	$\dfrac{\$1,500 - \$1,000}{30\ \text{mg/dL} - 25\ \text{mg/dL}} = \$100\ \text{per mg/dL}$
New medication	$1,500	30 mg/dL	

LDL: low density lipoprotein.

incorporates both the quality and quantity of life. A QALY is a health utility measure combining quality and quantity of life, as determined by some valuations process. One year at perfect health equals one QALY.[13] The advantage of using this method is that different types of health outcomes can be compared using one common unit (QALYs) without placing a monetary value on these health outcomes (like CBA). The disadvantage of this method is that it is difficult to determine an accurate QALY value. This is a relatively new type of outcome measure and is not understood or embraced by many providers and decision-makers. Therefore, this method is rarely seen in the pharmacy literature. One reason researchers are working to establish methods for measuring QALYs is the belief that 1 year of life (a natural unit outcome that can be used in CEAs) in one health state should not be given the same weight as 1 year of life in another health state. For example, if two treatments both add 10 years of life, but one provides an added 10 years of being in a healthy state and the other adds 10 years of being in a disabled health state, the outcomes of the two treatments should not be considered equal. Adjusting for the quality of those extra years is warranted. When calculating QALYs, 1 year of life in perfect health has a score of 1.0 QALY. If health-related quality of life (HR-QOL) is diminished by disease or treatment, 1 year of life in this state is less than 1.0 QALY. This unit allows comparisons of morbidity and mortality. By convention, perfect health is assigned 1.0 per year and death is assigned 0.0 per year, but how are scores between these two determined? Different techniques for determining scales of measurement for QALY are discussed below.

There are three common methods for determining these scores: rating scales, standard gamble, and time trade off (TTO). A rating scale consists of a line on a page, somewhat like a thermometer, with perfect health at the top (100) and death at bottom (0). Different disease states are described to subjects and they are asked to place the different disease states somewhere on the scale indicating preferences relative to all diseases described. As an example, if they place a disease state at 70 on the scale, the disease state is given a score of 0.7 QALYs.

The second method for determining patient preference (or utility) scores is the standard gamble method. For this method, each subject is offered two alternatives. Alternative one is treatment with two possible outcomes: either the return to normal health or immediate death. Alternative two is the certain outcome of a chronic disease state for life. The probability (p) of dying is varied until the subject is indifferent between alternative one and alternative two. As an example, a person considers two options: a kidney transplant with a 20% probability of dying during the operation (alternative one) or dialysis for the rest of his life (alternative two). If this percent is his point of indifference (he would not have the operation if the chances of dying during the operation were any higher than 20%), the QALY is calculated as 1 – p or 0.8 QALY.

The third technique for measuring health preferences is the TTO method. Again, the subject is offered two alternatives. Alternative one is a certain disease state for a specific length of time t, the life expectancy for a person with the disease, then death. Alternative two is being healthy for time x, which is less than t. Time x is varied until the respondent is indifferent between the two alternatives. The proportion of the number of years of life a person is willing to give up $(t - x)$ to have her remaining years (x) of life in a healthy state is used to assess her QALY estimate. For example, a person with a life expectancy of 50 years is given two options: being blind for 50 years or being completely healthy (including being able to see) for 25 years. If the person is indifferent between these two options (she would rather be blind than give up any more years of life), the QALY for this disease state (blindness) would be 0.5. Table 8–8 contains examples of disease states and QALY estimates for each disease state listed.

As one might surmise, QALY measurement is not regarded as being as precise or scientific as natural health unit measurements (like blood pressure and cholesterol levels) used in CEAs. Some issues in the measurement of QALYs are debated in the literature. One issue concerns whose viewpoint is the most valid. An advantage of having patients with the disease of interest determine health state scores is that these patients may understand the effects of the disease better than the general population, whereas, some believe these patients would provide a biased view of their disease compared with other diseases. Some contend that health care professionals could provide good estimates because they understand various diseases and others argue that these professionals may not rate discomfort and disability as seriously as patients or the general population.

Another issue that has been addressed regarding patient preference or utility-score measures is the debate over which is the "best" measure. Utility scores calculated using one

TABLE 8–8. SELECTED QALY ESTIMATES

Disease State	QALY Estimate
Complete health	1.00
Moderate angina	0.83
Breast cancer: removed breast, unconcerned	0.80
Severe angina	0.53
Cancer spread, constant pain, tired, not expected to live long	0.16
Death	0.00

SOURCES: From Kaplan RM.[12]

method may differ from those using another. Finally, utility measures have been criticized for not being sensitive to small, but clinically meaningful, changes in health status.

Example

An article by Kennedy et al.[14] assessed the costs and utilities associated with two common chemotherapy regimens (vindesine and cisplatin [VP], and cyclophosphamide, doxorubicin, and cisplatin [CAP]) and compared the results with the costs and utilities of using best supportive care (BSC) in patients with nonsmall cell lung cancer. The perspective was that of the health care system or the payer. Using the TTO method, treatment utility scores were estimated by members of the oncology ward. Although the chemotherapy regimens provide a longer survival (VP = 214 days, CAP = 165 days) than BSC (112 days), the quality of life TTO score was higher for BSC (0.61) compared with the chemotherapy regimens (0.34). When survival time is multiplied by the TTO scores, the use of BSC results in an estimated 0.19 QALYs, which is similar to VP (0.19 QALYs), but higher than CAP (0.15 QALY). The costs to the health care system for the three options are about $5000 for BSC, $10,000 for VF, and $7000 for CAP.* Cost-utility ratios are calculated similarly to cost-effectiveness ratios, except that the outcome unit is QALYs. Therefore the cost-utility ratio is about $26,000/QALY for BSC and about $44,000 to $52,000/QALY for the chemotherapy regimens. Because BSC is at least as effective, as measured by QALYs, and is less expensive than the other two options, a marginal (or incremental) cost-utility ratio does not need to be calculated. Marginal cost-utility ratios only need to be calculated to estimate the added cost for an added benefit, not when the added benefit comes at a lower cost.

Performing an Economic Analysis

Conducting a pharmacoeconomic analysis can be challenging. Resources (time, expertise, data, and money) are limited. Data used to construct a model may be impossible to obtain due to lack of computer automation. Comparative studies of drug treatments may not be available or poorly designed. Results of clinical trials may not apply at the institution performing the analysis due to lack of resources.

Methods for conducting a pharmacoeconomic analysis have been described. All four types of analyses described (CMA, CBA, CEA, and CUA) should follow 10 general steps. A modified practical approach to these steps based on the work developed by Jolicoeur et al.[15] will be reviewed.

---

*The authors reported median costs instead of average costs due to the abnormality of the cost data.

STEP 1: DEFINE THE PROBLEM

This step is self-explanatory. What is the question or objective that is the focus of the analysis? An example might be, "The objective of the analysis is to determine what medications for the treatment of urinary tract infections (UTIs) should be included on our formulary." Perhaps one of the drugs being evaluated is a new drug recently approved by the FDA. Should the new drug be added to the drug formulary? The important thing to remember in this step is to be specific.

STEP 2: DETERMINE THE STUDY'S PERSPECTIVE

It is important to identify from whose perspective the analysis will be conducted. As mentioned in the Assessment of Costs section, this will determine the costs to be evaluated. Is the analysis being conducted from the perspective of the patient or from that of the hospital, clinic, insurance company, or society? Depending on the perspective assigned to the analysis, different results and recommendations based on those results may be identified. If you are deciding on whether to add a new antibiotic to your formulary for treating UTIs, the perspective of the institution or payer would probably be used.

STEP 3: DETERMINE SPECIFIC TREATMENT ALTERNATIVES AND OUTCOMES

In this step, all treatment alternatives to be compared in the analysis should be identified. This selection should include the best clinical options and/or the options that are used most often in that setting at the time of the study. If a new treatment option is being considered, comparing it with an outdated treatment or a treatment with low efficacy rates is a waste of time and money. This new treatment should be compared with the next best alternative or the alternative it may replace. Keep in mind that alternatives may include drug treatments and nondrug treatments. For the UTI example, a new antibiotic would probably be compared with nitrofurantoin or sulfa drugs, or even the use of cranberry juice—old or gold standard therapy—but still the usual and most commonly used therapy. Today's expensive new chemical entities are very unlikely to cost less than the standard therapy, so they are often compared to the most recent, most expensive drug used as alternative therapy.

The outcomes of those alternatives should include all anticipated positive and negative consequences or events that can be measured. Remember, outcomes may be measured in a variety of ways: lives saved, emergency room visits, hospitalizations, adverse drug reactions, dollars saved, QALYs, and so forth. For the UTI example, cure rates would be the most important outcome.

STEP 4: SELECT THE APPROPRIATE PHARMACOECONOMIC METHOD OR MODEL

The pharmacoeconomic method selected will depend on how the outcomes are measured (see Table 8–1). Costs (inputs) for all four types of analyses are measured in dollars. When all outcomes for each alternative are expected to be the same, a CMA is used. If all outcomes for each alternative considered are measured in monetary units, a CBA is used. When outcomes of each treatment alternative are measured in the same nonmonetary units, a CEA is used. When patient preferences for alternative treatments are being considered, a CUA is used. For the UTI example, cure rates are a natural clinical unit measure, so a CEA would be conducted.

STEP 5: MEASURE INPUTS AND OUTCOMES

All resources consumed by each alternative should be identified and measured in monetary value. The cost for each alternative should be listed and estimated (see Assessment of Costs section). The types of costs that will be measured will depend on the perspective chosen in step 2. When evaluating alternatives over a long period of time (e.g., greater than 1 year), the concept of discounting should be applied. For the UTI example, if the perspective is an acute-care hospital, only inpatient costs of treatment are measured. If the perspective is that of the third-party payer, all direct medical costs for the treatment are included whether they are provided on an inpatient or outpatient basis.

Measuring outcomes can be relatively simple (e.g., cure rates) or relatively difficult (e.g., QALYs). Outcomes may be measured prospectively or retrospectively. Prospective measurements tend to be more accurate and complete, but may take considerably more time and resources than retrospective data retrieval. For the UTI example, cure rates attributed to the new product may be estimated from previous clinical trials, expert opinion, or measured prospectively in the population of interest.

STEP 6: IDENTIFY THE RESOURCES NECESSARY TO CONDUCT THE ANALYSIS

The availability of resources to conduct the study is an important consideration. Lack of access to important data can severely limit the validity of an analysis, as can the accuracy of the data itself. Data may be obtained from a variety of sources, including clinical trials, medical literature, medical records, prescription profiles, or computer databases. Before proceeding with the project, evaluate whether reliable sources of data are accessible or the data can be collected within the time frame and budget allocated for the project.

STEP 7: ESTABLISH THE PROBABILITIES FOR THE OUTCOMES OF THE TREATMENT ALTERNATIVES

Probabilities for the outcomes identified in step 3 should be determined. This may include the probability of treatment failures or success, or adverse reactions to a given treatment or alternative. Data for these can be obtained from the medical literature, clinical trials, medical records, expert opinion, prescription databases, as well as institutional databases. For the UTI example, probabilities of a cure rate for the new medication can be found in clinical trials or obtained from the FDA-approved labeling information. Probabilities of cure rates for the previous treatments (e.g., sulfas) can also be found in clinical trials or by accessing medical records. If prospective data collection is conducted, the probabilities of all alternatives will be directly measured instead of estimated.

STEP 8: CONSTRUCT A DECISION TREE

Decision analysis can be a very useful tool when conducting a pharmacoeconomic analysis (see the section on Decision Analysis for a step-by-step review). Constructing a decision tree creates a graphic display of the outcomes of each treatment alternative and the probability of their occurrence. Costs associated with each treatment alternative can be determined and the respective cost ratios derived. An example using a decision tree will be provided in Figure 8–2 in the Decision Analysis section.

STEP 9: CONDUCT A SENSITIVITY ANALYSIS

Whenever estimates are used, there is a possibility that these estimates are not precise. These estimates may be referred to as *assumptions*. For example, if the researcher assumes the discount rate is 5%, or assumes the efficacy rate found in clinical trials will be the same as the effectiveness rate in the general population, this is a best guess used to conduct the calculations. A sensitivity analysis allows one to determine how the results of an analysis would change when these best guesses or assumptions are varied over a relevant range of values. For example, if the researcher makes the assumption that the appropriate discount rate is 5%, this estimate should be varied from 0 to 10% to determine if the same alternative would still be chosen within this range. In order to vary many assumptions at one time, a *probabilistic sensitivity analysis* can be conducted that simulates many patients randomly being processed through the decision model using a range of estimates chosen for the analysis.[16]

This method will help determine the robustness of the analysis. Do small changes in probabilities produce significant differences in the outcomes of the treatment alternatives? Another example of a sensitivity analysis will be provided in the Decision Analysis section.

STEP 10: PRESENT THE RESULTS

The results of the analysis should be presented to the appropriate audience, such as P&T committees, medical staff, or third-party payers. The steps outlined in this section should be employed when presenting the results. State the problem, identify the perspective, and so on. It is imperative to acknowledge or clarify any assumptions.

Although none of the above models presented above are perfect, their utility may lead to better decision-making when faced with the difficult task of evaluating new drugs or technology for health care systems.

What Is Decision Analysis?

Decision analysis is a tool that can help visualize a pharmacoeconomic analysis. It is the application of an analytical method for systematically comparing different decision options. Decision analysis graphically displays choices and performs the calculations needed to compare these options. It assists with selecting the best or most cost-effective alternative. Decision analysis is a tool that has been utilized for years in many fields, but has been applied to medical decision-making more frequently in the last 10 years. This method of analysis assists in making decisions when the decision is complex and there is uncertainty about some of the information.

Discussions of the medical uses of decision analysis have been included in collections of pharmacoeconomic bibliographies,[17-21] and in such specific topic areas as CEAs,[22] CUAs,[23] CBAs,[24] CMAs,[25] policies,[26] formulary processes,[27] pharmacy practices,[28] and drug product development.[29]

STEPS IN DECISION ANALYSIS

The steps in the decision process are enumerated in greater detail in several articles,[30-33] and are relatively straightforward, especially with the availability of computer programs that greatly simplify the calculations.[34] Articles reporting a decision analysis should include a picture of the decision tree, including the costs and probabilities utilized. The steps in a decision analysis will be outlined using the UTI example. The steps involved in performing a decision analysis are provided below.

Step 1: Identify the Specific Decision (Therapeutic or Medical Problem)

Clearly define the specific decision to be evaluated (what is the objective of the study?). Over what period of time will the analysis be conducted (e.g., the episode of care, a year)? Will the perspective be that of the ill patient, the medical care plan, an institution/organization, or society? Specifying who will be responsible for the costs of the treatment will determine how costs are measured. For the UTI example, the decision was whether to add a new antibiotic to the formulary to treat UTIs. The perspective was that of the institution and the time period is 2 weeks.

Step 2: Specify Alternatives (e.g., Two Different Drugs or Treatments, A or B)

Ideally, the two most effective treatments or alternatives should be compared. In pharmacotherapy evaluations, makers of innovative new products may compare or measure themselves against a standard (read as older, more well-established) therapy. This is most often the case with new chemical entities. For pharmaceutical products, dosage and duration of therapy should be included. When analyzing costs and outcomes of pharmaceutical services, these services should be described in detail. For the UTI example, the use of the new medication (drug A) will be compared with that of a sulfa drug (drug B).

Step 3: Specify Possible Outcomes and Probabilities

Consequences and outcomes calculated in dollars yield a CPA; in natural medical units, such as mg/dL, a CEA. For each potential outcome, an estimated probability must be determined (e.g., 95% probability of a cure or a 7% incidence of side effects). Table 8–9 shows the outcomes and probabilities for the UTI example.

Step 4: Draw the Decision Analysis Structure

Lines are drawn to joint decision points (branches or arms of a decision tree), represented either as choice nodes, chance nodes, or final outcomes. Nodes are places in the decision tree where decisions are allowed; a branching becomes possible at this point. There are three types of nodes: (1) a choice node is where a choice is allowed (as between two drugs or two treatments), (2) a chance node is a place where chance (natural occurrence) may influence the decision or outcome expressed as a probability, and (3) a terminal node is the final outcome of interest for that decision. Probabilities are assigned for each possible outcome and the sum of the probabilities must add up to one. Most computer-aided software programs utilize a square box to represent a choice node, a circle to represent a chance node, and a triangle for a terminal branch or final outcome. Figure 8–2 illustrates the decision tree for the UTI example.

TABLE 8–9. OUTCOMES AND PROBABILITIES, UTI EXAMPLE

	Drug A	Drug B
Effectiveness probability	0.95	0.85
Side effect probability	0.05	0.15
Cost of medication	$120	$100
Cost of side effects	$50	$50

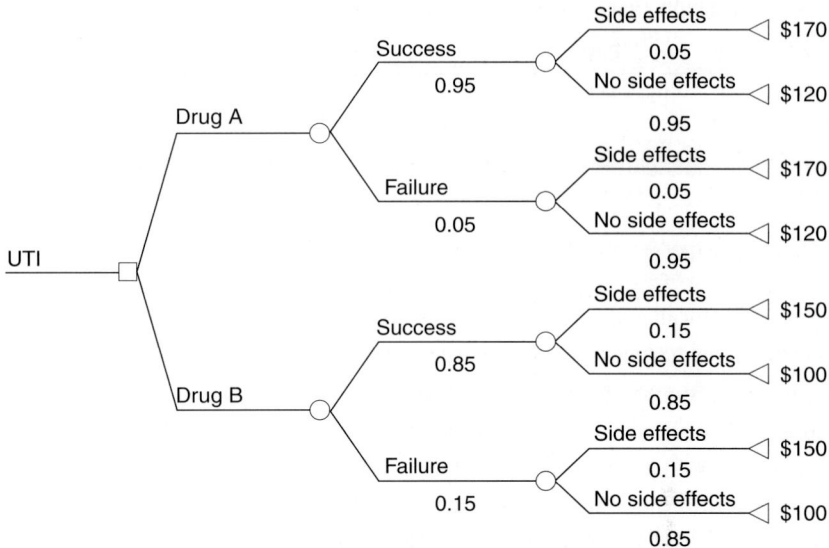

Figure 8–2. Decision tree for UTI example.

Step 5: Perform Calculations

The first consideration should be the PV, or cost, of money. If the study is over a period of less than 1 year, actual costs are utilized in the calculations. If the study period is greater than 1 year, then costs should be discounted (converted to PV). For each branch of the tree, costs are totaled and multiplied by the probability of that arm of the tree. These numbers (costs x probabilities) calculated for each arm of the option are added for each alternative. Example calculations are given in Tables 8–10, 8–11, and 8–12. The UTI example would be a cost-effectiveness type of study, so the difference in the cost for each arm would be divided by the difference in effectiveness for each arm to produce a marginal cost-effectiveness ratio (see Table 8–12).

Step 6: Conduct a Sensitivity Analysis (Vary Cost Estimates)

Because these models are constructed with our best guesses, a sensitivity analysis is conducted. The highest and lowest estimates of costs and probabilities are inserted into the

TABLE 8–10. DECISION ANALYSIS CALCULATIONS FOR DRUG A

Drug A	Cost	Probability	Probability × Cost ($)
Outcome 1	$120 + $50 = $170	0.95 × 0.05 = 0.0475	8.08
Outcome 2	$120	0.95 × 0.95 = 0.9025	108.30
Outcome 3	$120 + $50 = $170	0.05 × 0.05 = 0.0025	0.42
Outcome 4	$120	0.05 × 0.95 = 0.0475	5.70
Total		1	122.50

TABLE 8–11. DECISION ANALYSIS CALCULATIONS FOR DRUG B

Drug B	Cost	Probability	Probability × Cost ($)
Outcome 1	$100 + $50 = $150	0.85 × 0.15 = 0.1275	19.12
Outcome 2	$100	0.85 × 0.85 = 0.7225	72.25
Outcome 3	$100 + $50 = $150	0.15 × 0.15 = 0.0225	3.38
Outcome 4	$100	0.15 × .85 = 0.1275	12.75
Total		1	107.50

equations, to determine the best case and worse case answers. These estimates should be sufficiently varied to reflect all possible true variations in values. For the UTI example, the new drug (drug A) would be added to the formulary if the committee thought the added cost ($150) was worth the added benefit (one more successful treatment) (see Table 8–12). Some might not agree with the probability of the side effects of drug A; because the therapy is new, they may believe 5% may be an underestimate. If we increase this estimate to a 10% side effect rate for the new drug and recalculate the marginal cost-effectiveness ratio, the recalculated ratio would be $175 per added treatment success. Again, the committee would have to decide if the added cost is worth the added benefit.

Decision analysis is being used more commonly in pharmacoeconomic evaluations. The use and availability of computer programs[33] to assist with the multiple calculations makes it fairly easy for someone to automate their evaluations. Examples of software available for this purpose include Data TreeAge, DPL by Applied Decision Analysis, and DecisionPro. The prices for these software packages range from less than $100 for student versions to almost $1000 for professional versions. More examples of computer software, vendors, and prices can be found at <http://faculty.fuqua.duke.edu/daweb/dasw6.htm>>.[35]

Example

An article by Botteman et al.[36] used a decision tree analysis to model the cost-effectiveness of enoxaparin compared to warfarin for the prevention of complications (deep vein thrombosis, venous thromboembolisms, and postthrombotic syndromes) due to hip replacement surgery. Data for this model were obtained through published literature and expert opinion. The model was created to assess both short-term (immediately after surgery) and long-term (followed until death or 100 years old) costs and consequences. The perspective was that of the payer, and a discount rate of 3% was used for the long-term analysis. For the short-term

TABLE 8–12. MARGINAL COST-EFFECTIVENESS RATIO

	Alternative Costs of Drug and Treating Side Effects ($)	Effectiveness in Treating UTI (%)	Marginal Cost per Treatment Success
Drug A	122.50	95	$\dfrac{\$122.50 - \$107.50}{0.95 - 0.85} = \$150$
Drug B	107.50	85	

model, therapy with enoxaparin was more expensive (+$133 per patient), but had a better outcome (+0.04 QALY per patient). For the long-term model, therapy with enoxaparin saved money (–$89 per patient) and had a better outcome (+0.16 QALY per patient), and was therefore the dominant choice. Both univariate and probabilistic sensitivity analyses were conducted and reported.

Steps in Reviewing Published Literature

It is more likely that a practicing pharmacist will be asked to evaluate published literature on the topic of pharmacoeconomics, rather than actually conduct a study. When evaluating the pharmacoeconomics literature for making a formulary decision, or selecting a "best" product for your institution, a systematic approach to evaluating the pharmacoeconomics literature can make the task easier.

Several authors[15, 37–42] cite methodology to assist in systematically reviewing the pharmacoeconomic literature. If a study is carefully reviewed to ensure the author(s) included all meaningful components of an economic evaluation, the likelihood of finding valid and useful results is high. The steps for evaluating studies are similar to the steps for conducting studies, because the readers are determining if the proper steps were followed when the researcher conducted the study. When evaluating a pharmacoeconomic study, at least the following 10 questions should be considered.

1. Was a well-defined question posed in an answerable form? The specific questions and hypotheses should be clearly stated at the beginning of the article.
2. Is the perspective of the study addressed? The perspective should be explicitly stated, not implied.
3. Were the appropriate alternatives considered? Head-to-head comparisons of the best alternatives provide more information than comparing a new product or service with an outdated or ineffective alternative.
4. Was a comprehensive description of the competing alternatives given? If products are compared, dosage and length of therapy should be included. If services are compared, explicit details of the services make the paper more useful. Could another researcher replicate the study based on the information given?
5. What type of analysis was conducted? The paper should address if a CMA, CEA, CBA, or CUA was conducted. Some studies may conduct more than one type of analysis (i.e., a combination of a CEA and a CUA). Some studies, especially older published studies, incorrectly placed in the title of the article a reference to a benefit or effectiveness analysis, when many were actually CMA studies.

6. Were all the important and relevant costs and outcomes included? Check to see that all pertinent costs and consequences were mentioned. Compare their list to your practice situation.

7. Was there justification for any important costs or consequences that were not included? Sometimes, the authors will admit that although certain costs or consequences are important, they were impractical (or impossible) to measure in their study. It is better that the authors state these limitations, than to ignore them.

8. Was discounting appropriate? If so, was it conducted? If the treatment cost or outcomes are extrapolated for more than 1 year, the time value of money must be incorporated into the cost estimates.

9. Are all assumptions stated? Were sensitivity analyses conducted for these assumptions? Many of the values used in pharmacoeconomic studies are based on assumptions. For example, authors may assume the side effect rate is 5%, or that compliance with a regimen will be 80%. These types of assumptions should be stated explicitly. For important assumptions, was the estimate varied within a reasonable range of values?

10. Was an unbiased summary of the results presented? Sometimes, the conclusions seem to overstate or overextrapolate the data presented in the results section. Did the authors use unbiased reasonable estimates when determining the results? In general, do you believe the results of the study?

Example

An example of an evaluation is given below. Due to space limitations, a manuscript abstract rather than a full article will be evaluated. The names and details of the products are fictional.

Title: Pharmacoeconomic Analysis of Ultraceph and Megaceph

Background: Two new antibiotics were recently approved by the FDA—Ultraceph and Megaceph. Both have similar spectrums of activity. Ultraceph is dosed orally—50 mg once per day. Liver function affects Ultraceph, so monitoring is needed. Megaceph is also dosed orally—25 mg twice per day and is associated with a 1% chance of hearing loss, which is reversible if caught within the first 2 days of treatment.

Methods: The purpose of this study was to calculate the net benefit/cost when comparing Ultraceph and Megaceph. Costs paid by third-party payers were assessed. Costs of the medications, administration time, and lab monitoring were included as input costs. The average number of hospital days was assessed for patients on each medication. An estimated cost of $1,500 per hospital day was used to calculate the outcome costs.

Results: The net savings of using Ultraceph compared to Megaceph were $700 per patient. The average cost estimates of hospitalization varied from $500 to $2000 per day and results still favored Ultraceph (range of $200 to $950 net savings).

Conclusion: Although the costs associated with administering Ultraceph are higher than Megaceph, Ultraceph may allow patients to leave the hospital sooner, thus third-party payers may realize a net benefit.

EVALUATION

1. Was a well-defined question posed in an answerable form? Yes, the objective was stated in the first line of the methods section: "The purpose of this study was to calculate the net benefit/cost when comparing Ultraceph and Megaceph."

2. Is the perspective of the study addressed? Yes the perspective was stated when the authors wrote: "Costs paid by third-party payers were assessed."

3. Were appropriate alternatives considered? Yes, these medications had similar spectrums of activity.

4. Was a comprehensive description of competing alternatives given? Yes, alternatives and their dosing were clear—Ultraceph is dosed 50 mg once per day. Megaceph is dosed 25 mg twice per day.

5. What type of analysis was conducted? A CBA because net costs($) were compared to net savings($)

6. Were appropriate costs and consequences measured? With an abstract it is difficult to determine if certain specific costs and benefits were included, but the categories of costs measured (medications, administration time, and lab values) seem appropriate for the perspective given (third-party payer).

7. Was there justification for any important costs or consequences that were not included? No, but when these are mentioned it is usually in the text versus the abstract.

8. Was discounting appropriate? Conducted? Because of the short time frame it was not needed nor conducted.

9. Were assumptions stated—were they reasonable? Was a sensitivity analysis conducted on these assumptions? One assumption was that $1500 per day was a reasonable estimate for a hospital stay. A sensitivity analysis on this assumption was conducted—"The average cost estimates of hospitalization varied from $500 to $2000 per day."

10. Was an unbiased summary of the results presented? In an abstract, it is difficult to tell if parts of the article seemed biased—the abstract itself did not seem biased.

Many articles, several journals, and numerous texts have been devoted to pharmacoeconomics. Research and further development and refinement of the analysis tools are ongoing. It can be expected that the literature on pharmacoeconomics will continue to expand rapidly, not only for use in proving the value of new therapies, but invalidating the worth of standard therapies. Draugalis,[37] Baskin,[38] Greenhalgh,[39] and Mullins and Flowers[42] among others, cite references to assist readers in understanding and assessing economic analyses of health care as well as providing checklists (with examples and explanations) to evaluate published articles.

Selected Pharmacoeconomics Websites

Articles that provide an overview of the field of pharmacoeconomics, its changing methodologies, and recent advances can often be found readily at Internet sites devoted to this area of specialization. These sites usually highlight articles that are not necessarily drug or therapy specific, but many present an overview or validation of methodologies. Several pharmacoeconomic websites are included as references. They were selected because they all have multiple links to other pharmacoeconomic related sites.

- Canadian Coordinating Office of Health Technology Assessment <<http://www. ccohta.ca>>
- Cochrane Collaboration Home Page <<http://www.cochrane.org/index0.htm>>
- Department of Defense Pharmacoeconomic Center <<http://www.pec.ha.osd.mil/links.htm>>
- Institute of Health Economics <<http://www.ihe.ca>>
- International Society for Pharmacoeconomics and Outcomes Research <<http://www.ispor.org/links_index.asp>>

Educational opportunities in pharmacoeconomics have grown tremendously over the past 10 years, especially in U.S. Schools of Pharmacy.[43] A website that lists links to over 60 other websites that offer pharmacoeconomic education can be found at <<http://www.healtheconomics.com/education.cfm>>.[44]

Conclusion

Many pharmacy and therapeutics committees continue to be challenged with managing costs of pharmacotherapy. Pharmacoeconomic models can be useful tools for evaluating the costs of pharmaceuticals. The ability to objectively measure and compare costs may also produce better decisions about the choice of pharmaceuticals for a formulary. Decision analysis is one of the many tools finding increased utilization in the field of medicine, and pharmacoeconomics specifically. As the science of pharmacoeconomics becomes more standardized, rigorous comparisons among several papers on the same topic will be possible (and necessary).

Study Questions

1. Describe the differences in CEA, CBA, CMA, and CUA.

2. What are the steps in the decision analysis process?

3. Why is a sensitivity analysis performed as part of the decision analysis?

4. Would all articles presenting pharmacoeconomic studies contain essentially the same steps? Why?

REFERENCES

1. Centerwatch: Clinical trials listing service. [accessed 2004 Mar 9]. Available from: http://www.centerwatch.com/patient/ drugs/druglist.html.
2. Wang Z, Salmon JW, Walton SM. Cost-effectiveness analysis and the formulary decision-making process. J Manag Care Pharm. 2004;10(10):48–59.
3. Bootman JL, Townsend RJ, McGhan WF. Introduction to pharmacoeconomics. In: Bootman JL, Townsend RJ, McGhan WF, editors. Principles of pharmacoeconomics. 2nd ed. Cincinnati (OH): Harvey Whitney Books; 1996. p. 5–11.
4. Bungay KM, Sanchez LA. Types of economic and humanistic outcomes assessments. In: Grauer et al., editors. Pharmacoeconomics and outcomes: applications for patient care. 2nd ed. Kansas (MO): American College of Clinical Pharmacy; 2003.
5. Nadel HL. Formulary conversion from glipizide to glyburide: a cost-minimization analysis. Hosp Pharm. 1995;30(6):467–9, 472–4.
6. Farmer KC, Schwartz WJ, Rayburn WF, Turnball G. A cost-minimization analysis of intracervical Prostaglandin E$_2$ for cervical ripening in an outpatient versus inpatient setting. Clin Ther. 1996;18(4):747–56.
7. Mithani H, Brown G. The economic impact of once-daily versus conventional administration of gentamicin and tobramycin. PharmacoEconomics. 1996;10(5):494–503.
8. Bjornson DC, Hiner WO, Potyk RP, Nelson BA, Lombardo FA, Morton TA, et al. Effects of pharmacists on health care outcomes in hospitalized patients. Am J Hosp Pharm. 1993;50:1875–84.
9. Jackson LA, Schuchat A, Gorsky RD, Wenger JD. Should college students be vaccinated against meningococcal disease? A cost-benefit analysis. Am J Public Health. 1995;85(6):843–5.
10. Bloom BS, Hillman AL, LaMont B, Liss C, Schwartz JS, Stever GJ. Omeprazole or ranitidine plus metoclopramide for patients with severe erosive oesophagitis. PharmacoEconomics. 1995;8(4):343–9.
11. Law AV, Pathak DS, Segraves AM, Weinstein CR, Arneson WH. Cost-effectiveness analysis of the conversion of patients with non-insulin-dependent diabetes mellitus from glipizide to glyburide and of the accompanying pharmacy follow-up clinic. Clin Ther. 1995;17(5):977–87.
12. Kaplan RM. Utility assessment for estimating quality-adjusted life years. In: Sloan FA, editor. Valuing health care: costs, benefits, and effectiveness of pharmaceuticals and other medical technologies. Cambridge (NY): Cambridge University Press; 1995.

13. Pashos CL, Klein EG, Wanke LA, editors. ISPOR Lexicon. Princeton (NJ): International Society for Pharmacoeconomics and Outcomes Research; 1998. p. 73.

14. Kennedy W, Reinharz D, Tessier G, Contandriopoulos AP, Trabut I, Champagne F, et al. Cost-utility analysis of chemotherapy and best supportive care in non-small cell lung cancer. PharmacoEconomics. 1995;8(4):316–23.

15. Jolicoeur LM, Jones-Grizzle AJ, Boyer JG. Guidelines for performing a pharmacoeconomic analysis. Am J Hosp Pharm. 1992;49:1741–7.

16. Shaw JW, Zachry WM. Application of probabilistic sensitivity analysis in decision analytic modeling. Formulary (USA). 2002;37:32–34, 37–40.

17. McGhan WF, Lewis NJW. Basic bibliographies: pharmacoeconomics. Hosp Pharm. 1992;27:547–8.

18. Wanke LA, Huber SL. Basic bibliographies: cancer therapy pharmacoeconomics. Hosp Pharm. 1994;29:402.

19. Skaer TL, Williams LM. Basic bibliographies: biotechnology pharmacoeconomics I. Hosp Pharm. 1994;29:1053–4.

20. Skaer TL, Williams LM. Basic bibliographies: biotechnology pharmacoeconomics II. Hosp Pharm. 1994;29:1136.

21. McGhan WF. Basic bibliographies: pharmacoeconomics. Hosp Pharm. 1998;33:1270, 1273.

22. Duggan AE, Tolley K, Hawkey CJ, Logan RF. Varying efficacy of *Helicobacter pylori* eradication regimens: cost effectiveness study using a decision analysis model. BMJ. 1998;316:1648–54.

23. Messori A, Trippoli S, Becagli P, Cincotta M, Labbate MG, Zaccara G. Adjunctive lamotrigine therapy in patients with refractory seizures: a lifetime cost-utility analysis. Eur J Clin Pharmacol. 1998;53(6):421–7.

24. Ginsberg G, Shani S, Lev B. Cost benefit analysis of risperidone and clozapine in the treatment of schizophrenia in Israel. PharmacoEconomics. 1998 Feb 13;231–41.

25. Sesti AM, Armitstead JA, Hall KN, Jang R, Milne S. Cost-minimization analysis of hand held nebulizer vs metered dose inhaler protocol for management of acute asthma exacerbations in the emergency department. ASHP Midyear Clinical Meeting; 32: MCS-7: 1997; 1996 Dec 8–12; New Orleans, Louisiana.

26. Hinman AR, Koplan JP, Orenstein WA, Brink EW. Decision analysis and polio immunization policy. Am J Public Health. 1988;78:301–3.

27. Kessler JM. Decision analysis in the formulary process. Am J Health Syst Pharm. 1997;54:S5–S8.

28. Einarson TR, McGhan WF, Bootman JL. Decision analysis applied to pharmacy practice. Am J Hosp Pharm. 1985;42:364–71.

29. Walking D, Appino JP. Decision analysis in drug product development. Drug Cosmet Ind. 1973;112:39–41.

30. Rascati KL. Decision analysis techniques practical aspects of using personal computers for decision analytic modeling. Drug Benefit Trends. 1998 July; 33–36.

31. Richardson WS, Detsky AS. Users' guides to the medical literature. Part 7. How to use a clinical decision analysis. Part A. Are the results of the study valid? JAMA. 1995;273:1292–5.

32. Richardson WS, Detsky AS. Users' guides to the medical literature. Part 7. How to use a clinical decision analysis. Part B. What are the results and will they help me in caring for my patients? JAMA. 1995;273:1610–3.

33. Baskin LE. Practical Pharmacoeconomics. Cleveland (OH): Advanstar Communications; 1998.

34. Sacristán JA, Soto J, Galende I. Evaluation of pharmacoeconomic studies: utilization of a checklist. Ann Pharmacother. 1993;27:1126–32.

35. Decision tree and influence diagram software. [accessed 2004 Mar 9]. Available from: http://faculty. fuqua.duke.edu/daweb/dasw6.htm.

36. Botteman MF, Caprini J, Stephens JM, Nadipelli V, Bell CF, Pashos CL, et al. Results of an economic model to assess cost-effectiveness of enoxaparin, a low-molecular-weight heparin, versus warfarin for the prophylaxis of DVT and associated long-term complications in total hip replacement surgery in the United States. Clin Ther. 2002:24(11):1960–86.

37. Draugalis JR. Assessing pharmacoeconomic studies. In: Bootman JL, Townsend RJ, McGhan WF, editors. Principles of pharmacoeconomics. Cincinnati (OH): Harvey Whitney Books; 1996. p. 278–9.

38. Baskin LE. How to evaluate the validity and usefulness of pharmacoeconomic literature. In: Practical pharmacoeconomics. Cleveland (OH): Advanstar Communications; 1998. p. 95–102.

39. Greenhalgh T. How to read a paper: papers that tell you what things cost (economic analyses). BMJ. 1997;315:596–9.

40. Drummond MF, Richardson WS, O'Brien BJ, Levine M, Heyland D. Users' guides to the medical literature. XIII. How to use an article on economic analysis of clinical practice. A. Are the results of the study valid? Evidence-Based Medicine Working Group. JAMA. 1997;277(19):1552–7.

41. O'Brien BJ, Heyland D, Richardson WS, Levine M, Drummond MF. Users' guides to the medical literature. XIII. How to use an article on economic analysis of clinical practice. B. What are the results and will they help me in caring for my patients? Evidence-Based Medicine Working Group [erratum JAMA. 1997;278(13):1064]. JAMA. 1997;277(22):1802–6.

42. Mullins CD, Flowers LR. Evaluating economic outcomes literature. In: Grauer et al., editors. Pharmaco-economics and outcomes: applications for patient care. 2nd ed. Kansas City (MO): American College of Clinical Pharmacy; 2003.

43. Rascati KL, Drummond MF, Annemans L, Davey PG. Education in pharmacoeconomics: an international multidisciplinary view. PharmacoEconomics. 2004;22(3):139–47.

44. HealthEconomics.com. [accessed 2004 Mar 9]. Available from: http://www.healtheconomics.com/ education.cfm.

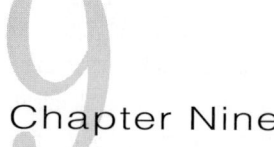

Chapter Nine

Evidence-Based Clinical Practice Guidelines

Kevin G. Moores

Objectives

After completing this chapter, the reader will be able to

- Define clinical practice guideline.
- Describe the role of clinical practice guidelines in pharmacy practice and the pharmacist's role in development and use of these guidelines.
- Identify various sources of published guidelines and organizations currently involved in guideline activities.
- Describe various intended purposes for the development and implementation of clinical practice guidelines.
- Explain the methodology for development of clinical practice guidelines.
- Describe the process of the systematic review of scientific evidence as part of the early steps involved in drafting clinical practice guidelines to assess benefits and harms of therapeutic interventions.
- Apply structured criteria to evaluate the validity of clinical practice guidelines.
- Identify the key issues in interpreting clinical practice guidelines and issues involved in their implementation.

Introduction

Evidence-based clinical practice guidelines are "systematically developed statements to assist practitioner and patient decisions about health care for specific circumstances."[1] Clinical practice guidelines are developed by a variety of groups and organizations including federal and state government, professional societies and associations, managed care organizations, third-party payers, quality assurance organizations, and utilization review groups. The purpose of the guidelines, development methods used, format of the documents, and the strategies for implementation vary widely. Considering the potential for clinical practice guidelines to influence thousands to millions of decisions on medical interventions, it is incumbent on all health care practitioners to be thoroughly familiar with criteria to judge the validity of guidelines, and be skilled in determining their appropriate application.

Development and implementation of clinical practice guidelines have many characteristics in common with traditional activities performed by drug information practitioners, such as evaluation of new drugs for formulary consideration, medication use evaluation, and quality improvement. Many of the skills required for guideline development are required of drug information practitioners, including clear, specific definition of clinical questions, literature search and evaluation, epidemiology, biostatistics, clinical expertise, writing, editing, formatting, and education. Drug information practitioners benefit from the use of clinical practice guidelines as information resources for their work, and based on their skills are logical professionals to participate in guideline development and implementation. Other pharmacists also find clinical practice guidelines to be useful in their practices.

The primary attraction for all health care practitioners in properly developed, valid practice guidelines is that they provide a concise summary of current best evidence on what works and what does not when considering specific health care interventions. New information and new technology in health care are developed at a rapid pace. It is very difficult for individual practitioners to systematically evaluate the benefits and risks of all new technology, including new medications. By presenting a summary of best evidence, guidelines assist the practitioner in decision-making for specific patients and also facilitate discussion of care options most consistent with individual patient needs and preferences. Guidelines may also enhance provider communication and continuity of care, especially when decisions are made by multiple providers in different care settings.[2]

There is a growing awareness in health care that a significant time lag occurs in getting research information into practice. There are several examples of treatments that have been well studied and proven effective that are substantially underutilized, and interventions that have been proven ineffective or harmful that continue to be provided.[3] One of the goals of development and implementation of evidence-based clinical practice guidelines is to help speed up the process of getting evidence into practice.

Clinical practice guidelines to assist with health care decision-making and to identify indicators for monitoring quality of care, are frequently mentioned in connection with efforts to improve quality and efficiency of services. The key issues in reorganizing the U.S. health care system are access to care, cost, and quality. Quality and safety are a major focus as evidenced by legislative proposals for specific requirements of health insurance coverage, critical recommendations in the report from the President's Advisory Commission on

Consumer Protection and Quality in the Health Care Industry,[3] and the conclusions of The Institute of Medicine National Roundtable on Health Care Quality.[4] In addition, The Institute of Medicine (IOM) has published landmark reports in the past few years regarding quality of care problems in the United States,[5] recommendations to improve the health care system,[6] and specific recommendations to focus on improvements in patient safety.[7] A central concept in these reports and recommendations relates to utilizing the best available evidence, providing decision support tools, use of informatics, and participation of patients in health care decisions and responsibilities. These concepts are also central to clinical practice guidelines.

Methods currently recommended as the most valid for development of clinical practice guidelines emphasize an evidence-based approach, formal quantitative techniques to calculate risks and benefits, and incorporation of the patient's preference. The concepts of an evidence-based approach and use of methods to grade the quality of evidence and strength of recommendations are critical elements that will be reviewed in more detail in this chapter in the sections on methodology for clinical practice guideline development and interpretation of guideline recommendations. The evidence-based health care movement and the implementation of continuous quality improvement (CQI) programs have stimulated growth in guideline development. There have also been advancements in methods of evaluation and summarizing the best available evidence (e.g., systematic reviews, meta-analyses, and decision analyses). Development of new information databases of systematic reviews, and new informatics resources facilitate the production of clinical practice guidelines and improve access to this information.

This chapter will present a review of the background for why clinical practice guidelines have become a common element in health care; describe the activities of selected major organizations involved with guidelines; review evidence-based methods for guideline development, evaluation, and implementation; describe interpretation skills for guideline recommendations; and provide directions to locate sources of guidelines and further information.

Evidence-Based Practice and Clinical Practice Guidelines

Evidence-based medicine (EBM) is a philosophy of practice and an approach to decision-making in the clinical care of patients. Sackett and colleagues have defined EBM as the "conscientious, explicit, and judicious use of current best evidence in making decisions about the care of individual patients."[8] The practice of EBM refers to integrating individual clinical expertise with the best available external clinical evidence from systematic research. EBM is often mistaken for, or reduced to, just one of its several components, critical appraisal of the literature. However, EBM requires both clinical expertise and an intimate knowledge of the individual patient's situation, beliefs, priorities, and values to be useful. External evidence must be used to inform, but not replace, individual clinical expertise. It is clinical expertise that determines if the external evidence may be applied to the individual patient and, if so, how it should be used in decision-making by the patient and the health care provider. The development and application of clinical practice guidelines is one of the tools used in EBM. In fact, David Eddy, who remains one of the most recognized individuals for development of EBM, writes that the first published use of the term *evidence-based* was in fact in the context of clinical guidelines.[9] An understanding of EBM is necessary to understand recommended methods for production and implementation of guidelines.

Physicians working at McMaster University in Hamilton, Ontario, first used the terminology *evidence-based medicine*. This group, called The Evidence-Based Medicine Working Group, published a description of what they considered a new paradigm for medical practice and teaching.[10] In that article they presented their views on changes that were occurring in medical practice relating to the use of medical literature to more effectively guide decision-making. They state that the foundation for the paradigm shift rests in the significant developments in clinical research over the past 30 years; particularly the randomized-controlled trial. Also considered important is meta-analysis as a method of summarizing the results of a number of randomized trials that may have profound effects on setting treatment policy.

The Evidence-Based Medicine Working Group cites the following changes that document the development of the new philosophy: (1) proposals to apply the principles of clinical epidemiology to day-to-day clinical practice; (2) numerous articles published instructing clinicians on how to access, evaluate, and interpret the medical literature; (3) growing demand for courses that instruct physicians on how to use the medical literature; (4) improvements in the format of journal articles; (5) textbooks with more rigorous review of available evidence; (6) new information resources like the American College of Physicians (ACP) Journal Club; and (7) the development of practice guidelines based on rigorous methodological review.

The practice of EBM has been described as focusing on five linked activities[11]: (1) express information needs in clearly defined answerable clinical questions, (2) conduct a systematic search for the best available evidence for the problem, (3) evaluate the validity and applicability of the evidence, (4) prepare a synthesis or summary of the evidence for decision-making and implement the decision in practice, and (5) evaluate performance and follow-up on any areas for improvement. Those who are familiar with the literature in drug information practice will recognize that these activities are remarkably similar to the systematic approach to drug information requests as outlined by Watanabe and colleagues over 30 years ago.[12] This process is still very similar to the approach to drug information questions today (see Chap. 2).

In 2000, the lead individuals in the Evidence-Based Medicine Working Group published a slightly modified description for what the practice of evidence-based care represents.[13] This description recognizes that not all practitioners will be "interested in gaining a high level of sophistication in using the original literature, and secondly, those who do will often be short of time in applying these skills." The modified description notes that sources of appropriately preappraised evidence can be used by "highly competent, up-to-date practitioners who deliver evidence-based care." Examples of preappraised evidence would include clinical practice guidelines and systematic reviews that have been produced with evidence-based methods. These authors note that skill in interpreting the medical literature is still necessary to judge the quality of the "preappraised" resources, to know when the recommendations in the preappraised resources are not applicable to selected patients, and to use the original literature when preappraised resources are unavailable.[13]

In his most recent review of the philosophy of EBM, Eddy describes an approach which is similar to the Evidence-Based Medicine Working Group.[9] Eddy refers to the Evidence-Based Medicine Working Group's original description of the practice as "evidence-based individual decision-making." He refers to a second approach to EBM as being "evidence-based guidelines." In this second approach he describes four important features: "first, the work of analyzing the evidence and developing a guideline, or other type of policy is done by small groups of specially trained people, usually sponsored by an organization. Second, they all use an explicit, rigorous process. Third, for all of them the 'product'—whether it is an evidence review, a guideline, or another type of policy—is generic. It is intended to apply to a class or group of patients defined by some clinical criteria, rather than to an individual patient. Fourth, their effects are indirect. That is, they are intended to enable, guide, motivate, or sometimes force physicians and other types of providers to deliver certain types of care to people; they do not directly determine the care provided to a particular patient."[9] Eddy goes on to explain that the most appropriate definition of EBM is a combination of these two approaches. The combination provides for medical practice that will achieve the most efficient and effective use of evidence.

Medical education has also taken on philosophies related to EBM and guidelines. International trends in continuing medical education were described in a series of seven articles published in the *British Medical Journal*.[14-20] The major themes of these articles include the following:

- Individual responsibility for health professionals to direct their own learning.
- Self-assessment and specific needs-directed education.
- Wider aspects of continuing professional development including computer literacy, literature appraisal, information management, problem solving skills, and EBM.
- Improved working and collaboration among different health professionals to achieve gains in quality and savings in cost.
- Innovative portfolio-based programs to capture learning issues and achievements that occur in everyday practice.
- Programs for better communications with patients and with other health care providers.

- Programs based on skill development rather than the traditional lecture format.
- Distance learning and use of technology to support learning.
- Focus on education that will affect behaviors and improve outcomes of care.
- Problem-based learning and small group activities.
- Quality improvement tools.
- Programs based on the theories of adult learning.

The U.S. IOM made recommendations for reform of health professions education in 2003.[21] In this report it was stated, "The committee believes that the following should serve as an overarching vision for all programs and institutions engaged in the clinical education of health professionals, and further that such organizations should develop operating principals that will allow this vision to be achieved. All health care professionals should be educated to deliver patient-centered care as members of an interdisciplinary team, emphasizing evidence-based practice, quality improvement approaches, and informatics."[21] This statement has been referred to as the five core competencies for health professionals. The recommendations provided in this report were a follow-up to the influential IOM report *Crossing the Quality Chasm* from 2001.[6] Examination of these five core competencies and the goals of evidence-based clinical practice guidelines demonstrate significant overlap.

Health care professionals face the complicated reality of constantly changing and increasing medical knowledge. What is required to practice effective, high quality medicine is not an encyclopedic memory, but the skills to acquire and critically assess the specific information that is necessary to make clinical decisions. The philosophy of EBM is consistent with the philosophy of clinical practice guidelines. The decision-making process of EBM is supported by access and use of clinical practice guidelines.

Guideline Development Methods

A thorough understanding of the methodology used for clinical practice guideline development is critical for pharmacists. Although relatively few pharmacists actually participate in guideline development, this understanding will prepare practitioners for involvement in appropriate evaluation and implementation of these guidelines. Evaluation of the quality of a guideline, and the appropriateness of its use in a given setting, depends primarily on an ability to distinguish methods that minimize potential biases in development. A strong indication of the quality of guideline development methods can be obtained by a quick scan to determine if the recommendations are based on focused clinical questions, the recommendations are specifically linked to evidence, the quality of the evidence and strength of recommendations have been graded, and evidence tables and a balance sheet are available. A lack of understanding of the requirements for guideline development could lead to inappropriate

interpretation, or acceptance of inappropriate levels of enforcement of biased guideline recommendations. Application of biased guidelines may result in provision of ineffective or
harmful therapy. Because of the central importance of guideline development methods, a significant portion of this chapter is devoted to this topic.

Several methods for developing practice guidelines have been described including
informal consensus development, formal consensus development, evidence-based guideline
development, and explicit guideline development.[22] For decades, informal consensus methods have been used as the basis of guideline development. These guidelines were produced following a meeting of an expert panel in which agreement was reached through
open discussion; sometimes producing recommendations in a single meeting. The actual
guideline document would often provide only the recommendation, with little background
on the evidence that was used or information on the methodology of the group. This practice made it difficult or impossible for readers to verify the accuracy of the recommendation
or that bias did not significantly influence the results. Informal consensus development
remains a common approach to developing practice guidelines because it is a relatively
fast, easy, and inexpensive process. However, this approach generally results in guidelines
of questionable quality. The fact that explicit methods for how the decisions were made are
often not provided leaves doubt about how consensus was reached. Treatment recommendations are notoriously fallible when they are the result of efficacy evaluations based primarily on opinion. In addition, the ability to implement such black box guidelines will be
seriously hampered based on the inability of the user to verify the accuracy and a resultant
lack of confidence.[22]

The formal consensus development process was once used by the National Institutes of
Health Consensus Development Program.[23] The National Institutes of Health (NIH) used a
structured 2.5-day conference in which guidelines are developed in closed session after a plenary session and open discussion, and are presented to an audience and press conference on
the third day.[22] In some instances, the usual 2.5-day format of the conference is not sufficient
and alternative formats are used.[24] It should also be noted that substantial advanced planning
occurs for presentations of up-to-date reviews of available evidence by experts. This process
provides more structure than informal consensus; however, it has been criticized for its
requirement to produce recommendations in a relatively short period, the absence of explicit
criteria, the variability in the type and degree of referencing of the recommendations to the
literature, and the inconsistent degree of labeling recommendations as to the level of certainty provided by empirical evidence.

Most recently the NIH has been using evidence-based methods for guideline development, for example, the Third Report of the National Cholesterol Education Program (NCEP)
Expert Panel on Detection Evaluation, and Treatment of High Blood Cholesterol in Adults
(Adult Treatment Panel III [ATP III]).[25] In keeping with evidence-based methodology, an
update to this guideline was published in July 2004 based on the results of five major studies
that were completed after the ATP III guidelines were released. These clinical trials provided

evidence regarding several significant issues pertaining to the benefits of cholesterol lowering. The purpose of the update was to "translate the scientific evidence into guidance that helps professionals and the public take appropriate action to reduce the risk for coronary heart disease (CHD) and cardiovascular disease."[26] Another example guideline produced with evidence-based methods by the NIH is the Seventh Report of the Joint National Committee on Prevention, Detection, Evaluation, and Treatment of High Blood Pressure (JNC 7).[27]

Guideline development procedures that can be considered evidence-based were first used in the late 1970s by the Canadian Task Force on Preventive Health Care (formerly knows as the Canadian Task Force on the Periodic Health Examination).[28] The U.S. Preventive Services Task Force (USPSTF) which was first convened by the U.S. Public Health Service in 1984, adapted the Canadian Task Force methodology and also uses a systematic evidence-based methodology to review the evidence of effectiveness of clinical preventive services.[29] The USPSTF efforts culminated in the 1989 *Guide to Clinical Preventive Services*. A second edition of the *Guide* was published in 1996. For the third edition of the *Guide*, recommendations are being released incrementally as they become available as periodic updates at the following website <<http://www.ahrq.gov/clinic/gcpspu.htm>>.

The most influential early publications on evidence-based guideline development methods were the writings of Eddy,[30-33] and the Manual for Clinical Practice Guideline Development prepared by the Agency for Health care Research and Quality (AHRQ) (the agency was known as the Agency for Healthcare Policy and Research [AHCPR] at that time).[34] Even though the AHRQ no longer produces guidelines directly, the methodology has been adopted, and in some cases slightly modified, by other groups. The AHCPR evidence-based guideline methodology is still recognized as a rigorous valid method. Most major guideline development programs in the United States, as well as those internationally, use an evidence-based process.[35] Examples of some of these organizations in the United States include the American College of Cardiology (ACC)/American Heart Association (AHA),[36] the American College of Rheumatology,[37] the American College of Chest Physicians (ACCP),[38] the American Academy of Pediatrics,[39] and the Infectious Diseases Society of America.[40] Prominent international guideline development groups have published methodologies that focus on evidence-based principles. These programs include the National Institute for Clinical Excellence (NICE) in the United Kingdom,[41] the New Zealand Guidelines Group (NZGG),[42] and the Scottish Intercollegiate Guidelines Network (SIGN).[43]

Considering that the AHRQ had a large role in the development of evidence-based guideline methods, additional information about this agency is helpful for understanding current issues regarding guidelines. This agency was created in November 1989, when Congress amended the Public Health Service Act. Under the terms of Public Law 101-239 (also known as Omnibus Budget Reconciliation Act of 1989, OBRA '89) this agency was given responsibility for supporting research, data development, and other activities to "enhance the quality, appropriateness, and effectiveness of health care services." The AHCPR was also charged with the responsibility to "arrange for" the development and periodic review and updating of

(1) clinically relevant guidelines that may be used by physicians, educators, and health care practitioners to assist in determining how diseases, disorders, and other health conditions can most effectively and appropriately be prevented, diagnosed, treated, and managed clinically; and (2) standards of quality, performance measures, and medical review criteria through which health care providers and other appropriate entities may assess or review the provision of health care and assure the quality of such care.[44] That legislation also reflected the increased importance of quality, safety, and access issues in national health policy and elevated the activities of the AHCPR to the level of a full Public Health Service (PHS) agency; on the same level as the Centers for Disease Control (CDC) and Prevention, the National Institutes of Health (NIH), and the Food and Drug Administration (FDA).

Between 1990 and 1996, the AHCPR supported panels produced 19 clinical practice guidelines. However, the agency discontinued the guideline development program in the fall of 1996 after political conflicts developed based on recommendations in some of these guidelines. It was also recognized that convening separate national panels to develop each guideline was expensive and time-consuming. The demand for evidence-based information far exceeded the resources that could be devoted to the guideline development program. Furthermore, the agency recognized that many professional organizations, health plans, and commercial firms were producing thousands of guidelines. Therefore, the agency initiated the *Evidence-Based Practice Program*, and now serves as a science partner with private- and public-sector organizations to develop evidence reports. Evidence reports are based on comprehensive reviews and rigorous analysis of relevant scientific evidence. These reports are intended for use as the scientific foundation for public and private organizations to develop tools (including guidelines, technology assessments, and quality indicators) for improving quality of care.

The methodology developed by the AHRQ has influenced all major guideline development programs. The description of guideline development methods provided in this chapter are based primarily on the early publications of guideline methods that were mentioned above, and the publications on guideline development methods from the ACCP,[38,45–47] the NICE in the United Kingdom,[41] the NZGG,[42] and the SIGN.[43] Each publication dealing with methods for evidence-based guideline development describes a multistep process (see Appendices 9–1 and 9–2 for examples of the steps described for different programs). Major steps common in the evidence-based guideline development process used by these major organizations include the following:

- Select an appropriate topic for creation of a guideline.
- Recruit appropriate multidisciplinary membership for a panel to be involved in development of the guideline.
- Define the clinical questions to be addressed.
- Determine the criteria for evidence that will be considered.
- Conduct a systematic search for the qualifying evidence.
- Perform a systematic evaluation and grading of the evidence.

- Prepare a synthesis of the evidence.
- Agree on procedures for a consensus process, or other procedures for making recommendations, in the absence of higher levels of evidence for decision-making.
- Formulate and grade recommendations based on the grade of evidence and balance of benefits, harms, and costs of treatment options.
- Draft the guideline document.
- Conduct peer-review and pilot testing of the guideline.
- Revise the guideline as appropriate.
- Create tools for implementation of the guideline.
- Establish a plan for follow-up and periodic updating of the guideline.

Additional details for each of these steps are described below. The description provided for evidence-based guideline development provided in this chapter incorporates the recommendations from several groups. Not all groups describe all procedures or methods included in this chapter. If the reader wishes to review the specific details of a single organization's procedures for guideline development, the references provided should be consulted. Readers who wish to examine other details of guideline development that are not addressed in this chapter, such as organizational details for coordination of the guideline development, group work planning, a development timeline, and other administrative steps, which are beyond the methodology issues discussed in this chapter, should consult the references provided. A systematic review of evidence represents a substantial amount of the work that goes into development of a clinical practice guideline; therefore, guides for creating a systematic review are also valuable for anyone involved in performing this work. Two such excellent guides are *The Reviewers' Handbook from the Cochrane Collaboration,*[48] and the *Centre for Reviews and Dissemination Guidance for those Carrying Out or Commissioning Reviews.*[49]

SELECT A TOPIC FOR GUIDELINE DEVELOPMENT

Selection of a topic for guideline development has aspects in common with selection of topics for a medication use evaluation program; or in a broader sense for any quality improvement program. Considering that guidelines are intended to improve the quality of care process and outcomes of care, it is important to consider the potential to achieve this improvement when a topic is chosen. As with a clinical management decision, the potential benefits of development and implementation of a guideline should be assessed. Disease conditions with the maximum potential for benefit from guideline development and implementation share common characteristics including the following:

- High prevalence.
- High frequency and/or severity of associated morbidity or mortality.
- Availability of high-quality evidence for the efficacy of treatments that reduce morbidity or mortality.

- Feasibility of implementation of the treatment based on expertise and other resources required.
- Potential cost-effectiveness.
- Evidence that current practice is not optimal.
- Evidence of practice variation.
- Availability of personnel, expertise, and resources to develop and implement the practice guideline.

As an example, the AHA/ACC identified the following reasons for developing evidence-based guidelines for cardiovascular disease prevention in women:[50]

- Cardiovascular disease remains the leading killer of women in the United States.
- Because Coronary Heart Disease (CHD) is often fatal, and two-thirds of women who die suddenly have no previously recognized symptoms, it is essential to prevent CHD.
- In the wake of the reports of the Women's Health Initiative and the Heart and Estrogen/Progestin Replacement Study (HERS) there is a heightened need to critically review and document strategies to prevent CHD in women.
- There has been an increase in the number and proportion of women that have participated in clinical trials which provides more evidence of efficacy of different treatment strategies.
- Because patients seen in clinical practice may have characteristics that are not similar to those of clinical trial participants it is necessary to evaluate the ability to apply these data in practice.

Individual guideline development programs will also use criteria for selecting a topic for guideline development that will maximize the potential benefit for the stakeholders that program serves. For an example of these criteria see Appendix 9–3; criteria for selecting topics used by the NICE in the United Kingdom.[51] In addition to the characteristics mentioned above, the potential to achieve improvements in care by implementing a guideline in a practice depends on characteristics related to the individual practice. For example, has a recognized leader been identified to promote implementation of the guideline within the organization and make sure it will proceed in a timely fashion? Also, achievement of improvement in care is more likely to be realized if there are systems in place to allow the change to be measured, and to provide feedback to individuals and to the implementation team.

RECRUIT APPROPRIATE MULTIDISCIPLINARY MEMBERSHIP FOR A PANEL TO BE INVOLVED IN DEVELOPMENT OF THE GUIDELINE

The development of a clinical practice guideline should be a multidisciplinary process. Ideally, all groups that have a stake in the development and implementation of a guideline are represented in the process. Participants should include physicians with special expertise in the condition being considered; primary care practitioners involved in treatment of patients with the identified condition; representatives of other health disciplines involved in providing care for the identified condition (e.g., physical therapy, respiratory therapy, nursing, pharmacy, occupational therapy, social work, and dentistry); experts in research methods applicable to the topic; individuals with expertise in conducting a systematic search for evidence; individuals with administrative, health services, economics, and other health care systems expertise; and patient representatives or caregivers. Organizational skills, project management, and editorial ability are also key to the success of a guideline program. As an example, the AHA/ACC selected the following panel membership to produce evidence-based guidelines for cardiovascular disease prevention in women[50]:

> "the leaders of each of the 13 AHA Scientific Councils were asked to nominate a recognized expert in cardiovascular disease (CVD) prevention with particular knowledge about women; the president of the AHA appointed at large members to fill gaps in specific areas of expertise; the AHA Manuscript Oversight Committee approved the chair of the expert panel; major professional or government organizations with a mission consistent with CVD prevention were solicited to serve as cosponsors and were asked to nominate one representative to serve on the expert panel; diverse professionals and community organizations were also suggested to endorse the final document after its approval by the AHA Scientific Advisory Coordinating Committee and cosponsoring organizations."[50]

Individuals being considered for membership on a guideline development panel should also be asked to declare potential conflicts of interest. Individuals with a potential conflict of interest may still be considered for participation on a panel depending on the type and degree of conflict, along with appropriate levels of management and disclosure.[52] Rigid complete exclusion of any possible conflict could result in guideline panels excluding the majority of individuals with the critical expertise needed. Surveys have shown the need for attention to this issue as guideline authors frequently have some relationship with pharmaceutical manufacturers.[53] The controversy that may occur has been manifest with challenges voiced regarding the sponsorship of guideline development and publication,[54] and potential conflicts of interest by panel members.[55] Public criticism of potential conflicts of interest by panel members involved in the NCEP Expert Panel on Detection, Evaluation, and Treatment of High Blood Cholesterol in Adults (ATP III), prompted a response from Barbara Alving, MD, Acting Director, National Heart, Lung, and Blood Institute (NHLBI). She issued a statement on July 29, 2004,[56] another on September 24, 2004,[57] and an 11-page letter on October 22, 2004,[58] to explain the development and review methodology used by the panel, defend the integrity of the process, and the scientific basis for the recommendations.

Expertise in guideline development methods that facilitate implementation of practice guidelines would also be valuable to the panel. Substantial research has been conducted in the past 10 years to identify methods of guideline implementation and guideline characteristics that facilitate adherence.[59] Recognized characteristics of guidelines that facilitate implementation include aspects of format, provision of clear unambiguous recommendations, and ability to incorporate the guideline recommendations into a decision support tool. These characteristics should be considered during the production process when possible. For example, significant progress has been made in translating document-based knowledge into systems or tools that can be conveniently integrated in the normal clinical workflow.[60] In order to accomplish this, Shiffman and colleagues (<<http://ycmi.med.yale.edu/GEM/>>) have developed a Guideline Elements Model (GEM) for translation of the typical document-based clinical practice guideline into a format that can be integrated into clinical workflow with computerized decision support systems.[60] This method attempts to deal with guidelines that lack explicit definitions, contain excessive ambiguity, do not consider sequencing or timing of interventions, do not account for important patient-specific variables, lack prioritization of key recommendations, and otherwise do not include all parameters that must be considered for decision-making. Attention to these details are needed for computer decision support systems because they work best when clear dichotomous responses can be made one at a time to reach the desired endpoint. Ambiguity, lack of prioritization, and lack of required variables present significant obstacles to computerized decision support systems. It is also worth considering that the process of decision-making in health care is not always well understood, and in some instances it may not be possible to create the explicit linear process just described. If that is the case, it may be necessary for the guideline panel to recommend reconsideration of the specific questions to be addressed by the guideline. Or, it may be necessary for the panel to make other specific recommendations about how to best implement the guideline in a way to facilitate adoption.

However, even with the advantages offered by information technology, there are potential barriers created by the technology itself which should be considered in guideline implementation plans.[61] Lyons and colleagues identified that physicians, nurses, and administrators perceive some aspects of the use of information technology for guideline implementation as facilitators and others as barriers. Information technology can facilitate guideline implementation because computerization may improve accessibility of some information, may facilitate documentation, assist with guideline updating, and provide useful decision support tools. However, there may be barriers to guideline implementation when there are problems with computer literacy, availability of equipment, and computer glitches or downtime. Lyons also identified that the different disciplines had opposing opinions on the overall importance and reality in the work place for some of these elements.[61] Consideration of these facilitators and barriers during the development process can ultimately improve the success of implementation.

Finally, techniques as simple as writing guidelines with concrete, precise behavioral terms (what, who, when, where, and how) may be effective to achieve guideline adherence.[62] Ensuring that the guideline development panel includes members with expertise to address each of these issues is important to maximize the desired endpoint; a well-constructed guideline that will be followed by practitioners and patients.

DEFINE THE CLINICAL QUESTIONS TO BE ADDRESSED

After the disease or condition is selected and the panel with applicable expertise is formed, the panel will accomplish the next step; further definition of the specific issues for which recommendations will ultimately be provided. The panel will consider what specific decision-making or action steps related to surveillance or screening for the disease, diagnosis, or treatment can be improved with specific recommendations. The decision-making points can be expressed as clinical questions. The definition of the clinical questions to be addressed by a guideline is a key step which provides direction for the activities to follow. The questions are important to provide direction to the systematic review of the literature, and also provide the outline for the recommendations that the guideline will provide. The importance of this phase cannot be overemphasized. Just as in the systematic approach to a drug information question, it is critical to first clearly define the question to be successful in searching for the necessary evidence, and subsequently be able to provide useful valid conclusions.

A clear description of the questions to be addressed by the guideline is also a good starting point for a practitioner to determine if a guideline could be useful in their practice. Depending on the overall goals of a guideline, questions may be about prognosis, the best diagnostic test, methods of screening, what forms of treatment or prevention are most effective, quantification of the potential harms of treatment, what comorbidities change recommendations, or what costs are associated with different management strategies. Many of the guideline development groups use the PICO format for framing the questions, which includes the following parts:

- Patients: Which patients are being considered for the question, how can they be described, and are there any subgroups that require special consideration? (Similar to inclusion and exclusion criteria in a clinical study, however, usually not as restrictive.)
- Interventions: Which intervention or treatment should be considered?
- Comparison: What are the main alternatives that should be compared with the intervention?
- Outcome: What is most important to the patient (e.g., mortality, morbidity, treatment complications, rates of relapse, physical function, quality of life, and costs)?

Another format for question framework used by some groups is PECOT. The additional part added for this question format is Time, (i.e., over what timeframe are the benefits or the outcomes of care expected to occur?) In this format the **E** represents Exposure: which may be treatment, a risk factor, or management approach of interest.

The clinical questions should define the relevant patient population, the management strategies that will and will not be considered, and the outcomes of care that the guideline intends to achieve. In addition, the guideline development panel should describe the care setting for use of the guideline, for example, primary care, secondary care, or tertiary referral centers. All the questions that are necessary for consideration of patient management in a given clinical scenario are delineated to make sure that the recommendations provided by the guideline will be of sufficient scope to avoid important gaps in decision-making. There is no specific standard for the number of questions required for each guideline; however, most guideline development groups state that if the number exceeds 30, or in some cases 40 questions, it may be necessary to break the guideline into subtopics.

In some instances, a preliminary review of the literature may be necessary to assist with delineation of the focused clinical questions to be considered in the guideline. Clinical experts in the field as well as patients provide critical input in formulating the clinical questions. The SIGN places particular emphasis on obtaining input from patients. They obtain published studies, both qualitative and quantitative, that reflect patients' and caregivers' experiences and preferences in relation to the clinical topic. The program manager presents a summarized report of these findings to the panel at their first meeting to underline the significance of patient needs and preferences in the guideline development.

DETERMINE THE CRITERIA FOR EVIDENCE

It is necessary to define the admissible evidence, i.e., the types of published or unpublished research to be considered so that an appropriate literature search may be performed. Key words from the focused clinical questions define the types of patients, interventions, comparators, and outcomes of studies that are considered to provide useful evidence. The guideline panel may decide that it will consider evidence from previous guidelines, meta-analysis or systematic reviews, and randomized-controlled trials. The panel may also decide to consider evidence from observational studies, diagnostic studies, economic studies, and qualitative studies. This direction is necessary for the information specialists that will conduct the search for evidence. Detailed criteria are also important in this step so that evidence will be retrieved and selected for inclusion in the review with a minimum of bias, so that the search is reproducible, and so that the entire process is as transparent as possible. In most cases, more than one person is involved in searching for evidence and selecting evidence for consideration in the review. Clear criteria must be used so that there is consistency among all individuals involved in this process. Inconsistency in the retrieval of evidence between evaluators would add a significant potential for bias in the review.

The process to define admissible evidence may also be revisited at a later stage of guideline development depending on the results of the initial search. It is conceivable, and in fact not uncommon, that based on the initial review of evidence, the questions may be modified or new questions formed, and a decision may be made to expand the scope of admissible evidence. Documentation of these decisions, and the reasons for any changes, is another indicator of a guideline that has been developed with rigorous methods. The Cochrane

Collaboration recommends the following considerations when a change in the review questions or criteria for admissible evidence is made:

- What is the motivation for the refinement?
- Was it made after you had seen and been influenced by results from a particular study or was it simply that you had not initially considered alternate but acceptable ways of defining the participants, interventions, or outcomes of interest?
- Are your search strategies appropriate for the refined question (especially any that have already been undertaken)?
- Is your data collection tailored to the refined question?[48]

CONDUCT A SYSTEMATIC SEARCH FOR THE QUALIFYING EVIDENCE

Evidence-based guidelines require that all relevant evidence is located and appraised; therefore, a thorough literature search must be conducted. Many of the guideline development groups will first conduct a search to identify previously completed guidelines or systematic reviews of the same or closely related questions. The literature retrieval process should include a search of the available bibliographic resources such as MEDLINE®, Current Contents, EMBASE, Science Citation Index, Cochrane Library, and CINAHL. A number of specialized databases exist and should be considered depending on the subject of the search. Also evidence may be obtained from citations listed in published bibliographies, textbooks, and any literature that may be identified by researchers and other individuals on the "expert" list that the panel may create. Specific keywords and other search constraints, for example MeSH (**Me**dical **S**ubject **H**eadings from MEDLINE®) terms, limits by publication year, language, randomized-controlled trials or other study types, and so forth should be recorded to allow verification of the process. Each retrieved article should then be judged for its relevance and compliance to criteria for inclusion as predetermined by the panel. When possible, it is helpful to have more than one reviewer judge the inclusion of studies. A log should be kept of excluded studies and the rationale for their rejection. The Centre for Reviews and Dissemination (CRD) has created a flow diagram to illustrate steps involved in selecting studies for inclusion in a systematic review (see Appendix 9–4). The CRD has also identified key points for consideration in this process (see Appendix 9–5).

A review of all the details regarding search strategies, such as controlled vocabulary searching, textword searching, truncation of terms, use of the vocabulary tree structures to explode select terms, and adjacency of terms are beyond the scope of this chapter. Most guideline development groups use highly trained methodologists and librarians to perform this critical search for evidence. A carefully planned and executed search is necessary to obtain a result that is very sensitive to avoid missing important evidence and at the same time as specific as possible to avoid the requirement to manually screen many irrelevant citations. The Cochrane Collaboration has developed detailed search strategies and filters for use in conducting searches for literature.[48] The Cochrane Collaboration has also made specific recommendations for guideline developers for documentation of the search process, for example for the search or an electronic data set the following should be documented:

- Title of database searched (e.g., MEDLINE®).
- Name of the host (e.g., SilverPlatter version 2.0).
- Date search was run (month, day, year).
- Years covered by the search.
- Complete search strategy used, including all search terms (preferably electronically cut and pasted rather than retyped).
- One or two sentence summary of the search strategy indicating which lines of the search strategy were used to identify records related to the health condition and intervention, and which lines were used to identify studies of the appropriate design.
- The absence of any language restrictions.[48]

Other details that should be documented include search methods for obtaining conference proceedings, hand searching of selected resources, whether the guideline developers contacted other methodologists or researchers to ask for references or to obtain information about unpublished studies, whether contact is made with product manufacturers for additional data, and any other efforts made to obtain published or unpublished evidence.

PERFORM A SYSTEMATIC EVALUATION AND GRADING OF THE EVIDENCE

There are a variety of methods for evaluating individual studies, many of which are discussed in other sections of this text. The purpose of this process is to identify issues with the trial design or any biases that would affect internal or external validity. Issues to consider include the basic trial design (i.e., randomized controlled clinical trial, cohort study, and case-control study), sample size, statistical power, selection bias, inclusion/exclusion criteria, choice of control group, randomization methods, comparability of groups, definition of exposure or intervention, definition of outcome measures, accuracy and appropriateness of outcome measures, attrition rates, data collection methods, methods of statistical analysis, confounding variables, unique characteristics of the study population, and adequacy of blinding. Formal methods may also be used to assign a quality score to each trial. Other factors are considered in the overall body of evidence, for example, are the results of different trials consistent with each other or is there significant heterogeneity. The amount of evidence is also an important consideration—how many individuals have been evaluated over what length of time. The amount of available evidence is particularly important in consideration of the safety of treatments. Potentially serious adverse events that occur infrequently will not be identified in a database that does not contain a sufficient sample size or in a sample population that is too narrowly defined.

Many additional issues of evaluation of evidence are provided in other chapters in this text and will not be repeated here. There are other resources available to provide assistance with methods for this critical process. Each of the guideline development manuals that have been described in this chapter include significant sections on evaluation of the evidence.[1,41-43] *The Reviewers' Handbook from the Cochrane Collaboration*[48] (available to download at <<http://www.cochrane.org/resources/handbook/hbook.htm>>), and the Centre for *Reviews and Dissemination Guidance for those Carrying Out or Commissioning Reviews*, are particularly useful for this purpose.[49] In addition, the AHRQ commissioned the Research Triangle Institute—University of North Carolina Evidenced-Based Practice Center to "prepare a report on methods or systems to assess health care research results, particularly methods or systems to rate the strength of the scientific evidence underlying health care practice, recommendations in the research literature, and technology assessments."[63] The overarching goals of this project were to "describe systems to rate the strength of scientific evidence, including evaluating the quality of individual articles that make up a body of evidence on a specific scientific question in health care, and to provide some guidance as to 'best practices' in this field today." This report can be obtained at <<http://www.ahrq.gov/clinic/ evrptfiles. htm#strength>> for a downloadable zip file, or <<http://www.ncbi.nlm.nih.gov/ books/bv. fcgi?rid=hstat1.chapter.70996>> for online access via the Health Services Technology/ Assessment Texts (HSTAT). HSTAT is a free, Web based resource of full text documents that provide health information and support health care decision-making.

Evaluation of the evidence, and grading of the recommendations, are critical aspects for users of guidelines to understand in order to appropriately interpret the recommendations. Because these aspects are critical to users of guidelines, a separate expanded section on the topic of Interpretation of Guideline Recommendations is provided in another section of this chapter.

PREPARE A SYNTHESIS OF THE EVIDENCE

The evidence from the selected studies should be summarized in a format that facilitates consideration of the characteristics and quality of individual studies, the consistency of the results between studies, the overall size of the evidence database, and the size of the treatment effects for benefits and harms. These key concepts for consideration in synthesis of evidence have been described by the CRD (see Appendix 9–6) The NICE has a standard format that they recommend for evidence tables (see Appendix 9–7). Most guideline development groups use a similar format. If the necessary evidence is available, it may be appropriate to perform a meta-analysis to present the summary estimate of the size of a treatment effect. Readers interested in a detailed description of meta-analysis may wish to consult the *Cochrane Handbook for Systematic Reviews of Interventions*.[48] Formal methods for grading the quality of the evidence should be used as described above. The level of evidence assigned to each study is included in the evidence table. A detailed description of a consensus recommendation for methods to grade the quality of evidence and strength of guideline recommendations is provided in the section on Interpretation of Guideline Recommendations in this chapter.

The SIGN group and the NZGG use a form to document how the evidence synthesis was used to reach guideline recommendations. This process is called considered judgment. See Appendix 9–8 for a representation of the considered judgment form.

Methods for incorporation of economic evidence in practice guidelines are not well developed. In some instances, the ability to employ economic evaluations from one setting to another is very limited. The SIGN stated in their March 2004 guideline developers' handbook that none of the approaches to incorporation of resource use were regarded as sufficiently well proven or appropriate for SIGN methodology.[43] The SIGN does, however, include published economic studies in evidence tables, and uses a structured method to evaluate this evidence. They also have a form similar to the considered judgment form mentioned above that can be used to present information relating to economic issues associated with guideline implementation. In addition, they may include a commentary on economic issues in the published guideline.

The NICE includes a six-page chapter on incorporating health economics in their guidelines development manual.[41] The NICE utilizes a health economist as a core member of their guideline development team. They use the process of cost-effectiveness analysis to maximize the health gain by incorporating both costs and health benefits in the analysis. NICE may utilize published economic evidence, or may carry out or commission a cost-effectiveness or cost-utility analysis (see Chap. 8 for further information on these analyses). Formal quality appraisal and synthesis of the economic evidence is also performed, just as it is with epidemiologic or clinical study data, using study-type specific checklists. In regard to economic analysis, NICE employs the following general principles:

- An economic analysis should be underpinned by the best-quality clinical evidence.
- There should be the highest level of transparency in the reporting of methods.
- Uncertainty (around both internal and external validity) should be discussed fully and explored by sensitivity analysis (and, where data allow, statistical analysis).
- Limitations of the approach and methods taken should be fully discussed.
- Conventions on reporting economic evaluations should be followed (see Drummond and Jefferson, 1996).*
- Analysis should be carried out in collaboration between the health economist and the rest of the guideline development group.[41]

Users of practice guidelines should examine the document for inclusion of economic information. The primary concern should be to identify the methods used for obtaining and

---

* Drummond MF, Jefferson TO. Guidelines for authors and peer reviewers of economic submissions to the BMJ. BMJ. 1996;313:275–83.

evaluating the economic information, and in what way, if any, the economic information was used in formulating recommendations for patient care.

AGREE ON PROCEDURES FOR A CONSENSUS PROCESS, OR OTHER PROCEDURES FOR MAKING RECOMMENDATIONS, IN THE ABSENCE OF HIGHER LEVELS OF EVIDENCE FOR DECISION-MAKING

In the absence of high levels of evidence, some guideline development groups will elect to state that the evidence for making a recommendation is inconclusive and will simply provide a summary of that evidence with no specific recommendation. Other guideline groups will consider a variety of consensus methods to derive a recommendation. There is no one method for consensus that is considered the standard for this process. For more information about consensus methods the reader may wish to review the material in the referenced guideline development guides,[41-43] or the NIH Consensus Development Program website at <<http://consensus.nih.gov>>.

The key aspect for users of a guideline is to note the description of consensus methods, and to be certain to distinguish guideline recommendations that are made on the basis of high levels of evidence as opposed to those based on consensus only. A variety of designations are used by different guideline development groups to make this distinction. See Appendix 9–9 for a table from the Ontario Guidelines Advisory Committee (GAC) which shows a variety of designations used by nine guideline development groups (<<http://gacguidelines.ca/pdfs/LevelsOfEvidenceChart.pdf>>). Guideline recommendations which are based on consensus opinion are generally considered the least reliable recommendations. They are suggestions for consideration and not standards for care.

FORMULATE AND GRADE RECOMMENDATIONS BASED ON THE GRADE OF EVIDENCE AND BALANCE OF BENEFITS, HARMS, AND COSTS OF TREATMENT OPTIONS

The details of this process are provided below in the section titled Interpretation of Guideline Recommendations. The specific recommendations in a guideline must be worded carefully, and must clearly communicate the confidence that the guideline panel has that the expected outcomes will be achieved if the recommendations are followed. Because many guideline users do not read the full guideline document, the recommendations should be written to stand alone as much as possible. NICE provides the following guidance regarding the wording of the recommendations (with slight modifications):

- Recommendations should stand alone.
- Recommendations should be action oriented.
- All recommendations should be assigned a grade (though these are not shown for the key priorities).

- Recommendations referring to drug use should use the generic drug name, avoid stating dosages, and indicate where the recommendation refers to off-label use.
- Tables can be used to present recommendations but only where this substantially improves clarity.
- Recommendations should take the patient into consideration and should try to avoid the use of words such as "subjects" rather than "people" or "patients."[41]

DRAFT THE GUIDELINE DOCUMENT

The basis of the draft document is provided by the evidence tables and the graded recommendations. A formal narrative summary should also be provided with all relevant details of decisions made in the development of the guideline. It is highly desirable for the finished guideline to include details of the scope of the guideline including target patient population, restrictions on the population, interventions considered, specific outcomes or performance measures, who are the intended users of the guideline (e.g., specialty and care setting), and the overall objective of the guideline. A clear description of authorship, sponsorship, and any potential conflicts of interest should be provided. A detailed description of all production methods used (as detailed in this chapter), decision-making methods, recommendations for consideration in applying the guideline in practice (e.g., patient variables, setting, provider, and estimates of how the effects of these factors will alter outcomes are helpful for users to apply the guidelines locally), comments about ongoing studies which may affect recommendations, and any plans for updating the guideline. A detailed structure for a guideline as recommended by NICE is provided in Appendix 9–10.

Considering publication length limitations, some guideline producers are using Internet websites to provide some of the details recommended for finished guidelines. For example, the AHA/ACC Evidence-Based Guidelines for Cardiovascular Disease Prevention in Women uses the following website to provide access to the evidence tables <<http://www.acc.org/clinical/consensus/CVD_women/index.htm>>.

It is also desirable for a guideline to be written in different formats and levels of detail for different audiences and purposes. Many guideline developers produce quick reference guides, which give the essentials of the recommendations without the detailed background. These documents are more convenient to use as quick reminders and decision aids in a patient care setting than a full guideline document. It is important however for users of the quick reference guides to review the full document before deciding that the guideline is one that is valid for their use, and to recognize any specific limitations in how they may wish to use that particular guideline. Another format that is useful is a guideline summary that may be used for a patient education purposes. As an example of the different formats, the Seventh Report of the Joint National Committee on Prevention, Detection, Evaluation, and Treatment of High Blood Pressure (JNC VII) was produced with a quick reference card (available at

<<http://www.nhlbi.nih.gov/guidelines/hypertension/jnc7card.htm>>). There are also two different versions of the guideline document: an express version[64] and the complete version.[27] These two versions of the guideline, as well as patient education materials, media and press materials, and files for use on a PDA, are also available for download at the NHLBI website <<http://www.nhlbi.nih.gov/guidelines/hypertension/index.htm>>.

In the system used by the former AHCPR, panel members were asked to provide review comments on the report to address flaws in the literature review process, specific studies or data that were overlooked, errors in interpretation of studies, errors in the assessment of individual decision points, or errors in the overall assessment of benefits and harms. Panel members may also be asked to comment on the need to reconsider any of the questions that the guideline is intended to address or whether any time-consuming, optional techniques not done need to be performed (e.g., meta-analysis, decision analysis, or focus groups) to make decisions, or to assess patient preference or values for certain procedures or outcomes. Very careful consideration is given to the wording of each recommendation and to obtaining agreement among panel members.

In preparation of the Seventh ACCP Conference on Antithrombotic and Thrombolytic Therapy, four editors (two methodologists and two content experts) worked with several authors for each chapter.[38] A number of drafts were prepared for each chapter with revisions recommended by each of the authors using a website to post recommendations to each other. At the conference, authors worked together to "finalize and harmonize" potentially controversial recommendations. Plenary meetings were also held to obtain feedback from other chapter authors for consideration of the guideline recommendations. "Authors continued this process after the conference until they reached agreement within their groups and with other group authors who provided critical feedback."[38]

Reaching clear decisions on recommendations for clinical practices is often difficult because the data are not adequate to clearly label the practice appropriate or inappropriate. Unfortunately, many practices fall into this gray zone category because of uncertainties about the benefits and harms, variability in patients and in their responses to treatment, and differences in patient preferences about the desirability of outcomes and aversion to risk. The use of rigid language in an effort to produce clear-cut recommendations can be dangerous, particularly when presented as simplistic algorithms that fail to recognize the complexity of medical decision-making and the need for individual clinical judgment. This danger can be avoided by describing uncertainty and providing broad boundaries for appropriate practice that allows for legitimate differences of opinion. Attempts to develop rigid guidelines when the data are not conclusive is clearly worse than having no written guidelines.

It is important to consider the information needs of the guideline's user. Practitioners will want specific, quantitative estimates of the relevant health outcomes if a recommendation is followed, a statement of the strength of the evidence and expert judgment supporting the guidelines, information on patient preferences, projections of cost, details of the reasoning behind the recommendations, and the ability to review the data independently if they so choose. Guidelines should be written such that they may be perceived as an explanation of the thinking process that is used in evaluating and applying the information. If guidelines are perceived as information only, they may be rejected as the "cookbooks" that practitioners fear guidelines will become. Such guidelines would also not achieve the educational goals to focus further research efforts (outcomes research or other) on gaps in the current evidence. The Manual for ACC/AHA Guideline Writing Committees Methodologies and Policies from the ACC/AHA Task Force on Practice Guidelines (<<http://www.acc.org/clinical/manual/ manual_index.htm>>) includes the following checklist for guideline authors to review the draft recommendations:

- Are the recommendations within the stated purpose and scope of the guideline?
- Are all recommendations cited and referenced (either in the text or in the evidence table)?
- Are all recommendations assigned a Classification of Recommendation and a Level of Evidence?
- Are clinically important and feasible recommendations made?
- Are areas of uncertainty and exceptions to the rule clearly identified?
- Are evidence tables and appropriate text provided to support recommendations, where applicable?
- Are recommendations and key clinical points displayed visually, when possible?[36]

Depending on the subject of the clinical practice guideline, more or less emphasis may be placed on the various sections of the guideline document. In addition, recommendations for future research may be included with the document. The process of developing practice guidelines often calls attention to the gaps in scientific information. The direction provided for future research is one of the important results of the practice guideline development process. Practice guidelines that fail to address research priorities may discourage innovation and negatively influence funding decisions for needed research in the involved area. For the few examples that exist in which clear answers are already provided by high-quality scientific evidence, waste of research resources may be avoided by stopping generation of data that would not increase understanding of a disease process or its treatment.

CONDUCT PEER-REVIEW AND PILOT TESTING OF THE GUIDELINE

Each guideline development group has its own methods for obtaining peer-review and feedback on the draft guidelines. In some cases, the peer-review is confined within that organization, in other groups specific requests will be made for review from targeted organizations, and in some guideline development groups open input from any interested party is sought by public notice. For example, SIGN holds a national open meeting which is widely publicized. This meeting is usually attended by 150 to 300 health care professionals and others interested in the guideline topic. The draft guideline is also available on the SIGN website for a limited time period to permit contributions to be submitted. Participation in the draft of the guideline can give a sense of ownership to the broader audience and may be a positive factor in the implementation of the guideline. SIGN also utilizes independent expert referees who are asked to comment on specific aspects of the guideline. In addition, they send the guideline for review by a non-health-care professional to get comments from the patients' perspective. See Appendix 9–11 for a figure representing the consultation and peer-review steps used by SIGN.

The next step may be pretesting the guideline in practice settings. The pretesting panel should be given clear instructions on the observations that would be considered most useful and be asked to keep written notes of their experiences, observations, and suggestions. A summary report of these observations is provided to the development panel. In the final revision steps, the panel should examine all review comments and pretesting results in an unbiased fashion. A disposition record that documents how each recommendation was handled and the rationale for inclusion or exclusion in the final document should be kept. However, not all groups conduct pilot testing. For example, SIGN considers that pilot testing is more appropriate at a local level and leaves this to be done by local groups as part of their implementation process.

The guideline development process may be viewed in the philosophy of CQI from several aspects. The methodology emphasizes building quality in the production process, use of scientific principles and data, and plans to conduct follow-up studies on the outcomes of the use of the guideline, which are then used to update and improve the guideline.

REVISE THE GUIDELINE AS APPROPRIATE

Based on feedback from the peer-review process and any pilot testing of the application of the guideline, revisions may be required for the guideline to meet its intended goals. As with many steps in the guideline development process, one of the keys in this step is documentation. The decisions and actions taken in response to the recommendations from external review should be carefully documented. It is particularly important if there are critical recommendations that the guideline panel decides to reject that the reason for that decision is documented.

CREATE TOOLS FOR IMPLEMENTATION OF THE GUIDELINE

It is helpful if the guideline developers create tools that will assist target groups in the implementation step. A variety of tools may be used including preparing various formats of the guideline for convenient use in the practice setting, creating guidelines that facilitate automated implementation, algorithms or flow charts that facilitate understanding of the use of the guideline, or educational programs. Much of the activities that the guideline development committee has performed in creating the guideline, careful wording of the recommendations, and the documentation of all procedures, is done with the end in mind, i.e., implementation. One of the simplest forms of implementation is to make the guideline accessible as freely and as widely as possible. Many of the guideline development groups make the guidelines available as electronic documents and post them for free access on a website.

ESTABLISH A PLAN FOR FOLLOW-UP AND PERIODIC UPDATING OF THE GUIDELINE

In most cases the guideline development group will determine a review interval for consideration to update the guideline. Depending on the topic and knowledge of ongoing studies, it may be reasonable to review the guideline after a period of between 2 and 5 years. However, if it is a topic in which rapid change may occur, more frequent review is necessary. In some instances, the guideline development group will designate a subgroup to monitor the literature and alert the entire group if new evidence becomes available that might necessitate revisions of the guideline recommendations. When it is time to consider updating a guideline, the careful records kept during the production of the previous edition are invaluable.

Interpretation of Guideline Recommendations

As mentioned previously, proper evaluation of a guideline and interpretation of the recommendations requires knowledge of methods for development. Interpretation of the recommendations in a guideline requires detailed understanding of the methods used for grading the quality of the evidence, the balance between the benefits and harms, and the strength of the recommendation. This can be difficult because a variety of grading systems are currently in use by different organizations producing guidelines which creates confusion. If the grading system for the recommendations in a practice guideline are not interpreted correctly, a significant amount of information is lost. In addition, if guideline developers use methods that do not account for all the important decision-making factors, the recommendations cannot be presented with the necessary details. The Grades of Recommendation Assessment Development and Evaluation (GRADE) working group has provided a proposal to standardize the grading methods for the quality of the evidence and the strength of recommendations in practice guidelines.[65] The working group believes that consistent judgments about the quality of evidence and strength of recommendations, combined with better communication about those judgments will be achieved by use of the GRADE system. Ultimately, it is believed that this will support better informed choices in health care.[65]

The quality of the evidence that forms the basis for recommendations is a key aspect for interpretation and use of a practice guideline. However, before deciding to implement a guideline recommendation it is also necessary for the user to have information for consideration of the balance between benefits and harms, and the ability to translate the evidence to specific circumstances (i.e., external validity). A system to communicate the strength of a recommendation should consider all of these factors. The designated strength of a recommendation should convey the amount of confidence one can have that adherence to that recommendation will do more good than harm.[65]

Substantial inconsistencies exist in the systems used by different guideline development groups to rate the quality or strength of evidence, and how that information is communicated within the guideline. Different systems may designate the same evidence and recommendation as II-a, B, C+, 1, Level III, or 2++ (see Appendix 9–9 for a comparison of the levels of evidence and grades of recommendation assembled by the Ontario GAC). Since most health care professionals will encounter guidelines from many different groups, these various grading systems are confusing and reduce their effectiveness in communicating the amount of confidence one should have in a given recommendation.[65]

The GRADE working group began as an informal collaboration of people who recognized the shortcomings of the present grading systems and wished to offer recommendations for improvement.[65] The GRADE working group has conducted an analysis of six prominent grading systems that are used by ACCP, Australian National Health and Medical Research Council (ANHMRC), Oxford Centre for Evidence-based Medicine (OCEBM), SIGN, USPSTF, and U.S. Task Force on Community Preventive Services (USTFCPS).[66] Based on this evaluation, there was general agreement that none of these six systems addressed all of the important concepts and dimensions considered necessary for guideline recommendations. See Appendix 9–12 for a description of the GRADE working group's comparison of the proposed system to the other systems evaluated, including comments about the advantages of the GRADE system.

The system proposed by GRADE starts with explicit definitions of what is meant by quality of evidence and strength of recommendation. "Quality of evidence indicates the extent to which one can be confident that an estimate of effect is correct. The strength of a recommendation indicates the extent to which one can be confident that adherence to the recommendation will do more good than harm."[65] Using the GRADE system requires sequential judgments about the following:

- The validity of the results of individual studies for "important" outcomes.
- The quality of evidence across studies for each important outcome.
- Which outcomes are "critical" to a decision.
- The overall quality of evidence across these "critical" outcomes.
- The balance between benefits and harms.
- The strength of recommendations.[65]

The GRADE system starts with clearly defined clinical questions and considers all outcomes that are important to patients. Each outcome is rated on a scale from low to high importance for a treatment decision as not critical, important, or critical. Critical outcomes are given more weight in the final recommendation than outcomes that are considered important. Outcomes that are considered not critical get little consideration.[65]

The quality of evidence for each outcome should be made on the basis of a systematic review using explicit criteria. The GRADE system recommends four key elements for consideration: (1) study design, (2) quality of study methods and execution, (3) consistency of results across studies, and (4) the directness of application of the results to the patients, interventions, and outcomes of interest. In terms of study design, randomized controlled trials have been considered to provide the highest level of evidence since the first efforts at grading evidence in health care were made by the Canadian Task Force on the Periodic Health Examination.[28] Over the years since that first hierarchy for evidence was described, there have been some refinements in designation of the quality of evidence. Basic study design does not tell the whole story of the quality of evidence. Randomization, when it is used correctly, has tremendous power to reduce the potential bias in the results. However, there are randomized controlled trials in which other aspects of the study design are seriously flawed, and there are observational studies (e.g., follow-up, case-control, interrupted time series, and controlled before and after) with very strong methods that may produce high quality evidence. Consideration of the quality of study methods must include criteria such as adequacy of allocation concealment, blinding, and follow up. The consistency of results between different studies can also add to the confidence that the results are valid. The "directness" of the results refers to the extent to which the subjects, interventions, and outcomes of a study are similar to the ones of interest for a given treatment recommendation. If study subjects differ from your patients in ways that may predict a different level of response based on factors such as age, gender, race, other comorbidities or severity of illness, the quality of evidence for your decision-making is not as great. In addition, studies using surrogate treatment outcomes, or intermediate outcomes, are not as reliable for estimation of ultimate treatment benefits. Surrogate outcomes include measurements like changes in bone mineral density rather than incidence of fractures, effects of a medication on the electrocardiogram (ECG) rather than mortality, changes in lipids rather than incidence of coronary artery disease events or mortality. Another example in which indirect evidence must be used is when there are no studies comparing different interventions directly and the evaluation must be made across different studies. This is a common problem with new drugs that have been studied only in comparison to placebo and not to other effective treatments. With this type of evidence comparison, it is difficult to determine which treatment is more effective, and it is even more difficult to estimate the size of a potential treatment difference.[65]

Based on consideration of the four components described above, the Appraisal of Guide-lines for Research & Evaluation (AGREE) system arrives at a grade of evidence in one of the following categories:

- High: Further research is very unlikely to change our confidence in the estimate of effect.
- Moderate: Further research is likely to have an important impact on our confidence in the estimate of effect and may change the estimate.
- Low: Further research is very likely to have an important impact on our confidence in the estimate of effect and is likely to change the estimate.
- Very low: Any estimate of effect is very uncertain.[65]

Beginning with basic study design, a randomized trial would start with a grade of high, a quasi-randomized trial would start as moderate, an observational study would be low, and any other form of evidence would be graded very low. From that starting level, the grade of evidence could be decreased based on the other components as follows: serious limitations to study quality (subtract one level), very serious limitations to study quality (subtract two levels), important inconsistency between results of different studies (subtract one level), some uncertainty about directness of the evidence (subtract one level), major uncertainty about directness of the evidence (subtract two levels), imprecise or sparse data (subtract one level), and high probability of reporting bias (subtract one level).[65] The working group sug-gested that data be considered sparse if "the results include just a few events or observations and they are uninformative." In the GRADE system, the data are considered imprecise "if the confidence intervals are so wide that an estimate is consistent with either important harms or important benefits." Reporting bias (also referred to as publication bias) is a common con-cern in a systematic review as it is well known that small negative trials are less likely to be published than positive trials. This results in a bias in favor of an intervention on the basis of just the evidence that has been reported. Factors that can result in an increase in the grade of the evidence are "a strong measure of association, i.e., a significant relative risk of >2 or <0.5, based on consistent evidence from two or more observational studies with no plausible confounders (add one level); very strong evidence of association, i.e., a significant relative risk of >5 or <0.2, based on direct evidence with no major threats to validity (add two levels); evidence of a dose response relationship (add one level); all plausible confounders would have reduced the size of the effect (add one level)."[65] All of these adjustments are cumulative, so that if more than one modifier exists for the quality of evidence, each modifier is applied.

The evidence for harms should be graded using the same system as the evidence for bene-fits. This creates somewhat of a challenge when making judgments about the balance of benefits and harms because the quality of evidence for harms is rarely on the same level as the evidence for benefits. One only has to look at the evidence for harms for rofecoxib (Viox®) to note that obtaining high-quality evidence about harm is a more difficult process. The magnitude of the balance of the benefits compared to the harms, as well as value judgments of the desirability of the benefits and harms, must also be considered for treatment recommendations. In addition, information should be provided to demonstrate how the evidence translates into specific circumstances, and what adjustments may be necessary for individuals with different baseline risks, or who are receiving treatment in different settings. The GRADE working group recommends the following definitions to categorize the trade off between benefits and harms:

- Net benefits: The intervention clearly does more good than harm.
- Trade-offs: There are important trade-offs between the benefits and harms.
- Uncertain trade-offs: It is not clear whether the intervention does more good than harm.
- No net benefits: The intervention clearly does not do more good than harm.[65]

Factors that should be considering in arriving at one of these designations include the estimated size and confidence intervals of the effect for the main outcomes, the quality of the evidence, ability to extrapolate the evidence to different patients or care settings, and uncertainty of the baseline risk of disease events in the population of interest.

Finally, the GRADE system assigns one of the following categories for a recommendation for an intervention:

- Do it (90 to 100% of people are likely to do it).
- Probably do it (60 to 90% of people are likely to do it).
- Maybe do it (40 to 60% of people are likely to do it).
- Probably do not do it (10 to 40% of people are likely to do it).
- Do not do it (0 to 10% of people are likely to do it).[65]

High grades of evidence, combined with net benefits and strong measures of association, would produce a recommendation of do it. High grades of evidence for no net benefits or possibly net harm would produce a recommendation of do not do it. Different grades of evidence and different categorization for the trade off of benefits and harms will produce recommendations between these extremes. For the intermediate strength of recommendation, individual patient values, different patient risk factors or circumstances, or different care settings will assume a more prominent role in the decision-making by the patient and the health care practitioner. The advantage of the GRADE system is that all of the evidence that is most important for making the decision has been judged with explicit criteria, the judgments are made transparent, evidence summary tables and balance sheets have been created, consequently facilitating the use of best evidence.

Although the system recommended by the GRADE working group may appear complex with the number of steps involved, it provides a balance of the need for simplicity with a need for full explicit consideration of important issues in clinical decision-making, as well as transparency for the judgments made in arriving at recommendations. A pilot study on the use of this system identified some issues that warrant further improvements in the system, but on balance it was considered to be clear, understandable, sensible, and met the criteria for providing the communication necessary for guideline recommendations.[67]

Examples of evidence profiles using the GRADE system and additional information about the GRADE working group are available on their website <<http://www.gradeworkinggroup. org/>>.

The majority of published guidelines do not currently use the GRADE system for recommendations. Therefore for each guideline that is used, the practitioner must carefully read the description of the grading scheme used by that particular guideline so that they will correctly interpret the strength of the recommendations, the quality of the evidence, and the balance between benefits and harms of the interventions considered.

Guideline Evaluation Tools

Prior to selecting a clinical practice guideline for implementation in a health care system, or for personal use by a health care professional, it is important that the quality of published guidelines be evaluated. Perhaps the most useful tool available for evaluation of a practice guideline is the one created by the AGREE collaboration. The purpose of AGREE is to improve the quality and effectiveness of clinical practice guidelines by establishing a shared framework for their development, reporting and assessment.[68] The AGREE collaboration involves an international group of researchers and policy makers from 13 countries. This collaboration has produced a structured instrument which can be used for critical appraisal of clinical practice guidelines. The AGREE instrument is designed to assess the methodology used for guideline development and how completely and clearly the process is reported.[68] For groups or individuals who wish to perform an assessment of a guideline, the AGREE instrument provides a tool that is structured, reliable, and reasonable to use.

In development of the AGREE instrument, quality was defined as "the confidence that the biases linked to the rigor of development, presentation, and applicability of a clinical practice guideline have been minimized and that each step of the development process is clearly reported."[68] It should be noted, the AGREE instrument does not assess clinical content, or the quality of evidence, it assesses the quality of the process of guideline development methods and the reporting quality. Individual items for consideration in developing the instrument were grouped into the following five quality domains: (1) scope and purpose, (2) stakeholder involvement, (3) rigor of development, (4) clarity and presentation, and (5) applicability. An initial set of 82 items was generated from previously validated appraisal instruments and other published literature. Based on coverage, overlap, and content validity, a working group within the collaboration reduced the list to 34 items. Further refinements were made after these items and a user's guide were pretested on two Dutch and two English guidelines. The AGREE partners and 15 international experts were then asked to comment on the clarity, comprehensiveness, relevance, and ease of use of the draft items and user's guide. In addition, each of the AGREE partners were asked to apply the instrument to two more guidelines. Following removal of overlapping items and revision of ambiguous items, there were 24 remaining items grouped into the five quality domains mentioned above. As part of the user's guide, a four-point scale was to be used to score each item: 1—strongly disagree; 2—disagree; 3—agree; and 4—strongly agree. An overall recommendation on whether the guideline should be used was also evaluated using the following three-point scale: 1—not recommended; 2—recommended with provisos or modifications; 3—strongly recommended.[68]

During development, the AGREE instrument was field tested twice; first by 194 appraisers using a structured protocol on a sample of 100 guidelines from 11 countries. At an AGREE workshop in spring 2000, the instrument was revised in response to the first field test. The second field test was based on a random sample of three guidelines per country (33 total) from the original 100 guidelines. In the second field test, 74 newly recruited appraisers used the instrument. Following field testing, a sixth quality domain was added to the instrument; editorial independence. The final form of the AGREE instrument includes 23 items grouped into six quality domains (see Appendix 9–13). A copy of the AGREE instrument, instructions for use, a training manual, and other details are available from the website <<http://www.agreecollaboration.org>>. Guideline users may benefit from using this instrument to evaluate the quality of guidelines before choosing to adopt them.

Although the AGREE instrument was developed with the primary intent of providing a tool for evaluation of a guideline by users, guideline developers may also use the AGREE instrument to ensure that the methods used to develop a guideline and the documentation provided with the guideline will meet minimum standards. In addition, if AGREE is adapted by editors of peer-reviewed journals it should provide a framework to improve the quality of reporting of published guidelines. This intent is similar to the Consolidated Standards of Reporting Trials (CONSORT) statement, which is well established for the reporting of randomized-controlled trials.[69] The full text of the article describing revisions to the CONSORT statement, a detailed explanation of the statement, the CONSORT checklist, flow diagram, and a glossary are available at the website <<http://www.consort-statement.org>>. The quality of reporting of randomized trials has been proven to increase with use of the CONSORT statement.[70]

Another collaborative effort to improve guideline quality and reporting standards is the Conference on Guideline Standardization (COGS). The purpose of COGS is to "define a standard for guideline reporting that will promote guideline quality and facilitate implementation."[71] Problems arise in guideline implementation if the guideline is developed with inadequate methods, or if there is inadequate documentation of the methods used. It is the intent of COGS to improve the quality of guideline development methods, and the quality of reporting as well. The COGS panel developed a checklist to be used prospectively by guideline developers to improve documentation.[71] As opposed to the AGREE instrument, the COGS checklist is intended more for use by guideline developers or publication editors, but it is still a useful checklist for practitioners when considering quality issues of a published guideline.

The COGS panel included representatives from medical specialty societies, government agencies, private groups that develop guidelines, journal editors, the National Guideline Clearinghouse (NGC), managed care representatives, informatics experts, and academicians. With this broad representation, the panel included input from the perspectives involved in guideline development, dissemination, and implementation. Items considered for inclusion on the checklist were rated for their importance for establishing validity and practical application of the guideline. Using a formal consensus process in the development of the checklist, 44 items were considered necessary for reporting in a guideline; 36 items were considered necessary for establishing guideline validity, 24 items were considered necessary for practical implementation, and some were considered necessary for both. After consolidating closely related items, the checklist contained 18 topics. The titles for these topics are overview of material, focus, goal, users/setting, target population, developer, funding source/sponsor, evidence collection, recommendation grading criteria, method for synthesizing evidence, prerelease review, update plan, definitions, recommendations and rationale, potential benefits and harms, patient preferences, algorithm, and implementation considerations.[71] For a more detailed description of each of these topics, please see Appendix 9–14.

Twenty-two organizations that produce guidelines were sent the COGS checklist to survey their opinions. Sixteen of the organizations (73%) responded that the checklist would be helpful for creating more comprehensive guidelines; 19 (86%) responded that documenting the items on the checklist would fit within their guideline development methods; 15 (68%) stated that they would use the proposed checklist, and 4 indicated that they might use it. One comment from organizations that expressed possible reluctance to using the checklist was regarding the need to produce guidelines that are succinct and brief in order to increase health professional acceptance. Guidelines that are brief may conflict with the need for comprehensiveness required by the checklist.[71]

Authors of the COGS checklist have also commented that it can have impact similar to the CONSORT statement as mentioned above for the AGREE instrument. The COGS checklist authors caution that, although this checklist can help improve guideline development, documentation, and reporting, it should not be used alone to judge the quality or adequacy of a guideline. Updates for the COGS checklist are planned to be published on their website at <<http://ycmi.med.yale.edu:8080/cogs/>>.

Implementation of Clinical Practice Guidelines

David Eddy stated in a lecture to the IOM "All the science in the world has no effect until it is implemented properly, and measuring performance is one of the most powerful tools for implementation."[72]

The most effective methods for implementing guidelines to achieve the desired effects of improved quality of care have not been determined. Institutional, organizational, local practice, political characteristics, and even individual practitioner characteristics should be considered when planning an implementation strategy for a practice guideline. It was previously believed that implementation strategies using multiple methods would be the most likely to succeed. In a systematic review of the adoption of clinical practice guidelines, variables that affected the success of implementation included qualities specific to the guidelines, characteristics of the health professional, characteristics of the practice setting, incentives, regulation, and patient factors.[73] The implementation methods shown to be weak were traditional CME and mailings. Audit and feedback was moderately effective, especially if it was concurrent, targeted to specific providers, and delivered by peers or opinion leaders. Strong methods were reminder systems, academic detailing, and the use of multiple intervention systems.[73]

However, the most current and extensive review of guideline dissemination and implementation strategies does not support the conclusion that multiple intervention methods are more effective.[59] Grimshaw and colleagues conducted a systematic review of 235 studies that reported 309 comparisons of strategies for guideline dissemination and implementation.[59] Overall, multifaceted interventions were involved in 73% of the comparisons. Eighty-four of the 309 comparisons (27%) were performed on a single intervention compared to no intervention or usual care. One hundred thirty-six (44%) of the comparisons were of multifaceted interventions compared to no intervention or a usual care group. Multifaceted interventions were compared to a control intervention, which was either a single intervention or an alternative multifaceted intervention, for 85 (27%) of the comparisons in the identified studies. Of the single interventions compared to no intervention, the most common strategies used and the percentage of all comparisons in the systematic review were reminders (13%), educational materials (6%), audit and feedback (4%), and patient-directed interventions (3%). The most frequent strategies used in multifaceted interventions and corresponding percentage of all comparisons were educational materials (48%), educational meetings (41%), reminders (31%), audit and feedback (24%), and patient-directed interventions (18%). For a more detailed description of these implementation strategies please see Appendix 9–15.[59]

The effect size of the interventions were described in one of four categories on the basis of the absolute difference in the post-intervention measures, which were generally process measures of care. The four categories of effect size were: small—an effect size

≤5%; modest—an effect size >5% and ≤10%; moderate—an effect size >10% and ≤20%; and large—an effect size >20%. Examples of the process measure of care included the frequency of prescribing a specific therapy, providing patient education, or test ordering that was in accordance with the guideline. Overall, 86% of interventions tested achieved positive improvements in process of care measures. There was considerable variation in the effect size of the interventions in different studies and in some studies between different interventions. The majority of interventions produced modest to moderate improvements in care. The lack of consistency of the differences between and within interventions did not permit any conclusion regarding the most effective strategy for guideline implementation. Multifaceted interventions were not found to be consistently more effective than single intervention strategies, and the number of components in the multifaceted interventions did not appear to be associated with effect size. The authors of this systematic review also noted that the overall quality of the methodology and reporting of the included studies were poor.[59]

This systematic review provides the best evidence available, and concludes that further research is required to develop and validate systems for estimation of the efficacy and efficiency of different strategies to implement patient, health professional, and organizational behavior change. Decision-makers will have to evaluate the choice for implementation strategies carefully. Local factors, potential facilitators and barriers to implementation are recommended for prominent consideration in this decision.[59]

The report of the systematic review by Grimshaw and colleagues is available at The National Coordinating Centre for Health Technology Assessment (NCCHTA) website at <<http://www.ncchta.org/fullmono/mon806.pdf>>. The NCCHTA Programme is part of the United Kingdom National Health Service. Individuals involved in planning an implementation strategy for a practice guideline would benefit from review of this report.

As noted above, barriers to guideline implementation should be considered when making plans for this effort. Cabana and colleagues conducted a systematic review of the literature regarding barriers to physician adherence to clinical practice guidelines.[74] For this review the authors conducted a search for articles published between January 1966 and January 1998 that focused on clinical practice guidelines, practice parameters, clinical policies, national recommendations or consensus statements, and that examined at least one barrier to adherence. A barrier was defined as any factor that limits or restricts complete physician adherence to a guideline. The full text of 423 articles was examined and 76 met the criteria for inclusion in the review. After classifying possible barriers into common themes, the authors identified seven general categories of barriers. Table 9–1 lists the seven categories of barriers and provides examples or a description of each barrier. The relative importance of different barriers will vary depending on the characteristics of the specific guideline, and on many local health care system characteristics. However, this review provides a "differential diagnosis for why physicians do not follow practice guidelines." Appropriate attention to these potential barriers in the planning and development of guidelines will facilitate successful implementation.

TABLE 9–1. SEVEN CATEGORIES OF BARRIERS

Barrier Category	Examples of Barriers Identified or Description of Barrier
Lack of awareness	Did not know the guideline existed
Lack of familiarity	Could not correctly answer questions about guideline content or self-reported lack of familiarity
Lack of agreement	Difference in interpretation of the evidence Benefits not worth patient risk, discomfort, or cost Not applicable to patient population in their practice Credibility of authors questioned Oversimplified cookbook Reduces autonomy Decreases flexibility Decreases physician self-respect Not practical Makes patient-physician relationship impersonal
Lack of self-efficacy	Did not believe that they could actually perform the behavior or activity recommended by the guideline, e.g., nutrition or exercise counseling
Lack of outcome expectancy	Did not believe intended outcome would occur even if the practice was followed, e.g., counseling to stop smoking
Inertia of previous practice	This barrier relates primarily to motivation to change practice, whether the motivation is professional, personal, or social. It was also noted that guidelines that recommend eliminating a behavior are more difficult to implement than guidelines that recommend adding a new behavior
External barriers	Patient resistance/nonadherence Patient does not perceive need Perceived to be offensive to patient Causes patient embarrassment Lack of reminder system Not easy to use, inconvenient, cumbersome, confusing Lack of educational materials Cost to patient Insufficient staff, consultant support or other resources Lack of time Lack of reimbursement Increased malpractice liability Not compatible with practice setting

An observational study of general practice in the Netherlands identified the following characteristics that influenced the use of guidelines: (1) specific attributes of the guidelines determine whether they are used in practice, (2) evidence-based recommendations are better followed in practice than those not based on scientific evidence, (3) precise definitions of recommended performance improve use, (4) testing the feasibility and acceptance of clinical guidelines among target groups is important, and (5) the people setting the guidelines need to understand the attributes of effective evidence-based guidelines.[75]

Computer-based clinical decision support (CDSS) is one method thought to facilitate guideline implementation. In 1998, a systematic review was published of controlled trials assessing the effects of CDSS systems. This systematic review indicated that CDSS can enhance clinical performance for drug dosing, preventive care, and other aspects of medical care, but was not convincing for effects on diagnosis.[76] The same research group published an updated systematic review of CDSS that produced only slightly different results.[77] One hundred studies published between 1998 and September 2004 met inclusion criteria for this updated review. Of the included trials, 88% were randomized; 49% of these were cluster randomized; and 40% used a cluster as the unit of analysis or adjusted for clustering. The methodological quality of the trials was noted to improve over time.

In the updated systematic review, there were 29 trials involving drug dosing or prescribing. Of 24 studies involving systems for single-drug dosing, 15 (62%) demonstrated improved practitioner performance with guidelines, and 2 of the 18 studies assessing patient outcomes showed positive improvement. Of the five systems using computer order entry for multidrug prescribing, four improved practitioner performance, but none improved patient outcomes. There were 40 studies of systems for disease management of conditions such as diabetes, cardiovascular disease prevention, urinary incontinence, human immunodeficiency virus infection, and acute respiratory distress. Thirty-seven of these studies evaluated practitioner performance with 23 (62%) demonstrating improvement. Only five (18%) of the 27 disease management trials evaluating patient outcomes demonstrated improvement. Of 21 trials of reminder systems for preventive care, 16 (72%) found improvements in practitioner performance according to practice guidelines. Of 10 trials that evaluated CDSS for diagnostic systems, only 4 (40%) found improvements in practitioner performance. Of the five trials of diagnostic systems that evaluated patient outcomes, none found improvement.[77]

Garg and colleagues also reported that improved practitioner performance was associated with CDSS systems that automatically prompted the practitioner to use the system compared to systems that required the practitioner to initiate system use. Improved performance was noted in 73% of trials of automated systems compared to 47% of user initiated systems (p = 0.02). It was also interesting to note that the best predictor of success of a CDSS was a study in which the authors were also the developers of the system. Studies conducted by the developer of the system were more likely to find success (74%), compared to 28% when the authors were not the developers (p = 0.001).[77] It is clear that as with other methods for implementation of guidelines and achieving performance or behavior change, further research is needed on use of CDSS to provide clear guidance on predictable success rates. Many individual factors will need to be considered in the decision-making for implementation of these systems.[78]

A randomized controlled trial of CQI and academic detailing to implement clinical guidelines for the primary care of hypertension and depression produced mixed results.[79] The authors concluded that both academic detailing and CQI interventions involve complex social interactions that produce varied implementation across the different organizations.

One of the first systematic literature reviews and evaluations of the effect of practice guidelines was published in 1993.[80] The authors of this study conducted an extensive literature search and identified 59 studies that they considered to have appropriate methods to evaluate the effect of guidelines on either physician behavior or patient outcomes. All but four of the studies showed some benefit from the guidelines; however, the magnitude of the benefit and the patient care significance was not impressive in all cases.

Guidelines represent an early application of decision support systems to facilitate providing quality clinical care. When done well, practice guidelines should contain all the necessary elements of routine care for most individuals with a specific condition. They should prompt consideration of what specific characteristics of an individual patient might warrant departures from the guideline. When effectively implemented, such systems save clinicians time. They should be assisted by computerized systems that, among other functions, can catalogue past histories, check orders for medications against measures of hepatic and renal function, and schedule reminders for screening tests or preventive services. They should be part of the continuous improvement of systems of care. Guidelines will not be perfect at the outset; systems that use them must be constructed so that experience can be applied to improve the guidelines, just as the guidelines indicate where care delivery can be improved.[81]

Sources of Clinical Practice Guidelines

There are several mechanisms to locate completed clinical practice guidelines or systematic reviews. The Web based NGC <http://www.guideline.gov>> is an initiative of AHRQ, created in cooperation with the American Medical Association and the American Association of Health Plans. The mission of the NGC is to provide an accessible mechanism for obtaining objective, detailed information on clinical practice guidelines and to further their dissemination, implementation, and use. Components of the NGC include structured abstracts about the guideline and its development; a utility for comparing attributes of two or more guidelines in a side-by-side comparison; synthesis of guidelines covering similar topics, highlighting areas of similarity and difference; links to full text guidelines where available and/or ordering information for print copies; an electronic forum for exchanging information on clinical practice guidelines, their development, implementation and use; and annotated bibliographies on guideline development methodology implementation and use. In order to be included in the NGC, the following criteria must be met:

1. The clinical practice guideline contains systematically developed statements that include recommendations, strategies, or information that assists physicians and/or other health care practitioners and patients make decisions about appropriate health care for specific clinical circumstances.

2. The clinical practice guideline was produced under the auspices of medical specialty associations; relevant professional societies, public or private organizations, government agencies at the Federal, State, or local level; or health care organizations or plans. A clinical practice guideline developed and issued by an individual not officially sponsored or supported by one of the above types of organizations does not meet the inclusion criteria for NGC.

3. Corroborating documentation can be produced and verified that a systematic literature search and review of existing scientific evidence published in peer-reviewed journals was performed during the guideline development. A guideline is not excluded from NGC if corroborating documentation can be produced and verified detailing specific gaps in scientific evidence for some of the guideline's recommendations.

4. The full text guideline is available on request in print or electronic format (for free or for a fee), in the English language. The guideline is current and the most recent version produced. Documented evidence can be produced or verified that the guideline was developed, reviewed, or revised within the last 5 years.[82]

The NGC provides a search function for identifying guidelines by disease, producer, bibliographic source, characteristics of the guideline, date, clinical specialty, objective, target population, and many other factors. The search engine allows the use of boolean operators, truncation, automatic concept mapping, textword searching, and multiple sort and display options. The NGC premiered in January 1999 with 286 guidelines and as of January 2005, it contained 1436 guideline summaries.

Many guidelines have been published in the peer-reviewed medical literature and can therefore be located in MEDLINE®. A variety of search techniques may be used, but the most efficient may be to search for *practice guideline* in the publication type field of the record, or use the MeSH term *practice guidelines* in conjunction with other terms for the specific disease or therapy of interest. Additional publication types in the NLM record that may be searched include the terms consensus development conference; consensus development conference, NIH; guideline; meta-analysis; and review, academic. Systematic review articles are also useful in preparation of clinical practice guidelines. The key differences with systematic reviews compared to the old forms of narrative review articles are that the systematic review begins with a focused clinical question, involves a comprehensive search for evidence, uses criterion-based selection that are uniformly applied to include evidence in the review, performs rigorous critical appraisal of the studies chosen, and provides a quantitative summary of the evidence.[83] Literature search strategies have been published for locating systematic reviews.[84,85]

The NIH Consensus Statements, NIH Technology Assessments, the USPSTF Guide to Clinical Preventive Services, AHRQ evidence reports, and other resources are available on

Health Services Technology Assessment Texts (HSTAT). HSTAT was developed by the NLM Information Technology Branch and can be accessed at <<http://www.ncbi.nlm.nih.gov/books/bv.fcgi?rid=hstat>>.

The Guidelines International Network (GIN) is an international not-for-profit association of organizations and individuals involved in clinical practice guidelines. Founded in November 2002, GIN has now grown to 52 member organizations including World Health Organization (WHO) from 26 countries. According to the GIN website "GIN seeks to improve the quality of health care by promoting systematic development of clinical practice guidelines and their application into practice, through supporting international collaboration." GIN's Guideline Library contains updated information about guidelines for specific health topics, tools and resources for guideline development, training materials, and patient or consumer resources. In December 2004, about 2700 programs were available at <http://www.g-i-n.net/>>. Some of the resources from this website require membership for access.

The Ontario GAC, a joint body of the Ontario Medical Association and the Ontario Ministry of Health and Long-Term Care with ex officio representation from the Institute for Clinical Evaluative Sciences, was formed in 1997. According to their website "The Committee mandate is to develop and recommend appropriate strategies for the implementation and monitoring of practice and referral guidelines, make recommendations for assisting in the implementation of prescribing guidelines, consult widely with the profession in the development of its recommendations." The GAC assess the methodological quality and clinical relevance of existing practice guidelines and recommends one for use by practicing physicians. The GAC also develops and recommends strategies for implementation and evaluation of guidelines. The GAC has established a network of key stakeholders to assist in the development, implementation, and evaluation of these strategies (<<http://gacguidelines.ca/>>). Also on their website is a group of links to guideline collections, guideline developers, research and education groups related to guidelines, and Canadian and International specialty societies.

The Turning Research Into Practice (TRIP) Database started in 1997 as a small search engine with a focus on medical articles considered evidence-based. The aims of the TRIP Database have remained the same since 1997—allow health professionals to easily find the highest-quality material available on the Web. Content areas in this database include evidence-based, clinical guidelines, and others. TRIP is a subscription-based product (<<http://www.tripdatabase.com/>>).

The Combined Health Information Database (CHID) at <<http://chid.nih.gov>> provides access to information from several federal agencies, e.g., the NIH, CDC, and complementary and alternative medicine. At present, CHID covers 11 topics. It is possible to search either individual topics or the entire database. The topics are AIDS, sexually transmitted disease, tuberculosis education, Alzheimer's disease, complementary and alternative medicine, deafness and communication disorders, diabetes, digestive diseases, kidney and urologic diseases, maternal and child health, medical genetics and rare disorders, oral health, and weight control.

As previously mentioned in this chapter, multiple professional organizations, academic centers, independent research centers, and government agencies are involved in development of clinical practice guideline activities. Updated information may be obtained by contacting these organizations directly and many have provided access to their guidelines on the Internet.

The Cochrane Library is based on the work of an international collaboration of health care providers and scientists who engage in preparing, maintaining, and disseminating systematic reviews of relevant randomized-controlled trials of health care.[86] This collaboration is named in honor of Archie Cochrane who in 1979 wrote, "it is surely a great criticism of our profession that we have not organized a critical summary, by specialty, adapted periodically, of all relevant randomized controlled trials." The Cochrane Library provides a collection of several databases: The Cochrane Database of Systematic Reviews (Cochrane Reviews), Database of Abstracts of Reviews of Effects (DARE), The Cochrane Central Register of Controlled Trials (CENTRAL), The Cochrane Database of Methodology Reviews (Methodology Reviews), The Cochrane Methodology Register (Methodology Register), Health Technology Assessment Database (HTA), NHS Economic Evaluation Database (NHS EED), About The Cochrane Collaboration, and the Cochrane Collaborative Review Groups (About). Full access to the Cochrane Library requires a subscription; however, abstracts of the systematic reviews are available at <<http://www.cochrane.org/reviews/index.htm>>.

The Cochrane Database of Systematic Reviews is a collection of highly structured and systematic reviews of research evidence in specific areas of health care. Data are often combined statistically (with meta-analysis) to increase the power of the findings from multiple studies. As of issue 1 of 2005, update this database includes over 2249 complete reviews and is growing. This database also includes another 1539 protocols (which are reviews that are in process).

The CENTRAL is a bibliography of controlled trials identified by contributors to the Cochrane Collaboration as part of an international effort to create an unbiased source of data for systematic reviews of the medical literature. Additional information about the Cochrane Collaboration is available at their website <http://www.cochrane.org/>. Links to Cochrane training resources (including the previously mentioned Reviewers' Handbook), and training resources from other organizations are available at these sites <<http://www.cochrane.org/resources/training.htm>> and <<http://www.cochrane.org/resources/revpro.htm>>.

The Internet has rapidly become a useful tool for access to health-care-related information. Many sites are potentially useful. Three excellent sites that are specifically designed to support EBM are the AHRQ website <<http://www.ahrq.gov/>>, the Health Information Research Unit at McMaster University (<<http://hiru.mcmaster.ca/>>), and the Centre for

Evidence-Based Medicine at Oxford (<<http://www.cebm.net/>>). These sites contain extensive information about systematic appraisal and use of evidence, worldwide projects for development of EBM including clinical practice guidelines, and links to many other quality sites.

Many activities conducted by professional organizations in pharmacy have principles in common with EBM and clinical practice guidelines. The American Society of Health-System Pharmacists (ASHP), in 1990 created a policy-recommending body called the Commission on Therapeutics. This commission develops therapeutic guidelines defined as "systematically developed documents that assist health care professionals on appropriate use of drugs for specific clinical circumstances."[87] With the publication of the ASHP Therapeutic Guidelines on Angiotensin-Converting-Enzyme Inhibitors in Patients with Left Ventricular Dysfunction,[88] the ASHP initiated an evidence-based style for its therapeutic guidelines.[89] The ASHP uses a process for preparation of the therapeutic guidelines similar to the one developed by the Agency for Health Care Policy and Research.

Another example of a therapeutic guideline from ASHP is on stress ulcer prophylaxis.[90] This extensive review used the most current methods for guideline preparation including decision algorithms and a decision tree for pharmacoeconomic analysis. The authors employed methods for assessing the literature by using evidence tables and categorized the recommendations according to the strength of evidence using a system based on recommendations from the Evidence-Based Working Group at McMaster. This system for defining levels of evidence takes into consideration the information provided in meta-analyses, the consistency of results across trials, and the bounds of the 95% confidence interval compared to the numerical threshold for clinically important benefit. In keeping with EBM ideals, an update representing the implications of recent studies in this area has been published.[91] In addition to therapeutic guidelines, ASHP produces Therapeutic Position Statements which are "concise statements that respond to specific therapeutic issues of concern to health care consumers and pharmacists, as approved by the board of directors" (<<http://www.ashp.org/bestpractices/index.cfm?cfid=5753/88&CFToken=42165878>>). More information about therapeutic guidelines and therapeutic position statements, and access to these documents is available at the ASHP website <<http://www.ashp.org/>>.

The American Pharmaceutical Association has published the APhA *Guide to Drug Treatment Protocols: A Resource for Creating & Using Disease-Specific Pathways*.[92] This resource includes specific drug treatment protocols and an extensive handbook on the guideline development process and many issues surrounding the use of evidence-based guidelines. This resource was developed by the APhA to assist health professionals with their efforts to develop, use, and measure patient outcomes with disease-specific drug treatment protocols. The APhA uses a multidisciplinary process to develop the guidelines based on scientific evidence published in the peer-reviewed literature. New protocols are being produced and released on a continuing basis.

Conclusion

Clinical practice guidelines have become a significant tool in health care with the focus on evidence-based practice. These guidelines fit well with the emphasis of CQI techniques. Guidelines have the potential to assist medical decision-making and ultimately improve the quality of care, improve patient outcomes, and make more efficient use of resources. Significant advances have been made in the methodology to produce valid guidelines. Information technology and greater understanding of optimal methods for implementation of guidelines will maximize their effect to improve quality of care. Pharmacists' active involvement in preparation and implementation of evidence-based clinical practice guidelines is vital to ensure that pharmaceutical care issues are addressed. A thorough understanding of evidence-based methodology will prepare the pharmacist to participate in this process.

Study Questions for Evidence-Based Clinical Practice Guidelines

1. Which of the following groups or types of organizations have been involved in development of clinical practice guidelines?
    a. Federal and state government
    b. Professional societies and associations
    c. Managed care organizations
    d. Third-party payers
    e. All of the above

2. Which of the following is a common characteristic of practice guideline development and traditional drug information practice activities?
    a. Decision-making and recommendations based on individual experience
    b. Assurance of cost savings
    c. Clear specific definition of clinical questions
    d. Lack of interdisciplinary participation
    e. All of the above

3. True or false. Clinical practice guidelines are intended to assist practitioner decision-making but are not intended to inform decisions made by patients.

4. Which of the following methods of guideline development is currently recommended as the most valid?
    a. Evidence-based
    b. Informal consensus

c. Formal consensus

d. a or c

e. None of the above

5. Which of the following are included in the five core competencies for health professionals as recommended in the Institute of Medicine report Health Professions Education: A Bridge to Quality?

a. Deliver patient-centered care

b. Participate in interdisciplinary teams

c. Emphasize evidence-based practice

d. Utilize informatics

e. All of the above

6. True or false. Clinical practice guidelines and evidence-based practice have a common philosophy in their origin.

7. Which of the following characteristics associated with a disease would suggest that it would be a good topic for development and implementation of a practice guideline?

a. Low prevalence

b. Evidence that current practice is optimal

c. Evidence of little variation in current practice

d. Availability of high quality evidence for the efficacy of interventions

e. Low frequency and severity of morbidity

8. True or false. The development of clinical practice guidelines ideally should involve a multidisciplinary process, but that is not considered particularly important for topics not intended for primary care.

9. True or false. Guideline development panels have in some instances been criticized for having a members with potential conflicts of interest.

10. Which of the following information does the GRADE working group recommend be incorporated with guideline recommendations?

a. Quality of evidence from studies

b. Balance of benefits and harms of interventions

c. The strength of the recommendation

d. a and c only

e. a, b, and c

11. The GRADE working group includes which of the following elements in designating the quality of evidence?

a. Basic trial design, e.g., randomized controlled trial

b. Quality of study methods and execution

c. Consistency of results across studies

d. Similarity of study subjects, interventions, and outcomes to target patients

e. All of the above

12. Which of the following is *not* true regarding the AGREE instrument for guideline evaluation?

a. It was created by an international panel of researchers and policy makers.

b. It provides a structured process for evaluating multiple aspects of quality in several domains.

c. It is intended for use by organizations but not individuals.

d. It focuses on the quality of the guideline development methods and reporting quality but not the clinical content.

e. It has been field tested for clarity, comprehensiveness, relevance, and ease of use.

13. Which of the following is true regarding the checklist created by the COGS?

a. It is intended primarily for users of guidelines but not for guideline developers.

b. It is intended to improve both development methods and quality of reporting.

c. Its intent and philosophy are significantly different from the CONSORT statement for randomized trial reporting.

d. Guidelines that are brief are most likely to be consistent with the criteria in the checklist.

e. It focuses on guideline development and reporting but does not consider issues with implementation.

14. Which of the following is *not* true regarding guideline implementation?

a. Implementation strategies that used multiple methods are the most effective and efficient way to achieve compliance.

b. Hundreds of studies have been conducted to evaluate implementation methods.

c. The most effective methods to achieve the desired effects on the quality of care are still undetermined.

d. Organizational, local practice, political characteristics, and individual practitioner characteristics may be important considerations.

e. There is significant variation in success between implementation interventions and with the same intervention from one organization to another.

15. Which of the following is true regarding studies of the effect of CDSS systems on patient care?

a. The best predictor of success of the system is that the study to evaluate success is conducted by the system developer.

b. Systematic reviews of these systems have shown enhanced clinical performance for drug dosing, preventive care, and diagnosis.

c. Very few studies of these systems used randomization procedures.

d. Most of the studies evaluate specific patient outcomes.

e. The success of the system is not dependent on automatic prompting or practitioner initiated use.

REFERENCES

1. Field JM, Lohr KN, editors. Guidelines for clinical practice: from development to use. Washington, DC: National Academy Press; 1992.

2. Jones RH, Ritchie JL, Fleming BB, Hammermeister KE, Leape LL. 28th Bethesda Conference. Task force 1: clinical practice guideline development, dissemination and computerization. J Am Coll Cardiol. 1997;29:1133–41.

3. President's Advisory Commission on Consumer Protection and Quality in the Health Care Industry. Quality first better health care for all Americans, 1998 [cited 1999 Jan 18]: [1 screen]. Available from: http://www.hcqualitycommission.gov/final/execsum.html

4. Chassin MR, Galvin RW. The urgent need to improve health care quality. Institute of Medicine National Roundtable on Health Care Quality. JAMA. 1998;280:1000–5.

5. Kohn LT, Corrigan JM, Donaldson MS, editors. To err is human: building a safer health system. Institute of Medicine. Washington, DC: National Academy Press; 1999.

6. Corrigan JM, Donaldson MS, Kohn LT, editors. Crossing the quality chasm: a new health system for the 21st century. Institute of Medicine. Washington, DC: National Academy Press; 2001.

7. Aspden P, Corrigan JM, Wolcott J, editors. Patient safety: achieving a new standard for care. Institute of Medicine. Washington, DC: National Academy Press; 2004.

8. Sackett DL, Rosenberg WM., Gray JA, Haynes RB, Richardson WS. Evidence-based medicine: what it is and what it isn't. BMJ. 1996;312:71–2.

9. Eddy DM. Evidence-based medicine: a unified approach. Health Aff. 2005;24:9–17.

10. Evidence Based Medicine Working Group. Evidence based medicine: a new approach to teaching the practice of medicine. JAMA. 1992;268:2420–5.

11. Sackett DL, Straus SE, Richardson WS, Rosenberg W, Haynes RB. Evidence-based medicine: how to practice & teach EBM, 2nd ed. New York: Churchill-Livingstone; 2000.

12. Watanabe AS, McCart G, Shimomura S, Kayser S. Systematic approach to drug information requests. Am J Hosp Pharm. 1975;32:1282–5.

13. Guyatt GH, O Meade M, Jaeschke RZ, Cook DJ, Haynes RB. Practice of evidence based care. Not all clinicians need to appraise evidence from scratch but all need some skills. BMJ. 2000;320:954–5.

14. Towle A. Changes in health care and continuing medical education for the 21st century. BMJ. 1998;316:301–4.

15. Davis D. Continuing medical education. Global health, global learning. BMJ. 1998;316:385–9.

16. Fox RD, Bennett NL. Learning and change: implications for continuing medical education. BMJ. 1998;316:466–8.

17. Bashook PG, Parboosingh J. Recertification and the maintenance of competence. BMJ. 1998; 316:545–8.

18. Holm HA. Quality issues in continuing medical education. BMJ. 1998;316:621–4.

19. Southgate L, Dauphinee D. Maintaining standards in British and Canadian medicine: the developing role of the regulatory body. BMJ. 1998;316:697–700.

20. Headrick LA, Wilcock PM, Batalden PB. Interprofessional working and continuing medical education. BMJ. 1998;316:771–4.

21. Greiner AC, Knebel E, editors. Health professions education: a bridge to quality. Institute of Medicine. Washington, DC: National Academy Press; 2003.

22. Woolf SH. Practice guidelines: a new reality in medicine. II. Methods of developing guidelines. Arch Intern Med. 1992;152:946–52.

23. Perry S. The NIH consensus development program. A decade later. N Engl J Med. 1987;317:485–8.

24. Guidelines for the planning and management of NIH consensus development conferences, 1995 [cited 1999 Feb 22]: [1 screen]. Available from: http://odp.od.nih.gov/consensus/about/process.htm

25. National Cholesterol Education Program (NCEP) Expert Panel on Detection, Evaluation, and Treatment of High Blood Cholesterol in Adults (Adult Treatment Panel III). Third report of the National Cholesterol Education Program (NCEP) Expert Panel on Detection, Evaluation, and Treatment of High Blood Cholesterol in Adults (Adult Treatment Panel III) final report. Circulation. 2002;106:3143–21.

26. Gundy SM, Cleeman JI, Merz CNB, Brewer HB, Clark LT, Hunninghake DB, et al. Implications of recent clinical trials for the national cholesterol education program adult treatment panel III guidelines. Circulation. 2004;110:227–39.

27. Chobanian AV, Bakris GL, Black HR, Cushman WC, Green LA, Izzo JL, et al. Seventh report of the Joint National Committee on Prevention, Detection, Evaluation, and Treatment of High Blood Pressure. Hypertension. 2003;42:1206–52.

28. Canadian task force on the periodic health examination: the periodic health examination. Can Med Assoc J. 1979;121:1193–254.

29. About USPSTF. U.S. Preventive Services Task Force. AHRQ Publication No. 00-P046,2003. Rockville (MD): Agency for Health care Research and Quality. [cited 2004 Nov 17]. Available from: http://www.ahrq.gov/clinic/uspstfab.htm

30. Eddy DM. Clinical decision-making: from theory to practice. Guidelines for policy statements: the explicit approach. JAMA. 1990;263:2239–40, 2243.

31. Eddy DM. Clinical decision-making: from theory to practice. Anatomy of a decision. JAMA. 1990;263:441–3.

32. Eddy DM. Clinical decision-making: from theory to practice. Practice policies: guidelines for methods. JAMA. 1990;263:1839–41.

33. Eddy DM. Designing a practice policy. Standards, guidelines, and options. JAMA. 1990;263:3077–81, 3084.

34. Woolf SH. Manual for clinical practice guideline development. AHCPR Publication No. 91-0007. Rockville (MD): Agency for Health Care Policy and Research, Public Health Service, U.S. Department of Health and Human Services; 1991.

35. Burgers JS, Grol R, Klazinga NS, Makela M, Zaat J; for the AGREE Collaboration. Towards evidence-based clinical practice: an international survey of 18 clinical guideline programs. Int J Qual Health Care. 2003;15:31–45.

36. Manual for ACC/AHA guideline writing committees: methodologies and policies from the ACC/AHA task for on practice guidelines [cited 2004 Nov 19]. Available from: http://circ.ahajournals.org/manual/index.shtml

37. American College of Rheumatology. Guidelines for the development of practice guidelines, 1998. [cited 2004 Nov 19]. Available from: http://www.rheumatology.org/publications/guidelines/guidesonguides.asp?aud=mem

38. Schunemann HJ, Munger H, Brower S, O'Donnell M, Crowther M, Cook D, et al. Methodology for guideline development for the seventh American college of chest physicians conference on antithrombotic and thrombolytic therapy. Chest. 2004;126(suppl 3):174S–8S.

39. American Academy of Pediatrics and American Academy of Family Physicians. Clinical practice guideline: diagnosis and management of acute otitis media. Pediatrics. 2004;113:1451–65.

40. Mandell LA, Bartlett JG, Dowell SF, File TM, Musher DM, Whitney C. Update of practice guidelines for the management of community-acquired pneumonia in immunocompetent adults. Clin Infect Dis. 2003;37:1405–33.

41. National Institute for Clinical Excellence. Guideline development methods: information for national collaborating centres and guideline developers, 2004. London: National Institute for Clinical Excellence [accessed 2004 Nov 21]. Available from: http://www.nice.org.

42. New Zealand Guidelines Group. Handbook for the preparation of explicit evidence-based clinical practice guidelines, 2001. Available from: http://www.nzgg.org.nz/development/documents/nzgg_guideline_handbook.pdf

43. Scottish Intercollegiate Guidelines Network. SIGN 50: a guideline developers' handbook. SIGN Publication No. 50 [cited 2004 Nov 21]. Available from: http://www.sign.ac.uk/guidelines/fulltext/50/index.html

44. Field JM, Lohr KN, editors. Clinical practice guidelines: directions for a new program. Washington, DC: National Academy Press; 1990.

45. Hirsh J, Guyatt G, Albers GW, Schunemann HJ. The seventh ACCP conference on antithrombotic and thrombolytic therapy. Evidence-based guidelines. Chest. 2004;126(suppl 3):172S–3S.

46. Guyatt G, Schunemann HJ, Cook D, Jaeschke R, Pauker S. Applying the grades of recommendation for antithrombotic and thrombolytic therapy. The seventh ACCP conference on antithrombotic and thrombolytic therapy. Chest. 2004;126(suppl 3):179S–87S.

47. Schunemann HJ, Cook D, Grimshaw J, Liberati A, Heffner J, Tapson V, et al. Antithrombotic and thrombolytic therapy: from evidence to application. The seventh ACCP conference on antithrombotic and thrombolytic therapy. Chest. 2004;126(suppl 3):688S–96S.

48. Alderson P, Green S, Higgins JPT, editors. Cochrane reviewers' handbook 4.2.2 [updated 2004 Mar; accessed 2005 Feb 5]. Available from: http://www.cochrane.org/resources/handbook/hbook.htm.

49. Khan KS, ter Riet G, Glanville J, editors. Undertaking systematic reviews of research on effectiveness CRD's guidance for those carrying out or commissioning reviews, 2nd ed. CRD Report No 4. Centre for Reviews and Dissemination, University of York, York, UK, 2001 [cited 2005 Feb 5]. Available from: http://www.york.ac.uk/inst/crd/report4.htm

50. Mosca L, Appel LJ, Benjamin EJ, Berra K, Chandra-Strobos N, Fabunmi RP, et al. Evidence-based guidelines for cardiovascular disease prevention in women. J Am Coll Cardiol. 2004;43:900–21.

51. National Institute for Clinical Excellence. Topic suggestion and selection. criteria for selecting topics for the advisory committee on topic selection [cited 2005 Jan 29]. Available from: http://www. nice.org.uk/pdf/topicsuggestionselectiocriteria.pdf

52. Fye WB. The power of clinical trials and guidelines, and the challenge of conflicts of interest. J Am Coll Cardiol. 2003;41:1237–42.

53. Choudhry NK, Stelfox HT, Detsky AS. Relationships between authors of clinical practice guidelines and the pharmaceutical industry. JAMA. 2002;287:612–7.

54. Curtiss FR. Consensus panel, national guidelines, and other potentially misleading terms. J Manag Care Pharm. 2003;9:574–5.

55. Van Der Weyden MB. Clinical practice guidelines: time to move the debate from the how to the who. Med J Aust. 2002;176:304–5.

56. Alving B. NHLBI clinical guidelines development. Statement from Barbara Alving, MD, Acting Director of the National Heart, Lung and Blood Institute [cited 2005 Jan 30]. Available from: http://www. nhlbi.nih.gov/new/press/04-07-29.htm

57. Alving B. Cholesterol guidelines: the strength of the science base and the integrity of the development process. Statement from Barbara Alving, MD, Acting Director of the National Heart, Lung and Blood Institute [cited 2005 Jan 30]. Available from: http://www.nhlbi.nih.gov/new/press/04-09-24.htm

58. Alving B. Letter to Mr. Merrill Goozner, Director, Integrity in Science Center for Science in the Public Interest. 2004 Oct 22. [cited 2005 Jan 30]. Available from: http://www.nhlbi.nih. gov/guidelines/ cholesterol/response.pdf

59. Grimshaw JM, Thomas RE, MacLennan G, Fraser C, Ramsay CR, Vale L, et al. Effectiveness and efficiency of guideline dissemination and implementation strategies. Health Technol Assess. 2004;8(6) [cited 2005 Jan 29]. Available from: http://www.ncchta.org/fullmono/mon806.pdf and http://www. ncchta.org/fullmono/mon806a.pdf

60. Shiffman RN, Michel G, Essaihi A, Thornquist E. Bridging the guideline implementation gap: a systematic document-centered approach to guideline implementation. JAMIA. 2004; 11: 418–26.

61. Lyons SS, Tripp-Reimer T, Sorofman BA, DeWitt JE, Boots-Miller BJ, Vaughn T, et al. VA QUERI Informatics paper. Information technology for clinical guideline implementation: perceptions of multidisciplinary stakeholders. JAMIA. 2005;12:64–71.

62. Michie S, Johnston M. Changing clinical behaviour by making guidelines specific. BMJ. 2004;328: 343–5.

63. West S, King V, Carey TS, Lohr KN, McKoy N, Sutton S, et al. Systems to rate the strength of scientific evidence. Evidence Report/Technology Assessment No. 47 (Prepared by the Research Triangle Institute-University of North Carolina Evidence-based Practice Center under Contract No. 290-97-0011). AHRQ Publication No. 02-E016. Rockville, MD: Agency for Health care Research and Quality; 2002.

64. Chobanian AV, Bakris GL, Black HR, Cushman WC, Green LA, Izzo JL, et al. The seventh report of the Joint National Committee on Prevention, Detection, Evaluation, and Treatment of High Blood Pressure: the JNC 7 report. JAMA. 2003;289:2560–72.

65. Atkins D, Best D, Briss PA, Eccles M, Falck-Ytter Y, Flottorp S, et al. for the GRADE working group. Grading quality of evidence and strength of recommendations. BMJ. 2004;328:1490.

66. Atkins D, Eccles M, Flottorp S, Guyatt GH, Henry D, Hill S, et al. Systems for grading the quality of evidence and the strength of recommendations I: critical appraisal of existing approaches.

BMC Health Serv Res. 2004;4:38 [Epub ahead of print]. Available from: http://www.biomedcentral.com/1472-6963/4/38

67. Atkins D, Briss PA, Eccles M, Flottorp S, Guyatt GH, Harbour RT, et al. The GRADE* working group. A pilot study of a new system for grading the quality of evidence and the strength of recommendations [cited 2005 Jan 31]. Available from: http://www.gradeworkinggroup.org/publications/Grade_pilot_study_2004_01_20.pdf

68. Cluzeau F, Burgers J, Brouwers M, Grol R, Makela M, Littlejohns P, et al. Development and validation of an international appraisal instrument for assessing the quality of clinical practice guidelines: the AGREE project. Qual Saf Health Care. 2003;12:18–23.

69. Moher D, Schulz KF, Altman DG, for the CONSORT Group. The CONSORT statement: revised recommendations for improving the quality of reports of parallel-group randomized trials. Ann Intern Med. 2001;134:657–62.

70. Moher D, Jones A, Lepage L. Use of the CONSORT statement and quality of reports of randomized trials: a comparative before-and-after study. JAMA. 2001;285:1992–5.

71. Shiffman RN, Shekelle P, Overhage M, Slutsky J, Grimshaw J, Deshpandey AM, et al. Standardized reporting of clinical practice guidelines: a proposal from the conference on guideline standardization. Ann Intern Med. 2003;139:493–8.

72. Eddy DM. Performance measurement: problems and solutions. Health Aff (Millwood). 1998;17(4): 7–25.

73. Davis DA, Taylor-Vaisey A. Translating guidelines into practice. A systematic review of theoretic concepts, practical experience and research evidence in the adoption of clinical practice guidelines. CMAJ. 1997;157:408–16.

74. Cabana MD, Rand CS, Powe NR, Wu AW, Wilson MH, Abboud PAC, et al. Why don't physicians follow clinical practice guidelines? A framework for improvement. JAMA. 1999;282:1458–65.

75. Grol R, Dalhuijsen J, Thomas S, Veld C, Rutten G, Mokkink H. Attributes of clinical guidelines that influence use of guidelines in general practice: observational study. BMJ. 1998;317:858–61.

76. Hunt DL, Haynes RB, Hanna SE, Smith K. Effects of computer-based clinical decision support systems on physician performance and patient outcomes: a systematic review. JAMA. 1998;280:1339–46.

77. Garg AX, Adhikari NK, McDonald H, Rosas-Arellano MP, Devereaux PJ, Beyene J, et al. Effects of computerized clinical decision support systems on practitioner performance and patient outcomes. A systematic review. JAMA. 2005;293:1223–38.

78. Wears RL, Berg M. Computer technology and clinical work. Still waiting for Godot. JAMA. 2005;293:1261–3.

79. Horowitz CR, Goldberg HI, Martin DP, Wagner EH, Fihn SD, Chirstensen DB, et al. Conducting a randomized controlled trial of CQI and academic detailing to implement clinical guidelines. Jt Comm J Qual Improv. 1996; 22:734–50.

80. Grimshaw JM, Russell IT. Effect of clinical guidelines on medical practice: a systematic review of rigorous evaluations. Lancet. 1993;342:1317–22.

81. Chassin MR. Is health care ready for six sigma quality? Milbank Q. 1998;76(4):565–91, 510.

82. Inclusion Criteria. Washington, DC: National Guideline Clearinghouse [updated 2005 May 23; cited 2005 May 23]. Available from: http://www.guideline.gov/about/inclusion.aspx

83. Cook DJ, Mulrow CD, Haynes RB. Systematic review: synthesis of best evidence for clinical decisions. Ann Intern Med. 1997;126:376–80.

84. Hunt DL, McKibbon KA. Locating and appraising systematic reviews. Ann Intern Med. 1997;126:532–8.

85. Montori VM, Wilczynski NL, Morgan D, Haynes RB; for the Hedges Team. Optimal search strategies for retrieving systematic reviews from MEDLINE®: analytical survey. BMJ. 2005;330(7482):68. Epub Dec 24, 2004.

86. Sackett DL. The Cochrane Collaboration [editorial]. ACP J Club. 1994;120(suppl 3):A11.

87. Practice Standards of ASHP 1993-1994. Bethesda (MD): American Society of Hospital Pharmacists, 1993.

88. American Society of Health-System Pharmacists. ASHP therapeutic guidelines on angiotensin-converting-enzyme inhibitors in patients with left ventricular dysfunction. This official ASHP practice standard was developed through the ASHP Commission on Therapeutics and approved by the ASHP Board of Directors on Nov 16, 1996. Am J Health Syst Pharm. 1997;54:299–313.

89. Cooke-Ariel H. Promoting use of angiotensin-converting-enzyme inhibitors. Am J Health Syst Pharm. 1997;54:264.

90. American Society of Health-System Pharmacists. ASHP therapeutic guidelines on stress ulcer prophylaxis. Am J Health Syst Pharm. 1999;56:347–79.

91. Allen ME, Kopp BJ, Erstad BL. Stress ulcer prophylaxis in the postoperative period. Am J Health Syst Pharm. 2004;61:588–96.

10

Chapter Ten

Clinical Application of Statistical Analysis

Karen L. Kier

Objectives

After completing this chapter, the reader will be able to

- Describe the importance of understanding statistics in completing and evaluating scientific studies.
- Define the various levels of data.
- Determine whether the appropriate statistics have been performed and provided in a study.
- Interpret the statistical results provided in a research study to determine whether the authors' conclusions are supported.

Biostatistics is an area essential to understanding biomedical and pharmacy literature. This chapter will provide a basic understanding of biostatistics for the reader who has little or no statistical background. The focus will be on describing concepts as they relate to evaluating medical literature rather than discussing the mathematical formulas and various statistical procedures. Understanding statistics will enhance the pharmacist's ability to interpret the biomedical literature and draw conclusions from research studies.

Before discussing the types of statistics that are used in medical literature, it may be helpful to review information about the design of studies and type of data collected. When using statistical tests, assumptions are often made that require knowledge of the research design and the methods used by the researchers. The first part of this chapter will review some basic concepts about populations, samples, data, and variables. The second part will discuss specific types of descriptive and inferential statistics. This chapter should be used in conjunction with Chaps. 6 and 7 because many of the concepts are interrelated.

Basic Concepts

POPULATIONS AND SAMPLES

A population refers to all objects of a particular kind in the universe, while a sample is a portion of that population. The measurements that describe a population are referred to as parameters, while those measurements that describe a sample are considered statistics. The sample statistic is an estimate of the population parameter. When investigating a particular issue, one must describe the population to be studied. In most practical situations, it is impossible to measure the entire population; rather, one must take a representative sample. For example, if one wanted to study the effect that a calcium channel blocker agent has on blood glucose levels in insulin-dependent diabetes mellitus subjects, then insulin-dependent diabetes patients would be the study population. In order to study this group, the researchers would have to take a representative sample from all insulin-dependent diabetic patients.

To make appropriate and accurate inferences about the study population, the sample must be representative of the population. Samples must be selected from the population appropriately or the data may not actually reflect the population parameters. One of the most common methods for selecting a representative sample is called a simple random sample. When making inferences from the study population by using a sample of the population, it is important that the study sample be selected at random. Random, in this case, does not imply that the sample is drawn haphazardly or in an unplanned fashion, but that each member of the population has an equal probability of being selected for the sample. Referring back to the example of diabetes, each insulin-dependent diabetic patient theoretically has an equal chance of being selected into the sample from the population. There are several approaches to selecting a simple random sample; however, the most common is the use of a random numbers table. A random numbers table is a set of integers between 0 and 9 that have been selected at random without any trends or patterns. At any point in the table, it is equally likely that any digit between 0 and 9 would be selected. Choosing a number in this fashion is analogous to pulling numbers from a hat. In using a random numbers table, a point is selected within the table as the starting point and the numbers are then used in order from that point.

Depending on the type of study design, a simple random sample may not be the best means for determining a representative sample. Sometimes it may be necessary to separate the population into nonoverlapping groups called strata, where a specific factor (e.g., gender) will be contained in separate strata to aid in analysis. In this case, the random sample is drawn within each strata. This method is called a stratified random sample. For certain types of research, a particular factor is important in the study group. An example would be when gender or ethnic background are important factors within the study. In order to assure that gender or ethnic background are properly represented in the study, a method of stratifying is done so that these demographics appear in necessary numbers within the study sample. By creating the stratified groups, the researcher is assured that these groups will be appropriately represented. In stratified random sampling, a simple random sample is still performed within each group or strata. An example would be if a researcher is interested in knowing about the effects of aspirin therapy in the prevention of an acute myocardial infarction, but wants to make sure that both males and females are represented. The researcher could opt to stratify the sample so that they enroll both males and females in equal numbers for the study. Many researchers do not use this technique when starting their studies because of editorial concerns about randomization, but by not stratifying, they give up the ability to make conclusions regarding certain subsets of the population when analyzing their results.

Another means of randomly sampling a population is a method that is known as random cluster sampling. It may not be practical to sample all pharmacists in the United States about their patient counseling practices; therefore, the researchers may opt to randomly select 5 states from the 50 states; the five states would represent the clusters to be sampled. The clusters could represent different regions of the United States, especially if the researcher felt that there may be differences based on geographic regions. A researcher may also feel that there could be differences in rural versus urban practices and want to make sure that the clusters contain these aspects as well. The researchers would then select their sample from the pharmacists within these five states, or clusters, for their study.

Another method often used is referred to as systematic sampling. This technique is used when information about the population is provided in list format, such as in the telephone book, election records, class lists, or licensure records. With systematic sampling, one name is selected near the beginning of the list and every nth name is then selected thereafter. For example, the researchers may decide to take every 10th name from the first name selected. It should be noted, however, that some statisticians and researchers do not consider this type of sampling to be truly random.

In review, the sample describes those individuals who are in the study. The population describes the entire group of people to whom the study refers. The ideal situation is one in which the sample drawn and studied adequately represents or estimates the population being studied.[1]

VARIABLES AND DATA

A variable is a characteristic that is being observed or measured. Data are the values assigned to that variable for each individual member of the population. There are two types of variables: independent and dependent. Some statistical textbooks will refer to a third type of variable called a confounding variable. Within a study, the dependent variable is the one that changes in response to the independent variable. The dependent variable is the outcome of interest within the study. In the previous example involving the effect of a calcium channel blocker on blood glucose, blood glucose would be the dependent variable; the independent variable is the intervention or what is being manipulated (the calcium channel blocker in the example). A confounding variable is one that can confuse or cloud the study variables. In the calcium channel blocker example, the subjects' diet needs to be controlled as a confounding variable because of the influence diet has on blood glucose levels.

Discrete versus Continuous Data

Discrete variables can have only one of a limited set of values. Discrete variables can also be described as being able to assume only the value of a whole number. For example, in studying the number of seizures that patients experienced with certain tricyclic antidepressants (TCAs), it would only be practical to describe seizures as whole numbers. It would not be possible for a patient to have half of a seizure. On the other hand, continuous data may take on any value within a defined range. This would include things like time, temperature, length, and blood glucose. Blood glucose is usually only reported in whole numbers, which seems to be a discrete variable. However, blood glucose can be measured in fractions of whole numbers. If using very sensitive laboratory equipment, glucose could be measured as accurately as 80.3 mg/dL. It is important to understand the difference between discrete and continuous variables, since this is a determining factor in selecting the appropriate statistical procedure.

Scales of Measurement

There are four recognized levels of measurement: nominal, ordinal, interval, and ratio scales. Each of these scales has certain distinguishing characteristics that are important in determining which statistical procedure should be used to analyze the data.

A nominal variable, sometimes called the classificatory variable, consists of categories that have no implied rank or order. Nominal data fit into classifications or categories, such as male or female and presence or absence of a disease state.

An ordinal variable is similar to a nominal variable in that the data are placed into categories. However, ordinal variables do have an implied order or rank. It is important to note that the differences between the categories cannot be considered equal. Examples of this type of data include ranks assigned in the military or grade levels in school (sophomore vs. senior). In medicine, an example would be a pain scale, where the patient may be able to tell you it hurts more, but not exactly how much more. In such a case, the patient may be asked to classify the pain as none, mild, moderate, severe, or unbearable.

Interval and ratio variables are also similar, because they both have constant and defined units of measurement. There is an equal distance or interval between values. Both of these variables imply that a value is greater than, less than, or equal to another variable. For example, blood glucose of 80 mg/dL is the same interval from 70 mg/dL as it is from 90 mg/dL. Each mg/dL is at an equal distance or interval from the next; likewise, each mg/dL is greater than, less than, or equal to all other mg/dL measurements. The difference between interval and ratio variables is that the ratio scale has an absolute zero. Be careful in confusing an absolute zero with an arbitrary zero point that is set. The classic example of this difference is that of the Celsius scale for temperature, which has an arbitrary zero that has been set at the freezing point for water, and the Kelvin scale, which has an absolute zero that represents the absence of molecular motion. This difference is really not essential when determining the type of statistical test to perform. Interval and ratio variables are analyzed using the same statistical procedures.[2]

Descriptive and Inferential Statistics

Statistics allow description and interpretation of data. There are two major ways that we can use statistics to describe data. The first is called descriptive statistics and is used to present, organize, and summarize data. Descriptive statistics are usually considered a very basic way to present data and focus on describing the data. This information can give clues as to the appearance of the data. In comparison, inferential statistics provide the ability to generalize the results from the study to the appropriate population.

DESCRIPTIVE STATISTICS

Descriptive statistics are often defined as a means to summarize a collection of data in a clear and understandable way. This summarization can be done either numerically or graphically. Mean, median, mode, and standard deviation are all types of numerical representation of descriptive statistics. Graphical representation can include such things as bar graphs, pie charts, and histograms. The descriptive statistics are often organized, summarized, and presented in tables or graphic form. Some things to consider when reviewing data in this format include the following:

1. The table or graph should be easy to read and understand.
2. The title should be clear and concise, as well as accurately describe the data being presented.
3. The units of measure on all scales, axes, rows, or columns should be easily visible and understandable.
4. The scales should be of equal interval or space without exaggerating one part of the scale; if an axis is shown with a break in the intervals, it should be clearly marked; often a break will be noted by two slash marks at that point.

5. Codes, abbreviations, and symbols should be defined in the text of the paper or explained in a footnote with the graph or table.

6. If comparisons are made between data or groups, the comparison should be done on equivalent scales.

Sometimes when evaluating a graph taken from an article, it can be helpful to graph the information on graph paper using a standard scale. By using a standard scale or re-graphing the data, it may offer the reader a different perspective on how the data look for comparison purposes.

MEASURES OF CENTRAL TENDENCY

Measures of central tendency are sometimes referred to as measures of location. These descriptive measures are helpful in identifying where a set of values are located. The most common measures of central tendency are the mode, the median, and the arithmetic mean. In a normal distribution of values, the mean is equal to the median and the mode. The central tendency value that is used depends on the scale of measurement for the variable being studied.

The mode is defined as the most frequently occurring value or category in the set of data. A data set can have more than one mode; a data set with two modes is referred to as bimodal, with three modes being referred to as trimodal, and so on. The mode is the measure of central tendency for nominal data. Remember that nominal data are categories with no specific order or rank. Therefore, the only appropriate measure of central tendency is the category that contains the most values.

The median is the middle value in a set of ranked data; in other words, it is a value such that half of the data points fall above it and half fall below it. In terms of percentiles, it is the value at the 50th percentile. The median is the appropriate measure of central tendency when describing ordinal data. Likewise, it can be useful in describing interval or ratio data as well because it gives some perspective on whether the data may be skewed or pulled away from the mean. Sometimes extreme values (outliers) can have a significant impact on the mean value but will have little or no impact on the median value. Therefore, a comparison of the mean and median values can give an insight into whether outliers influenced the data.

The mean or arithmetic mean is the most common and appropriate measure of central tendency for data measured on an interval or ratio scale. It is best described as the average numerical value for the data set. The mean is calculated by adding all the data points and dividing this number by the sample size. In the calcium channel blocker example, the mean would be the average blood glucose value for the study group.

There are other measures of central tendency, such as the geometric mean, however they are much less likely to be seen and will not be discussed further.

MEASURES OF VARIABILITY

Measures of variability, another type of descriptive statistic, are also referred to as measures of dispersion. The most common measures of variability are the range, interquartile range, standard deviation, and variance. In analyzing data, the measures of variability are useful in indicating how close the data are to the measure of central tendency. In other words, how scattered are the data from the median and/or mean? Data points that are widely scattered from the mean give a different perspective than data points very close to the mean. The mean value could be equal for two groups, but the variability of the data can give a different picture. When evaluating the biomedical literature, this point can be crucial in interpreting the results of a study. In evaluating nominal data, there is no measure of dispersion. The best option is to describe the number of categories studied.

The range can be used to describe ordinal, interval, and ratio data. The range is the difference between the highest data value and the lowest data value. In the calcium channel blocker example, if the highest blood glucose was 357 mg/dL and the lowest was 54 mg/dL, the range would be equal to 303 mg/dL. In medical literature, authors often provide the range by indicating the lowest to the highest values without actually calculating the difference for the reader (i.e., the blood glucose range was from 54 to 357 mg/dL). Although the range is an easy number to calculate, the measurement is not very useful in describing or comparing data.

The interquartile range is another measure of dispersion that can be used to describe ordinal, interval, and ratio data. This range is a measure of variability directly related to the median. The interquartile range takes the data values within the 25 and 75% quartiles. Therefore, the interquartile range deals with the middle 50% of the data. This value is less likely to be affected by extreme values in the data, which plagues the usefulness of the range.

The two best measures of dispersion with interval and ratio data are the standard deviation and variance. The relationship between the standard deviation and variance is that the standard deviation is the square root of the variance. The standard deviation is often preferred over the variance because it is the measure of the average amount by which each observation in a series of data points differs from the mean. In other words, how far away is each data point from the mean (dispersion or variability) or what is the average deviation from the mean? In medical literature, the standard deviation and mean are often reported in the following fashion: mean ± standard deviation. In comparing two groups with equal means, the standard deviation can give an idea of how much the individuals in each group were scattered from the mean value. It is important when evaluating the literature to look at the standard deviation in comparison to the mean. How much variability existed among the subjects in the study? A larger standard deviation means that there is more variability among the subjects versus a smaller standard deviation, which shows less variability and is often preferred. Another important concept to keep in mind when evaluating the standard deviation is that 65% of all data points will be within one standard deviation of the mean, while 95% and 99% will be within two and three standard deviations of the mean, respectively.

The coefficient of variation is another measure used when evaluating dispersion from one data set to another. The coefficient of variation is the standard deviation expressed as a percentage of the mean. This value is calculated by dividing the standard deviation by the mean and multiplying this value by 100. This index is useful in comparing the relative difference in variability between two or more samples or determining which group has the largest relative variability of values from the mean. For example, if a reader was interested in comparing two different blood pressure regimens from two different studies, one could use the coefficient of variation. In this case, a pharmacist could look at comparing a beta blocker to a calcium channel blocker and ask the question as to of which one of these therapies most consistently lowers blood pressure in all study subjects. If the coefficient of variation was 67% for the beta blocker and 33% for the calcium channel blocker, one could make a reasonable judgment that there was less variability in blood pressure control with the calcium channel blocker in comparison to the beta blocker even though the drugs were not studied within the same sample of individuals. One caution is that when comparing one study to a different study, it does not assure equality among the materials and methods for the studies. The drug literature evaluation chapters (Chaps. 6 and 7) go on to explain this concept further.

MEASURES OF SHAPE

Two descriptive measures that refer to the shape of a distribution are the coefficient of skewness and the coefficient of kurtosis; both used to describe the distribution of interval and ratio data. Skewness is the measure of symmetry of a curve. These descriptive measures are usually not described in the biomedical literature, but rather are used by researchers to evaluate the distribution properties of their variables. These distribution properties can be helpful in determining the type of statistical tests that best suit the research. Skewness tells how well each half of the curve or distribution relates to the other half of a normal distribution; if each half is equal in shape and size to the other half, they are mirror images of each other. The skewness is an indicator of where the data lie within the distribution. A distribution is said to be skewed to the right or have a positive skew when the mode and median are less than the mean. A distribution that is skewed to the left, or has a negative skew, is one in which the mode and median are greater than the mean. As stated previously, the mean is extremely sensitive to outlying values and can be skewed (pulled) to the left or the right by those very low or very high values, respectively. This shows the importance of looking at other indicators, like the median, and statistical software that might give printouts with indicators like kurtosis or skewness. Kurtosis refers to how flat or peaked the curve appears. A curve with a flat or board top is referred to as platykurtic, while a peaked distribution is described as leptokurtic. A platykurtic curve often is an indicator of more variability in the data, with it spread out over a larger range. Likewise, a leptokurtic distribution has less variability and has a number of data points surrounding the mean. A normal distribution or curve has a kurtosis value of 0 with the mean, median, and mode all being the same value.[2]

RATIOS, PROPORTIONS, AND RATES

Ratios, proportions, and rates are frequent terms used in the medical literature. A ratio expresses the relationship between two numbers, such as the ratio of men to women who suffer from multiple sclerosis (MS). A proportion is a specific type of ratio in which the numerator is included in the denominator and the value is expressed as a percentage. For example, the percentage of men with MS would be the number of men with MS in the numerator divided by the number of people in the population with MS (this number would include the men in the numerator). A rate is a special form of proportion that includes a specific timeframe. The rate is equal to the number of events in a specified period divided by the population at risk in a specified period. The rate for MS would be the number of cases during a specified timeframe, such as 1 year, divided by the total population in that timeframe. The reason the total population is used as the denominator is that the population is the group at risk for the disease.

INCIDENCE AND PREVALENCE

Incidence and prevalence are two measures used to describe illness within the population. Both measures are frequently used in the literature pertaining to epidemiology and public health. The incidence rate measures the probability that a healthy person will develop a disease within a specified period. In essence, it is the number of new cases of disease in the population within a specific period. Prevalence, on the other hand, measures the number of people in the population who have the disease at a given time. Incidence and prevalence differ in that incidence refers to only new cases and prevalence to all existing cases, regardless of whether they are newly discovered.

$$\text{Incidence rate} = \frac{\text{Number of new cases of a disease}}{\text{Population at risk}} \text{ per a given timeframe}$$

$$\text{Prevalence} = \frac{\text{Number of existing cases of a disease}}{\text{Total population}} \text{ per a given timeframe}$$

Incidence indicates the rate at which new disease occurs in a previously disease-free group over a specified timeframe, while prevalence describes the probability of people having a disease within a specified timeframe. It is important to look at both incidence and prevalence when describing diseases. Prevalence varies directly with incidence and the duration of the disease. In a disease with a rapid recovery or rapid death, the duration is short and the prevalence low. With a drug treatment that has a profound effect on prolonging life without curing the disease, prevalence will be high but the incidence may be low. A good research article will describe both incidence and prevalence, as well as specify the timeframe studied.

RELATIVE RISK AND ODDS RATIO

Relative risk and odds ratio are two measures of disease frequency. Both measures compare the incidence of disease when a specific factor is present or absent. An actual risk (such as relative risk) can only be measured by using a cohort type of study design (see Chap. 7). A cohort study design is an observational study design that usually starts with a large number of healthy subjects and follows their exposure to different factors over time. The large sample sizes seen with cohort study designs is what allows a researcher to calculate actual risk, rather than estimating it from a much smaller sample that would be seen in a case-control study design. The relative risk is defined as the incidence rate among those exposed to a particular factor divided by the incidence among those not exposed to the same factor. The relative risk is an appropriate measure in a cohort study. Prospective studies allow for defining populations at risk and, therefore, allow calculation of the excess risk caused by exposure to a particular factor.

If a cohort study design is not practical or is not chosen by the researchers, a case-control study design (see Chap. 7) is used and the odds ratio, an estimator of relative risk, is calculated. A case-control study is also an observational study design that recruits subjects into the study who have the outcome of interest (cases) to a group of individuals who do not have this particular outcome (controls). After cases and controls are identified, the researchers assess whether the subjects have been exposed to the risk factor being studied. For example, one could look at the development of lung cancer as the outcome while assessing the risk factor of exposure to second-hand smoke. The use of this case-control design would allow the researchers to "estimate" the risk (odds ratio) of the development of lung cancer in subjects exposed to second-hand smoke. In using the odds ratio as an estimator of relative risk, one must assume that the control group is representative of the general population, the cases are representative of the population with the disease, and the frequency of the disease in the population is small. The odds ratio is calculated by multiplying the number of cases with the disease and exposed to the factor by the number of cases without the disease and not exposed to the factor, and dividing this number by the number of cases with the disease without exposure to the factor multiplied by those cases without the disease but exposed to the factor. The table that follows may clarify this calculation.

		Disease	
		Present	**Absent**
Factor	Exposed factor	A	B
	Not exposed	C	D

$$\text{Odds ratio} = \frac{A \times D}{B \times C}$$

The odds ratio is commonly referred to in the medical literature, as well as in the lay press. When reading a study that refers to an odds ratio, it is important to understand the interpretation of the value. For example, if a study indicates that the odds ratio is 10 for developing prostate cancer if one uses tobacco, then the study shows us that a tobacco user is 10 times more likely to develop prostate cancer than a nonuser of tobacco. Some things to keep in mind when looking at an odds ratio is that it is an estimate and that available cohort studies with relative risk described are likely to be more accurate, and confidence intervals should always be given anytime an odds ratio or relative risk is reported in the literature.

SENSITIVITY, SPECIFICITY AND PREDICTIVE VALUES

Sensitivity, specificity, and predictive values are measures of the effectiveness of a test procedure. Sensitivity and specificity are the two indices used to evaluate the accuracy of a test. The following definitions will help in understanding these important measures:

- True positives (TP) are individuals with the disease who were correctly identified as having the disease by the test.
- False positives (FP) are individuals without the disease who were incorrectly identified as having the disease by the test.
- True negatives (TN) are individuals without the disease who were correctly identified as disease free by the test.
- False negatives (FN) are individuals with the disease who were incorrectly identified as disease-free by the test.

Sensitivity is the probability that a diseased individual will have a positive test result and is the true positive rate of the test.

$$\text{Sensitivity} = \frac{\text{Disease with positive test}}{\text{All diseased}}$$

$$\text{Sensitivity} = \frac{\text{True positives}}{\text{True positives} + \text{false negatives}}$$

Specificity is the probability that a disease-free individual will have a negative test result and is the true negative rate of the test.

$$\text{Specificity} = \frac{\text{Disease-free with negative test}}{\text{All disease-free}}$$

$$\text{Specificity} = \frac{\text{True negatives}}{\text{True negatives} + \text{false positives}}$$

In designing research studies involving a diagnostic test procedure or a screening test, the authors need to indicate a standard level that they will use as a cutoff for their screening. In setting their cutoff level, they determine who is to be identified with the disease and those patients who will be omitted without disease. In making this judgment they need to decide the cost of classifying individuals as FN and FP. For example, if a researcher is trying to screen for early diabetes mellitus, they might want to set the cutoff for blood glucose to be lower (i.e., fasting blood glucose of 110 mg/dL) realizing that they will probably see several FPs. The practitioner has to make the judgment on whether it is better to miss some potential individuals with early disease or to identify some people who on further testing test negative for diabetes. Additional costs may be incurred when additional testing needs to be done as well as consideration needs to be given to the emotional costs of patients falsely believing they potentially have a serious disease.

Predictive values are also calculated as a measure of the accuracy of a test procedure. Predictive value can be expressed as a function of sensitivity, specificity, and the probability of disease in the general population. Researchers can use the predictive values to determine a good research tool for studies. A method or tool with a high predictive value will often be more valuable as a screening test than other methods with lower predictive values.[3]

$$\text{Positive predictive value} = \frac{\text{Diseased with positive test}}{\text{All with positive test}}$$

$$\text{Negative predictive value} = \frac{\text{Disease-free with negative test}}{\text{All with negative test}}$$

DISTRIBUTIONS

All types of data can be organized in a manner that allows the observer to view general patterns and tendencies in the data. Data can be organized such that the values construct a frequency distribution. If the variable is continuous, there are an infinite number of possible values that graph as a continuous frequency distribution. Whereas, if the variable is discrete, the frequency distribution is limited in the number of possible values. The type of distribution can be helpful in determining the appropriate statistical test. For example, a normal distribution or the assumption of a normal distribution is a requirement for using parametric statistical tests in analyzing data. Probability distributions, like the binomial and the Poisson (see next section), are analyzed using specific formulas that evaluate the probability of an event occurring. This is often referred to as the success or failure of an event.

Probability Distribution

A probability distribution is a graphed representation of the probability values from the event or study. Probability values deal with the relative likelihood that a certain event will or will not occur, relative to some other events. The binomial distribution and the Poisson distribution are two forms of probability distributions.

Binomial Distribution

Many discrete objects or events belong to one of two mutually exclusive categories. For example, in describing gender, people can be categorized into either the male or female group. All people belong to one of these two groups, but cannot belong to both (mutually exclusive). The binomial distribution shows the probabilities of different outcomes for a series of random events, which can have only one of two values.

Properties of the binomial distribution include the following:

1. The event or trial occurs a specified number of times (analogous to sample size).
2. Each time the event occurs, there are only two mutually exclusive outcomes.
3. The events or trials are independent, meaning that one outcome has no effect on the next outcome of events.

Poisson Distribution

The Poisson distribution is another form of a discrete probability distribution. This distribution is used to predict the probabilities of the occurrence of rare, independent events or determine whether these events are independent when the sample size is indefinitely large. For example, the Poisson distribution could predict radioactive counts per unit of time. This is rarely ever used in the pharmacy or biomedical literature. The reader is not likely to see many studies that refer to this type of distribution.

Normal Distribution

In distinct contrast to the probability distribution is the more commonly used normal distribution. The frequency distribution histogram of a continuous variable often forms a symmetric, bell-shaped curve referred to as a normal distribution. The normal distribution is one of several continuous probability distributions with the following characteristics:

1. The mean, median, and mode all have the same value (see Figure 10–1).
2. The curve is symmetric around the mean.
3. The kurtosis is zero.
4. The tails of the distribution get closer and closer to the x-axis as the values move away from the mean, but the tails never quite touch the x-axis.

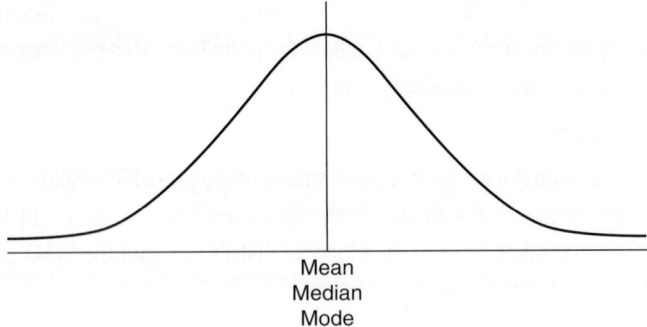

Figure 10–1. Mean, median, and mode of normal distribution.

5. The distribution is completely defined by the mean and standard deviation.
6. One standard deviation above and below the mean includes 68.26% of the values in the population; two standard deviations above and below the mean include 95.46% of the values, while three standard deviations include 99.73%.
7. The area under the normal curve is, by definition, 1.

It is statistically very important to know whether a variable is normally distributed in the population or approaches a normal distribution. The type of statistical test that is selected to analyze data often makes an assumption about the variables being normally distributed. This can be a key in interpreting the medical literature, which will be discussed later in the chapter. Did the researchers assume a normal distribution or was their variable normally distributed in the population? This is often difficult for the reader to evaluate when reviewing a study and should be provided as part of the materials and methods provided by the researchers in their overview of the study.

Standard Normal Distribution

Among the infinite number of possible normal distributions, there is one normal distribution that can be compared to all other normal distributions. This distribution is called the standard normal distribution. The standard normal distribution has a mean of 0 and a standard deviation and variance of 1 (see Figure 10–2). The tails of the distribution extend from minus infinity to positive infinity. When converting normal distributions to the standard normal, the variables are transformed to standardized scores referred to as z scores. A standard z score is a means of expressing a raw score in terms of the standard deviation. The raw score is so many standard deviation units from the standard mean score of 0, which would correlate to the number of standard deviation units that the score was from the mean score of the original distribution. Researchers can use the standard normal distribution to take their raw data and put it into standardized scores. Often by doing this, the authors can make comparisons between data sets that may be on different scales or have different values. By standardizing the data, a comparison can be made using a standard or equivalent scale. Therefore, differences between the data sets may

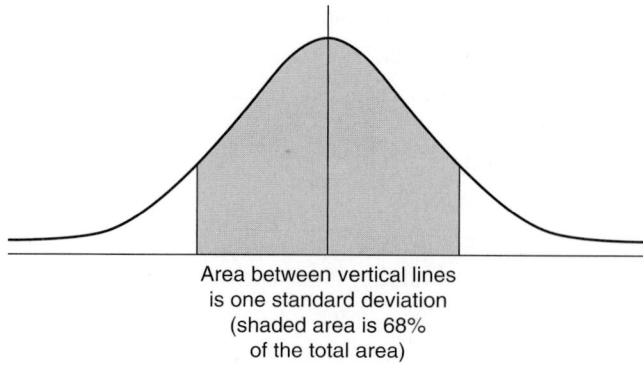

Area between vertical lines
is one standard deviation
(shaded area is 68%
of the total area)

Figure 10–2. Area of one standard deviation.

be more easily detected and understood. In the rare case that an author would provide the actual data set as part of their study, one could take the raw data and standardize it to a scale in another study. For example, a study that used a 0 to 10 visual analog scale (VAS) for pain therapy could be compared to another study that used a 0 to 5 scale that was not specifically the VAS. The pain data could be compared once both scales were standardized to provide similar results.

Statistical Inference

Inferential statistics are used to determine the likelihood that a conclusion, based on the analysis of the data from a sample, is true and represents the population studied.

CENTRAL LIMIT THEOREM

An essential component of using inferential statistics is knowing whether the variable being studied is normally distributed in the population. In most cases, researchers do not really know this fact. So, in order to use various statistical tests appropriately, an assumption is made that the variable or item being studied is normally distributed in the population. This is where the central limit theorem takes on a critical role in determining the type of statistical tests that can be applied. If the central limit theorem is correctly applied, the researchers do not really need to know if the study variables are normally distributed.

The central limit theorem states that when equally sized samples are drawn from a non-normal distribution, the mean values from those samples will form a normal distribution. With repeated sampling of size n samples, the mean value from each one of these samples when plotted will form a normal distribution. Therefore, the central limit theorem states that with a large enough sample size, an assumption can be made about the distribution being normal. A large enough sample size, according to the central limit theorem, is usually considered greater than 30. One should be careful and not confuse the issue of large enough for statistical purposes (central limit theorem) and large enough of a sample to be representative of the population, including large enough to be powered to detect differences in the data. For further review of the issues related to sample size and power to detect clinical differences in data, refer to Chaps. 6 and 7.

When looking at the distribution of the sample means as is done with the central limit theorem, the standard deviation of the sample means can be calculated. This standard deviation of the sample means is referred to as the standard error of the mean (SEM). The SEM is equal to the standard deviation divided by the square root of the sample size. The standard deviation reflects how close the values cluster to the sample mean, whereas the SEM indicates how close the repeated samples' mean scores are from the population mean. It is important in evaluating the medical literature to distinguish between the standard deviation and the SEM. Researchers often use the SEM to show variability instead of appropriately using the standard deviation. Obviously, the SEM will be a smaller number than the standard deviation, which makes the data look less variable and more appealing. Unfortunately, it is the wrong measure of dispersion.[4]

PARAMETRIC VERSUS NONPARAMETRIC TESTING

After determining whether a variable is normally distributed or the researchers have applied the central limit theorem, it is important to focus on whether the research requires a parametric or nonparametric test. Often in the statistical methods used within the medical literature, the use of a parametric or nonparametric test is inappropriately applied. In most cases, a parametric test is used when a nonparametric method should have been applied. The essential aspect is to ensure the assumptions are met for performing that statistical test.

When selecting a statistical test for evaluating data there are several assumptions that one makes about the variable or variables. The type of assumptions made determine whether the data are to be analyzed by parametric or nonparametric statistical testing. If an erroneous assumption has been made, often the inappropriate statistical test has been performed.

Basic assumptions for a parametric test include the following:

1. The variable is normally distributed or an assumption is made based on a large enough sample size to consider the variable normally distributed (central limit theorem).
2. The variable is continuous or, if it is discrete, it at least approximates a normal distribution.
3. The variable is measured on an interval or ratio scale.

If the data do not meet these basic assumptions, a nonparametric test rather than a parametric test should be used to analyze the data. Nonparametric tests are considered to be distribution-free methods and are also useful in analyzing nominal and ordinal scale data.

The key to understanding the major differences between parametric and nonparametric tests is that parametric statistical tests require interval or ratio level data and nonparametric tests can be used for nominal and ordinal data. A researcher may have interval or ratio level data, but may still not meet the first assumption for parametric testing. In this case, interval or ratio data would have to be analyzed using a nonparametric test (parametric and nonparametric tests will be described later in this chapter).[4-7]

HYPOTHESIS TESTING

A hypothesis is a contention about some outcome that the researcher is interested in studying. Further information on developing a hypothesis can be found in Chap. 6. A hypothesis may or may not be true, but is assumed to be true until otherwise proven differently with evidence; it is a contention about a population. The null hypothesis is the hypothesis of no difference, meaning that the assumption is made that there is no difference in the purported outcome between the different study groups, and the alternate hypothesis (often referred to as the research hypothesis) is the hypothesis of difference (an outcome difference exists between the study groups). A study is performed to determine whether this contention is true. A representative sample is drawn from the population to estimate the population parameters. These estimates are then tested to see whether the contention is indeed true or false. In answering this contention, statistical or significance testing is performed.

When establishing the hypothesis, the researchers often need to determine whether they are writing a hypothesis that involves a one-sided or two-sided test. When writing a hypothesis it is necessary for the researcher to determine whether he or she is looking for any difference, whether it is greater or smaller, or whether the difference will only occur in a single direction. If the researcher is looking for any difference, it is considered a two-sided test. A specific difference in only one direction uses a one-sided test. The previous example using a calcium channel blocker would be a two-sided test, because the study is testing whether the calcium channel blocker had either raised or lowered blood glucose. If the researcher had been interested specifically in a calcium channel blocker causing only an increase in blood glucose in insulin-dependent diabetics, this would have been a one-sided test. Two-sided tests are considered to be statistically stronger, because they are harder to prove and are the test of choice for clinical trials.

ERRORS

It is essential that researchers establish how much error they are willing to accept before the initiation of the study. Refer to Chap. 6 for a review of Type I and Type II errors and their acceptable values.

SIGNIFICANCE

Once alpha (Type I) error has been established and the data collected, a researcher is interested in knowing whether to accept or reject the null hypothesis. Once the appropriate statistical test has been selected, a p value is calculated. The p value is the probability of obtaining a result as extreme or more extreme than the actual sample value obtained given that the null hypothesis is true. Some statisticians refer to the p value as the actual probability of an alpha error.

If the p value is less than the alpha value established (usually 0.05, although it may be 0.01 or even 0.001), the null hypothesis is rejected and the difference between the groups is considered statistically significant. If the p value is equal to or greater than the alpha value established, the null hypothesis is accepted and the difference between the groups is not considered statistically significant. The smaller the p value, the greater the statistical significance. The smaller the p value, the less likely that the test statistic occurred by chance and that an actual difference exists between the groups. Researchers should include the actual p value in their reports.

Establishing a confidence interval, which will sometimes be used by researchers instead of expressing p values, can also test significance. The p value is a probability of the outcome of the study occurring by chance alone, while the confidence interval is a range of values in which there is confidence that the population parameter being measured is actually contained. Generally, either a 95% or 99% confidence interval is reported. When a study is observing the differences between two treatments, a difference in the mean values can be reported by a confidence interval. In theory, if the difference in mean values were calculated between all possible study groups in the population, the 95% confidence interval would contain the true difference 95% of the time. As an example, a study may have reported that drug A decreased blood pressure an average of 8 mm Hg more than drug B with a confidence interval (this could be either a 95% or 99% confidence interval, depending on what the authors set) of a −4 to 16 mm Hg decrease in blood pressure. In this example, because the confidence interval contains a value of 0, it is not possible to reject the null hypothesis (stating there is no difference between the two treatments). This is where readers must use their professional judgment. This is an excellent example of how results are statistically significant, but readers may question the clinical significance of the values. Refer to Chaps. 6 and 7 for further discussions of this topic.

It is important when evaluating significance to keep in mind that statistical significance does not always correlate to clinical significance. What is proven statistically may not make a difference clinically. For example, with a large enough sample size, the researchers may have been able to prove that a calcium channel blocker caused a statistically significant difference in blood glucose in insulin-dependent diabetes mellitus patients. However, on examining the data, they may have found that the difference in blood glucose was 5 mg/dL. Clinically is this a significant difference? Probably not. Other things that may be taken into consideration when evaluating clinical and statistical significance include costs, adverse effects, quality of life, and actual morbidity and mortality numbers within the study.

STATISTICAL TESTS

Once the basic assumptions have been considered, it is time to determine whether the appropriate statistical tests have been used. The statistical tests will be covered in the order in which they are most commonly seen in the literature. Whenever a parametric test is reviewed, the nonparametric equivalent will also be discussed. Refer to Table 10–1 to help put the statistical tests into perspective.

Most statistical hypothesis testing includes the following sequence of steps. It is essential when evaluating the medical literature to determine whether the researchers have followed these steps.

1. Clearly state the research question.
2. Consider the characteristics of the sample and the variables in question. On what scale is the variable measured? What is the distribution of the variable? Is it known or can a normal distribution be assumed?
3. State the null hypothesis and the alternative hypothesis. Do the data require a one-sided or two-sided test?
4. Set alpha and beta errors.
5. Based on your answers to numbers 2, 3, and 4, what type of statistical test should be used (see Table 10–1)?
6. After data collection, calculate the test statistic.
7. Determine the p value or the confidence interval in order to accept or reject the null hypothesis.

TABLE 10-1. OVERVIEW OF STATISTICAL TESTS

Type of Data	Two Independent Samples	Two Related Samples (Paired/Matched)	Three or More Independent Samples	Three or More Related Samples (Paired/Matched)
Nominal	Chi-square	McNemar		Chi-square
Ordinal	Mann-Whitney U	Sign test Wilcoxon signed ranks	Kruskal-Wallis	Friedman
Interval or ratio	Parametric t-test	Parametric paired t-test	Parametric ANOVA	Parametric ANOVA Repeated measures
	Nonparametric Mann-Whitney U	Nonparametric Wilcoxon signed ranks	Nonparametric Kruskal-Wallis	Nonparametric Friedman

COMPARING TWO GROUPS

Parametric Tests

t-Test for Independent Samples

The t-test for independent samples (also referred to as the Student's t-test) is a statistical method used to test for differences between the means of the two independent groups. The null hypothesis assumes that the means of the two populations are equal. This test statistic can be used to compare two groups of equal sample size or two unequal sample size groups. The equations differ slightly but both rely on the following assumptions.

Assumptions:

1. The two samples are random samples drawn from two independent populations of interest.
2. The measured variable is approximately normally distributed and is continuous.
3. The variable is measured on an interval or ratio scale (for example, the effect on blood glucose levels or a difference in white blood cell counts).
4. The variances of the two groups are similar; this is known as the requirement of homogeneity of variance. This can be difficult sometimes for the reader to determine. This really needs to be described in the materials and methods section by the researcher. Otherwise, the reader will have to look at demographic data provided by the authors to determine how similar the study groups really are. Studies that do not provide this type of information should be questioned.

A t-test can still be performed if there is a violation of the last assumption. If the variances are shown to be different, a t-test that does not pool the variances is used.

t-Test for Matched or Paired Data

If there is a violation of the first assumption, a different type of t-test is performed. In medical research, paired or matched data are often used. Matching or pairing data is a good way to control for issues that may confound or confuse the data. In pairing data, the same subject is used to collect data for both groups. In many instances, a crossover design is used so that the same subject receives all treatments. A good example of paired data is a pretest, and posttest design. For example, if a group of students are given a pretest, testing their therapeutic knowledge prior to rotations, and then provided a posttest after rotations, a researcher would pair their pretest scores with their posttest scores for statistical purposes. In matching data, the subjects from one group are matched on certain factors or conditions relevant to the study to a subject in the other group. For example, in the study with the calcium channel blockers and diabetes, the researcher may find it helpful to match age, gender, and age at first diagnosis between the two groups. Therefore, the data from the two groups are no longer independent because they have been matched or paired. In addition to matching subjects between groups, researchers can also use a crossover design that allows the same subject to receive more than one treatment within a study. The researchers will use the same study subject as their own control as part of the crossover design. When this design is used it is similar to the pretest/posttest design and also requires a paired t-test. When the first assumption is violated and the samples are no longer independent, a paired t-test is the appropriate statistical test.

A common error often made by researchers is the use of the t-test when they are studying more than two groups (comparing two groups at a time). The t-test can be used only when comparing two groups. When looking at more than two groups other tests such as ANOVA are appropriate.[8–10]

Nonparametric Equivalents to t-Tests
For Independent Samples
Mann-Whitney U Test

The nonparametric Mann-Whitney U test can be used when data are measured on an ordinal scale, are not normally distributed or when the variable is discrete. In this situation, the t-test is not appropriate to compare the samples, but the Mann-Whitney U test can be used in its place.

For Matched or Paired Samples
Sign Test

The sign test is a nonparametric test used with paired or matched ordinal data. The sign test involves determining if there is a positive (+) or negative (−) difference between the pairs (i.e., which treatment was better or worse than the other). The test involves determining if the probability of the + and −− values is actually occurring. If the sign test is statistically significant, it shows that a larger portion of the data were either positive (one treatment was better than the other) or negative (one treatment was worse than the other). Otherwise, if the sign test is not statistically significant, then the treatment groups would be deemed equal.

Wilcoxon Signed Ranks Matched Pairs Test

This nonparametric test can be used when data are matched or paired, but do not meet assumptions 2, 3, and 4 for the parametric paired t-test. When paired or matched data are measured on an ordinal scale or the variable is not normally distributed within the population, the Wilcoxon signed ranks test can be used as the test statistic. This test is often preferred over the sign test because it reflects the magnitude of difference between the pairs. This test actually requires a rank order of the differences of the pairs and provides a rank order of the positive and negative differences.[7–10]

COMPARING MORE THAN TWO GROUPS

Parametric

Analysis of Variance (ANOVA)

The null hypothesis of ANOVA assumes that the means of the various groups being compared in the study are not different. In testing the null hypothesis, it is not possible to simply compare the mean of each group with every other mean, but rather it is necessary to use the ANOVA to partition the variance in a set of data into various components. The test then determines the contribution of each of these components to the overall variation. The components compared include the total variance for the complete data set, the variance within each group of the data set, and the variance between each group within the data set. The error within each group is called the error variance. The total variance is compared to the error variance. If there is a large difference in this comparison, it is attributed to a difference between groups, which can be related to the treatment or intervention. In certain types of ANOVA designs, the main effect of a variable can be contrasted with interactions between variables. The main effect is the effect of the variable by itself on the outcome and an interaction is defined as two variables whose relationship with each other explains the outcome.

The test statistic calculated for ANOVA is the F statistic. As with the t-test, there are several different types of ANOVA testing that depend on the experimental design. The assumptions for all types of ANOVA are the same.

Assumptions:

1. Each of the groups is a random sample from the population of interest.
2. The measured variable is continuous.
3. The variable is measured on a ratio or interval scale.
4. The error variances are equal.
5. The variable is approximately normally distributed.

The first assumption cannot be violated. If assumptions 2 through 5 cannot be met, one should consider a nonparametric test equivalent, such as the Kruskal-Wallis or Friedman test.

Types of ANOVA Tests

Completely Randomized Design ANOVA with Fixed Effects

This test involves a random assignment of subjects to various treatment groups, but the investigator chooses the treatments for each group. For example, if researchers wanted to compare the cardiovascular side effects of tricyclic antidepressants (TCAs), patients would be randomly assigned to groups, but the researchers would assign which TCA each group would receive.

Completely Randomized Design ANOVA with Random Effects

This test includes random assignment of subjects with random treatment effects. Compared to the previous example, the patients would be randomly assigned to groups and the treatment with TCAs would be random as well.

Randomized Complete Blocks Design ANOVA

This test is also referred to as a two-way ANOVA without replication. Individuals are blocked or grouped according to the characteristic whose variance one wishes to identify. The treatments are chosen for each group. With the TCA example, individuals in the study would be blocked based on a specific characteristic, such as their cardiovascular side effect profile (electrocardiogram [ECG] changes), and then the researchers would assign treatments with TCA after the side effect profile was controlled (blocked).

Randomized Complete Blocks Design ANOVA with Repeated Measures

With this test, the same individual is used for the repeated measurement. This is similar to the paired t-test, but more than two measurements are involved. This test would be the same, as the preceding example, except each patient would receive each treatment. In other words, each patient would serve as his or her own control and receive all treatments.

Factorial Design ANOVA

When two or more factors interact with each other to produce either synergistic or antagonistic effects, the factorial design is appropriate. This test is also referred to as the two-way ANOVA with replication. If the TCA example was taken one step further, the effect that benzodiazepine therapy had on the TCA-induced cardiovascular side effects would be studied using this design. In this example, there are two factors that need to be considered in the statistical test. One factor is the cardiovascular side effects and the other is the effect of benzodiazepine therapy. This statistical test looks at the interaction of cardiovascular side effects with benzodiazepine therapy and how that changed the results related to treatment with a TCA. For example, the researcher might want to know if benzodiazepine offered any protective effect against cardiovascular side effects when a patient was taking a TCA.

Types of Post Hoc Comparisons

After getting a significant ANOVA result, a researcher knows that there is a difference among the means of the different groups. Sometimes this is all that is necessary for the research. At other times, the researcher may be interested in knowing which group is different from the others. To answer this question, the researcher can do several post hoc comparisons to compare the means of the groups two at a time. This is very different from performing separate t-tests between each group (a common medical literature error). Rather than using separate t-tests, there are several types of post hoc comparison tests that can be used with ANOVA. The reason post hoc tests are used rather than separate t-tests is that the post hoc tests correct for the multiple error rates that would be associated with running the separate t-tests.

It is important to realize that some post hoc tests are more conservative than others, meaning they have less error associated with them. Post hoc procedures are very complex tests and there are subtle differences between the various tests. Readers who want to understand more about post hoc tests would be advised to find a good textbook devoted to just ANOVA testing. The following tests are all post hoc procedures that may be cited in the literature: Bonferroni correction, Scheffé method, Tukey Least Significant Difference, Dunnett, and Newman-Kuels.[8–10]

Nonparametric Tests

The following tests are forms of nonparametric statistics that can be used when assumptions for parametric testing cannot be used. These are essential tests for ordinal and/or nominal data and when normal distribution cannot be assumed.

Kruskal-Wallis One-Way ANOVA

This is the nonparametric counterpart to the ANOVA with a completely randomized design. When data do not fit the assumptions for a parametric test, this would be a reasonable nonparametric alternative. The data need to be at least measured on an ordinal scale. Nominal data are not appropriate for this type of statistical test. In addition, the samples must still be drawn from independent populations (meaning they should not be paired or matched).

Friedman Two-Way ANOVA

This is the nonparametric counterpart to the randomized complete block design. Like the Kruskal-Wallis, the data need to be of at least an ordinal scale.[8–10]

DESCRIBING THE RELATIONSHIP BETWEEN TWO OR MORE VARIABLES

Correlation and Regression

Correlation and regression are used when there is an interest in exploring the relationship between two or more variables. These analyses are applied to data to quantify and define the relationship between the variables. An example may be the relationship between estrogen use and cervical cancer. Correlation analysis allows for a quantitative measurement indicating the strength of the relationship between two variables. Correlation helps to determine whether there is an association between two variables and also indicate the strength of the association. In this description, association is one way of saying that one variable changes in a consistent manner when the other variable changes. Correlation analysis does not assume a cause and effect relationship. For example, creatinine and blood urea nitrogen (BUN) may vary in relationship to one another, but BUN does not go up because creatinine goes up. Instead, both are going up because of increasing renal failure. In comparison, regression analysis is used to mathematically describe the relationship, such as predicting one variable from other variables. Regression analysis or linear regression usually assumes some type of cause and effect relationship. In regression analysis, the independent variable or variables explain the dependent variable. When more than one independent variable is analyzed the technique is known as multiple linear regression.

Correlation

In correlation analysis, the following questions are asked:

1. Are the two variables related in some consistent and linear fashion?
2. What is the strength of the relationship between the two variables?

The measure of the strength of the relationship is the correlation coefficient, often referred to as Pearson correlation coefficient or Pearson product moment coefficient. The sample correlation coefficient is usually symbolized by a small r.

The null hypothesis for correlation analysis is that r will be equal to 0, meaning that there is no correlation or linear relationship. If r is not equal to 0, some relationship exists. The value of r is important in determining the strength of the relationship and is a dimensionless number that varies from 0 (no relationship) to positive or negative one (strongest relationship). Therefore, if r is close to 0, a weak relationship exists; if r is closer to positive or negative 1, a stronger relationship exists. A positive 1 depicts a perfect positive linear relationship, indicating that as one variable changes the other changes in the same direction. Likewise, a negative 1 indicates a perfect negative linear relationship in which as one variable changes the other changes in an inverse fashion.

Assumptions:

1. Random sample from the population of interest.
2. Variables are normally distributed.
3. Variables measured on an interval or ratio scale.
4. If a relationship exists, the relationship is linear.

Remember that correlation does not mean causation. Two variables may be correlated, but that does not mean that one variable can be predicted from the other variable.

Regression

In regression analysis, the hypothesis is that there is a functional relationship that allows prediction of a value of the dependent variable corresponding to a value of the independent variable. Mathematically, a regression equation is developed that indicates that the dependent variable is a function of the independent variable. This concept is frequently seen in pharmacy-related information: for example, the relationship between the dose of gentamicin and the blood level of gentamicin. A graph can be drawn with the data and a linear regression line can be predicted from the graph. Therefore, regression analysis approximates an equation that describes the linear relationship between two variables (regression equation) and constructs a line through the data points in a graphic presentation (regression or least squares line). Regression analysis answers the question of what proportion of the variance in the dependent variable is explained or described by the independent variable. In regression analysis, the coefficient of determination, also known as r^2 (the square of the correlation coefficient), is the indicator of explained variance. The coefficient of determination describes the proportion of variance in the dependent variable explained by the independent variable. The coefficient of determination varies from 0 to 1, and the closer to 1, the greater the amount that variance in the dependent variable is explained by the independent variable. An example would be how much does hypertension explain the variation in left ventricular hypertrophy (LVH)? In looking at left ventricular size, how much of this size change can be related to or explained by the individual's blood pressure? For example, researchers could discover that 60% of the changes that occur in left ventricular size are directly related to the individual's blood pressure.

Assumptions:

1. The independent variable is fixed and does not represent a random variable in the population.
2. Dependent variable is normally distributed.
3. Observations are independent.

Simple Linear Regression

Simple linear regression is when there is only one dependent variable with only one independent variable being analyzed. Within this test, the independent variable is analyzed to determine how much it explains the change or variance in the dependent variable. The example above of LVH and hypertension is representative of a simple linear regression. It would help answer the question, how much does hypertension explain or predict LVH?

Multiple Linear Regression

Multiple regression is similar to simple linear regression, except that there is one dependent variable with more than one independent variable. Multiple regression is used when a more complex problem exists that involves multiple variables to predict the dependent variable. An example of multiple regression would be the effect that stress and vitamin intake has on blood glucose levels. One of the problems to be aware of in multiple regression is the possibility that the independent variables may be intercorrelated, such that one independent variable has some relationship with another independent variable. A correlation analysis is often done to determine whether the independent variables are correlated to one another. If a relationship exists between the independent variables, it is often referred to as multicollinearity. In the example of LVH, researchers may be interested in more than just the relationship to blood pressure. They may also want to consider the relationship of LDL cholesterol, exercise capacity, and blood pressure. The study may indicate that blood pressure explains 60%, LDL cholesterol 20%, and exercise capacity 8%. This would help the researchers to understand the relationship these variables have in explaining changes in left ventricular size. It would also demonstrate that blood pressure is a stronger factor than LDL cholesterol or exercise capacity. Notice that these numbers do not add up to 100%. This outcome is common in regression analysis, where other factors explain partly but not all of the changes. Often the researchers do not know what the other factors are, or additional factors may need to be included in future studies to determine their contributions. Sometimes when doing regression analysis, a certain study variable may not explain any variance or less than 2% of the variance; this variable is considered to be unrelated or not predictive of the outcome (dependent variable).[6,8–10]

Nonparametric Tests for Correlation and Regression
Correlation Tests
Nominal Data

There are three nonparametric measures of association for nominal data. These include the contingency coefficient, the phi coefficient, and Cohen's kappa coefficient. When looking at the correlation or association between nominal variables, the tests involve the degree of frequency expressed within categories. The contingency coefficient involves the use of chi-square. It is actually the square root of the chi-square statistic divided by the chi-square statistic added to the sample size. One noted problem with this measure is that even with a perfect relationship, the coefficient will never be one. The phi coefficient is a ratio of the quantities found in a 2×2 contingency table. The 2×2 contingency table has four cells labeled from a to d. The equation for phi is $(ad – bc)/bc$. The kappa coefficient also involves the 2×2 contingency table. This measure adjusts for error in data. So the equation for kappa is equal to the observed agreement (from the table) minus chance agreement divided by 1 minus the chance agreement. The kappa coefficient is often considered the most desirable measure for a 2×2 table. Usually researchers who use nominal data will just use descriptive data to discuss the results of the study, it can add strength to the data when these coefficient measures are used. These measures help the reader to make some inferences about the strength of the association between the study variables. They provide a better way to show some cause and effect rather than just looking at data presented as mere percentages. For example, a reader might find it helpful to know that the coefficient shows a strong correlation between the study variable and the outcome versus knowing that 52% of the sample responded to the medication.

Ordinal Data

There are three nonparametric measures of association for ordinal data. The three measures are Spearman rank correlation, Kendall tau coefficient, and Kendall W coefficient. Spearman's r or Spearman's rank r is the nonparametric equivalent to Pearson's r. When data are measured on an ordinal scale or when other parametric assumptions are not met, Spearman's r would be the appropriate test. Spearman correlation is based on the differences in the ranks of paired data. Kendall's tau can be used for the same type of data as one would use Spearman's r. However, Kendall's tau does not require the mathematical calculations that Spearman's requires. Kendall's tau relies on counting the ranks and comparing them to see if they are in the right order. Kendall's W is utilized when there are multiple observations. For example, if you were looking to see the extent of agreement between three different observers of faculty teaching, you may have observations from the students, from the department chairs, and from peer faculty members. Kendall's W allows for the sum of the ranks of the different observers. This helps the reader to understand how consistent the multiple observers were in rating the outcome. This is especially crucial in study designs that require multiple observers to evaluate fairly subjective data. If all of the observer ranks were similar to one another, the reader would be able to put more faith in the outcomes than if the observer ranks varied widely from one another.

Nonparametric Regression Tests
Logistic Regression

Logistic regression is similar to linear regression. The difference is that logistic regression does not require the dependent variable or outcome variable to be measured on an interval or ratio scale. In the medical literature, the dependant variable is often measured on an ordinal scale. In this case, logistic regression would be preferred to linear regression. Logistic regression can be used when assumption 2 of linear regression is not met. Logistic regression can be performed as simple logistic regression (one dependent variable and one independent variable) or as multiple logistic regression (one dependent variable and more than one independent variables). Logistic regression also provides odds ratios for the data determining outcome measures of risk. For example, a researcher would like to consider what factors (independent variables) cause an increased risk of myocardial infarction (ordinal scale dependent or outcome variable) in male adults less than 40 years of age. A researcher might consider factors such as cholesterol level, exercise activity, and family history as important independent variables. The researcher could use logistic regression to analyze the data. Logistic regression would be able to provide the reader with how each one of these variables contributed to the outcome of acute myocardial infarction. In addition, this method gives the odds ratio for each variable. This gives the reader some perspective on which of these variables might be the most important factor in the whole equation.

Log-Linear Analysis

Log-linear analysis is used to analyze categorical variables to determine if an effect exists among the variables. Log-linear analysis treats all variables as categorical variables. Log-linear analysis tries to determine if there is an association between the dependent variable, the independent variables, and the interaction of independent variables. As with certain ANOVA models, log-linear analysis allows the researcher to look at the main effects of each variable and likewise, analyze the interaction effects between the variables. In considering the example provided above for logistic regression, the advantage of log-linear analysis would be the ability to establish interactions between the variables. For example, how does one's family history interact with one's cholesterol values to determine the outcome of acute myocardial infarction.

Analysis of Covariance

Analysis of covariance (ANCOVA) is a technique that is used to analyze independent variables that include both categorical data and interval level data. ANOVA and regression are two methods that can be used for interval level data. ANCOVA provides a way to combine ANOVA and regression techniques when research involves categorical independent variables. ANCOVA can be a useful test when researchers want to adjust for baseline differences among the different treatment groups or therapies. An important assumption that must be met prior to doing ANCOVA is that there is no relationship between the covariate and the treatment variables. A good example of a study design that would lend itself to an ANCOVA test would be if a researcher wants to determine what effect three different calcium channel blockers may have on left ventricular ejection fraction, controlling for the independent variable of gender. Gender would be the covariate and the treatment would be the drug therapy. The assumption would be made that gender was not correlated with the drug therapy of a calcium channel blocker. In addition, ANCOVA can be performed with multiple covariates within a particular study design. In the previous example, the study may have also included ethnic background as a covariate.[5,7,10]

OTHER NONPARAMETRIC TESTS

Chi-square

Chi-square is the most commonly reported and used nonparametric statistical test. This test can be used with one or more groups and compares the actual number within a group to the expected number for that same group. The expected number is based on theory, previous experience, or comparison groups. Chi-square tests are used to answer research questions related to rates, proportions, or frequencies. Chi-square analysis is an appropriate test for evaluating nominal and ordinal data; however, it is probably most useful in analyzing nominal data (i.e., categorical data such as male and female). When evaluating ordinal data, other methods that preserve the ranking may be preferred over chi-square.

Assumptions:

1. Frequency data.
2. The measures are independent of one another.
3. Categorization of the variables or that the variables are best described by placing them into categories.

Contingency Tables

Categorical data are often arranged in a table consisting of columns and rows with individual data fitting into one of the designated squares. The rows represent the categories of one variable and the columns represent the categories of the other variable. The chi-square test is essentially the comparison of the expected frequencies in each cell compared to the actual or observed frequencies in those same cells. If the frequencies from the observed to the expected are significantly different, the independent variable had some effect on the dependent variable. This chi-square test is also known as the chi-square test of association. The most common contingency table is the 2×2 table. An example is cigarette smoking and its effect on lung cancer. The rows would be cases with lung cancer and controls without lung cancer. The columns would be exposure to the risk factor cigarette smoking or nonexposure to the risk factor cigarette smoking. The 2×2 contingency table would appear as the following:

		Lung cancer	
		Yes	No
Cigarette smoking	Yes	Number of patients	Number of patients
	No	Number of patients	Number of patients

The researcher would then compare the expected with the observed to determine whether cigarette smoking contributed to lung cancer.[7,10]

Other Methods of Inference for Categorical Data

Fisher Exact Test

Sometimes in performing a study, a cell within the matrix will have an expected frequency of less than five or the sample size may be small; the most appropriate type of analysis for this case is called a Fisher Exact Test. This situation usually occurs when the number of people being studied or the number of individuals who are expected to have a particular outcome is small. It is important to remember that it is the expected cell frequency and not the actual cell frequencies observed that will determine whether the Fisher exact test should be used. A researcher should be able to calculate the expected cell frequency before collecting the data.

McNemar's Test (Paired or Matched Data)

The usual chi-square test cannot be used for paired or matched data, because this violates the assumption of independence. Therefore, when matched or paired nominal data are collected as part of the research design, the appropriate statistical test is McNemar test. In the lung cancer study, if the subjects were matched for gender, paired data would be placed in the contingency table and a McNemar test could be performed.

Mantel-Haenszel Test

The Mantel-Haenszel test is necessary when analyzing stratified data. In performing research, it may often be necessary to stratify data based on some factor that may be confounding or confusing the data. In the lung cancer example, what would the effect be of passive smoke on the rate of lung cancer? Were any of the nonsmokers or smokers also exposed to passive smoke? In this case, the researchers would stratify the data based on exposure to passive smoke. Therefore, the data would be presented as two separate 2 × 2 contingency tables. One table would be for passive smoke exposure and the other for no exposure to passive smoke.[7,10]

Other Nonparametric Tests

SURVIVAL ANALYSIS

There are four basic assumptions that must be met prior to doing survival analysis. They are the following:

1. Each person must have an identified starting point and each subject at this point should be as similar as possible in the diagnosis of the illness (i.e., length of Type I diabetes since diagnosis).
2. A clearly defined outcome or endpoint.
3. Dropout rates should be independent of the outcome (i.e., loss to follow-up).
4. The diagnostic and therapeutic practices did not change during the observational period.

Survival analysis is done with observational studies in which the outcome variable may have significant variability in the time it takes to reach the defined outcome. This outcome could be a time period that a subject takes to develop the disease state of interest or it could be an outcome such as death. This outcome could occur at anytime within the study time-frame or sometimes may not occur at all within the allocated time for the study. Sometimes within these observational study designs, enrollment may take place over a specified period of time (i.e., 3 months or 3 years). Not all subjects enter at time 0. In addition, subjects may also drop out of the study or be lost to follow-up. Typically when these situations happen, survival analysis is preferred and used to analyze these types of data because survival analysis will place each subject at time 0 and follow them until the designated outcome is met or the study ends, whichever comes first. Some common examples of this type of study analysis would include things like the timeframe to develop complications as it relates to diabetes or 5-year survival rates for cancer after treatment with chemotherapy or radiation.

There are two methods of looking at survival data. The first is referred to as the actuarial method for survival analysis. This method takes fixed time periods or endpoints. So a researcher could pick fixed time periods, such as 6 months, 1 and 2 years. With this method, the number of patients who have survived to these endpoints are counted. This method does not account for actual days, months, or years of survival, just who reaches that endpoint. So a subject could die at 5 months and 29 days and not be included in the 6-month analysis. The second technique is called the Kaplan-Meier survival analysis. The advantage to this method is that the actual length of time is measured for the endpoint or outcome. In the previous example, the subject who died at 5 months and 29 days would be in the analysis. Kaplan-Meier is considered to be superior to the actuarial method, especially when the sample size is less than 50.

Cox's Proportional Hazards Model

Adjusting survival data based on subject differences at the beginning of the study can be accomplished in one of two ways. If a researcher is concerned about group differences as it relates to a covariate that is a dichotomous variable (such as gender), then a Mantel-Haenszel test can be performed by stratifying for the variable. If a researcher is concerned about group differences at baseline that relate to a covariate that is measured on a continuous scale then Cox's proportional hazards model is used. This technique allows researchers to look at survival data and adjust for differences in the groups such as age or blood levels. In many cases, Cox's proportional hazards model can provide a better analysis of survival data by controlling for confounding issues or by showing differences in survival by baseline characteristics. For example, since survival data can depend on so many different factors than just treatment type, a researcher would use Cox's proportional hazards to try and control for as many confounding issues (such as tumor size, tumor staging, age of patient, and other comorbid conditions) so that they could identify what affect the treatment had on the cancer survival outcome.

MULTIVARIATE ANALYSIS

Multivariate analysis is a means to study multiple dependent variables simultaneously versus the univariate techniques previously described in this chapter, which allow for only one dependent variable to be analyzed at a time. The multivariate technique is a superior technique for handling multiple dependent variables, rather than performing multiple univariate tests to determine the significance of each dependent variable independent of each other. In the calcium channel blocker example, the researcher may be interested in two outcomes of the drug therapy. The outcomes or dependent variables could be systolic blood pressure and blood glucose levels. With the univariate t-test, these two dependent variables would be analyzed separately from each other. Whereas, a multivariate technique would be more appropriate because often the two dependent variables when measured for the same person can be correlated to each other.

Discriminate Function Analysis

Discriminate function analysis is used when the researcher wants to account for differences among the variables. This analysis is also a multivariate technique that has multiple dependent variables. What discriminate function analysis tries to do for the researcher is to indicate which variables are the most important ones in explaining the differences in the groups. Therefore, it tries to find the variables that best discriminate between the groups. This technique can be used with two or more than two groups. Wilks lambda is used to test for statistical significance (establish a p value). Discriminate function analysis can be done after finding a statistically significant value for data analyzed using other statistical tests. This type of test can help to discriminate which variables explained the differences noted. This statistical test has gained some popularity because of its ability to take multiple study variables and statistically pull out the most essential variables to describe the data. This method should be looked at as a means to eliminate nonessential variables and find a way to focus on the ones that really explain or describe the data. An example would be if a pharmacy college wanted to see what variables predict which graduates pursue residency programs. The college could collect different variables about their students over a period of time and then look at those who chose residencies and those who did not. By doing a discriminate function analysis, they would be able to better predict what variables or factors appeared to explain a student's desire to do a residency versus those variables that explained why someone did not chose a residency option.

Factor Analysis

Factor analysis is a multivariate technique that can be used to explore patterns in data, confirm researchers' suggested hypotheses, or reduce correlated variables into related factors. A factor is an underlying related phenomena that more than one variable may help to explain. In factor analysis, a model is developed that explores the relationship of the variables to the factors and the factors to the dependent (outcome) variables. This model can be developed by the researcher prior to undertaking the research as part of a theory (*a priori*) and then be used to test the accuracy of the proposed (hypothesized) model. In addition to trying to prove a hypothesized model, factor analysis can be used to develop a model after the factor analysis has been done by the researcher depending on the statistical reporting of the tests. For example, a researcher may be trying to identify what factors affect a pharmacist's ability to counsel a patient. Researchers may decide that there are three factors that they feel influence patient counseling by the pharmacist. They title these factors as patient demographics, pharmacy setting, and communication skills. The researcher may decide to measure the following variables to help explain the factor described as pharmacy setting: the number of prescriptions waiting, FTE technician help, number of phone lines into the pharmacy, location of the pharmacy within the store, and/or the public's access to the pharmacist. After measuring each of these variables, the statistical program will produce a correlation matrix for the variables and also give what is termed *factor loadings*. This matrix and factor loading table provide a means to determine which variables explain a certain factor. The researcher can then decide if their model is sound or if another model should be constructed and tested. The researcher can now design a model based on these known factors and then gather data again to see how well the model works. On testing the model again, the researcher might find that although the model explains some of the aspects of the pharmacy setting other factors maybe necessary or are missing from the equation. The researcher would then have the option of evaluating different factors and continue to refine the model based on factor analysis.[10]

OTHER TYPES OF STUDY DESIGN WITH STATISTICAL ANALYSIS

Meta-Analysis

Meta-analysis is a technique used to perform a study by combining previously published or unpublished data. The researchers combine data from multiple sources (independent clinical trials) and reanalyze the data hoping to strengthen the conclusions. This study design is used to increase the power of a study or improve the effect size (clinical detectable difference) by combining studies. It can be helpful when clinical trials may conflict in their conclusions.[12] Sacks et al. have published six major quality points for meta-analysis studies. These include looking at the (1) study design, (2) ability to combine the data from the studies selected, (3) control bias within studies, (4) statistical analysis, (5) sensitivity analysis, and (6) application of the results from combined studies.[13] It is essential that the authors of the meta-analysis provide explicit criteria for how a study ended up in their analysis. From a statistical standpoint, meta-analysis involves very complex statistical techniques. When looking at a meta-analysis, it is important to analyze two areas. The first is to determine if they did a test of homogeneity. This test tells the reader if the outcome variables used in the different studies were very similar. In other words, did each study that was being combined into the analysis have similar characteristics as it related to the outcome variables? The second area is to determine if they did sensitivity analysis. As with the test of homogeneity, sensitivity testing is also extremely valuable in determining as a reader if the meta-analysis was sound. Sensitivity analysis is a means for the researchers to determine if certain trials were excluded or included in the study, how would it change the results they found. How would the inclusion or exclusion of trials affect the outcome variables or would it change the test of significance? It is a means to show the reader that the results would have been the same regardless of the inclusion or exclusion criteria of the related studies. Many types of bias can also adversely affect a meta-analysis design. The reader is referred to the drug literature evaluation chapters for the discussion of bias. One way that researchers have found to detect and quantify bias in a meta-analysis has been by using funnel plots. A funnel plot is a graphing of the trials effect size versus the sample size. The results are then plotted against a measure of precision, such as the standard deviation or variance. A funnel shaped plot will form as the precision or similarity of the studies increase. If a funnel shape does not appear or if there is asymmetry in the plot, this may indicate discordance among the different study results selected for the meta-analysis. In general, a good meta-analysis will present homogeneity tests and sensitivity analysis.

Conclusion

Statistics are an integral part of evaluating the medical literature. Understanding the various assumptions is essential to the basic foundation of statistical testing. The reader is encouraged to look at the medical literature and determine whether the basic assumptions have been met. Once this issue has been resolved, refer to Table 10–1 and decide whether the appropriate statistical test was chosen. The correct selection of a statistical test is an integral part of assuring that the research conclusions are accurate. Keep in mind that this chapter is by no means comprehensive for all types of statistical tests. The field of statistics is rapidly changing and different techniques continue to be developed and validated.

Study Questions

1. A researcher is looking at the effect that high pH soil has on the color of soybean leaves. The colors are classified as light green, dark green, blue-green, and yellow-green. What kind of measurement variable is leaf color?

2. A researcher is evaluating 60 patients using a crossover design to determine whether propranolol or hydrochlorothiazide is more effective in managing isolated systolic hypertension. What is the appropriate statistical test to analyze whether there is a difference in the mean blood pressure when using propranolol and hydrochlorothiazide?

3. A researcher has completed a cohort study on the effects of fertilizer on the development of breast cancer in women who live or work on farms. Will the researcher be calculating relative risk or an odds ratio?

4. A study has been performed that evaluates the effect that smoking has on the development of lung cancer. The researcher is looking at smokers versus nonsmokers who did or did not develop lung cancer. However, the researcher wants to stratify the data to look at the effects of passive smoke. What statistical procedure would be best for this type of research question?

5. A study was performed that evaluated the difference in platelet count after patients were treated with heparin, low molecular-weight heparin, and warfarin. Three hundred patients were enrolled and randomly assigned to one of the three treatment groups. What is the best statistical procedure to evaluate the difference between the mean platelet counts?

REFERENCES

1. Gaddis ML, Gaddis GM. Introduction to biostatistics: part 1, basic concepts. Ann Emerg Med. 1990;19:86–9.
2. Gaddis GM, Gaddis ML. Introduction to biostatistics: part 2, descriptive statistics. Ann Emerg Med. 1990;19:309–15.
3. Gaddis GM, Gaddis ML. Introduction to biostatistics: part 3, sensitivity, specificity, predictive value and hypothesis testing. Ann Emerg Med. 1990;19:591–7.
4. Gaddis GM, Gaddis ML. Introduction to biostatistics: part 4, statistical inference techniques in hypothesis testing. Ann Emerg Med. 1990;19:820–5.
5. Gaddis GM, Gaddis ML. Introduction to biostatistics: part 5, statistical inference technique for hypothesis testing with nonparametric data. Ann Emerg Med. 1990;19:1054–9.
6. Gaddis ML, Gaddis GM. Introduction to biostatistics: part 6, correlation and regression. Ann Emerg Med. 1990;19:1462–8.
7. Daniel WW. Applied nonparametric statistics. 2nd ed. Boston (MA): PWS-Kent Publishing Company; 1990.
8. Munro BH, Page EB. Statistical methods for health care research. 2nd ed. Philadelphia (PA): J.B. Lippincott Company; 1993.
9. Elston RC, Johnson WD. Essentials of biostatistics. 2nd ed. Philadelphia (PA): F.A. Davis Company; 1993.
10. Norman GR, Streiner DL. Biostatistics: the bare essentials. Chicago (IL): Mosby; 1993.
11. Hampton RE. Introductory biological statistics. Dubuque (IA): Wm. C. Brown Publishers; 1994.
12. Mancano MA, Bullano MF. Meta-analysis: methodology, utility, and limitations. J Pharm Pract. 1998;11(4):239–50.
13. Sacks HS, Berrier J, Reitman E, Ancona-Berk VA, Chalmers TC. Meta-analyses of randomized controlled trials. N Engl J Med. 1987;316:450–5.

11

Chapter Eleven

Professional Writing

Patrick M. Malone

Objectives

After completing this chapter, the reader will be able to

- State reasons both for and against writing professionally.
- Describe the various steps of professional writing.
- Identify the order for authors in a professional paper.
- Describe the importance of knowing the audience.
- Describe the various writing styles and their differences.
- Explain where to find a publication's requirements for submission.
- Describe what an article proposal consists of and why it is used.
- Explain the need for practice to develop good writing skills.
- List the components of both a research and review paper.
- Explain the general guidelines for writing.
- Describe the peer-review process.
- Explain the absolute importance of revision.
- Explain the steps in creating a newsletter or website.
- Describe how to prepare audiovisual materials for a poster or platform presentation and place those items on a website.
- Describe techniques for creating an abstract for an article.
- Describe how to correctly cite an article in a bibliography.

Introduction

A common thought when considering the topic of professional writing is "That doesn't apply to me, I'm not writing for a journal." But professional writing is certainly not limited to journal articles or books. It includes writing evaluations of medications for consideration on a hospital formulary, preparing written policies and procedures for the preparation of an intravenous admixture, reporting the results of the latest sale to the home office, preparing a written evaluation of a technician or clerk, writing in a chart, writing a term paper for a class, preparing slides or posters for presentation, and many other things. Essentially any time a professional takes pen, pencil, chalk, typewriter, word processor, or any other writing implement in hand to fulfill professional duties, it is considered professional writing. Although the format changes, the general principles remain the same. So whether the object is to write the ultimate book on the practice of pharmacy or to type a label, a pharmacist must know how to write professionally.

Although some may say the purpose of writing is "to keep my job" or "to pass this course," there are, generally, four larger purposes for the existence of written material. That material serves to inform, instruct, persuade, or entertain. The first three items are those usually considered in professional writing, although including the fourth, whenever possible, will help convince people to read what has been written.

There are also some advantages to professional writing besides those mentioned above. For example, writing is often good for promotion in many jobs. In academia, there is always the concept of "publish or perish." Even pharmacy technicians are encouraged to write as a means of advancement.[1] Also, writing gives the authors the opportunity to share their knowledge or ideas, obtain gratification or satisfaction,[2] and improve their knowledge. It may even lead to some fame or notoriety in a field.

Unfortunately, there are disadvantages to professional writing, too. The major problem is that any significant amount of writing often involves a lot of potentially frustrating work because few people are natural writers. The author must practice to become proficient at writing, which will involve false starts, numerous drafts, roadblocks, and other problems.[3] If that is not enough, writing exposes a person to criticism and possible rejection. Although at one time authors were paid to publish articles, today it is not unheard of that authors may actually have to pay to have their article published.[4,5] At best, the direct financial rewards are likely to be few, unless a best-selling novel is produced. Indirectly, writing may lead to pay increases and promotions. However, because writing is a professional necessity, it can be made easier by following the correct procedures, which will be covered in this chapter.

Steps in Writing

As each of the steps in professional writing are covered in this section, the emphasis will be on writing items likely to be encountered in a practice setting, although additional steps necessary when writing for publication will be mentioned.

PREPARING TO WRITE

The first step in writing is to know the purpose—why something needs to be written in the first place. It is necessary at this time to have a good idea of the expected endpoint, which is a good idea, no matter what is being done. For example, someone learning to plow a field with a tractor may be concentrating on the ground near the tractor and end up wandering all over the field, thinking he or she was going straight. However, by concentrating on going to a specific point on the far end of the field, rather than looking just in front of the tractor, the row will probably be plowed fairly straight. Throughout this whole process it is necessary to keep in mind that endpoint, to keep from wandering all over the place. If the item being written is for publication, rather than something required for work, it will also be necessary to pick the topic and, perhaps, submit an article proposal (see Figure 11–1). Although the writing is considered to be more important than the idea, it is still important to have a good idea or important topic before starting.[6] It should also be pointed out that in the case of clinical trial results, it can be important to publish articles showing that something did not work, although in the past such topics have often been avoided.[7] The topic should be of interest and/or importance to the prospective readers. It can even cover an old topic, as long as the topic is covered in greater depth, in a new way, or is addressed to a different group.

It is also necessary to decide whether there needs to be a coauthor. This may be easy to resolve, depending on who is working on the project. However, even if no one else has been involved, it may be a good idea to look for a coauthor. An inexperienced writer would benefit from working with an experienced author, and working with someone will give a different perspective and, hopefully, lessen the work for each person. Finally, it is sometimes a necessity to include coauthors for political reasons (as in "Would you prefer to share the credit or work nights and holidays for the rest of your life?"). Although this last reason should not exist, it does. A variety of other problems with authorship credit are also seen.[8,9] The best that may be fought for under the circumstances may be that everyone must do part of the writing[10] and that authors be listed in the order of their contributions to the project. This does not always happen.[11,12] In some cases, pharmaceutical manufacturers may want "ghost writers" to write an article for the researchers, but even they agree that original authors must prepare the first draft of editorials or opinion pieces, although non-English speaking authors may be assisted by others after that.[13] The "ghost writers" should also be appropriately acknowledged.[7] Although arguments may be made,[14–20] there is no valid reason for people to be listed as an author in excess of their contribution to the writing and submission of the work for publication.[21–25] The only exception would be if the publisher has other specific rules. For example, some journals may want to list "contributors" with an explanation of what they contributed (e.g., writing, origination of study idea, and data collection). Generally, all of the following must be met for an individual to be given credit as an author:[23,24]

- Conception and design of the study, or analysis and interpretation of the data in the study.
- Writing or revising the article.
- Final approval of the version that is published.

Although relatively few professionals write articles for journals or books, those who do need to follow an occasional step in addition to those outlined in the main text of this chapter. One difference is the potential need to write an article proposal to the publisher. This simply is a letter asking the publisher whether he or she would be interested in possibly publishing something on a particular topic written by the person who is inquiring. As might be expected, this step is generally not necessary if writing a description of original research, but would be important when writing a review article or even a descriptive article. The letter should contain certain information, which will be described below, and be addressed to an appropriate editor. If at all possible, it is also a good idea to talk to an editor before submitting your proposal. For example, the proposal for the first edition of this book originated after a discussion with the editor at the Appleton & Lange booth in the ASHP Midyear Clinical Meeting Exhibitor's Area.

In the written proposal, the prospective author should first briefly explain the basic idea that is to be covered in the article or book, including a working title. Similarly, a description of the approach the author wishes to take in covering the subject should be described. Although this description should be kept brief, it must provide enough information for the publisher to determine whether the topic and approach are even appropriate for their journal. In the case of a book, it is important to include a table of contents that is descriptive enough to be useful to reviewers who will be advising the publisher on the need for such a book. Related to that need, it is also necessary to describe why the proposed article or book will be important to the publisher's customers. This is the sales pitch. It is necessary to briefly show that there is nothing similar, or as good, currently available in the literature for the audience being addressed.

Although the above is the meat of the proposal, there are several other items that should be included. These include the time necessary to complete the article/book (be realistic), the approximate length of the work, and a statement of the authors' qualifications, including any previous publications.

There are several good reasons for submitting a proposal. The first is simply to avoid work if the editor decides that there is no need for such a publication (although an author should not hesitate to send the proposal to another publisher, if it still seems that the topic is important). Second, and perhaps most important, it allows the editor(s) to make suggestions. By following those suggestions, an author is more likely to be successful in getting the work published. Finally, if the idea is accepted, the acceptance letter will provide motivation.

Figure 11–1. Article proposal to publishers.

Things that do not qualify a person to be listed as an author include:[24,23]

- Acquisition of funding
- General supervision of the research group

Individuals that do not meet the first qualifications should be listed in the acknowledgments section. Also, the primary author should be able to explain the order the authors are listed in and journals may require one or more authors to be "guarantors," who will be taking responsibility for the work as a whole.[25]

It should also be mentioned that there can be too many authors and acknowledgments.[26] Some scientific papers list many, many authors for a particular paper, and the number of authors has grown over the years.[27] It is obvious that 20 authors could not have written a three-page paper. Some of this may be a result of job requirements that include publishing a certain number of articles, leading to demands by individuals to get their name listed on any article they can. Again, authors should contribute to the written work in some significant way, as defined above. In some cases, it may be necessary to just name the group performing the research, with a few of the most responsible individuals specifically named, and list others as acknowledgments, sometimes by group, institution, or type of contribution.[23,26,28] Others may be listed as "clinical investigators," "participating investigators," "scientific advisors," "data collector," or other appropriate titles.[25]

Before the first word is written, it is necessary to know the audience, which involves knowing the type of person who will be reading the final document and where it will be published. Keep in mind that the word "published" was picked for a specific reason. Whether the final product appears in *New England Journal of Medicine*, the "IV Room Policy and Procedure Book," or even the label on a prescription vial, it is "published." It is necessary to aim the work toward the audience. At a broad level, written work should not be submitted for possible publication in a journal that does not cover the topic; it is no more appropriate to submit an article on preparation of cardioplegic solutions to *Journal of Urology* than it is to type a monthly fiscal report on prescription labels.

More specifically, it is necessary to aim both the writing style and depth of information toward the audience. If something is written for physicians, it is not likely to be understood by laypeople. Conversely, items written for laypeople may not satisfy the needs of physicians. It is certainly appropriate to have a secondary audience in mind. For example, a report written for physicians may be of interest to pharmacists and nurses. However, make sure that the secondary audience is not served at the expense of the primary audience.

In regard to writing style, there are three types normally used by pharmacists and other health care professionals: "pure technical style," "middle technical style," and "popular technical style" (Table 11–1).[29]

TABLE 11–1. TYPES OF TECHNICAL WRITING

Pure technical style—used by professionals addressing other professionals in the same field
Middle technical style—used by professionals addressing professionals in other fields
Popular technical style—used by professionals addressing laypeople

Pure technical style is used by business or technical professionals when they are writing for other professionals in the same or similar fields. For example, an article published in *American Journal of Health-Systems Pharmacy* would normally be written in this style. There are several characteristics of this style. First, the authors can use technical jargon, because they can expect the readers will understand it. Second, it is written in formal English. Third, it is written in the third person; words such as I, we, us, and you are eliminated. Finally, there is a general lack of slang or contractions. The great majority of writing done by pharmacists will be in this style, because it is usually other pharmacists who will be reading their work.

Middle technical style is very closely related to pure technical style. This style is used by authors when they are writing for readers with a variety of technical backgrounds, with everyone having some unifying factor. For example, a report regarding a pharmacy department's quality assurance activities might be presented to the hospital's pharmacy and therapeutics committee. That committee is made up of physicians, nurses, hospital administrators, and other professionals. Although each has a background that makes their membership on the committee appropriate, not all of them would understand what a HEPA filter is, as would most hospital pharmacists. Therefore, it is necessary to better explain, or sometimes avoid, some technical areas. Otherwise, this writing style is very similar in most respects to pure technical style.

Finally, popular technical style is used in anything meant for the general public. Common language is used throughout. For example, a patient information sheet would need to be written in this style. A widely available example would be the articles on medical subjects that have appeared in *Reader's Digest* over the years. Information that is written in this style will use less complicated words and be less formal in its presentation.

It should be pointed out that usual technical writing differs greatly from what most people learn in high school English class or college composition courses. Although there is often a tendency to protest the formality of professional writing styles at first, the reality of the situation is that those styles must be followed for a piece of written material to be accepted.

The next step is to know the requirements of the publisher. Whether the work is for the department's policy and procedure manual or a journal, chances are that there is a format that needs to be followed. In the case of a journal, directions on the format to follow will be published at least once a year, usually in the first journal of the year. Also, specific guidelines are followed by a number of professional journals, both for general format and statistical reporting. Many journals have approved those guidelines and expect that all work submitted for publication will follow them. They are referred to as the "Uniform Requirements for Manuscripts Submitted to Biomedical Journals."[25] This standardization makes it easier on the prospective author; one style can be learned and followed, regardless of the journal. Other publications that can be helpful are *Scientific Style and Format: The CBE Manual for Authors, Editors, and Publishers* prepared by the Council of Biology Editors (CBE—now known as the Council of Science Editors, although the book uses the old name), *The American Medical Association Manual of Style, The MLA Style Manual,* and the *Publication Manual of the American Psychiatric Association.*

In the case of reports, policy and procedure manuals, and similar documents, it is best to see what has been done in the past. If this is the first time a particular item is being prepared, it is advisable to try to see what has been done in other places, and prepare something similar that meets the perceived needs. If writing something for work, do not be afraid to try to improve the format to make it more usable. However, be aware that it may be necessary to get any changes in format approved by the appropriate individual(s) or committee(s). Whenever possible, follow the "Uniform Requirements"[25] format used by the medical journals, because it is the standard for biomedical writing.

GENERAL RULES OF WRITING

Once the preparation is completed, it is time to start writing. Unfortunately, there is no easy way to learn how to write professionally; it just requires a lot of practice. However, a number of rules can be followed (Table 11–2). This section covers some of the general rules, with information on how to prepare specific items (e.g., introduction, body, conclusion, references,

TABLE 11–2. CHECKLIST IN PREPARATION OF WRITTEN MATERIALS

Do research first.
Put yourself in the reader's position.
Use proper grammar and spelling.
Make the document look "professional."
Keep things simple and direct.
Keep the document short.
Avoid abbreviations and acronyms.
Avoid the first person (e.g., I, we, and us).
Use active sentences.
Avoid slash construction (e.g., he or she and him or her).
Avoid contractions.
Cite other references wherever appropriate (and get permission to do so where appropriate).
Cover things in whatever order is easiest.
Get everything down on paper before revising.
Edit, Edit, Edit!

and abstracts) being covered later. The first step is to organize the information before starting to write. At the risk of sounding like a high school English teacher, it is still true that this step should include preparing an outline.[3] In the past, that was an onerous task that few performed. However, with modern word processing software, the outline actually becomes part of the finished product, so it does not amount to any significant extra work. Minimally the different sections should be listed to create some order to the layout of the work (remember, keep in mind the endpoint). Overall, the goal is to prepare a document that is clear, concise, complete, and correct. The two latter items depend, to a large part, on preparation. The former items, however, can be helped by following some simple rules.

The first two rules actually apply to the organization step. First, do sufficient research before getting started. Research in this regard, means obtaining whatever information—whether records, articles, performance evaluations, or anything else—necessary to prepare the item. Although it is likely that additional research will be necessary to fill in the "fine points" at some point in the process, most information should be gathered ahead of time. It is impossible to be organized if there is nothing collected, and a document that is not organized will generally not be worth much. The second rule is to put yourself in the reader's position. What does that reader want and how does he or she want it presented?

Although it should not need to be stated, it is very important to use proper spelling and grammar. This is easier than in the past, because high-end word processing programs can check both; however, it is still necessary to double check, because the computer is likely to overlook things. For example, a properly spelled, but incorrect, word will be missed (e.g., "two" instead of "to," "trail" instead of "trial," and "ration" instead of "ratio"). Unfortunately for some writers, appearances count greatly. The writer may know more about a particular subject than anyone else, but if poor grammar and spelling permeate the document, it is unlikely that anyone will read or believe the information presented.[30] It will be dismissed as probably wrong, based on grammar and spelling alone. In a case where the finished product will be published in a language other than the writer's native language, the writer should have the work read and edited by someone for whom the language is his or her native tongue. It should also be mentioned that the writing should try to be entertaining. Although professional writing tends to be a bit dry, an attempt should be made to make it as enjoyable and easy to read as possible, although it is necessary to be cautious with humor and stay within limits of professionalism and good taste. It should also be unpretentious, direct, and accurate.[31]

Related to this, the document should look presentable. Some students are well known for turning in papers that are crumpled, creased, torn, dirty, or, at least prior to the common use of computers, practically dipped in correction fluid. That is not professional and must be avoided. Fortunately, that problem appears to have been lessened with the use of word processors. The sad truth is that people will assume that if an author was sloppy with the appearance of the document, he or she was probably sloppy with the information. That may not be so, but that assumption will kill a good but sloppy document.

When writing it is best to keep things as simple and direct as possible.[32–35] This has been referred to as the KISS (Keep It Simple, Stupid) principle. There is a temptation to use big words that sound impressive, but doing so is more likely to confuse than impress. Related to that, keep the paper as short as possible.[36] Also, consider whether tables, figures, or graphs would make the document simpler and easier to understand. This can be particularly useful with documents containing a great deal of data that may be organized through the use of tables.

When writing, avoid using abbreviations or acronyms. If it is necessary to do so, state the full form of the word or term the first time it is mentioned in the document, followed by the abbreviation in parenthesis (e.g., acquired immunodeficiency syndrome [AIDS]). The only exceptions to this rule are units of measurement (e.g., mL and mg). Units of measurement should be expressed in the metric system. Clinical chemistry and hematologic measurements should be in terms of the International System of Units (SI). If a document is long, subheadings should be used. This can be part of the outline step as mentioned earlier.

Several rules apply to the wording that is used in professional writing.[29] First, completely avoid writing in the first person, and avoid the second person wherever possible. It is not a bad idea, at least at first, to ask the word processor to find all occurrences of *I, we, us,* and *you.* If those words are found, try to rewrite the sentence to avoid them. Also, it is preferable to avoid using the passive voice throughout;[37] again, a grammar checker can help. Avoid both contractions and slash construction (i.e., *and/or, he/she* [use *he or she*], and *this/that*). Finally, in this politically correct era, avoid sexism. That includes words like *he* or *she,* although it is not always appropriate or desirable to delete those terms. For example, using *he* in a case report of a patient with testicular cancer is quite appropriate. It is also inappropriate to use *their* instead of *his or her* to get around the problem.

When writing, be sure to give credit where it is due. This just does not mean making sure the listed authors wrote part of the document. It includes endnoting all information obtained from one or a limited number of sources. If there is extensive quoting, permission to do so should be obtained by writing to the person or organization holding the copyright on the material. Endnoting in the past was something everyone dreaded. They waited until the end, because the articles should be cited in the order they appear in the document. By that time it was difficult to go back and do it. Now, however, it is much easier with modern word processors; it is possible to insert the citations as the document is prepared and let the software worry about making sure that they are in the correct order.

Related to the endnoting, everything that is stated should be supported by objective evidence. When writing a paper based on scientific literature, that evidence must be shown in the endnoting. To reemphasize, any unreferenced statement of fact is for all practical purposes worthless. However, it is necessary to make sure information is extracted from the original article and expressed properly. Some writers will improperly twist facts, whether inadvertently or not, to support their assertions.[38]

Finally, work through the document in whatever order seems easiest.[3] In preparing a drug evaluation for a pharmacy and therapeutics committee, a stack of 50 articles might be used. At first, the stack may look like an impossible task, but after sorting the articles into groups that correspond to the sections, start with the shortest stack or the easiest information. By the time the document is finished, the writer may be surprised to find out that they were all fairly short, easy stacks.

At first, a writer should simply try to make sure that all of the information is down on paper.[3] Once that occurs, go back and revise, and perhaps reorganize the document. Waiting a few days before revising the document can be very beneficial. After some time away from the project, errors practically jump off the page. It is also a good idea to have someone else who has not been involved with the writing, read the document. Something that seems quite clear to the author may not actually be clear at all. Also, the author may be mentally inserting words or even sentences that were inadvertently omitted. Having someone edit the document can be humbling but helpful. Be sure to provide the product in a format that will make things easier for the person reviewing the document. A typed, double-spaced manuscript will make it easy to read and provide room for comments. Even better, it is now possible to send electronic versions of a document out for review directly from the word processor. The reviewer can put in comments or suggested wording changes electronically and then return the document. The writer can then go through the document making changes or simply accepting proposed changes with the click of a mouse. Often, the use of the electronic reviewing mechanism will be quicker, easier, and provide much clearer suggestions.

The three most important things in real estate may be "location, location, location," but the three most important things in writing are "edit, edit, edit." It is not sufficient to settle for "good enough"—do your best. Look at it this way: the boss or editor is only going to do so much editing before giving up. The trick is to make sure that the document is well prepared and does not need that much editing.

SPECIFIC DOCUMENT SECTIONS

A typical document consists of three main parts—the introduction, body, and conclusion. In the case of a clinical study, it is recommended to follow the "IMRAD" structure, which divides a paper into Introduction, Methods, Results, and Discussion.[25] Other parts, such as references, tables, figures, and abstracts may also be necessary. These will be discussed in later sections and in the appendices of this chapter. It should also be noted that a number of the points in Chaps. 6, 7, and 10 are applicable to writing, as are the contents of the websites for the International Committee of Medical Journal Editors (<<http://www.icmje.org>>), Consolidated Standards of Reporting Trials (CONSORT) statement (contains checklist for contents of clinical trial) (<<http://www.consort-statement.org>>)[39] [along with the Standards for Reporting of Diagnostic Accuracy (STARD) initiative for reporting diagnostic accuracy—<<http://www.consort-statement.org/stardstatement.htm>> and the Quality of Reporting of Meta-Analysis (QUOROM) statement for meta-analyses[40]—<<http://www.consort-statement.org/QUOROM.pdf>>], Conference on Guideline Standardization (COGS) standards (<http://gem.med.yale.edu/cogs/statement.do>>), and the Good Publication Practice for Pharmaceutical Companies (<http:// www.gpp-guidelines.org>>), and should be considered along with this material. A variation on the CONSORT statement for trials that study safety has been proposed, but is not yet finalized.[41] An example question layout is shown in Appendix 11–1.

Introduction

With the probable exception of policy and procedure documents, the two most important paragraphs in any document are the first and last. It is vital to start out strong, to encourage the reader to continue reading. Otherwise, the work will end up in that stack of articles everyone has that they "intend to read someday." That first paragraph should also inform the reader of what they can expect in the rest of the document; it should be similar to a road map that shows what is to be accomplished in the document. The introduction should have a clear objective for the existence of the document. Many people neglect the need for a clear objective, which leaves the reader to flounder and wonder whether there really is a purpose to the document. In a research article, the introduction will also contain the hypothesis being investigated. In a policy and procedure document, it may simply be a description of what the remainder of the document will cover. The introduction should also contain background information about the topic that provides a good information base for the reader. The amount of background information has to be a balance—enough to show the reader that the writer has done an appropriate amount of research, but yet not so exhaustive as to bore or overwhelm the reader with unnecessary details.[42] Overall, the introduction should be short but contain properly referenced background material and show the reader where the document is headed.

The introduction should generally not be a conclusion; some people are so anxious to jump to the end that they put the conclusion first. Admittedly, the BLOT concept (bottom line on top) has its purpose in some documents (e.g., policy and procedures and formulary monographs), but that should be a conscious decision. If the introduction amounts to a conclusion, many people will read no further, making the remainder of the document a waste of time and paper.

Body

The body of the document contains all of the details. In a research article, the body may be divided into the methods, results, and, possibly, discussion sections, although the latter section may be incorporated into the conclusion. Details of what should be included are covered in Chap. 6. In other documents, the body will probably be divided into whatever sections are appropriate or logical. A number of rules can be followed in preparing the body of a document.

The first rule is that while it is important to be concise, all necessary information must be presented. Again, keep an eye on the desired endpoint, and do not stray from the subject unless it is absolutely necessary. Including unnecessary information, even if it is interesting, will tend to confuse or obscure the important points. Also, be sure to provide a balanced coverage of the material and avoid unsupported bias.[7]

It is important to cover the information in a logical order, so that it flows easily from one point to another. A common mistake, when learning to write professionally, is to skip back and forth between subjects. For example, someone might insert a point about dosing in the middle of indications, when dosing is discussed at another point in the document.

Material that can identify patients should be left out of any work, unless it is absolutely necessary to include. If that is not possible, informed consent must be obtained[25] and pertinent legal procedures must be followed (see Chap. 12). The authors should also disclose any approval of the study by institutional review boards and their following of other rules related to protection of study subjects, both human and animal.[25]

The writer should also put the information in his or her own words. Perhaps out of lack of confidence, a number of professionals are tempted to simply quote other authors word for word. However, by presenting the information in their own words, writers demonstrate that they actually understand the topic. Remember, though, that if the information is taken from a particular source, even if it is reworded, the original author should be given credit via endnotes.

It is necessary to expand on the topic discussed in the previous paragraph because there seems to be much confusion about it and there are many cases where the rules against copyright infringement and plagiarism are broken. Plagiarism can be considered the copying of another's words or ideas without properly giving credit. Copyright violations consist of copying another's work, even with appropriate quotations and citation, without permission. They are similar; however, it is possible to commit either plagiarism or copyright violations without committing the other.

Sometimes those infractions are rather blatant, such as the cases documented in the newspapers about students downloading papers from the Internet and presenting them as their own or simply retyping a previously published article. (Interestingly, an attempt to prevent this can be seen on the Internet at <<http://www.plagiarism.com>>, <<http://www. plagiarism.org, http://www.turnitin.com>>, or <<http://www.powerresearcher. com>>).[43] Other times, the infringement is quite accidental. For example, it was once brought to the attention of the famous science fiction writer, Isaac Asimov, that a short story that he wrote was similar to an article that had been published 10 years previously.[44] Dr. Asimov went back and found the article and read it, realizing as he did so that he had read it when it first came out and had forgotten about it. When he wrote his story 10 years later, he did not at all realize that portions of it could be considered plagiarism. Although he had no intention of infringing on the other author's work, Dr. Asimov made sure that the story was never reprinted and even wrote an article discussing the problem. This shows how easy it is to inadvertently cross the line into copyright infringement or plagiarism, and there are many examples that would fall in between the extremes given above.[45] Therefore, it is necessary for the author to be on guard and to try to prevent the problem in the first place. A few general rules can act as a guide.

- When copying wording directly from another's work, it should be in quotations (or otherwise shown to be a quote) and a citation should appear to give credit to the original author(s). Also, if a significant amount of a work published in the last 100 years is quoted, it is probably necessary to get permission from the copyright holder, which may require paying a fee.[46] Exactly what is a "significant amount" is debatable; however, it would be best to err on the side of asking for permission if a quotation is more than a few sentences. Reproducing an entire chart, table, figure, and so on should normally require asking for permission. A letter to the copyright holder will solve problems; publishers often also have forms to request permission. Some special cases need to be mentioned. First, U.S. government documents are not copyrighted, so only quotation marks and citations are necessary. Second, if it is impossible to locate a copyright holder (e.g., the publisher went out of business without transferring copyrights), the writer should at least be able to document a thorough effort to obtain permission. Finally, there are special legal requirements for use of copyrighted materials in online education, covered in the Technology, Education, and Copyright Harmonization (TEACH) Act. Further information on this can be found in Chap. 12 and also at <<http://www.usg.edu/legal/copyright>>.
- Extensive quotations should be avoided. After all, if a writer cannot put something in his or her own words, does that person truly understand the material? In any writing, there really is very little reason to provide quotations. The author should try to put things in his or her own words whenever possible.
- Paraphrased information should have the original publication(s) cited, if it comes from one or a limited number of sources.
- Extensive paraphrasing, particularly without citations, may be considered plagiarism (i.e., copying the ideas of others).
- When citing an article, cite the one that the material comes from. If the material came from a review article, cite that article, not the original study that was not consulted. It is worth mentioning that in the case of unusual information, reading and citing the original study is preferable to just using a review article, because the review may be inaccurate.
- Be sure to follow publishers' rules or licenses, which may be stricter and may not allow any reproduction of material.

In preparing certain documents (written answers to questions, for example), there may be very little information available. Perhaps only one or two research articles will have been written on the topic. If so, it will often be desirable to summarize the articles in detail, including most of the information presented in an abstract (see Appendix 11–2). In general, the information presented will summarize how many and what type of patients (i.e., inclusion and exclusion criteria), the drug or procedure being investigated, the results (e.g., efficacy and adverse effects), and the author's conclusions. It is also important to point out any noticeable flaws in the paper. An example would be:

Smith and Jones performed a double-blind, randomized comparison of the effects of drug X and drug Y in patients with tsutsugamushi fever. Patients were required to be between 18 and 70 years old, and could not have any concurrent infection or disorder that would affect the immune response to the disease (e.g., neutropenia and AIDS). Twenty patients received 10 mg of drug X, three times a day for 15 days. Eighteen patients received 250 mg of drug Y, twice a day for 10 days. The two groups were comparable, except that the patients receiving drug X were an average of 5 years younger (p < .05). Drug X was shown to produce a cure, both in terms of symptoms and cultures in 85% of patients, whereas drug Y only produced a cure in 55.5% of patients. The difference was statistically significant (p < .01). No significant adverse effects were seen in either group. Although it appears that drug X was the better agent, it should be noted that drug Y was given in its minimally effective dose, and may have performed better in a somewhat higher or longer regimen.

A list of material to be covered in a review of an article similar to that above is found in Table 11–3.

Conclusion

A conclusion should be placed at the end of the body of the document, except for certain documents (e.g., policy and procedures). This conclusion should follow logically from the

TABLE 11–3. ITEMS TO INCLUDE IN WRITTEN REVIEW OF A JOURNAL ARTICLE

Items to Include	Examples
Main author of article and a reference number	Johnson et al.[2] Smith and associates[24]
Type of article	Clinical study, case report, case series, review, meeting abstract
Research design (if appropriate)	Blinding, randomization, experience report, descriptive report
Purpose of the report	
Description of group studied	Size of groups, age, sex, disease state(s), other pertinent demographic characteristics
Any important confounding factors	Smoking, age, general health
Description of treatment being studied	Drug, dose, administration route, dosing interval, treatment duration
What was measured as an indicator of effect	
Results	Efficacy, adverse effects
Author conclusions	
Strengths and weaknesses of the study	See Chaps. 6 and 7

information presented and should serve to summarize that information. Remember, the conclusion should also correspond with the objective stated in the introduction.[47] It is also worth noting that in clinical consultations, a common mistake is to write the conclusion in a general manner, rather than addressing the specific patient in question, which is what the reader wants to hear about. The author must remember to address the specific patient's situation.

Many writers are tempted to avoid formulating a conclusion. Various reasons include not feeling qualified to make a conclusion for the reader, not wanting to restate what has already been stated, laziness, and so on. This is improper. The readers need something to bring their thoughts together at the end, and the author is in the perfect position to provide this closure. However, the author should also be careful to avoid extrapolating beyond the information available.

Other Items

If items are endnoted, the references should be found following the conclusion (see Appendix 11–3 for more information on how to prepare a bibliography). Use of bibliographic software, such as Reference Manager (ISI ResearchSoft, Carlsbad, CA—<<http://www.refman.com>>), ProCite (ISI ResearchSoft, Carlsbad, CA—<<http://www.procite.com>>), or EndNote (ISI ResearchSoft, Carlsbad, CA—<<http://www.endnote.com>>) can be helpful in this process.[13] Other items may also be necessary depending on the document, such as tables, graphs, figures, and so forth. They will not be dealt with here other than to say that those items should supplement or clarify (not distort or misrepresent) and not duplicate material in the text portion of a piece of written work. Also, it is worth mentioning that many computer programs make the preparation of professional-quality graphs and figures easy and often allow embedding the artwork in the word processing document itself, when allowed by the circumstances.

SUBMISSION OF THE DOCUMENT

Once the document is completed, proofread, and edited, it is ready to be submitted, whether that is to a boss or a journal. In the latter case, you will need to include a cover letter that serves as an introduction to the document. In the former case, it will be possible to be less formal. Also, it should be noted that when submitting an item to a journal it may be necessary to include transfer of copyright forms, conflict of interest disclosures (including financial),[10,48-50] or other items that will be found in the directions for authors for that journal (usually found in the first issue of each year and on the publication's website). The conflict of interest may be reported by the publisher in the final publication, but that is variable.[51] In addition, be sure to precisely follow the journal's "Instructions for Authors" to improve chances for acceptance.[52] It is also worth a word of warning that articles should very rarely, if ever, be submitted to more than one journal at the same time (note: prior publication of an abstract does not mean that submission of a full article is duplication and publication in a second language is often considered acceptable).[7,10,53] If duplicate submission is felt to be appropriate and/or necessary, the rules outlined in the "Uniform Requirements" must be followed.[25] Also, the article should not be broken down into many small articles and submitted over time, unless submission as a whole would result in a publication that would be too long or complex.[54]

REVISION

In many cases, revision of the document will be necessary. This may be due to a difference in opinion or different perception of need. Although an author should never change a document to say something he or she believes is wrong, minor revisions are often necessary to improve clarity or make the document more appropriate in some other manner. The comments given with the request for revision are likely to be helpful,[55] and they should be taken seriously. Even if it is felt that the person who read and commented on the paper is wrong, all concerns should be addressed. If a comment is truly wrong, it may still indicate that the work was not clear in a particular area and needs some other appropriate revision to clarify the material. Changes should be made based on the comments, and completed within the time limits necessary.

Sometimes, however, a document may be rejected entirely. This can be for any of the following reasons:[29]

- The document is not up to standards (too much work for the boss or editor to correct).
- The idea or research the document is based on is too weak.
- The idea is inappropriate for that publication forum.
- A similar article has been prepared (and possibly published) by someone else in that forum recently.

In the case of the first item, major revisions would be necessary before resubmitting to the boss or a journal. The second reason may also prompt major revisions, or even cause an author to stop working on the document. An article submitted to a journal but rejected for the last two reasons is not necessarily bad. It may be possible to submit it to another journal after only minor changes.

GALLEY PROOFS

A term well known to authors who have published articles or books is galley (or page) proofs. This is a copy of the final article as it is to appear when published. It is the responsibility of the author(s) to carefully check to make sure there have been no mistakes made in typesetting. Although it may seem like a lot of work, everything must be checked, including the references, which frequently contain errors.[56–61] This step is necessary to prevent problems later. Although documents ready for the copy machine at work are generally not referred to as galley proofs, it is still necessary to carefully check those items.

Referees

Although this term is more familiar to sports fans, referees (also referred to as reviewers) are used in writing. These are the individuals to whom journals send submitted articles for review and comment. This is also referred to as the peer-review process. On a local level, reviewers are the people that a writer may ask to look at a report before the boss gets it. Whatever arena, whether local or international, a person should also be willing to be a reviewer at that level. To be a reviewer for a journal, a person usually can simply write a letter stating interests, qualifications, and experience to the editor of the journal, and ask to be considered for the journal's reviewer list. If the person has adequate credentials, the journal will usually be happy to have that person as a reviewer.

Anyone who is a reviewer should be up front about such things as lack of expertise, conflict of interest,[50] or inability to complete a review within a reasonable time, and should be willing to step aside as a reviewer of a particular paper if those are problems.[62] Also, a reviewer should treat anything submitted to him or her as a confidential document.

It should be pointed out that people who act as a reviewer for a paper should follow the procedures discussed in Chaps. 6 and 7. Specific directions will also be received from the editor and may involve preparing comments for both the editor (to discuss matters, such as ethics, with the editor alone) and for the author (this latter document is also used by the editor). It may be required that the latter be signed or unsigned. Also, as with any quality assurance procedure, the reviewer should treat it as an opportunity to provide constructive, as opposed to destructive, criticism.[63] Finally, for those who are reviewers for journals, it is recommended to get new people involved in the process, such as residents or new practitioners, so that they can learn how to be a reviewer.[64]

It is beyond the scope of this chapter, but if further information is needed on being an editor of a biomedical journal, the reader should consult the website of the World Association of Medical Editors (<<http://www.wame.org>>).

Specific Documents

NEWSLETTERS AND WEBSITES

Newsletters have been considered to be a part of any pharmacy practice, but have probably been encountered most frequently in hospitals as a method for communicating pharmacy and therapeutics committee actions and other drug-related topics to the medical, pharmacy, nursing, and other health care provider staffs. Newsletters have also been seen from community pharmacies[65,66] (addressed to patients and/or physicians), nursing homes, drug companies, pharmacy organizations, and government or regulatory bodies. Wherever newsletters are found, their reason for existence is likely to be one or more of the following reasons: to communicate information to a target group, advertisement, and/or compliance with legal/ accreditation standards.

In many cases, newsletters are now replaced by a website. Such sites can serve the same purposes, but can also have some specific advantages and disadvantages. For example, websites take very little effort for distribution, because all they take is a computer on the Internet, which can actually be provided by an Internet service provider (ISP) for a few dollars a month. Also, the material can take a greater variety of forms, including audio and video. The website can actually be used to sell products, including prescriptions. Within institutions, the material can be kept available for health care providers to review for an indefinite time period, thereby preventing problems when somebody wants another copy of some old article or when the nurses are trying to make sure that they have all of the publications for an accreditation visit. In regards to disadvantages, it does have to be noted that consulting a website does take more effort, because it does not just fall into people's hands when they open their mailboxes. Also, some people do not use the Internet and would, therefore, not be able to consult the site.

Whatever the reason for the existence of a newsletter or website, the same set of steps generally apply to their preparation.[67-71] These steps will be covered individually in the remainder of this section.

Define the Audience

Who will, or at least should, be reading the newsletter or accessing the website? It may be physicians, pharmacists, nurses, other health care professionals, the lay public, other groups, or some combination of these. The target group(s) will have an effect on decisions made in the other steps.

Define the Goals of the Newsletter or Website

The goal can be any of the reasons mentioned previously, but generally includes informing and educating the reader, and also to report news (including changes in policies and procedures, laws, and so forth). Websites can also be used to directly sell products or gather information.

Identify Constraints

No matter what kind of newsletter or website is produced, there are always going to be constraints that will limit what it can contain and how good it will be. One of the first constraints is time. It seems like every year people are busier and have less time to do things that they want or need to do. This includes preparing a newsletter or keeping up a website (must be done continuously), which can take a significant amount of time if it is done right. It will be necessary to have time to write, type, edit, typeset, and perform other functions in publishing the newsletter and all of those things have to be done in time to get the finished result to the printer, so that it can be ready for distribution on time. With a website, it is necessary to write the material, figure out the layout or organization, and prepare it on the computer. It is generally best, when beginning publication of a newsletter, to have it come out at longer intervals. If the newsletter is well received, it is found that there is enough time, and there is sufficient material, publication frequency can be increased. Overall, it is better to find it necessary to speed up publication frequency, rather than spread it out (people might get the idea the newsletter ceased publication).

Another constraint is the people that can or will be involved with publishing the newsletter or website, particularly the editor-in-chief and/or webmaster. This is a case where the phrase, "many hands make light work" may be applicable. If a group of dependable people are willing to work together to make sure the articles get written, the job may be easier. Generally, there are two extremely hard parts to publishing a newsletter or website, neither of which is the actual writing. One of them is coming up with topic ideas; the other is to make it look good. If others are at least willing to help here, it can be a great aid to the editor of the newsletter. If at all possible, people from all groups served by the newsletter should be asked for topics, if not entire articles. If a pharmacist is in charge of the newsletter or website, some other possible places for help include an institution's public relations department, if available, and clerical help (to do the typing, formatting, copying, distribution, and so forth). Keep an eye on the time necessary for pharmacy staff to produce the newsletter or website, because this is likely to be the most costly item.

The third constraint is financial. As has been said, "There is no such thing as a free lunch." This also applies to newsletters and websites. There is always some cost involved. Although personnel costs are likely to be the largest expense, the computer equipment and printing or duplication charges (for newsletters) can be significant. If the printing is to be done by an outside agency, it is best to check on such items as the effect of order size (number of copies) and type of paper (e.g., plain vs. glossy, $8\frac{1}{2} \times 11$ vs. 11×17 vs. A4, and colors), stapling or binding on the cost. It is preferable to get bids from at least three printers. Another item to consider is method of delivery (e.g., personal vs. first-class mail vs. second-class mail). All of these items do add up and, depending on the budget, it may be necessary to sell advertising space to cover the costs.

Finally, it is necessary to look at what equipment is available. In the past, it was necessary to either typeset or have a somewhat amateuristic cut and pasted typewritten newsletter; however, nearly everyone now has a computer and letter quality output device available. If at all possible, the use of a high-end word processing program or desktop publishing program with a laser or inkjet printer will allow production of a high-quality, professional newsletter quicker and at a lower cost. This equipment may be all that is necessary for a website, assuming that the computer has some type of Internet connection. Although a number of web programs are now available for little cost, and are the preferable solution, many times it is possible to just use a word processor or web browser to create and maintain the website.

Newsletter/Website Design

As a child of the 1960s, it was easy during and shortly after college to believe substance was more important than appearance. Being older and (hopefully!) wiser (or at least more cynical), it now is noticeable that many people do not bother looking at the substance if the appearance is poor or unprofessional. Therefore, one of the most important things is to make the publication look appealing.[72,73] People tend to throw away newsletters that look sloppy or unprofessional, and do not bother with websites that are not exciting, easy to use, and "neat." Even if the publication looks good it may[74-76] or may not[77,78] have any impact on physicians; but without looking professional it is highly unlikely to even have a chance.

A few general rules can help to make a newsletter or website more appealing. These will be covered in the remainder of this section. However, for a more in-depth look at this subject, the reader is directed to references specializing in the subject.[79,80] A particularly detailed book is available on the Internet at <<http://www.usability.gov/pdfs/guidelines.html>>.[81]

One of the first rules is to keep the publication consistent. This means not only from month to month, but also from page to page. This does not mean that improvements cannot be made from time to time. Nor does it mean that each page has to look exactly like the previous one. Instead, it means that it should have its own style that is recognizable by the reader, and that the various pages must fit with one another. The easiest way to do this, with either a newsletter or website, is to create a template, style sheet, or theme (these terms overlap somewhat). Many pieces of software make this possible for either type of publication. A template is a file that contains material that appears the same from issue to issue—the term is often associated with a newsletter. Examples of this can be the newsletter's masthead (first page heading), the listing of editors, footers at the bottom of each page, number of columns, and so on. A theme should be similar to a template, but may be used more frequently when discussing a website. Style sheets are a definition of how specific paragraphs or other parts of the newsletter or websites will look (they would often be incorporated into the template or theme). For example, a style might be called "Heading 1," and by using this style for each article's title, the look remains the same from page to page, and issue to issue. This style can include such items as what the font looks like (e.g., typeface, font size, bold, italic, underlined, superscript, and subscript), and what the paragraph looks like (e.g., left justified, right justified, centered, line spacing, and space before or after), in addition to other items (e.g., whether the section is to be located in a particular part of the page and borders). A style manual should be established or at least a commercially available style manual, such as the *American Medical Association Manual of Style*, should be used. Whatever the editor(s) establish should be reasonably simple and elegant (i.e., do not get carried away—a couple of different fonts on a page are fine, but 10 fonts look terrible). In the case of websites, it might be useful to consult the publication *Elements of E-text Style,* which is available at <<http://wiretap.area.com/Gopher/Library/Classic/estyle.txt>>.

A second rule is to use appropriate software and equipment. A high-end word processor or desktop publishing program and a laser printer can be used to produce the master copy of the newsletter for reproduction.[82,83] This can allow a pharmacy to turn out a product that looks typeset at a fraction of the cost. As mentioned, there are a variety of low (or no) cost website software tools. Some are specific (Microsoft FrontPage is probably the most popular and highest rated), whereas others are incorporated into word processors, web browsers, or other software. Also, just using a text editor is possible, although that tends to be much more difficult.

A third rule is to make the newsletter or website look "good." For example, use white space properly. Do not just crowd in as much material as possible on the page. The reader will have a hard time following if it is too crowded, and may just give up. Layout really is a difficult problem, and requires at least a little artistic ability to do well. If lack of artistic ability is a problem, it is probably a good idea to look over other newsletters or websites from various sources to try to come up with ideas concerning what looks good. Minimally, most newsletters should at least be set up in two columns to allow easier reading. Other, more artistic, items to consider are asymmetrical layout (not having the two sides of each page look the same from a distance, perhaps using a narrow column for graphics or titles along one edge), different column widths, "teasers" (statements taken from the text that may pique the curiosity of the reader enough to read the article), surrounding boxes and columns with rules, and artwork/graphics.[84] The programs used to prepare either newsletters or websites can also have samples that can be used to prepare a professional looking end product.

Next on the list for newsletters is to design a masthead. As mentioned, the masthead is essentially the part of the first page of the newsletter that gives the name of the publication, volume, issue, date, and so on. This may be at the top of the page or down one side of the first page. It is a good idea to consider having this done professionally, because it is a one-time expense and can be a major factor in the appearance of the newsletter. Sometimes it is good to have a multicolored masthead that is preprinted on blank stock paper. The newsletter text can then just be photocopied onto the paper and look much more professional. Material to be put into the masthead, or at least be included somewhere in the newsletter includes the newsletter name (be descriptive, but do not get cute—remember this is a professional newsletter), name and address of the pharmacy/organization, names of editor and editorial staff (give credit or blame where it is due), and frequency of publication. The name of the publication, along with some way of identifying the issue and page, should be placed on every page of the newsletter, so that the source of information can be identified if the page is photocopied or torn out.

Much of the material in a masthead should also be contained on the home page, if not every page, of a website. Again, getting professional design help, at least at first, may be of value. Also, following the guidelines of the Health on the Net Foundation Code of Conduct (<<http://www.hon.ch/HONcode/Conduct.html>>) in designing the web page is appropriate.

In general, software themes available will help create a professional looking site, if professional help is not available. However, some specific items that need to be considered for a website include:[85,86]

- Provide information that is good, credible, timely, and original. Share everything possible.
- Custom tailor information to take into account user preferences.
- Break up tables for readability.
- Use graphics effectively, but sparingly (they may take too long to download, annoying the reader). Graphics should be no more than 20 kilobytes in size.
- Related to the previous item, optimize the other aspects of the page to improve download times.
- Make the page easy to read—good contrast between the text and background, not too busy.
- Use self-generating content—make the site interactive.
- Web pages should be well organized—both the pages by themselves and how the pages are interconnected on the site.
- Consider selling things, if appropriate.
- Make sure everything works, from all likely browsers.

In designing the newsletter or website, effort should also be placed in deciding on a name. A local or institutional newsletter will often have a name related to the organization and the purpose of the newsletter. A website may be similarly named, but there is an opportunity to go farther. In this case, the Uniform Resource Locator (URL) should be considered. This is the address of the website on the intranet and/or the Internet. An institution may already have a registered URL, and the pharmacy web page may simply be under that name (e.g., <http://www.yourorganizationname.org/pharmacy>>). However, independent community pharmacies can also register an unused name on the Internet and have that address (e.g., <http://www.johnspharmacy.com>>).

It has been alluded to, but it is necessary to make a very specific decision on how the newsletter is to be printed. While typesetting still produces the best looking newsletter, it is quite easy to get a good-looking final product using a good photocopy machine. Also, even if the pharmacy produces the original copy on its computer, the file can be taken to a service bureau that can essentially produce a typeset copy. It is necessary to determine the paper to be used (glossy paper is not going to be used if you are photocopying). Most newsletters are $8\frac{1}{2} \times 11$ in. in size, but that does not mean the paper is that size. It is better to use 11×17 in. paper for multipage newsletters and just fold the sheets. That looks much better than simply stapling the corner. Also, it is possible to take a disk with the newsletter file on it to some professional printers for them to print good-looking final copies.

Newsletter/Web Page Content

Before getting into items that a newsletter or website should or can contain, it is necessary to discuss some general rules that deal with any article.[87]

First, it is a good idea to have a number of short articles, rather than one long article.[73,88] People will take a look at a short article and mentally decide they have the time to read it, whereas a long article may be dismissed immediately ("If I'm going to read something that long, it will be out of *New England Journal of Medicine!*") or put aside to read "when I have time." (Does house dust actually come from publications on the bottom of that "read some-day" pile disintegrating from old age?) As a matter of fact, some recommend that newsletters should not exceed two pages (one sheet, front and back)[87] and one hospital cut their newsletter to one page (for P&T News) and replaced the remaining articles with a page to fit into a Drug Therapy Pocket Guide that consisted of useful tables (e.g., sodium content and neutralizing capacity of different antacids).[89] Related to the above, use catchy titles to draw the reader into reading the article right then.

Use proper writing techniques, as described earlier in this chapter. Be clear, concise, and complete—do not waste the reader's valuable time. Also, be unbiased—support the article with facts. Be positive—talk about 90% compliance, rather than 10% noncompliance.

Finally, be sure that the newsletter or website is properly edited. Have multiple people read and edit the newsletter or web pages before publication. Having more people read it makes it more likely that simple mistakes will be noticed and corrected. In particular, the editors should check for spelling, grammar, and readability. Also, it is a good idea to have people from each target group as editors, particularly physicians.[90]

The actual content of a newsletter or website is one of the two most difficult areas for the editor that were mentioned in the Identify Constraints section (the other being that the newsletter should look good). Coming up with new ideas on a regular basis can be rather difficult. A list of possible areas to cover are included in Table 11–4. If at all possible, material that was prepared for a different audience can be recycled for the newsletter or website readers. For example, material from the pharmacy and therapeutics committee meeting might be turned into a short review of a drug. Whenever possible, the material presented should be topics not available to the audience from another source, or material that is prepared in a format that will be of greater value to the readers than that same topic area as presented by other publications. Whatever the topics used, it is a good idea to survey the readers on a regular basis to make sure that their needs are being met.

Newsletter Distribution

All of the above work will be for nothing if the readers do not get the newsletter. A good distribution system must be developed. Sometimes it can be as simple as sticking the newsletters in individual mailboxes, setting out piles of newsletters, or using interorganizational

TABLE 11–4. NEWSLETTER OR WEBSITE TOPICS[67,68,73,87]

Adverse drug reactions
Calendar of events
Clinical "pearls"
Effects of external events on jobs
Job-related information
New information sources
New legal or regulatory requirements
New services
News from other departments
Organization's stand on issues
Personnel policies
Pharmacoeconomics
Pharmacy and therapeutics committee actions and news (major area to be covered)
Productivity improvement
Professional announcements
Review of drugs/drug classes
Quality assurance

---

mail systems. If it is necessary to use the post office, it would be a good idea to check on the possibility of second class or bulk mail, which can save money. Newer innovative distribution methods are by electronic mail[91] or other computerized methods.[92] Community pharmacies may also distribute their newsletters by providing copies to physician waiting rooms or noncompeting businesses (e.g., banks, barber shops, beauty shops, and day care centers), or even including them with monthly statements.[66] Whatever method used, it is important to make sure the readers actually get the newsletter. Also, make sure they get the newsletters on a regular "cycle," so that they know when to anticipate the arrival of the publication.

PRESENTATIONS

Some time during a pharmacist's career, he or she may have the opportunity to give a formal presentation. This could be simply at where he or she works or at a national meeting. Although it is well known that fear of public speaking is an extremely common occurrence, a speaker who prepares should do well. The problem may simply be fear of the unknown. Having some simple directions may be of immense help. Overall, the main concern should be to know the topic. If someone knows enough to be asked to talk, chances are that person will know quite a bit about a topic, or will be able to learn enough about the topic. Alternately, the potential presenter may volunteer to give a presentation on a topic he or she is interested in or has done a lot of work about (e.g., a new method to practice or a new practice area). After that, most of the concern will deal with looking good. This includes a variety of items, many of which involve professional writing, and will be dealt with in the remainder of this section.

In cases where a person is asked to speak, a proposal will need to be submitted. This describes the proposed topic, which should be of interest to the target audience. The directions given by the organization preparing the meeting will need to be followed. Beyond that, the skills described earlier in this chapter or the appendicies will need to be used.

Next, it may be necessary to write an abstract that the organization providing the presentation forum will use to inform potential attendees about the presentation. Each organization may have a format for abstracts, which should be followed. As to what should appear in the abstract, the writer might use the information presented in Appendix 11–2. Admittedly, an abstract should usually be prepared after the presentation is done to best reflect what will be said. However, abstracts may be requested more than 6 months before the presentation, so in this case it will serve more as a planning document. Actually, it is probably best to create a brief outline of the presentation (at least the topics to be covered) and then write the abstract.

Along with the abstract, it may be necessary to prepare learning objectives to describe what the attendee will be able to do as a result of participating in the program. The objectives should state that behavior in objective, measurable terms. For example, an objective may state that the attendee can "explain," "list," or "identify" something. It will not say that the attendee "knows," "understands," or "learns," because those are not measurable. The objectives should relate directly to the program and should be adequately broken down to cover the different areas of the presentation. Refer to the beginning of any of the chapters of this book for examples of objectives.

Occasionally, the presenter may be requested to provide self-assessment questions. Often these will be multiple choice or true/false, to simplify assessment. Those questions should be clearly stated and measure that the attendee has met the objective. Efforts should be made to make the questions clear. Also, they should avoid the use of "not" or "except," because these terms can lead to confusion. Writing good questions can be extremely difficult, so testing the questions out on others before the presentation may help improve the quality.

The speaker may also have to prepare a brief biography to be used in his or her introduction. This includes a few items about his or her background, such as title and current position. Also, some information that gives the audience an idea of why that speaker is qualified to make a presentation is useful.

Presentations can usually be broken down into platform or poster presentations. The former is a more formal, oral presentation that typically requires some sort of audiovisual component and is often presented in a room set up for an audience. The latter requires the presenter to place a summary of the material to be presented on a poster (or series of small posters) that will be displayed on a bulletin board-type display (usually provided by the organization) that will be 3 to 4 ft. high and 6 to 8 ft. wide. In that situation, the attendees can walk through a group of such presentations, stopping to look at any that appeal to them and ask the presenter questions.

Many of the rules described in the main part of this chapter relate to preparing the information to be presented, including slides, posters, and other audiovisual materials. However, a few other rules need to be mentioned.

- The presenter should learn the circumstances under which the presentation is to be given. That includes whether it is a platform or poster presentation.
- The presenter should determine what equipment is to be provided (e.g., slide projector, overhead projector, microphone, and size of poster presentation board).
- If the presenter needs other items, they should be made clear to the organization. For example, it is common for presenters to want to use computer slide projection equipment, which may present certain technical requirements for both the equipment and support people. Also, the presenter may need such things as power outlet strips, extension cords, wireless microphones (many good speakers "wander" and are frustrated by a podium microphone that requires them to stand in one place behind a podium), Internet connection, connections from a computer to the room sound system, BlueTooth, USB connection, CD-ROM, videotape player, cables, and other items. The presenter should take into account his or her own needs and desires, in addition to those of the audience. It is necessary to be very specific, since the people organizing the meeting may not understand the requirements. For example, if the speaker requests an Internet connection, he or she may think he or she is getting a T1 connection that will work well with a graphics-intensive presentation, but may arrive to find a phone line that will be totally inadequate. Also, even the resolution of a computer projector or type of connector for a network may need to be specified.
- If the speaker is doing a poster presentation, he or she normally will need to remember to bring pushpins to mount the poster on the provided display board.
- The audience should be taken into account. One common complaint when a speaker flies in for a presentation is that they may not know anything about local circumstances, including simple social skills that are expected (e.g., foreign countries). It is best if the speaker tries to find out more about the audience and the situation, adjusting the presentation to take those items into account.[93]
- If necessary, the set up of the room should be specified (e.g., theater style, discussion tables, and screen placement).

All of the above should be double checked at the location of the presentation after arrival, but in plenty of time to correct any problems. Speakers may also want to take advantage of a "Speaker Ready Room" that many organizations offer to check out slides and prepare for their presentation. As a side note, checking in with those arranging the presentation is necessary so that they will not be worried about your arrival and they will be able to clear up any last minute items.

The speaker then needs to prepare the presentation, doing appropriate research and preparation, using skills described earlier in this chapter and in the following sections. The presentation should also be rehearsed adequately. The next steps will discuss preparation of audiovisual materials, which can enhance the audience's ability to understand and retain the material.[94,95]

Platform Presentations

When giving platform presentations it is usually necessary to prepare audiovisual materials and, possibly, handouts. This was once rather difficult and expensive. Often a graphic artist would be necessary to prepare good-looking slides. Presenters might have settled for slides prepared by a drug company or may have tried to type and photograph simple slides. In some cases, simple handwritten overhead projector transparencies would be used. However, the availability of presentation programs has made the preparation of professional quality audio-visual materials a much easier task. There really is no excuse to have less than professional-looking slides because of these programs. Overhead slides should only be used to allow recording of items during a discussion; there is little, if any, reason to use them in a formal presentation.

Most office software suites (e.g., Microsoft Office) have very powerful tools to create slides and other materials. These also have professionally designed "templates" that provide good layouts for materials, including color and background choices. The programs may also guide the user to follow general rules, such as avoiding a "busy" slide that will be unreadable from the back of a large room.[96] Also, the programs can be used to do everything from creating simple slides to multimedia extravaganzas—the former being learned in a few minutes, with the more advanced features available for those who need or desire them. Be aware, however, that it is necessary to limit yourself to those features that truly add to the presentation and it is best to avoid having fancy effects in slides just for the sake of the effects.[96] Instead of concentrating on the technology, it is best to concentrate on the message.[97] That will also have the advantage of having fewer things that might go wrong in a presentation.

When starting to prepare audiovisuals, it is necessary to determine what type of equipment and situation will be found at the presentation. The most desirable type of audiovisual is the use of a computer with a projector and appropriate software to give the presentation. It is also possible to project slides from a personal digital assistant (PDA) that is properly equipped,[98] although the presentation will likely be unable to use any advanced features, such as the embedding of multimedia items.[99] The use of computers equipped with presentation software poses various advantages, including lower cost for the presenter, the ability to make last minute changes to slides before the presentation, the ability to include audio and video in the presentation slides, and the capability to embed Internet links into the presentation. When information or software is available on the network or the Internet, it can be demonstrated. Also, in cases where a discussion ensues, it is possible for the presenter to use a word processor, presentation program, or other software to record items on the screen for users to read during or after the session. It is even possible, using a web page creation program (e.g., Microsoft FrontPage), to not only record the information on the screen during the presentation, but to also make it immediately available on the Internet at the end of the program. Some disadvantages include the cost of the equipment for the organizing group, the need for greater technical skills by both the presenter and organizing group, the potential for technological problems (e.g., a computer that refuses to boot, a corrupted data disk, and an Internet connection that does not work), and it may be necessary for the presenter to bring his or her own notebook computer with appropriate software and data. Fortunately, the technical support people for professional meetings are becoming much more familiar with the equipment and the equipment itself is often more dependable.

When preparing the slides themselves, the presenter will have to prepare an outline to guide what is to be presented and determine the information to be presented in each slide. Some general rules can be mentioned.

- Limit each slide to a particular topic. Sometimes this will be an overview, but specifics should be limited to a discrete topic. One or two minutes of presentation material per slide is appropriate. If it is necessary to refer back to a previous slide, just make a duplicate that is inserted at the appropriate location.
- Keep things simple. The program may be able to do many things (e.g., 20 fonts in 16 million colors), but they may not be desirable. Typically use one font (perhaps with bold or underline in a few specific places for emphasis) and limited graphics.
- Limit the amount of information presented on each slide.[96] A rule of thumb is no more than about five bulleted points per slide and no more than about five words per bulleted point. Any more than that quickly becomes confusing or unreadable. Generally, if someone in the back of the room has to squint or it takes more than 10 seconds to take in a slide, there is too much information on it.[100] It has been theorized that a portion of the blame for the loss of the space shuttle, *Columbia*, was due to the information necessary for NASA engineers being hidden in small print on an extremely busy slide.[101] While the consequences for most presentations are not nearly as large, it is still important that slides enhance the provision of the appropriate information, rather than obscure it.
- Consider using a "theme" in the program that will provide colors that go together well and contrast enough to be legible. Colors and color combinations have to be carefully considered because they may have emotional overtones or, in cases of color-blind attendees, may not even be distinguishable.[102]
- Consider graphics. They can make the slide more pleasing to the eye, but they also need to be as simple as possible. If cartoons are included to entertain the audience,

make sure they are related to the talk and, preferably, help to make a point. Also, pictures of landscapes or the presenter's institution may be desired by the presenter, but serve only to distract from the presentation and should be avoided.

- Consider embedding sound or video in the presentation, if it adds to the presentation. That sounds difficult, but may be done with a few clicks of the mouse.
- Embed links to appropriate websites in the presentation.
- Save the presentation several ways. Even if it is on the computer hard drive, it may become corrupted or the computer can break. Perhaps also bring it on a floppy disk, so that someone else's computer can be borrowed if necessary. It usually now preferable to consider "burning" the presentation to a recordable (or read/write) CD-ROM or DVD, which will not be sensitive to magnetic fields that might have affected the original disk, or to carry the presentation on a USB storage "key" device. Also, in case the computer to be used in the presentation does not have presentation software, it might be necessary to use the feature in many presentation software packages that creates a run-time presentation that does not require the actual software. In some cases, putting the slides on a web server in presentation format may work, although accessing the slides and web pages over the Internet can be a risky proposition. Also, as mentioned previously, the presentation might be given using a PDA device.

Other items to consider include the following:

- When presenting, if traditional 2×2 slides are used, bring them in a projector carousel tray that is labeled with the name and address of the speaker and with the title of the presentation. Check the slides before the meeting to make sure that they are in the correct order and are in the correct orientation. Also, be sure to check to make sure there will be a slide projector, since the use of traditional slides is becoming very rare.
- Make sure to carry the presentation materials personally and do not check them as luggage, since they may be lost. Also, be careful not to damage the materials being carried.
- Try to make the presentation interactive—ask the audience questions and take input.
- In all but a very small room be sure to use the microphone. Speakers may not want to be bothered or may feel it is a sign of weakness to use a microphone, but they need to remember that the microphone is there to help the audience, not the speaker, and should be used so that everyone in the back of the room can hear over the ventilation system.
- Keep to the slides, if at all possible, but do not read the slides—use the slides as a jumping point to your oral presentation information and to organize your thoughts.[96]
- Do not read a prepared script. Actors and politicians can read such scripts and sound natural, but most speakers cannot do so. Instead use the slides (preferable) or a simple outline. The presentation program will allow easy preparation of handouts and speakers notes that can be used.

- Be prepared for technological disaster.[97] Even when using something as simple as an overhead projector, the bulb can burn out. When using more equipment and more complex equipment, the potential for equipment failure rapidly increases. Whenever possible, have backup equipment, but also have a backup plan so that the presentation can proceed without any equipment.

It may be desirable to prepare a handout for the audience, in which case, the presenter can consider the following styles:[103]

- *Outlines*—A reference document that gives the audience a guide to where the speaker is going in text form. This can often be prepared by importing the slide content from the presentation software to a word processor. Some presentation programs will also prepare the document itself.
- *Full-text handouts*—This is essentially a transcription of the speech. While helpful as a reference document, it is probably of more use to politicians when they wish to avoid being misquoted. This is seldom seen in pharmacy, because the presenter will not be able to make last minute changes and the audience will likely read ahead and become bored. Interestingly, a comment heard when such documents are presented is that "the speaker did not know the material, because all she (or he) did was read the handout," even though the speaker was the one who wrote it!
- *Slide reproductions*—This is becoming more popular and easy; presentation programs allow easy slide handout preparation. This does give the attendee all of the information, including graphics, but will likely require more paper.
- *Partial-text handouts*—This can be something of a combination of the above, where only a portion of the talk is on the handouts.

In any of the above, it is good to consider the following:[103]

- Consider whether it is necessary to provide references or supplemental readings.
- Make sure that the handout follows the order of the presentation. If it does not, the attendee may become confused and annoyed.
- Make it look good, using skills mentioned elsewhere in this chapter. By all means, allow plenty of room for the attendee to take notes.

The speaker may also use the handout as a set of speaker notes, but care should generally be taken to avoid just reading the handout to the audience, except in the case of full-text handouts, for the reasons previously mentioned.

The skills necessary to give the presentation itself are beyond the scope of this chapter that deals with the preparation and distribution of written material. New presenters may wish to read a book or pamphlet on how to give effective talks. Also, Toastmasters International (<<http://www.toastmasters.org>>) is a group that will help individuals develop speaking skills. Many institutions have a chapter of this organization. These aids will provide guidance on such skills as what level of sophistication to use in speaking, how to stand (e.g., "do not hide behind the podium" and making eye contact), what language to use, how to use humor and other techniques to entertain the audience, how to address questions (including so called "sniper" questions that tend to disrupt speakers due to level of difficulty and how they are thrown into the middle of the presentation),[104] how to avoid distractions by having everyone turn off phones and pagers,[105] and so forth. Also, some of the references used in preparation of this chapter provide many additional suggestions.[94,103]

Poster Presentations

Preparing a poster requires the presenter to first determine what is to be included. Typically, the information will be similar to that found in an abstract, but with an expansion of the various sections. There are likely to be tables, bulleted points, and figures. Overall, the information to be presented must be brief, so that it can be read within a couple of minutes by an individual passing by the display. Therefore, large amounts of text are undesirable. A poster presentation will not likely contain nearly as much information as a formal journal article, but will contain many of the same sections. It will serve as a place for discussion to begin between the presenter and interested individuals.

Preparing posters was at one time a very difficult prospect. A good-looking poster required either the use of graphic services or many hours using rub-on letters. This has changed with the availability of presentation and high-end word processing/publishing software on computers.

Some people prefer to use essentially the same presentation programs as would be used for slides. The individual "slides," which may be longer than could possibly fit on a typical 2×2 slide, will then be printed on a color printer and mounted on poster board. An assortment of these "slides" will then be pinned to the board provided at the meeting. This is easy to do, but does require carrying and mounting many individual pieces. Also, it tends to limit the size of items on the presentation and may not lend itself to allowing the most professional looking presentation. A final disadvantage is that any one-page handouts will have to be prepared separately.

Another possibility is the preparation of a large, one-piece poster that is typically about 3×6 ft. Although the final poster must be printed by a graphics firm (e.g., printer and architectural drawing firm), the cost can be reasonable to produce a very good-looking poster. The initial preparatory work can also be done by such firms, but it is less expensive to do this yourself. The software necessary would be either a desktop publishing software (e.g., Adobe PageMaker and Microsoft Publisher) or a high-end word processor (e.g., Microsoft Word and WordPerfect). Essentially, what needs to be done is to lay out the page in these programs so that it is in landscape format (i.e., sideways from the normal typed page). The top of the page will have a centered title in large print, with the author names, institution, city, and so on centered in a smaller font below the title. Often, it is desirable to place graphics to one or both sides of that information, such as the symbol for the authors' institution(s). Under that, the page may be divided up into three or so columns and the information laid out in a logical order, including tables and figures. It may be desirable, once finished, to print out the final copy in two sizes. One can be a copy that fits on typical $8^{1}/_{2} \times 11$ in. paper, which can be reproduced and distributed to interested individuals at the meeting. The second may be on larger paper (e.g., 11×17 in.) if there is a suitable high-quality printer available. The graphics firm can use this and/or the data file on a disk to create the final poster. Using the data file may be less expensive, but it will be necessary to contact and work with a graphics firm before preparing the file to make sure that the file is prepared with a program and in a format that can be used by the graphics firm.

Whatever method is used, the final product will need to be transported to the meeting (poster tubes are available for little or no cost from many graphics firms). It is preferable to carry such posters on airplanes, because they may be crushed in the baggage areas. The presenter should also remember to bring pushpins to mount the presentation at the meeting. The presenter should show up early enough for the presentation to have the material mounted to the bulletin board before meeting attendees are allowed in the area and will be expected to remain with the presentation to answer questions for the assigned time. Although many people may be the authors of a presentation, it is not uncommon that only one or two actually attend the meeting and give the presentation.

Web Posting

After a presentation, consider making the material available on the Internet. Some organizations are now making at least some presentation materials available that way. Of course, copyright restrictions may prevent individuals from posting the material, but technology makes it easy when it is allowable. Text documents, such as posters, are easily placed on a website. However, even full slide presentations can be placed on a website, using streaming audiovisual. A variety of software, such as RealVideo or Microsoft PowerPoint and Producer, can be used to prepare such streaming presentations that can include slides and an audiovisual recording of the presenter. This can even be done concurrently with the presentation (live streaming), with a recording being made for later viewing. The equipment needs are relatively minor (i.e., recent computer, presentation software, microphone, and inexpensive computer video capture device [e.g., Logitech QuickCam] for recording). For the actual Internet streaming, the appropriate streaming software, running on a file server, is necessary. For those who do not have the appropriate streaming software just placing the slides themselves, as a downloadable file or in presentation format, can be an easy process using the original software used to prepare the slides. Even the simplest website can then be used to give access to the material.

Conclusion

Professional writing is a skill necessary for every pharmacist. It simply consists of following the accepted rules for writing that have been established by the profession to prepare a written item that is clear, concise, complete, correct, and in the appropriate format.

REFERENCES

1. Thordsen DJ. Preparing an article for publication. J Pharm Technol. 1986;5:268–75.
2. Moghadam RG. Scientific writing: a career for pharmacists. Am J Health Syst Pharm. 2003;60: 1899–1900.
3. Armbruster DL. Starting the writing process. J Pediatr Pharmacol Ther. 2003;8(3):210–1.
4. Fye WB. Medical authorship: traditions, trends, and tribulations. Ann Intern Med. 1990;113:317–25.
5. Gannon F. Ethical profits from publishing. EMBO Rep. 2004;5(1):1.
6. Nahata MC. Publishing by pharmacists. DICP Ann Pharmacother. 1989;23:809–10.
7. Wager E, Field EA, Grossman L. Good publication practice for pharmaceutical companies. Curr Med Res Opin. 2003;19(3):149–54.
8. Wilcox LJ. Authorship: the coin of the realm, the source of complaints. JAMA. 1998;280:216–7.
9. Hoen WP, Walvoort HC, Overbeke AJPM. What are the factors determining authorship and the order of the authors' names? A study among authors of the Nederlands. Tijdschrift voor Geneeskunde (Dutch Journal of Medicine). 1998;280:217–8.
10. Committee on Publication Ethics (COPE). Guidelines on good publication practice. Cope Report; 2002. p. 48–52.
11. Shapiro DW, Wenger NS, Shapiro MF. The contributions of authors to multiauthored biomedical research papers. JAMA. 1994;271:438–42.
12. Flanagin A, Carey LA, Fontanarosa PB, Phillips SG, Pace PB, Lundberg GD, et al. Prevalence of articles with honorary authors and ghost authors in peer-reviewed medical journals. JAMA. 1998;280:222–4.
13. Wager E. Raising the quality of publications: now we have GPP! Qual Assur J. 2003;7:166–70.
14. Peterson AM, Lowenthal W, Veatch RM. Authorship on a manuscript intended for publication. Am J Hosp Pharm. 1993;50:2082–5.
15. Carbone PP. On authorship and acknowledgments [letter]. N Engl J Med. 1992;326:1084.
16. Hart RG. On authorship and acknowledgments [letter]. N Engl J Med. 1992;326:1084.
17. Pinching AJ. On authorship and acknowledgments [letter]. N Engl J Med. 1992;326:1084–5.
18. Canter D. On authorship and acknowledgments [letter]. N Engl J Med. 1992;326:1085.
19. Rennie D, Yank V, Emanuel L. When authorship fails. A proposal to make contributors accountable. JAMA. 1997;278:579–85.
20. Fathalla MF, VanLook PFA. On authorship and acknowledgments. N Engl J Med. 1992;326:1085.
21. The International Committee of Medical Journal Editors. Statement from the International Committee of Medical Journal Editors. JAMA. 1991;265:2697–8.
22. Hasegawa GR. Spurious authorship. Am J Hosp Pharm. 1993;50:2063.

23. Rennie D, Flanagin A. Authorship! Authorship! Guests, ghosts, grafters, and the two-sided coin. JAMA. 1994;271:469–71.

24. International Committee of Medical Journal Editors. Uniform requirements for manuscripts submitted to biomedical journals. Med Educ. 1999;33:66–78.

25. International Committee of Medical Journal Editors. Uniform Requirements for manuscripts submitted to biomedical journals: writing and editing for biomedical publication [Internet]. Philadelphia (PA): International Committee of Medical Journal Editors, 2003 Nov [cited 2004 Apr 2]. Available from: http://www.icmje.org/index.html

26. Kassirer JP, Angell M. On authorship and acknowledgments. N Engl J Med. 1991;325:1510–2.

27. Drenth JPH. Multiple authorship. The contribution of senior authors. JAMA. 1998;280:219–21.

28. Kassirer JP, Angell M. On authorship and acknowledgments [letter]. N Engl J Med. 1992;326:1085.

29. McConnell CR. From idea to print: writing and publishing a journal article. Health Care Superv. 1984;2:78–94.

30. Burnakis TG. Advice on submitting papers. Am J Hosp Pharm. 1993;50:2523.

31. Higa GM. Scientific publications and scientific style. W V Med J. 1995;91:198–9.

32. Crichton M. Medical obfuscation: structure and function. N Engl J Med. 1975;293:1257–9.

33. Jones DEH. Last word. Omni. 1980;2(12):130.

34. Hamilton CW. How to write effective business letters: scribing information for pharmacists. Hosp Pharm. 1993;28:1095–1100.

35. Albert T. The fear of writing—it's not as hard as pharmacists seem to think. Pharmaceut J. 2003;270:55–6.

36. Baker SJ. Getting published. Aust J Hosp Pharm. 1994;24(5):410–5.

37. Hamilton CW. How to write and publish scientific papers: scribing information for pharmacists. Am J Hosp Pharm. 1992;49:2477–84.

38. Ingelfinger FJ. Seduction by citation. N Engl J Med. 1976;295:1075–6.

39. Moher D, Schulz KF, Altman D. The CONSORT statement: revised recommendations for improving the quality of reports of parallel-group randomized trials. JAMA. 2001;285:1987–91.

40. Moher D, Cook DJ, Eastwood S, Olkin I, Rennie D, Stroup DF. Improving the quality of reports of meta-analyses of randomised controlled trials: the QUOROM statement. Lancet. 1999;354: 1896–1900.

41. Ioannidis JPA, Evans SJW, Gøtzsche PC, O'Neill RT, Altman DG, Schulz K, et al. Better reporting of harms in randomized trials: an extension of the CONSORT statement. Ann Intern Med. 2004;141:781–8.

42. Talley CR. Perspective in journal publishing [editorial]. Am J Hosp Pharm. 1993;50:451.

43. Ware J. Cheat wave. Yahoo! Internet Life. 1999;5(5):102–3.

44. Asimov I. Gold: the final science fiction collection. New York: HarperPrism; 1995.

45. Willful infringement [cited 2004 Aug 9]. Available from: http://www.willfulinfringement.com/.

46. Ardito SC, Eiblum P, Daulong R. Conflicted copy rights. Online. 1999;23(3):91–5.

47. Gousse G. Advice on submitting papers: I. Am J Hosp Pharm. 1993;50:2523.

48. World Association of Medical Editors. WAME policy statements [Internet]. Chicago (IL): World Association of Medical Editors, 2004 Apr 7 [cited 2004 Apr 14]. Available from: http://www.wame.org/wamestmt.htm

49. International Committee of Medical Journal Editors. Conflict of interest. Am J Hosp Pharm. 1993;50:2398.

50. Davidoff F, DeAngelis CD, Drazen JM, Hoey J, Horton R, et al. Sponsorship, authorship, and accountability. Lancet. 2001;358:854–6.

51. Krimsky S, Rothenberg LS. Financial interest and its disclosure in scientific publications. JAMA. 1998;280:225–6.

52. Laniado M. How to present research data consistently in a scientific paper. Eur Radiol. 1996; 6:S16–8.

53. DeAngelis CD. Duplicate publication, multiple problems. JAMA. 2004;292:1745–6.

54. Stead WW. The responsibilities of authorship. JAMIA. 1997;4:394–5.

55. Garfunkel JM, Lawson EE, Hamrick HJ, Ulshen MH. Effect of acceptance or rejection on the author's evaluation of peer-review of medical manuscripts. JAMA. 1990;263:1376–78.

56. Evans JT, Nadjari HI, Burchell SA. Quotation and reference accuracy in surgical journals. JAMA. 1990;263:1353–4.

57. Roland CG. Thoughts about medical writing. XXXVII. Verify your references. Anesth Analg. 1976;55:717–8.

58. Biebuyck JF. Concerning the ethics and accuracy of scientific citations. J Anesthesiol. 1992;77:1–2.

59. McLellan MF, Case LD, Barnett MC. Trust, but verify. The accuracy of references in four anesthesia journals. Anesthesiology. 1992;77:185–8.

60. de Lacy G, Record C, Wade J. How accurate are quotations and references in medical journals. Br Med J. 1985;291:884–6.

61. Doms CA. A survey of reference accuracy in five national dental journals. J Dent Res. 1989;68:442–4.

62. Hasegawa GR. How to review a manuscript intended for publication. Am J Hosp Pharm. 1994;51:839–40.

63. Hoppe S, Chandler MJJ. Constructive versus destructive criticism. Am J Health Syst Pharm. 1995;52:103.

64. Baker DE. Peer-review: personal continuous quality improvement. Hosp Pharm. 2004;39:8.

65. Seltzer SM. Desktop publishing in a drug store? Am Druggist. 1987:196:64, 66.

66. Srnka QM, Scoggin JA. 10 ways to distribute newsletters to build sales volume. Pharm Times. 1984:50;71–2, 74.

67. Making the media. The pharmacy newsletter. Hosp Pharm Connection. 1986;2(3):11–2.

68. Kaldy J. Effectively creating a pharmacy newsletter. Consult Pharm. 1992;7(6):700, 697–8.

69. Goldwater SH, Haydon-Greatting S. How to publish a pharmacy newsletter. Am J Hosp Pharm. 1991;48:2121, 2125.

70. Almquist AF, Wolfgang AP, Perri M. Pharmacy newsletters—the journalistic approach. Hosp Pharm. 1988;23:974–5.

71. Schultz WL, Dendiak ST. Pharmacy newsletters: a needed service. Hosp Pharm. 1975;10(4):146–7.

72. Plumridge RJ, Berbatis CG. Drug bulletins: effectiveness in modifying prescribing and methods of improving impact. DICP Ann Pharmacother. 1989;23:330–34.

73. Appearance and content attract newsletter audience. Drug Util Rev. 1988;4(4):45–8.

74. Lyon RA, Norvell MJ. Effect of a P&T Committee newsletter on anti-infective prescribing habits. Hosp Formul. 1985;20:742–4.

75. Fendler KJ, Gumbhir AK, Sall K. The impact of drug bulletins on physician prescribing habits in a health maintenance organization. Drug Intell Clin Pharm. 1984;18:627–31.

76. May JR, Andrusko KT, DiPiro JT. Impact and cost justification of a surgery drug newsletter. Am J Hosp Pharm. 1984;41:1837–9.

77. Ross MB, Volger BW, Bradley JK. Use of "dispense-as-written" on prescriptions for targeted drugs: influence of a newsletter. Am J Hosp Pharm. 1990;47:2519–20.

78. Denig P, Haaijer-Ruskamp FM, Zijsling DH. Impact of a drug bulletin on the knowledge, perception of drug utility, and prescribing behavior of physicians. DICP Ann Pharmacother. 1990;24:87–93.

79. Parker RC. Looking good in print, 4th ed. Scottsdale (AZ): The Coriolis Group, LLC; 1998.

80. Baird RN, McDonald D, Pittman RK, Turnbull AT. The graphics of communication. methods, media and technology, 6th ed. New York: Hartcourt Brace Jovanovich College Publishers; 1993.

81. Koyanl SJ, Bailey RW, Nall JR. Research-based web design & usability guidelines [monograph on the Internet]. Department of Health and Human Services, 2003 [cited 2004 Oct 15]. Available from: http://www.usability.gov/pdfs/guidelines.html

82. Don't let cost prohibit publication of pharmacy-related newsletter. Drug Util Rev. 1988;4(4):48–9.

83. Utt JK, Lewis KT. Using desktop publishing to enhance pharmacy publications. Am J Hosp Pharm. 1988;45:1863–4.

84. Pfeiffer KS. Award-winning newsletter design. Windows Mag. 1994;5(8):208–18.

85. What makes a great website? [cited 1999 May 13]: [1 screen]. Available from: http://www.webreference.com/greatsite.html

86. Tweney D. Don't be a slow poke: keep your site up to speed or lose visitors. InfoWorld. 1999;22;21(12):64.

87. Tullio CJ. Selecting material for your newsletter. Hosp Pharm Times. 1992;58(Oct):12HPT–16HPT.

88. Journalism pro offers editing tips for effective pharmacy newsletters. Drug Util Rev. 1988;4(4): 49–50.

89. Mitchell JF, Cook RL. Pharmacy newsletters: time for a new approach. Hosp Formul. 1985;20:360–5.

90. Ritchie DJ, Manchester RF, Rich MW, Rockwell MM, Stein PM. Acceptance of a pharmacy-based, physician-edited hospital Pharmacy and Therapeutics Committee newsletter. Ann Pharmacother. 1992;26:886–9.

91. Craghead RM. Electronic mail pharmacy newsletters. Hosp Pharm. 1989;24:490.

92. Mok MP, Castile JA, Kowaloff HB, Janousek JR. Drugman—a computerized supplement to a hospital's drug information newsletter. Am J Hosp Pharm. 1985;42:1565–7.

93. Speaking abroad. How to prepare when you're presenting over there. Presentations. 1999;13(6): A1–15.

94. Spinler SA. How to prepare and deliver pharmacy presentations. Am J Hosp Pharm. 1991;48:1730–8.

95. Simons T. Multimedia or bust? Presentations. 2000;14(2):40–50.

96. Buchholz S, Ullman J. 12 commandments for PowerPoint. Teaching Prof. 2004;18(6):4.

97. Zielinski D. Technostressed? Don't let your gadgets and gizmos get you down. Presentations. 2004;28–35.

98. Malone PM. Slides, files and keeping up. Adv Pharm. 2004;2(2):175–80.

99. Goldstein M. PDA presenting has come a long way, but still has drawbacks. Presentations. 2003:22.

100. Endicott J. For the prepared presenter, fonts of inspiration abound. Presentations. 1999;13(4):22–3.

101. Bullet points may be dangerous, but don't blame PowerPoint. Presentations. 2003:6.

102. The psychology of presentation visuals. Presentations. 1998;12(5):45–51.

103. Engle JP, Firman SC. Perfecting pharmacist presentation skills. Am Pharm. 1994;NS34(7):60–4.

104. Simons T. For podium emergencies. Presentations. 2003:24–9.

105. Hill J. The attention deficit. Presentations. 2003:27–32.

12

Chapter Twelve

Legal Aspects of Drug Information Practice

Martha M. Rumore

Objectives

After completing this chapter, the reader will be able to

- Describe the legal issues related to the provision of drug information (DI).
- Determine the applicability of various legal theories that impose liability on pharmacists providing DI.
- Describe how pharmacists can help protect themselves from malpractice claims resulting from the provision of DI.
- Review the Doctrine of Drug Overpromotion as it pertains to the 1997 Food and Drug Administration (FDA) Modernization Act (FDAMA).
- Identify the liability concerns inherent with off-label drug use and informed consent.
- Describe U.S. copyright law and the Digital Millennium Copyright Act (DMCA).
- Identify copyright, liability, and privacy issues arising from the Internet.
- Formulate a plan to deal with the major provisions of the Health Insurance Portability and Accountability Act (HIPAA) of 1996.
- Explain the legal issues involved with industry support for pharmaceutical educational activities.

An understanding of the legal aspects of DI can help the practitioner in day-to-day practice, as well as provide some possible ways to protect himself or herself in the legal system. This chapter is intended to examine legal issues and should not be considered legal advice.

There are myriad legal issues confronting the various facets of DI. These legal issues crossover a number of traditional legal specialties, including computer law, advertising law, privacy law, intellectual property law, telecommunications law, and tort law. This chapter provides an overview and discussion of the key legal issues involving intellectual property rights, torts, privacy, and advertising and promotion that may arise in the provision of DI.

More than 35 years after the genesis of DI services, the legal duties of pharmacists providing DI are still evolving. Today, most pharmacy curriculums include DI, realizing that whether a student specializes in DI or not, it is an integral part of pharmacist-supervised patient care. Pharmacists can and will be held liable for their conduct relating to DI. This chapter begins with an examination of the expanded liability of the DI specialist, which is defined as those pharmacists who either work in drug information centers (DICs) or who spend the majority of their working day providing DI. The liability inherent in the provisions of DI to patients as an integral component of pharmacist-supervised patient care is then examined and recommendations for prevention and mitigation of liability are provided for the non-DI specialist. The chapter then explores copyright, privacy, unique legal issues pertaining to the Internet, direct-to-consumer advertising, off-label use, as well as industry support for educational activities.

Tort Law

DI practice is a specialized discipline of pharmacy. Despite the clear prevalence of pharmacist-staffed DICs, the legal obligations of the DI specialist remain unclear. Specialists are held to the highest degree of care by the law. Because of the DI pharmacists' greater expertise in the area of DI, it is likely that the courts would expand their legal and professional liability beyond that of other pharmacists. The liability of the DI specialist versus generalist differs for a number of reasons, the most obvious of which are the nature of the information provided and the recipients of the information. In the provision of pharmaceutical care, pharmacists are providing information to patients, whereas the DI specialist is often providing DI to other health professionals.

Functions such as online searching, monitoring or recommending drug therapy, patient counseling, participation in clinical studies and pharmacy and therapeutics (P&T) committees, drug use evaluation, and identifying adverse drug experiences entail legal obligations of proper performance. Willig has stated[1]:

> If you voluntarily offer and create a higher standard of careful practice, the public has a legal right to assume that pharmacists can and will consistently perform according to that standard.

Minimal practice standards for specialists have been put forth to delineate functions and activities that may be considered essential to the provision of DI services and the expected competencies of DI specialists. Position papers and standards of the American Society of Health-System Pharmacists (ASHP) and Joint Commission on Accreditation of Health care Organizations (JCAHO), as well as DI curriculum standards, remove any doubt about the level of expertise needed for DI specialists and standards for DICs.[2,3] Minimal standards of performance and a consistent level of competence must be assured by pharmacists promoting or offering this service regardless of the practice site. Although there are no standards to accredit DICs, professional standards of performance may be used by courts as an objective measuring tool for the standard of care.

In the latter part of the nineteenth century, the locality rule or community rule was followed. This doctrine stated that the local defendant practitioner would have his or her standard of performance evaluated in light of the performance of other peers in the same or similar communities.[4] This is no longer the case and a DIC in New York City will be held to the same standard as one in a rural area. Creation of standards of practice and the disappearance of the locality rule have made it easier for plaintiffs to prevail.

In addition to the DI specialist, the pharmacy profession is assuming an increased legal responsibility to provide DI in the daily practice of pharmaceutical care. Although the physician has been considered the learned intermediary, responsible for communicating the manufacturer's warnings to the patient, the Omnibus Budget Reconciliation Act of 1990 (OBRA '90) may be shifting this responsibility to the pharmacist. Failure to counsel or warn cases are showing an increasing trend in pharmacist liability.[5] Recent cases demonstrate the pharmacist's duty to warn of foreseeable complications of drug therapy is becoming a recognized part of the expanded legal responsibility of pharmacists.

Where the patient is at higher risk than the general population, the courts have uniformly found liability. There are many such cases against physicians for failure to disclose material risks of medical procedures or treatments to their patients.[6-8] Today, there is some question as to when a pharmacist provides DI, whether they be generalists or DI specialists, are held to the same standards as physicians when determining standard of care.

Traditionally, physicians remain responsible for their patients and must exert "due care"; that is, a physician who knows or should have known that information provided was improper may be held liable for negligence. Currently, most litigation concerning pharmacists involves negligence. Therefore, it is safe to assume that a legal cause of action pertaining to the provision of DI will be founded on the theory of negligence as the direct or proximate cause of personal injury or death. Malpractice liability based on negligence refers to failure to exercise the degree of care that a prudent (reasonable) person would exercise under the same circumstances. Elements of negligence include the four Ds: (1) duty breached, (2) damages, (3) direct causation, and (4) defenses absent. To establish a negligent failure, actual conduct must be compared to what is considered standard professional conduct. Typically, this is accomplished by introducing evidence of the relevant professional standards or testimony from expert witnesses such as pharmacy school faculty or other

DI practitioners. Once the duty of care is established, the plaintiff would need a preponderance of evidence to prove that (1) the information provided was materially deficient, (2) the deficient information was a proximate cause of injury suffered (or at least a substantial contributing factor), (3) the recipient reasonably relied on the information provided, (4) the information deficiency was due to failure to exercise reasonable care, and (5) the pharmacist knew or should have known that the safety or health of another may have depended on the accuracy of the information provided.

Expanding on the first element of negligence, duty breached, it is important to be aware of the fact that the duty must be a legal duty, not a moral or ethical duty. Although there are many ethical dilemmas pertaining to the provision of DI by pharmacists and they can sometimes give rise to a cause of action, an ethical breach is not necessarily a legal breach. Similarly, conduct that is considered unprofessional in the broad sense (e.g., rudeness) is distinct from legal duty. An example of an ethical breach that could result in liability for the pharmacist would be a breach of patient confidentiality, if that disclosure caused damages (e.g., loss of employment or the misuse of information gained in the course of employment).

In a study of DI requests, calls from consumers raised more ethical issues than calls from health professionals.[9] For example, should a pharmacist respond to a drug identification request for someone else's medication? Is the situation different if the medication is a drug of abuse and the inquiry is from a parent, relative, teacher, or police officer? Current law provides little guidance for disclosure of DI for questionable purposes and pharmacists must exercise independent professional judgment and assume legal responsibility for that judgment, when exercised.

It is necessary to expand on the fourth element of negligence, which is reasonable care. Reasonable care is that which would be considered acceptable and responsible. Suppose a patient develops a reaction that is believed to be caused by a drug, and the pharmacist is consulted to find any case reports of this drug causing the reaction. If the case is available online, but not in print, and the pharmacist had access to online databases, but did not consult them, was the pharmacist required to do so? Did the pharmacist exert reasonable care? What if the pharmacist searched MEDLINE®, but not *Exerpta Medica* databases, or vice versa, and thereby failed to retrieve the case? Should the pharmacist have searched both? There are no clear answers here. Who can say what a reasonable search might have been on a given day? However, using outdated references or old editions of textbooks would more likely constitute an inadequate search. In a German case, a court held a patent information service to be responsible for not having used updated materials.[10]

In a highly publicized case involving a clinical trial being conducted at Johns Hopkins University, a researcher conducted an incomplete search for lung damage from hexamethonium on PubMed®, which was searchable only back to 1966 and an open web search.[11] Although articles published in the 1950s and other sources such as TOXLINE and POISINDEX® warned of such dangers, the researcher had not consulted these references, resulting in a patient's death.

Recent cases against pharmacists have held that pharmacists who gain information about the unique susceptibility of a patient are liable for failure to warn of the risks. In *Dooley v. Everett*, the court held the pharmacist liable for failing to warn a patient on theophylline of the interaction with erythromycin that produced seizures and consequent brain damage.[12] Similarly, in *Hand v. Krakowski*, the pharmacist failed to alert either the patient or physician of the drug interaction between the patient's psychotropic drug and alcohol.[13] The fact that the medication profile indicated that the patient was an alcoholic created a foreseeable risk of injury and, therefore, a duty to warn on the part of the pharmacist.

In *Baker v. Arbor Drugs, Inc.*, the court ruled that by advertising its drug interaction software, the defendant pharmacy voluntarily assumed a duty to use its computer technology with due care. The pharmacy technician had overridden the drug interaction between tranylcypromine sulfate (Parnate®) and clemastine fumarate/phenylpropanolamine hydrochloride (Tavist-D®) that the system detected from the patient's medication profile. The patient committed suicide after suffering a stroke from the combination.[14]

There are a number of ways in which tort liability can attach to the provision of DI: incomplete information, inappropriate quality information, outdated information, inappropriate analysis, or dissemination of information.

INCOMPLETE INFORMATION

Is the pharmacist liable when the DI provided is incomplete? Should the pharmacist provide all the medication information via a DI sheet or patient package insert (PPI)? There have been several cases against pharmacists for failure to dispense mandatory PPIs for certain drugs that later caused harm. In *Parkas v. Saary*, the court addressed the issue of whether the pharmacist's failure to dispense the Food and Drug Administration (FDA)-mandated PPI for progesterone was the proximate cause of the congenital eye defect that occurred.[15] Because congenital defects, but not eye deformities, were specified in the PPI, failure to provide the PPI could not be proven to be the proximate cause. Therefore, judgment was in favor of the pharmacy. In *Frye v. Medicare-Glaser Corporation*, the pharmacist counseled the patient regarding drowsiness with Fiorinal®, but failed to provide a warning not to consume alcohol. The patient died, presumably as a result of combining the drug with beer. Here, the DI provided was incomplete. The trial court did not find the pharmacist had a duty to warn in this instance.[16] However, it is important to realize that this case was decided before OBRA '90 was in effect.

More recent cases are finding pharmacists have a responsibility for patient counseling and drug therapy monitoring.[17] In *Sanderson v. Eckerd Corporation*, the pharmacist was liable for "voluntary undertaking" to act in the absence of a duty, where the pharmacy's computer was inappropriately used by the pharmacist in detection of an adverse reaction and the pharmacist failed to warn the patient of the potential for an adverse reaction.[18] In *Horner v.*

Spalitto, the court imposed a duty on a pharmacist to alert the prescriber when the dose prescribed is outside the therapeutic range.[19] In *Happel v. Wal-Mart Stores*, the pharmacy's computer system was overridden, and the pharmacist failed to warn a patient allergic to aspirin and ibuprofen of the potential for cross-allergenicity with ketorolac.[20] The court found the pharmacist has a duty to warn when a contraindicated drug is prescribed. In *Morgan v. Wal-Mart Stores*, the court held that pharmacists have a duty beyond accurately filling a prescription "based on known contraindications, that would alert a reasonably prudent pharmacist to a potential problem."[21] However, the court did not find for the plaintiff opining that pharmacists do not have knowledge that desipramine may cause hypereosinophilic syndrome.

Clearly, these cases demonstrate an expansion of pharmacists' duties from the nondiscretionary standard of technical accuracy to a discretionary standard which requires pharmacists to perform professional functions, that is, from a technical model to a pharmaceutical care model. Knowledge of or access to DI is becoming an important factor that courts consider in determination of the pharmacist's duty to warn.

Conversely, while pharmacists are in a position to provide DI, providing the patient with all information may have a detrimental effect. In fact, it is the FDA's position that the information contained in professional labeling can be safely used only under the supervision of the licensed prescriber. It has, therefore, been the practice not to provide the patient with the professional labeling unless the patient specifically requests it. With regard to the duty to disclose to the patient low percentage risks, the court rulings have been inconsistent. One court has allowed strict liability against a pharmacy. In *Heredia v. Johnson*, the pharmacist dispensed an otic solution without warning of the risk of tympanic membrane rupture and the need to discontinue the drug if certain symptoms appeared. The plaintiff claimed that because of the lack of warning, he suffered from severe and permanent injury including brain damage.[22] However, in *Marchione v. State*, a prison inmate alleged lack of informed consent based on the failure of the prison doctor to inform him about the side effects of prazosin (Minipress®), which caused permanent impotence. The physician argued that his duty was only to warn of severe or frequent side effects. The *Marchione* court concluded that the physician need not disclose a list of 31 remote drug side effects. The side effect had a reported incidence of only two or three cases out of several million prescriptions and was, therefore, rare. The plaintiff also did not have any unique risk factors that would increase the likelihood of the reaction occurring.[23] The courts seem to look at risk factors unique to the patient in deciding whether the health professional is required to indicate the likelihood of occurrence of the risks.

Brushwood and Simonsmeier[24] delineate two responsibilities with regard to patient counseling: risk assessment and risk management. Risk assessment is judgmental and occurs before prescribing when a decision is made to accept or forego drug therapy. Although this has traditionally been the responsibility of the physician, the current scope of pharmacy practice is expanding as a growing number of states permit independent,

dependent, and collaborative prescribing.[25] Each level of prescriptive authority is characterized by a specific level of liability. For example, independent prescribers are professionally accountable for their own prescribing decisions. Dependent prescribing, which involves the delegation of authority from an independent prescriber as is typical of therapeutic interchange and drug therapy management protocols in health care facilities, involves a shared accountability. Similarly, in collaborative prescribing where there is a collaborative practice agreement that allows pharmacists to initiate and/or modify patients' medication regimens pursuant to an approved protocol, both the physician and pharmacists share accountability.[26] In addition, employers would remain vicariously liable for the actions and decisions of their staff.

Risk management occurs after prescribing, is nonjudgmental, and assists the patient in proper drug use to maximize benefits and minimize potential problems.[27,28] Drug risk management, but not drug risk assessment, information should be provided to patients. The drug management information provided to patients should be accurate and in a form that the patient understands.

Hall and Honey[29] divided the risks associated with a particular drug into two groups, inherent or noninherent. Inherent risks are unique to the drug and usually identified in the package insert, but do not include probable or common side effects. Noninherent risks are created by the particular drug in combination with some extrinsic factor about which the pharmacist should reasonably know, and include maximum safe dosages, interactions, patient characteristics influencing pharmacokinetics, and probable or common side effects. The responsibility of the pharmacist to provide DI about noninherent risks is expanding.

What liability does the pharmacist incur for information outside of the package insert? Physicians may prescribe drugs as they see fit, without adhering to the specific therapeutic indications or dosing guidelines within the labeling. The FDA regulates the manufacture and promotion of drugs, not the practice of medicine. However, it has been held that a physician's deviation from the package insert was prima facie (i.e., not requiring further support to establish validity, on its face value) evidence of negligence if the patient's injury resulted from the failure to adhere to the recommendations.[30] However, the states appear to be split on whether recommendations in a package insert are *prima facie* evidence of the standard of care. It would be prudent for the pharmacist to consult the package insert when responding to an inquiry and include such information in the response, especially if the response is contrary to what is contained in the package insert.

A recent disciplinary action by a state pharmacy board highlights the importance of checking the package insert or conducting a literature search concerning the proposed use of a product. In *re Michael A. Gabert*, a pharmacist received a prescription for 5% silver nitrate for bladder instillation. The pharmacist contacted a DIC and was told there was no literature supporting the proposed use of the product. The pharmacist then asked the physician what support he had for such use and the physician referred to a published Mayo Clinic Newsletter.

The pharmacist did not ask to see a copy of the newsletter, or have a copy of it for the pharmacy records. Significant patient harm resulted when the solution was instilled into the patient's bladder. The Mayo Clinic Newsletter pertained to silver argyrol, not silver nitrate.[31]

INAPPROPRIATE QUALITY INFORMATION

It has long been recognized by law that false information provided to another could result in harm to the recipient if the recipient acted relying on the false information. Although negligent misrepresentation has not been applied to DI, there is no guarantee that it will not be in the future.[32] The relevant law is the *Restatement (Second) of Torts, §311, Negligent Misrepresentation Involving Risk of Physical Harm*, which states:

> One who negligently gives false information to another is subject to liability for physical harm caused by action taken by the other in reasonable reliance upon such information …. Such negligence may consist of failure to exercise reasonable care in ascertaining accuracy of the information, or in the manner in which it is communicated.[33]

The DI itself may be faulty for one or more reasons: it may be outdated, it may simply be wrong, it may be incomplete and, therefore, misleading, or none may have been provided because of an incomplete search or incompetent searcher. Information negligence may occur because of (1) parameter negligence (failure to consult the correct source) or (2) omission negligence (consulting the correct source, but failure to locate the correct answer[s]). A study evaluated the accuracy of a drug identification response by 56 DICs. Only approximately 30% correctly identified the investigational drug product; 67% could not make the identification; most importantly, 3.6% (two DICs) made an incorrect identification. The study found inconsistencies in responses of DICs.[34] Another study evaluated the quality of DI responses provided by 116 DICs to multiple queries. The correct response rates varied from 5% for a question pertaining to erythromycin for diabetic gastroparesis to 90% for a drug interaction question pertaining to didanosine-dapsone. For three patient-specific questions, the percentages of centers eliciting vital patient data were 5%, 27%, and 86%. The findings suggest that many DICs continue to fail to elicit patient-specific information necessary for informed responses and focus instead on procedural and technical matters.[35] As an illustration, recently, despite the peer-review process all too familiar to authors, the structure of bilirubin was found to be incorrect in an article as well as the three leading biochemistry textbooks in the United States.[36]

Can pharmacists providing DI be held responsible for retrieving information that is itself inaccurate? What responsibility does the information producer incur for errors in information sources? An unskilled searcher or one with insufficient searching knowledge may not find correct or complete information, which can lead to the wrong answer. The fault can lie anywhere in the information dissemination chain, publication, collection, storage, retrieval, dissemination, or utilization. Although very few cases have been brought before courts concerning the liability of print or online information sources, there is some case law to guide. The issue concerns strict liability.

Strict liability applies where a defective product proximately causes physical harm. Where the service rendered is deemed to be a professional service, the courts exhibit a reluctance to impose strict liability. With exceptions, persons physically injured because of their reliance on defective and unreasonably dangerous information have only negligence as a cause of action, and only against the author, not the publisher[37]; only if the publisher is negligent or offers intentionally misleading information could it be held liable. This was tested in *Jones v. J.B. Lippincott Co.*, where a nursing student was injured after consulting and relying on a nursing textbook that recommended hydrogen peroxide enemas for the treatment of constipation. The courts rejected the plaintiff's claim that strict liability should be applied to the publisher.[38] Similarly, in a German case, a misprint in a medical textbook resulted in the injection of 25% rather than 2.5% sodium chloride solution, injuring a patient. Again, the court rejected strict liability for the publisher on the basis that any medically educated person should have noticed the misprint.[39] In *Roman v. City of New York*, the plaintiff sued for an alleged misstatement in a booklet distributed by a planned parenthood organization that resulted in a "wrongful conception." The court found that "a publisher cannot assume liability for all misstatements, said or unsaid, to a potentially unlimited public for a potentially unlimited period."[40] In *Winter v. G.R Putnam's Sons*, two persons required liver transplants after collecting and eating poisonous wild mushrooms. They had relied on an *Encyclopedia of Wild Mushrooms* in choosing to eat the mushrooms that caused this severe harm.[41] The court refused to hold the publisher liable and found that a publisher has no duty to investigate the accuracy of the information it publishes.

In *Delmuth Development Corp. v. Merck & Co.*, the plaintiff claimed lost sales because of the publication of erroneous information in the *Merck Index*. The court considered the duty of a publisher to a reader to publish accurate information in a compendium.[42] The court noted a publisher's right to publish without fear of liability is guaranteed by the First Amendment and societal interest. It further held that even if it had a duty to publish with care, the plaintiff could not claim it suffered damages because of reliance on this information.

In *Libertelli v. Hoffman La Roche, Ltd. & Medical Economics Co.*, the plaintiff became addicted to diazepam (Valium®) and sued the publisher of the *Physician's Desk Reference* (PDR).[43] The claim was based on the absence of warnings in the PDR regarding the addictive nature of the drug. The court dismissed the case against the publisher. Under a long line of cases, a publisher is not liable for matters of public interest if it has no knowledge of its falsity. Although some effort should be made to verify search results, the pharmacist cannot be held responsible for knowing and verifying the contents of all sources, whether in print or online. However, checking a second reference to verify information is prudent.

Strict liability would appear applicable to software that is licensed without significant modification as a standard packaged system, as has been found with defective medical computer programs.[44] Pharmacists providing DI should be aware of computer-related lawsuits involving defects (or bugs) in software that caused erroneous results. These cases are resulting in greater damage awards based on consequential (i.e., special as opposed to actual) damages suffered. An example of consequential damages would be damage to a firm's reputation. Perhaps, the most widely cited software-related accidents involve malfunctioning computerized radiation machines where overdosages have caused patient deaths.[45] Radiation overdosages from faulty software continue to occur today; grim reminders of the problems faced by reliance on software.[46] In one particularly relevant case, the court held that the National Weather Service was liable for the deaths of four fishermen off Cape Cod, Massachusetts. The Weather Service had forecasted calm weather because of faulty software. Although the verdict was overturned on technical grounds, the U.S. District Court let stand the precedent holding an entity liable for information it provides.[47]

In another case, *Jeppesen*, an information provider, was held liable for an airplane crash caused by faulty data from the Federal Aviation Administration on flight patterns. A pilot used one of the faulty charts and crashed into a mountain, killing the crew and destroying the plane. The company paid $12 million in damages.[48] The court held the information provider strictly liable because the charts were considered a product. In *Jeppesen*, the mass production and mass marketing of the charts rendered them a product. Similarly, in *Greenmoss Builders v. Dun & Bradstreet*, the issue involved the erroneous listing of Greenmoss Builders as a company in bankruptcy in Dun & Bradstreet Business Information Report database. A jury awarded $350,000, including $300,000 in punitive damages. The case was appealed all the way to the Supreme Court, where Dun & Bradstreet lost the case.[49]

In *Daniel v. Dow Jones & Co., Inc.*, where a subscriber brought action against a provider of a computerized database alleging that he relied on a false news report in making investments, the court found that the subscriber did not have a "special relationship" with the database provider necessary to impose liability for negligent misstatements. First Amendment guarantees of freedom of the press also protected the provider from liability.[50]

INAPPROPRIATE ANALYSIS/DISSEMINATION OF INFORMATION

Is liability for DI a rhetorical supposition or a real possibility? The responsibility of pharmacists providing DI goes beyond that of mere information intermediary, the person in between the information producer and the user. Published studies for DICs have reported that 41 to 83% of requested information is patient-specific or judgmental in nature.[51] In addition to liability for negligent information retrieval and dissemination, the pharmacist's role involves information interpretation, evaluation, and giving advice. This role falls into a consultative model and differs greatly from that of librarians. Librarians are not equipped to give advice. The pharmacist's role as evaluator and interpreter of the information creates a duty sufficient to sustain liability.

The paucity of case law in the area does not negate liability. The issue deserves consideration because of the potential for harm caused by the DI provided by the pharmacist. There have only been two cases involving poison information centers, one of which also was a DIC. In Reben v. Ely, the plaintiffs filed suit against the DIC for injuries sustained by inadvertent administration of cocaine solution instead of acetaminophen to a 10-year-old patient. The local pharmacy had colored the 10% cocaine solution red and labeled it red solution to thwart abuse. When the nurse realized the mistake, she contacted the Arizona Poison and DIC. The pharmacist described the symptomatology of cocaine overdose, but did not go far enough in recommending that the patient seek emergency room care. The patient developed seizures and cardiopulmonary arrest with brain damage that will require lifetime nursing care. At the trial, the expert witness testified that the DIC operated below the standard of care. The issue was not erroneous information, but whether the center went far enough in its responsibility in handling the call. The plaintiff was awarded $6.5 million; the DIC was held liable for $3.6 million.[52]

In another case, a lawsuit named a poison information center that was called for assistance when a student died after swallowing a toxic substance during a laboratory experiment. The poison center was named in the $2.5 million suit because it refused to release proof of its claim that the person who called had given the wrong name for the solution that the student drank.[53]

From a liability standpoint, there are disadvantages to the formal combination of poison control and DICs. For example, poison inquiries usually require immediate answers in critical situations without written documentation and sometimes without supporting references.[54,55] The outcomes of poisonings (e.g., overdoses and suicide attempts) are more likely to result in patient morbidity and mortality and require medical backup for acute treatment decisions. Some states (e.g., Arkansas, Oregon, Washington, Arizona, and New Jersey) have statutory provisions for joint poison control and DICs. In several of these states, such as Arkansas, immunity from personal liability in judgment (in contrast to carelessness or inadvertence) would not be actionable as malpractice unless a lack of due care can be shown. However, not all DICs are so protected from liability.

Defenses to Negligence and Malpractice Protection

Even if the plaintiff can establish all the necessary elements of negligence, legal defenses can avoid or reduce liability. Some defenses might include a statute of limitations, comparative or contributory negligence, informed consent, or governmental immunity. It is important to keep in mind that there may be differences in both types of defenses to negligence and insurance coverage for individuals and employers. Further information on defenses will be described in the following sections.

DEFENSES FOR INDIVIDUALS

Under informed consent, the defendant could assert that the patient knowingly assumed the risk for a new or experimental therapy or regimen. However, the risks that the patient assumes do not include negligence on the part of the physician or pharmacist. Delegation of authority does not mean abdication of responsibility. Under vicarious liability, a pharmacist who has not been personally negligent could be held responsible for the negligence of others. Supervision and adequate training of subordinates (e.g., interns, externs, residents, and other employees) are essential. Incompetence and substandard training of these individuals can lead to liability. An example might include a breach of confidentiality (e.g., revealing someone has a loathsome disease) by one of these employees.

Comparative negligence is the allocation of responsibility for damages incurred between the plaintiff and defendant, based on the relative negligence of the two. Concurrent negligence is the wrongful acts or omissions of two or more persons acting independently, but causing the same injury. Under comparative or concurrent negligence, the pharmacist may also be held liable either alone or together with the information requestor (e.g., physician and nurse) for inaccurate information or information that does not ensure maximal protection for the patient. Vicarious liability is the imputation of liability on one person for the actions of another. Through the doctrine of vicarious liability, a pharmacist could become associated with professional liability actions as part of a case against a hospital or physician.

In the landmark case *Harbeson v. Parke Davis*, a federal court ruled that the doctrine of informed consent required a physician to furnish a patient contemplating pregnancy with information concerning the teratogenicity of the phenytoin she was taking. The physician had a duty to provide information reasonably available in the medical literature, but failed to do so. Even though the physician was not aware of the potential effects of phenytoin, studies were reported in the medical literature.[56] This case represents the only case in which a lack of a literature search resulted in liability.

Cases of vicarious liability are not new to medical malpractice. Physicians have been found negligent for the negligence of nurses, therapists, and others working under their supervision. Significantly, no cases were found where physicians were found negligent from the negligence of pharmacists working under them. If a physician requests DI, he or she would also be held liable if a patient suffers because the search was deficient or the information incorrect. For example, in the *Harbeson* case, if the physician had requested the pharmacist to search for information about the teratogenicity of phenytoin and no references were found because of a faulty search, the pharmacist would share in the negligence together with the physician. The institution would probably also be named as a party in such legal action.

From a legal standpoint, does charging a fee increase liability for the DI provider? Fee-based providers would appear to be at greater malpractice risk, especially if the relationship is a contractual one. If any of the contractual expectations are not met, the client has a contractual cause of action against the DIC. The courts will look to the terms of the agreement and the reasonable expectations of the parties. However, where bodily injury results, tort law may impose liability even where the defective information is given gratuitously and the DI provider derives no benefit from giving it.

Does providing DI services to consumers increase liability exposure? Many DICs provide services to consumers; some via a hotline or health information line via the Internet. Several studies have reported that more ethical questions to DICs arise from consumers than any other group.[57-59] Such ethical questions may involve drug abuse and toxicologic effects, the safety of drugs in pregnancy or nursing, experimental therapy, or the appropriateness of prescribing decisions. A decision to comment on a physician's therapeutic recommendations, even if factually correct and in the patient's best interest, may result in a legal liability. The answers to this and other questions that the pharmacist providing DI encounter may experience (Table 12–1) are not found in the legal precedent.

DEFENSES FOR EMPLOYERS

Is the provider the hospital or the university where the DIC is located or the pharmacist providing the DI? The vast majority of DICs are located in hospitals and universities. In addition, many pharmaceutical companies have DI departments staffed by pharmacists who handle inquiries on the company's products. There also exist independent information brokers who have liability under contract law, as well as tort law. The employer-employee relationship is a significant factor under either common law *respondeat superior* doctrine or, alternatively, a theory of negligent hire or supervision. Respondeat superior refers to the proposition that the employer is responsible for the negligent acts of its agents or employees. The injured party may also sue the employer for its negligence in hiring or supervising the employee. Under a negligent hire theory, it must be shown that the employee was unfit for the position and that a reasonable, pre-employment interview or post-employment supervision would have discovered this fact.[60]

TABLE 12–1. LEGAL QUESTIONS PERTAINING TO DRUG INFORMATION PRACTICE

Should the DI consult be placed in the patient's chart?

Does the theory of warranty apply to therapeutic recommendations?

How should oral responses to DI inquiries be handled?

What is an unreasonable delay in responding to the DI inquiry?

Does providing DI services to the public open the door to liability?

What is the liability for discontinuing DI services?

What is the liability of drug choice decisions based on economic criteria?

Is the pharmacist providing DI responsible for soliciting information necessary to properly consider the question?

Although the person who provides the information is liable for the harm caused by it, the employer may also be held liable in the absence of sovereign or charitable immunity. For pharmacists providing DI employed by the government (e.g., Veteran's Administration [VA] or Public Health Service [PHS]), there are statutes providing governmental immunity, also called sovereign immunity, from civil liability. Such immunity, however, will not protect an intentionally or grossly negligent person.

Even if the lawsuit is nonmeritorious, DICs affiliated with hospitals or universities provide another "deep pocket" for contribution to the settlement. With exceptions, suing the pharmacist alone would fail to provide a windfall settlement for plaintiffs. The board of directors/trustees of the hospital or university or director of the DIC or pharmacy department where the DIC is located would be jointly liable. Joint and several liability refers to the sharing of liabilities among a group of people collectively and also individually. If the defendants are jointly and severally liable, it means that the injured party may sue some or all of the defendants together, or each one separately, and may collect equal amounts or unequal amounts from each. In states where joint and several liability applies, the pharmacist provides additional assurance that there will be sufficient assets to recover. The DI provider will be held responsible for the standard of care in the response to DI inquiries and may be found negligent.

PROTECTING AGAINST MALPRACTICE

Methods to protect against lawsuits include contracts covering financial arrangements, adequate documentation, disclaimers, and insurance.[61] For example, a disclaimer can be placed on the results of online searches stating that the data being provided are from a source believed to be reliable and factually correct.[62] The best way to avoid omission negligence is to learn from experience, anticipate mistakes that may appear in databases, and keep abreast of changes in DI sources. Even if the delivery of false information is the result of inaccurate information itself, the pharmacist would likely be named as a defendant if the database producer were sued.

Adequate documentation may spell the difference between refuting or not refuting an unfounded claim of malpractice. Such documentation includes responses to inquiries, as well as a record of steps taken in a search. Designing and following procedures to document the research process can help avoid negligence. In *Fidelity Leasing Corp. v. Dun & Bradstreet, Inc.*, the court looked at the operation procedures and adherence to them in that particular instance to determine liability for providing false information.

The key to provision of quality DI in an information service is the availability of current, objective information. Procedures should be in place to ensure that data is continually reviewed and updated. Quality assurance (QA) standards for the timeliness, thoroughness, and accuracy of information could also insulate against liability. QA programs, although they exist, are inconsistent among DICs.

Problem areas common to DICs, regardless of practice site, include files not updated and incomplete documentation of responses to requests. With regard to inquiries about adverse reactions, details of the adverse event should be taken and reported to the FDA-reporting program. Cases may be clinically urgent and the physician or nurse may have a patient waiting. Response via e-mail, even with alerts attached, is not prudent in such situations as there is no guarantee that the caller is at the desk to receive such e-mails. All statements made should be traceable to the literature. Additionally, information should be confirmed with other references to ensure consistency between various resources. DICs should address at least some of the items in Table 12–2.

Insistence on a good educational background for entry-level positions followed by the continuing education of DI professionals, certification in online training courses, and good interpersonal communication skills may also protect against malpractice. It is important to keep abreast of changes in sources of DI via regular advanced training, conferences, and reading. All courses in DI should teach situations in ethical conflict that will assist in the decision-making and value judgments encountered in the provision of DI.

TABLE 12–2. QUALITY ASSURANCE AS A LIABILITY-REDUCING FACTOR

Identify scope of activities and personnel requirements.

Develop and follow policies and procedures or formal call triaging protocols.

Keep standard operating procedure manual available for consultation.

Avoid violations of statutes and regulations.

Do not recommend an unapproved use or dose; if a use differs from the labeling, the requestor must be so notified.

Do not recommend a use or dose of a drug based solely on foreign literature or animal studies.

Never extrapolate pediatric dosages from adult dosages.

Maintain knowledge of the current literature, new drug applications and supplemental approvals, labeling changes, and new warnings.

Do not present inadequate data or ignore contrary data.

Avoid overly enthusiastic or exaggerated efficacy and safety claims; do not attempt to diagnose or treat acute poisoning—direct such inquiries to a poison control center or an emergency room.

Know the circumstances of the case and appropriate background information (e.g., knowledge of causality criteria, laboratory findings, concurrent drugs are necessary for adverse drug reaction inquiries; special care is needed for drug identification questions, especially in view of the surge of counterfeit drugs).

Responses of new employees, students, residents should be checked—document, document, document.

Maintain reasonable response time; if necessary prioritize requests.

Obtain peer concurrence or outside professional consultation, if necessary.

Develop a QA mechanism to ensure that service is maintained at a high level of quality (e.g., periodic audits or surveys).

Maintain up-to-date files and reference texts (e.g., files should be randomly checked to be sure they contain articles at least as recent as 2 years old).

Internet specific—check currency, authorship, publisher, length of time site has existed, site reviews, links to/from other sites, biases/objectiveness, intended audience, quality of the writing, references provided, and who maintains the site. (See Chap. 5 for further information regarding evaluating Internet websites.)

Under the tort law doctrine of respondeat superior, both the pharmacist providing DI and the employer are jointly and severally liable for the damages. This enables the plaintiff to have access to the pharmacist's personal assets where the employer's assets are not sufficient to cover an adverse judgment. Professional liability insurance provides protection to cover exactly this kind of liability. Consideration should be given to obtaining professional indemnity insurance for the DI pharmacist.

Most policies now provide coverage on either an occurrence or claims-made basis. Occurrence means any incident that occurs during the policy period, no matter when the claim is filed, within the applicable statute of limitations. Claims-made policies cover only claims that are filed while the policy is active. To cover claims that are filed after a claims-made policy is terminated, the DI pharmacist can purchase tail coverage from the insurer. It is important to be aware of the limitations and exclusions in these policies. Many do not require the carrier to obtain the consent of the insured before settling a claim. In these policies, the right to protect one's reputation may conflict with the economic interest of the insurer to dispose of the claim as inexpensively as possible. Therefore, it is imperative that individuals obtain insurance coverage policies separate from those of their employers. Most common exclusions are coverage for dishonest, fraudulent, criminal, or malicious acts; property damage; and personal injury coverage. In these cases, the pharmacist faces such liability alone, and in certain situations can be ruined financially.

Finally, limiting language in subscriber contracts (i.e., exculpatory clauses) may serve to restrict monetary awards in certain circumstances. Such clauses could be included in either contracts for subscribers or signed on acceptance of responses to inquiries. A provision could be included that specifically disclaims any responsibility to a third party who might rely on the information. Written information (e.g., a bulletin) should carry a disclaimer specifying that the information provided is issued on the understanding that it is the best available from the resources available to the service at a particular time.

An attorney could draft a standard agreement providing that the application of the research by the recipient would not be subject to any implied warranty of fitness for that purpose. However, certain jurisdictions have held that contracts that purport to exculpate a party from negligence will be subjected to strict judicial scrutiny. Courts in certain jurisdictions have declared contracts that attempt to exempt a party's willful or grossly negligent conduct to be void. Further, no exculpatory clause will protect a pharmacist who is grossly or intentionally negligent.

Labeling and Advertising

The FDA defines labeling as written or oral information used to supplement or explain a product, regardless of whether the information accompanies the product. As such, even literature, textbooks, reprints of articles, and scientific seminars may constitute labeling. Labeling requires full disclosure. Advertisements, on the other hand, require a fair balance, meaning there must be a discussion of both benefits and risks, so as not to be misleading, and substantial evidence from clinical trials must be included for comparative claims.[63]

There are at least three key areas of labeling and advertising liability: the learned intermediary rule, which is a defense of a failure to warn action; the doctrine of overpromotion, under which adequate warning is alleged to have been diluted by communications failing to adequately convey the full impact of the warning; and promotion of off-label or non-FDA-approved indications.

DIRECT-TO-CONSUMER DRUG INFORMATION AND EROSION OF THE LEARNED INTERMEDIARY RULE

In 1997, the FDA relaxed the standards for direct-to-consumer (DTC) television advertising.[64] DTC advertising involves magazine, TV, and web-based advertisements, suggesting the use of various prescription drugs for medical conditions the viewer might experience and also suggesting the viewer ask their physician if the medication would be appropriate for them.

Today, prescription drug advertising is a multibillion dollar industry. Prescription drug advertising is governed by the Food, Drug & Cosmetic Act (FDCA) and 21 U.S.C. §331, which prohibits the misbranding of a prescription drug.[65] The primary regulation aimed at pharmaceutical product advertising is found at 21 C.F.R. § 202.1, which pertains to all "advertisements in published journals, magazines, other periodicals, newspapers, and other advertisements broadcast through media such as radio, television, and telephone communication systems." These regulations specify that prescription drug advertisements cannot omit material facts, and must present a fair balance between effectiveness and risk information. Further, for print advertisements, the regulations specify that every risk addressed in the product's approved labeling must also be disclosed in the advertisements. The regulations further require that the advertisement contain a summary of "all necessary information related to side effects and contraindications" or "provide convenient access to the product's FDA-approved labeling and the risk information it contains." DTC advertising of off-label uses of prescription drugs is prohibited.[66]

There is evidence that DTC advertising is becoming more aggressive.[67] The FDA has cited unsubstantiated safety claims and minimization of risk, including "websites that omit or bury important safety information," as areas of particular concern.[68] In some cases, the advertising does not focus on a product but rather on patient education. One company has developed a campaign to bring mental health educational forums to college campuses featuring free screenings for depression. In another case, a 24-hour TV network directed to a captive audience (i.e., hospitalized patients) was launched. As federal regulations require patient education, this programming may be used by hospitals for patient education. Other manufacturers offer monetary rewards or gifts (e.g., free exercise video) to patients who visit their physician regarding the product, or offer a rebate or sweepstakes opportunity if the patient completes a questionnaire. Manufacturers are also sending out video press releases about drugs that are often aired as news stories. Many ads provide an 800 number to encourage consumers to seek additional information about the products; others offer free videotapes, brochures, and information packets discussing the product.[69] There also exist DI search tools for use directly by consumers, e.g., PDR.net (<<http://www.pdr.net>>).[70]

The advent of DTC advertising bypasses the advice of the physician. In 1999, the first lawsuit was brought against a pharmaceutical company in connection with DTC advertising. Other DTC cases have followed where the plaintiff's bar has made some footholds in convincing courts to abandon the learned intermediary doctrine, greatly impacting pharmaceutical product liability law.[71]

In *Perez v. Wyeth Laboratories Inc.*,[72] the New Jersey Supreme Court created an exception to the learned intermediary doctrine on the ground that foundational tenets of the doctrine are no longer applicable in the context of DTC advertising. The Court wrote, "...we believe that when mass marketing of prescription drugs seeks to influence a patient's choice of a drug, a pharmaceutical manufacturer that makes direct claims to consumers for the efficacy of its product should not be unqualifiedly relieved of a duty to provide proper warnings of the dangers or the side effects of the product." *Perez* involved Norplant®, an implantable contraceptive that provided contraception for up to 5 years, but was removable. The plaintiffs alleged personal injury and failure to warn of the contraceptive's side effects, including removal complications, which resulted in pain and scarring. The plaintiffs asserted that, based on the mass advertising campaign directly to women, the pharmaceutical manufacturer had a duty to warn patients directly. According to the majority in *Perez*, the learned intermediary doctrine has four theoretical premises: (1) a reluctance to undermine the doctor-patient relationship, (2) an absence for the need for the patient's informed consent, (3) the inability of drug manufacturers to communicate with patients, and (4) the complexity of the subject matter. The Court asserted that each of these bases, except the fourth, is obviated in DTC advertising of prescription drugs. According to *Perez*, when direct advertising influences a patient to request a particular drug, and the physician does not adequately consult with the patient, "neither the physician nor the manufacturer should be entirely relieved of their respective duties to warn."[73]

It is important for pharmacists providing DI to be aware of the emerging legal issues relating to DTC advertising, such as erosion of the learned intermediary doctrine and the shifting of liability to pharmaceutical manufacturers. Additionally, the erosion of the learned intermediary rule, as demonstrated in *Perez*, and shifting of liability away from physicians has broad implications for pharmacists. Increasingly, the courts are holding that the pharmacist has a duty to warn patients and intervene on their behalf. In 1991, Pharmacists Mutual reported no claims involving drug utilization review. In 1999, drug review claims accounted for 9% of all pharmacist liability claims. A 2002 study found that drug review claims were continuing in a straight-line increase.[74]

Multiple constitutionality issues have been raised regarding any government interference with DTC advertising of prescription drugs. In *Thompson v. Western States Medical Center*, the U.S. Supreme Court upheld the rights of pharmacists to advertise compounded prescription drugs.[75] In doing so, the Court held that the Food and Drug Administration Modernization Act (FDAMA) prohibition of the promotion or advertisement of compounded drugs by pharmacists violated the First Amendment and that proposed restrictions would limit the First Amendment rights of pharmaceutical manufacturers as well as the fundamental rights of patients to receive the information.

In any event, pharmacists must remain vigilant to ensure that DTC advertising does not promote false expectations. Clearly, DTC advertising achieves its goals of encouraging consumerism, whereby patients go to seek prescription information from health professionals. DTC advertisements increasingly lead patients to seek information that will confirm or refute the manufacturer's claims that differentiate a product from its competitors. When confronted with the influences of such advertising, pharmacists are on the front lines educating patients regarding these products, including the cost effectiveness of prescription drug options. Pharmacists have a responsibility to provide objective information, to educate the patient, and to serve as a DI resource.[76]

DOCTRINE OF DRUG OVERPROMOTION

The doctrine of overpromotion is based on the liability where an adequate warning is alleged to have been diluted by communications that do not adequately convey the full impact of the warning and so overpromoting such drugs that members of the medical profession prescribe it when it was not warranted.

On August 9, 2003, Prescription Access Litigation Project filed the first class action lawsuit against a pharmaceutical company in connection with DTC ads. The class action was brought for allegedly deceptive advertising and overpricing of Claritin®.[77] Plaintiffs alleged that the company's DTC advertisements overstated the limited efficacy of its product and that the company deliberately left out any information about the drug's efficacy. Another DTC lawsuit involves Paxil™, one of the top selling drugs in the world.[78] Mass joinder lawsuits (where highly individualized claims are litigated in an aggregated class action style, even though they would not satisfy the prerequisites for class action status) have been filed in about 15 states against the maker of the drug whereby plaintiffs allege the drug causes withdrawal symptoms, such as severe nausea and other psychologic problems, and that the company failed to tell plaintiffs, their physicians, or the public of this adverse effect.[78]

If the adverse reaction is not listed in the labeling, the health care prescriber (e.g., the physician) is exonerated, leaving the pharmaceutical company liable. Examples include cases involving neuropathy and polyneuropathy from HMG CoA reductase inhibitors.[79]

As evidenced by these DTC cases, there is no doubt that there has been a narrowing of the learned intermediary doctrine in pharmaceutical liability litigation and the use of the doctrine in failure to warn claims.

OFF-LABEL USE AND INFORMED CONSENT

Off-label use involves using medications for indications not specifically approved by the FDA. It is an accepted principle that once the FDA approves a drug for marketing, a physician's discretionary use of that product is not restricted to the uses indicated on the FDA-regulated labeling. This is particularly important in the areas of oncology and acquired immunodeficiency syndrome (AIDS) where a significant portion of drug use is off label. While patients and medical innovation, in general, benefit from having their doctors informed about off-label uses, off-label use information from manufacturers has been restricted. In fact, manufacturer promotion of off-label use constitutes misbranding under the Food Drug Cosmetic Act (FDCA.)[80]

Under the 1997 FDAMA, the FDA attempted to strengthen regulation of information pertaining to off-label uses.[81] One requirement under FDAMA is that the FDA review the material to be disseminated to ensure that it does not pose a significant risk to public health and is not false and misleading.[82] Recently, however, the authority of the FDA under the FDAMA to regulate the promotion of off-label uses has been successfully challenged.[83] In favoring the commercial free speech doctrine, the court ruled that the FDA had to permit drug company-sponsored advertisements for off-label use, as long as they were directed at physicians and not consumers.[84] The court found that the regulations implementing the FDAMA were more extensive than necessary.

Moreover, medical science liaisons are permitted to provide off-label information in response to unsolicited medical inquiries. The types of nonpromotional information that can be provided include general education, report of a clinical trial, follow-up to a question originally posed to a sales representative, and advice for formularies. Problematic are responses to inquiries that are not really unsolicited or formulary advice that borders on preapproval promotion (known as new product "seeding").[85] Additionally, pharmaceutical companies may freely distribute to health professionals copies of articles from peer-reviewed professional journals or reference textbooks containing discussions of off-label product usage. However, sales representatives are not permitted to use this information to promote the company's products. The FDA may require disclosures of significant financial relationships between the faculty and industry.

Researchers continually conduct studies to determine new uses for already marketed drugs and effective combinations of drugs for new indications with the results being published in the literature. Additionally, with up to 40% of all prescriptions being for off-label use, off-label use comprises a large component of providing DI.[86] These queries are often from physicians seeking evidence to support a particular off-label use. Problems arise when the off-label use is not really off-label, but rather, crosses the line and is experimental (in which case an Investigational New Drug Application and/or Institutional Review Board [IRB] approval for study is required).[86]

Medicare is required to cover off-label drugs used in cancer treatment when the use is supported by a citation in at least one of the following reference books: the *American Hospital Formulary Service (AHFS) Drug Information* or the *U.S. Pharmacopoeia Drug Information* and two or more peer-reviewed articles published in respected medical journals.[87] Following these guidelines for DI queries pertaining to an off-label use would appear to be a prudent practice. Similarly, in providing responses to DI requests pertaining to off-label uses (including usages of off-label dosages), it is prudent to provide complete information, so that a decision may be made whether the information is enough to warrant a particular off-label use. For example, letters to the editor or abstracts would not be complete information. When there is another drug on the market with an approved-label use for the same indication that the off-label product is being considered, the response to the DI request should mention that labeled alternative.[88] Moreover, it is also important to be cognizant of the implications of disseminating off-label information could have in the context of patent safety and liability. Responding to consumer requests for information about off-label uses is not advised, simply because, unlike health professionals, most often they are not in a position to evaluate the literature and extrapolate to a particular situation.

Off-label use of pharmaceuticals has resulted in liability. Recently, for example, physicians have been the targets of lawsuits involving coadministration of insulin with rosiglitazone (Avandia®) before the combination was approved by the FDA and included in the labeling.

While there is no question that patients should be advised if a proposed treatment is truly investigational or experimental, off-label use is not necessarily experimental or investigational, and informed consent is not necessary whenever an off-label use is proposed.[89] Federal informed consent regulations governing investigational drugs do not apply to off-label use.[90] State informed consent laws vary but usually require discussion of the nature, risks, benefits, and alternative modes of treatment. For example, the New York statute states:

> Lack of informed consent means the failure to the person providing the professional treatment or diagnosis to disclose to the patient such alternatives thereto and the reasonably foreseeable risks and benefits involved as a reasonable medical... practitioner under similar circumstances would have disclosed, in a manner permitting the patient to make a knowledgeable evaluation.[91]

Actions for informed consent are, therefore, limited to the nondisclosure of medical information. However, failure to disclose the FDA status does not raise a material issue of fact as to informed consent.

Liability Concerns for Internet Information

Information about diseases is already one of the most popular categories on the Internet. More than 25% of the Internet's content involves health care and medical information.[92] The surfer can now expect to find full prescribing information for most heavily marketed drugs. The situation is complicated by links to investigational products or investigational uses and vice versa. The question is whether this is promotion of off-label uses.[93]

Liability concerns arise in the area of whether a manufacturer's website content is considered labeling or advertising. It appears to be necessary to distinguish between Internet promotions directed to health professionals and consumers. DTC advertising on the Internet is considered labeling, rather than advertising and, as such, the FDA has principal authority to regulate it.[94]

On February 4, 2004, the FDA issued new industry guidelines, entitled *Help-Seeking and Other Disease Awareness Communications by or on Behalf of Drug and Device Firms* and *Brief Summary: Disclosing Risk Information in Consumer-Directed Print Advertisements*. While these guidelines are intended to improve the brief summaries of side effects that must be included in DTC advertising, they do not address Internet ads. The FDA has not issued guidelines on DTC advertising via the Internet. In fact, the FDA has stopped work on a planned guidance on Internet drug promotional activities because the Internet is changing so rapidly. The FDA now believes existing regulations can be followed.[66] For example, a drug's black box warning should be configured "prominently" on the Internet. A person should not have to click multiple times to get this important information.

Additionally, there are liability risks inherent in DTC advertising via the Internet, mainly because the risks are ill-defined by sparse FDA guidance and judicial precedence commingled with jurisdictional and extraterritoriality issues.

QUALITY OF INFORMATION

What about information obtained from the Internet and electronic journals? Is there a possibility of pharmacist liability occurring via cyberspace? The Internet contains a growing hodgepodge of sources with little organization and uneven credibility. In fact, material on the Internet may contain innocent mistakes and/or deliberate fraud, as well as outdated material. Failure to search comprehensively may occur based on the search strategy and the failure to realize that pre-Internet or old non-electronic material exists.[95] For, e-books (e.g., online textbooks) with their own built-in search engine (e.g., Merck Manual) there is a possibility of patient harm occurring where the computer malfunctions. Currently, there is inadequate law and no means for ensuring the accuracy of information posed on the Internet. Because the Uniform Commercial Code does not seem to apply, legislation may be necessary. It is possible for information to be false, misleading, corrupted by an outside source, or otherwise harmful to the readers to apply it to their specific situation. There is a potential for misinformation to be disseminated, while the reader unknowingly assumes the information to be accurate and true via the Internet and related technologies.

The Health Summit Working Group, which consists of professional societies including the American Society of Health-System Pharmacists (ASHP), and the Health on the Net Foundation are currently working to improve the quality of DI on the Internet. The Health Summit Working Group is developing an interactive tool to use in evaluating quality of DI on the Web available at <<http://hitiweb.mitretek.org/hswg>>. Also, the application of the National Information Infrastructure to consumer health information is one of the priorities of the federal government. Examples of website QA criteria are included in Table 12–2 and are found in Chap. 5.

Both the American Medical Association and the American Medical Informatics Association have issued guidelines for physicians using e-mail to communicate with patients.[96] These guidelines, available at <<http://www.amia.org/pubs/other/email_guidelines.html>> and <<http://www.ama-assn.org/apps/pf_new/pf_online?f_n=browse&doc=policyfiles/HnE/E-5.026.HTM>>, encourage physicians to be cautious when using e-mail because of the possibility of liability due to misunderstanding and privacy concerns.[97] Perhaps in the near future, health insurers will cover calls made to online pharmacists providing DI, much the same way as Medicare now covers teleconferencing. The Internet is at the forefront of future practice, where pharmacists will consult with each other, thereby learning from one another and benefiting their DI clients and patients.[98]

TELEMEDICINE AND CYBERMEDICINE

Legal issues are emerging from e-health technologies, such as telemedicine and cybermedicine programs. Telemedicine is defined as the use of telecommunications and interactive video technology to provide health care services to patients who are at a distance. Cybermedicine is a broader concept that includes the marketing, relationship creation, advice, prescribing, and selling pharmaceuticals and devices in cyberspace. Therefore, telepharmacy is a subset of telemedicine and the terms are used interchangeably here. As telemedicine and cybermedicine expand, questions regarding liability for pharmacists providing DI on the Internet will need to be addressed. For example, health professionals, such as pharmacists, are licensed by states. Which state law applies when the pharmacist is located in New York, the patient is in Florida, and the website is maintained by a company in California? Who is liable for technical problems that make it impossible for the information to be received in a timely manner or for breaches of confidentiality caused by those who would invade private files? Already some sites offer fee-based live physician offices and nurse triage services (e.g., Optum Online) for self-diagnosis and health screening. Additionally, some DICs provide information over the Internet.

Although the courts have yet to test liability for medical malpractice involving the practice of pharmacy or medicine on the Internet, such a case is bound to surface soon. The most important determination of whether there is such malpractice is whether or not a health care provider-patient relationship has been created by the consultation in the absence of physical contact. Hard copy printouts of Internet discussions would be discoverable before trial and could be uncovered in the defendant's computer files by a plaintiff's attorney. It is likely that where a physician consults with a pharmacist for DI via telemedicine, the pharmacist will not be deemed to have established a pharmacist-patient relationship. Telephone consultations between physicians are most analogous and have not been held to create a physician-patient relationship.[99] This is largely because of the public policy interest of promoting consultations, professional association, and education, as well as the assumed limited information conveyed to the consulting physician. However, in view of advancing technology where the patient's entire medical history and test results are available on the computer, this situation may change, especially where a consultation fee is involved. Also, where a pharmacist posts a website and is paid to provide DI, the courts will surely find such cybermedical consultation to create a pharmacist-patient relationship.

Although there have been several lawsuits for false information on online bulletin boards (e.g., USENET News and CompuServe), the basis of these lawsuits has been defamation, not malpractice.[100,101] The offering of general medical advice and judgments online (e.g., chat rooms) does not appear to be creating a formal physician-patient relationship. Nor does it appear that the giving of generic advice will generate liability for either the provider or the publisher. If the information is fraudulent or quackery, then courts do have authority under both state and federal computer statutes to stop the activity. Similarly, Internet (or telephone) medical call centers, or triage services used by some health care plans can expect to be held liable when misdiagnosis occurs. On the other hand, liability is lessened where Internet discussions resemble an academic conference between health care providers, rather than a formal consultancy. Similarly, the issuance of a disclaimer in writing with the original subscription and with each message written may help insulate from any liability.

Some websites now carry disclaimers to protect the authors from liability. The limitation of the remedies available should be displayed prominently. A cap equal to the price of the service sold may be included. The following is an example: "Please read this agreement entirely and carefully before accessing this website. By accessing the site, you agree to be bound by the terms and conditions below. If you do not wish to be bound by these terms and conditions, you may not access or use this site. Our maximum liability to you under all circumstances will be equal to the purchase price you paid for any goods, services, or information." This statement is then followed by disclaimers pertaining to accuracy, currency, copyright, no medical advice, no warranties, a disclaimer of endorsement, disclaimer regarding liability for third-party content, and a general disclaimer of liability including negligence with a statement that the user assumes all responsibility and risk for use.[102] It may also be desirable to include a provision that any dispute will be brought in the city of the site owner's principal place of business.

FRAUD AND ABUSE

Another consideration pertains to fraud and abuse laws, such as the antikickback laws.[103] The antikickback statute prohibits physicians participating in the Medicaid and Medicare programs from submitting any false remuneration, "including any kickback, bribe, or rebate" to induce referrals of patients.[104] Certain aspects of e-health promotional and marketing tools, such as per click payment arrangements, are particularly susceptible to violation of the antikickback statute. The violation occurs because the health care provider is receiving remuneration based on the referral rate provided by the fee charged per click. Likewise, promotional banners on a health care organization or pharmacist's website that link to a pharmacy or other type of patient care items are most likely in violation because the referring provider is receiving a benefit (i.e., per click arrangements involve the payment of a fee based on clicking a particular link on a website) in exchange for referrals.[105] Similarly, the provision of free e-mail services, online publications, computer equipment, or other types of computer ventures are in violation of the antikickback statute, when these companies sell items or services reimbursable under Medicaid or Medicare programs.

Another area of uncertainty pertains to the handling of links between web pages. A link is any component of a web page that connects to another web page. The issue of whether pharmaceutical manufacturers will be liable for material posted on sites they have not sponsored but have merely linked to their own is yet to be decided in the courts.

At least according to cases over the past few years, mere hyperlinking does not constitute copyright or trademark infringement.[106] Copyright law does not require that permission be obtained for linking, if there is copyrighted graphic material, you will be reproducing and displaying copyrighted material you do not own. You need the copyright owner's permission to use the graphic image, unless your use of the graphic is fair use (fair use is discussed further under the section for copyright law). Where the information being linked to is violating the copyright law, it is also possible that a website owner who links to a site containing infringing material may be liable for contributory copyright infringement. Contributory copyright infringement is established when a defendant, with knowledge of another's infringing activity, causes or materially contributes to the infringing conduct.

Moreover, whether deep linking (i.e., bypassing the home page and linking to an internal page of the linked site) is copyright infringement is currently unclear.[107] However, if a web page specifically states, "ask permission before linking," it is possible that linking to the site without the owner's permission may be trespass or breach of contract where there are terms of use that were agreed to.[108]

Additionally, certain businesses, who do not want their valuable content associated with or connected to certain sites, have brought legal action under theories of trademark, defamation, disparagement, unfair competition, false advertising, invasion of privacy, and other laws. In *Playboy Enterprises, Inc. v. Universal Tel-A-Talk, Inc.*, an X-rated website linked to the Playboy website.[109] Playboy sued and proved that users of the site may be confused as to whether Playboy sponsored or endorsed the adult site. Playboy also proved that its trademark bunny logo would be blurred or tarnished by the association with the adult site. Also, most recently, in *Coca-Cola Co. v. Purdy*, the Court entered judgment for several well-known trademark owners on their infringement claims where an antiabortionist used a host of domain names incorporating their famous marks.[110] The antiabortionist linked the domain names (e.g., *mycoca-cola.com*) with a website associated with *abortionismurder.com*. According to the decision, "the quick and effortless nature of 'surfing' the Internet makes it unlikely that consumers can avoid confusion through the exercise of due care."[111]

The practice of using framing to incorporate third-party content into a website is also an area of unsettled law. The framing site can surround the framed pages with its own advertising, logos, or promotions. Framing may trigger a dispute under copyright and trademark law theories because a framed site arguably alters the appearance of the content and creates the impression that its owner endorses or voluntarily chooses to associate with the framer.[112] However, liability for framing has not been fully or clearly resolved by the courts.[113]

Advances in technology may render this dilemma moot. Technology now exists to keep undesired links or frames off a website. In any event, it is advisable not to link to or frame another website without the express permission of that site. However, if a website owner is concerned about liability for links or frames, a prominently placed disclaimer may be added. Additionally, if you want others to obtain permission before linking to your site, post a "request permission" notice and require users to agree to the terms by clicking "I agree" on your home page.

The Internet raises a variety of legal issues, most of which are unresolved but evolving. Future goals should be for pharmaceutical manufacturers to promote their products to consumers more responsibly, for the FDA to regulate DTC advertising more effectively, and for the medical and pharmacy communities to educate the public about prescription drugs more constructively.

Intellectual Property Rights

COPYRIGHT

A copyright is a property right in an original work of authorship that is fixed in tangible form.[114] A copyright holder in a work is granted certain exclusive rights to control use of the work created. The exclusive rights subsist on fixation of a work. The current copyright law is codified at 17 U.S.C.A. § 101 *et seq*. A work of authorship must be original in order to qualify for copyright protection. This requirement has two facets: first, the author must have engaged in some intellectual endeavor of his own and not just have copied from a preexisting source. Second, the work must exhibit a minimal amount of creativity. Copyright protection covers both published and unpublished works. Also, the fact that the previously published work is out of print does not affect its copyright. Works of authorship under copyright and items not entitled to copyright are found in Table 12–3.

Pharmacists providing DI must have a working knowledge of copyright law, both to avoid liability and to protect their own literary works. Under the 1976 Copyright Act, an author is protected as soon as a work is recorded in some concrete way. The process of registering for a copyright involves depositing material with the Copyright Office to be reviewed by an examiner, followed by publication with a copyright notice, usually the symbol ©. Under the Copyright Term Extension Act of 1998, such work is protected until 70 years after the death of the author or for 95 years for corporate copyright holders. However, in February 2004, the Supreme Court granted *certiorari* (i.e., a discretionary writ issued by an appellate court demanding that a lower court deliver a case record for review. Most cases that reach the Supreme Court do so by Writ of Certiorari) to hear a case involving the constitutionality of the statute.[115] The author or copyright owner has the exclusive right to make copies of the work, control derivative works or adaptations, and sue for damages and injunctive relief (an injunction is a judicial remedy issued in order to prohibit a party from doing or continuing to do a certain activity) against infringers. Public domain works may be copied and distributed without copyright permission. Works of the U.S. government (e.g., General Accounting Office [GAO] reports, Congressional Record, and FDA releases) are considered part of the public domain.

Ownership of copyright usually rests with the author at the time the work is created. The exception is a "work made for hire," (i.e., "a work prepared by an employee within the scope

TABLE 12–3. COPYRIGHT PROTECTION

Works of authorship entitled to copyright protection include the following:
  Literary works
  Musical works, including any accompanying words
  Dramatic works, including any accompanying music
  Pantomimes and choreographic works
  Pictorial, graphic, and sculptural works
  Motion pictures and other audiovisual works
  Sound recordings
  Architectural works
Not entitled to copyright protection:
  Ideas, concepts, principles, or discovery
  Procedures, processes, systems, methods of operation
  Mere compilations of facts

---

of the employment relationship) or is a work specially ordered or commissioned for use as a contribution to a collective work, as part of a motion picture or other audiovisual work, as a translation, as a supplementary work, as a compilation, as an instructional text, as a test, as an answer material for a test, or as an atlas, if the parties expressly agree in a written instrument signed by them that the work shall be a work made for hire."[116] Another exception is the first-sale doctrine, which, in effect, permits intralibrary loan of materials. Under the first-sale doctrine, a person who legitimately owns a copy of a work is one who purchased the work or otherwise acquired ownership of the work with the permission of the copyright owner, and has the full authority to "sell or otherwise dispose of the possession of that copy."[117]

Since the Berne Convention in 1989, the copyright formalities of registration and notice have lost almost all their legal significance. Registration, although not mandatory, affords the copyright claimant certain advantages. For example, it prevents an infringer from pleading "innocent infringement." Similarly, the only substantive legal effect of copyright registration is that attorney fees and statutory damages are only recoverable for postregistration infringements, that is, U.S. authors must register before bringing suit. But for works prior to 1989 and the Berne Convention, copyright can be lost if notice was omitted and that omission was not cured within 5 years of publication by registration and affixation of notice to the remaining copies.

Under the fair use provision of the 1976 Copyright Act, if a use is fair, permission of the copyright owner need not be received nor royalties paid. Fair use is determined by a four-pronged test: (1) nature and character of use, (2) nature of the work, (3) the proportional amount copied, and (4) most importantly, the effect on the market for the copied work.[118]

The first factor in the fair use analysis is the nature and character of the use. Uses for research, teaching, scholarship, and news reporting are more likely to be considered fair than strictly commercial. In addition, there is a narrow special exemption for educators. The mere fact that the use is educational and not for profit does not insulate the use from a finding of infringement.

The second factor in the fair use analysis is the nature of the work. This factor centers on whether a copyrighted work is creative or informational, and whether it is published or unpublished. The scope of fair use is greater when the copyrighted work is informational, because it is generally recognized that there is a greater need to disseminate factual material than works of fiction or fantasy.[119] An unpublished work is given greater copyright protection than a published work and is, therefore, less likely to be subjected to a valid assertion of fair use.[120] In *Harper & Row Publishers, Inc. v. Nation Enterprises, Nation* obtained an unauthorized manuscript of ex-President Ford's memoirs before they were published in book form under a contract with Harper & Row. The fact that President Ford's memoirs had not yet been published by the time *Nation* published them was a deciding factor.[121] That is, in looking at the nature of the work, an unpublished work seems to be entitled to greater protection than a published work.

The third factor is the amount copied. There does not appear to be a minimal amount or threshold quantity (e.g., five sentences) standard where fair use will be presumed. Although the statute itself does not set the maximum standards for educational fair use, Classroom Guidelines have been agreed on by educational, author, and publisher organizations.[122] Multiple copies for classroom use, but not to exceed in any event more than one copy per pupil in a course, are permissible, provided each copy bears a copyright notice and meets the test of (1) brevity, (2) spontaneity, and (3) cumulative effect. For example, to meet the test of brevity, the Classroom Guidelines prohibit multiple copying of complete articles longer than 2500 words. They prohibit copying excerpts longer than 1000 words or 10% of the work, whichever is shorter. For motion media, up to 10% or 3 minutes, whichever is less, in the aggregate of a copyrighted motion media work may be reproduced or otherwise incorporated as part of an educational multimedia project. To meet the test of spontaneity, the copying must be at the instance and inspiration of the individual teacher, where the teacher's decision to use the work in class does not allow for a timely reply to request for permission. To meet the cumulative effect requirement, the copying must be for only one course in the school, and except for current news periodicals, newspapers, and current news sections of periodicals, only one article or two excerpts therefrom, may be copied from the same author, or three excerpts from the same collective work or periodical volume. Additionally, the copying must be for only one class term; and no more than nine instances of such multiple copying for one course during one class term. In other words, the copied material may only be used for one semester and permission for longer use must be obtained. Further, students may not be charged for the copy beyond the actual cost of photocopying.

In *Association of American Publishers v. New York University*, the issue was the production and distribution of custom-made anthologies sold to students. Although the Classroom Guidelines allow students to make single copies for personal use, the court found infringement when anthologies were sold for profit.[123] The action was settled with the adoption of certain procedures by New York University.

The fourth factor in a fair use analysis is the impact the infringing work will have on the market or potential market of the copyrighted work. The Supreme Court has decided that all four factors of the fair use test should be given equal weight.[124] Under the Copyright Act of 1976, these four fair use factors provide a broad and flexible defense against copyright infringement.

Fair use is an equitable defense to copyright infringement, determined by the courts on a case-by-case basis. Unfortunately, in court decisions on educational photocopying to date, the ruling in almost every case has been against fair use. Copying by nonprofit medical libraries has been held to be a fair use where the photocopying of medical journals by federal nonprofit institutions was made solely for the purpose of medical research. In *Williams & Wilkins Co. v. United States*, the library was copying a single copy for each request and the court found that "medical science would be seriously hurt if such library photocopying were stopped."[125] In *Williams & Wilkins*, the copying of medical journals was by two governmental libraries, i.e., the National Institutes of Health and the National Medical Library, a repository of much of the world's medical literature.[126] The public benefits of fair use apparently held considerably more weight than any commercial considerations presented before the courts. However, where the photocopying of medical journals by scientists occurred in a large for-profit company, the court decided the making of unauthorized copies of copyrighted articles published in scientific journals for use by research scientists was not fair use. The court determined that the publishers had created through the Copyright Clearance Center, Inc., a viable market for institutional users to obtain licenses to allow photocopying of individual articles. However, in *Princeton University Press v. Michigan Document Services, Inc.*, the court held that a copy shop selling course packs, which are compilations of various copyrighted and uncopyrighted materials such as journal articles, sample test questions, course notes, and book excepts, infringed the copyrights of several publishers.[127] In deciding this was not a fair use, the court noted that the copying was substantial and commercial. Similarly, in *Basic Books v. Kinko's Graphic Corp.*, the court held that a copy shop's reproduction and sale of course packs to students was not a fair use of the copyrighted material.[128] Recently, the court has ruled that there is only a limited copyright protection available to a compilation of works written by another author. In *Silverstein v. Penguin Putnam*, the plaintiff had compiled a collection of 122 unpublished Dorothy Parker poems.[129] He presented the compilation to Penguin, which rejected it and subsequently inserted the poems into a new edition of Parker's work published by Penguin. The court held that Silverstein would not be entitled to injunctive relief as he did not hold the copyrights on the poems, as his efforts to gather the poems were not protectable in copyright. Additionally, the court looked at Silverstein's arrangement of the poems and found that Penguin did not copy his arrangement.

Copyright infringement requires a showing of copying, which can be proven circumstantially by demonstrating that the defendant had access to the copyrighted work and that the defendant's work is substantially similar to that work. Copyright infringement for purposes of commercial advantage or private financial gain is punishable under 18 U.S.C. § 2319. Although the Act allows for damages of as much as $100,000 per infringement, innocent infringers (e.g., educators and universities) may be entitled to a remission of statutory damages. They are only liable for actual damages, such as profits earned by the infringer or profits denied to the copyright holder. This provision lowers the incentive for the publishing industry to sue. Recently, publishers have resorted to unsavory tactics in their attempts to control educational copying, such as the sending of letters threatening to sue copy shops for infringement unless they agree to pay royalties.

Newsletter copying is strictly prohibited and violators risk not only the statutory damages ($100,000), but can be subject to criminal penalties. These newsletters require a fee to be paid to the Copyright Clearance Center, even for internal or personal copying and offer rewards to those who report violations. For example, Washington Business Information, Inc.

has won major payments in infringement actions against pharmaceutical manufacturers for photocopying its *Food & Drug Letter.*

Section 201(c) of the Copyright Act has produced electronic copyright issues for free-lance articles and photography in electronic databases. Specifically, a series of cases involved whether or not permission is required from authors to place their articles on commercial databases or in the electronic public domain (e.g., MEDLINE®). In *New York Times v. Tasini,* the U.S. Supreme Court ruled that publishers cannot republish printed works on CD-ROMs and in electronic databases without obtaining permission from authors.[130] *Tasini* should not have much of an impact on new work, as most publisher agreements now address electronic publication rights. Problematic, however, are older works published without a written agree-ment. The publishers argued unsuccessfully that the use of the articles in a database was no different from issuing a microfilm or microfiche copy of a newspaper. However, permitting electronic republication of an entire issue of a newspaper, magazine, or newsletter without further payment to authors, remains unresolved.[131] Rather than attempt to contact free-lancers and offer compensation for articles, some database producers have already begun to purge their databases of freelance contributions.

Additionally, a bill has been proposed that would create a new form of copyright liability for intentionally inducing infringement.[132] The bill would amend the Copyright Act to add the basic provision that intentionally inducing infringement is akin to infringement. The term intentionally induces is defined to mean aids, abets, induces, or procures, and intent may be shown by acts from which a reasonable person would find intent to induce infringement including commercial value. It appears that the purpose of the amendment is to prohibit use of software that is used to infringe copyright of music recordings.[133]

Photocopies fall within the sphere of the Copyright Act. When sending copies of original articles, a statement to the effect that the copies are only for personal or private use must be made. The most effective way for any DI facility to protect itself against copy infringement lawsuits is to copy the page with the copyright notice and stamp the first page of the copies with a statement that the enclosed document is protected by copyright, thus putting the burden of responsibility on the recipient of the one copy. Such a notice might state, "This material is subject to the United States Copyright Law (17 U.S. Code): unauthorized copying may be prohibited by law."

The Computer Software Act of 1980 amended the Copyright Act to extend protection to computer software. However, copyright laws do not provide sufficient protection for infor-mation transmitted over the Internet and other information networks. Although copyright protection applies when copyrighted material is converted into a digital form, the havoc that cyberspace can wreak on copyright owner's rights cannot be overestimated. A debate is currently raging over whether existing copyright law can successfully adapt to the Internet.

On October 3, 2002, Congress enacted the *TEACH Act*, fully revising §110(2) of the U.S. Copyright Act governing the lawful uses of existing copyrighted materials in distance education. The TEACH Act defines the conditions and circumstances on which educators may clip pieces of text, images, sound, and other works and include them in distance education. If a particular use does not fit these conditions, one may still consider whether the use is a "fair use."[134]

Access to works on the Internet does not automatically mean that these can be reproduced and reused without permission or royalty payment and, furthermore, some copyrighted works may have been posted on the Internet without authorization of the copyright holder. With the ease of retrieval of material electronically, copyright holders are likely to uncover those who are violating their copyright. Publishers who did not previously press for royalty payments for copying of small segments of works can now trace the borrowing of snippets of text and create systems of payment and collection. Research downloading, with deletion of material after use, appears to be a fair use of the material. However, downloading to create a personal database and avoid payment of connect fees and higher user fees is illegal, unless covered under special agreements between the database owner and subscriber. Further, although the Berne Convention is the principal copyright treaty, there is no such thing as an international copyright. The treaty obligates signatory countries to extend the protection of their copyright law to foreigners whose works are infringed within their borders.[135]

DIGITAL MILLENNIUM COPYRIGHT ACT (DMCA)

The DMCA, enacted in 1998, limits copyright liability for Internet service providers (ISP), such as America Online, stemming from infringing material posted by users under certain circumstances, including linking to infringing material.[136] In *CoStar Group, Inc. v. LoopNet, Inc.*, the court did not find an ISP liable as a direct infringer when it passively copied and stored copyrighted material at the direction of users in order to make that material available to other users on their request.[137] However, immunity from liability for ISPs is not presumptive, but granted only to "innocent" service providers who can prove they do not have actual or constructive knowledge of the infringement. The moment the ISP becomes aware that a third party is using its system to infringe, i.e., via notification from the copyright holder, the Act shifts responsibility to the ISP to disable, or remove links to, the infringing matter. At the same time the DMCA imposes copyright infringement liability on persons who use or manufacture technology that circumvents copyright protection mechanisms (e.g., digital locks and passwords) and on those who would tamper with digitized copyright management information.[138]

Current copyright law denies protection to compilations of facts unless such facts are arranged or organized with some minimal element of originality. Even then, it is the creative aspect of such arrangements or organization that may be protected and not the underlying facts themselves. Legislation has been repeatedly introduced, advocated primarily by large database companies, aimed at codifying into law a new unique form of intellectual property protection for databases. The situation is different in Europe where the European Union (EU) 1996 Database Directive grants copyright protection for the selection and arrangement of information in a European database, and calls downloading and hyperlinking unfair extraction of information.

Related to copyright infringement is plagiarism and fictitious reporting. Plagiarism involves not providing the source for material, while fictitious reporting involves sourcing things that do not exist. However, the definition of plagiarism is subjective and vague. History, facts, and ideas are not copyrighted, although they may be plagiarized. Additionally, there is no fixed number or percentage of words that can be used without exposure to charges of plagiarism.[139] Verbatim quotes are permitted, provided it falls within the fair use protection. Software and web-based technologies (e.g., Turnitin detector) now exist that can scan millions of documents almost instantly to compare what has been written before to what is being written today. Further information on plagiarism is contained in Chap. 11.

Privacy

HEALTH INSURANCE PORTABILITY AND ACCOUNTABILITY ACT OF 1996

Information security concerns are at the forefront of legal issues involved in electronic communications, specifically, questions of authenticity and confidentiality or privacy of the contents of the message.

Today an individual's health information is often used for payment, QA, research, peer-review, accreditation, and a multitude of other purposes. In realizing that this creates significant privacy and security concerns, Congress enacted the Health Insurance Portability and Accountability Act of 1996 (HIPAA).[140] HIPAA's security standards are intended to protect the security of the environment in which health care information is maintained and transmitted. For pharmacies, the security standards are applicable only to electronic protected health information, not paper, facsimile, or telephone transmissions.

HIPAA's privacy standards govern the use and disclosure of protected health information. Both provisions must have been implemented by April 20, 2005. Many aspects of HIPAA fall outside the scope of this chapter.

Individually identifiable health information is information, including demographic data, that relates to the individual's past, present, or future physical or mental health or condition; the provision of health care to the individual, or the past, present, or future payment for the provision of health care to the individual, and that identifies the individual or for which there is a reasonable basis to believe it can be used to identify the individual.[141] Individually identifiable health information includes many common identifiers, such as name, address, birth date, and social security number.

However, there are no restrictions on the use or disclosure of de-identified health information.[142] De-identified health information neither identifies nor provides a reasonable basis to identify an individual. There are two methods for de-identifying protected health information: the statistical method and the safe-harbor method via removal of certain identifiers.[143] De-identified data sets, which separate individuals' identities from their protected health information, are becoming increasingly available through the Centers for Medicare and Medicaid Services and the National Institutes of Health.[144] These data are proving useful for outcomes and medical error research not associated with the original data collection protocol.

Under HIPAA, a covered entity may engage in research activities in four ways: (1) by using or disclosing only de-identified information, (2) by obtaining an authorization from the individual to use and disclose the information for research purposes, (3) by obtaining a waiver of an authorization from an IRB, or (4) by representing that the use or disclosure is solely of the protected health information of decedents. Clinical investigators are most likely to choose option 3.[145]

It is important to keep in mind that the HIPAA Privacy Rule is not intended to disrupt or discourage adverse event reporting or DI in any way. In fact, HIPAA specifically permits covered entities, such as pharmacists, physician, or hospitals, to report adverse events and other information related to the quality, effectiveness, and safety of FDA-regulated products to both the manufacturers and directly to the FDA. Under this exception, a pharmacist need not obtain an authorization from a patient before notifying a pharmaceutical company and the FDA that the patient had an adverse reaction to a drug manufactured by the drug company.[146]

There are several other situations in pharmacy practice where HIPAA compliance issues may be triggered. For example, in clinical case reports, whether for publication or teaching purposes, the patient should only be referred to via his or her initials, age or sex (e.g., RM) a 35-year-old female. HIPAA permits a pharmacist to counsel individuals other than the patient (e.g., a friend, family member, or neighbor picking up the patient's prescription) even though some of the patient' s protected health information may be revealed in such a situation. However, the regulation is clear that such disclosures must be limited and should only be made when the provider believes it is in the patient's best interest. For example, there can be no doubt that disclosing that the medication picked up is for treatment of HIV infection would not be necessary. Under HIPAA, personal representatives, defined as individuals legally authorized under state or other applicable law to make health care decisions on behalf of a patient, are to be treated in the same way as a patient. However, in some cases the personal representatives authority is limited to a specific matter, such as treatment for a life-threatening illness. In these cases, the personal representative may only access protected health information directly related to that illness. Additionally, many states have enacted laws that protect persons with illnesses that are seen as particularly stigmatizing, such as HIV, mental illness, and drug addiction. The Public Health Service Act and implementing regulations govern the confidentiality of substance abuse records maintained by federally-assisted drug and alcohol abuse programs.[147]

Similarly, a parent is considered the personal representative of a minor child and can access the minor's health records. Exceptions exist when the minor consents to health care and consent of the parent is not required under state or other law, or when the minor obtains health care at the direction of a court, or when the minor is emancipated. Other exceptions exist if a provider believes that a patient or minor is subject to abuse, neglect, or domestic violence by the personal representative.[148]

HIPAA also requires that pharmacies make a good faith effort to obtain a patients' acknowledgment that they have received a copy of the Notice of Privacy Practices. The notice describes how the pharmacy uses and discloses protected health information to carry out treatment, payment or health care operations, and the patient's rights. The notice is to be distributed to patients on or before the first treatment encounter. Where the prescription is being picked up by someone other than the patient, the pharmacy must attempt to deliver the notice to the patient. Examples of a good faith effort include providing the notice in the prescription bag or mailing the notice to the patient together with some type of return receipt means. However, the pharmacy is not in violation if the return receipt is not returned. The pharmacy need only document its efforts.[149]

In the DI arena, HIPPA allows disclosure of patient information for treatment, payment, and health care operations. Examples of health care operations include quality management, QA, outcomes evaluation, development of clinical guidelines, peer-review, and credentialing. While not specifically mentioned, DI would appear to fall under both treatment and health care operations. In most instances, HIPAA should not affect DI requests from health care providers as patient identity is usually not required or is provided via medical record number only. However, when patient identifying information is communicated, protection of information within the DIC (or pharmacy) is an important HIPAA requirement. Policies and procedures governing use and disclosure of confidential information should be in place. These policies should include guidance on training and strategies for mitigating risks during all stages of DI request processing (receipt, triage, and response). For example, procedures should be in place to verify the identity of the requestor of information. Patient information security safeguards should be in place, for example, requiring personal identifiers to be removed as soon as feasible, physical controls, software controls, and formal oversight.[150]

Under HIPAA pharmacists will be held accountable for handling confidential information properly. Civil and criminal penalties for violating patient confidentiality exist.

COMMUNICATION PRIVACY

The Telephone Consumer Protection Act sets rules prohibiting unsolicited commercial faxes. A new Federal Communication Commission (FCC) regulation implementing the Act requires businesses and nonprofit groups to get signed written permission from clients or members before faxing unsolicited materials containing advertisements.

Privacy is also an issue on the Internet (e.g., e-health sites) where the dominant privacy issue arises from the growing practice of data collection. Some websites are interactive; that is, they may require the patient to complete a survey or will send visitors a prescription refill reminder. These sites then link to privacy policies that address any concerns prospective patients may have about filling out an online survey. Disclosure of an online privacy policy together with an opt out feature can provide assurances about the protection of consumer privacy and personal information. The policy should also address passive disclosure of information, e.g., from cookies (a feature which allows Web servers to recognize a specific user or computer to access the website) or Web server logs. Unfortunately, e-health sites were not included under HIPAA. Some of these e-health Internet sites violate their own privacy policies and transfer patient-identifiable information to third parties.[151]

E-mail use in health care has developed without encryption and HIPAA does not directly address e-mail in any of its standards. However, because e-mail may involve protected health information in electronic form, both HIPAA's privacy and security rules apply. The security of unencrypted e-mail is low. Passwords, firewalls, and other conventional network security should exist to secure electronic DI communications.[152]

A number of broad consumer privacy bills have been introduced in Congress aimed at consumer surveys, mandated opt-in consents, and other privacy-enhancing technological features.[153] Many of these bills implicate DTC advertising such as interactive websites which inherently have invasion of privacy liability issues.

There has also been litigation in this area. In re *Pharmatrak, Inc. v. Privacy Litigation,* the plaintiffs alleged that numerous pharmaceutical companies secretly intercepted and accessed their personal information through the use of computer cookies and other devices,[154] in violation of state and federal laws such as the Electronic Communications Privacy Act.[155]

Industry Support for Educational Activities

Many pharmacists attend conferences, sometimes funded by pharmaceutical companies, to further their professional education. Dialogue between health professionals and the pharmaceutical industry is an opportunity to pass along scientific and educational information, and product risks and benefits. Such dialogue encourages and supports medical research, while providing the health professional with an opportunity to address questions, discuss issues, and offer expertise.

GUIDELINES AND GUIDANCE

The FDA, the American Council for Continuing Medical Education (ACCME), and the Pharmaceutical Research and Manufacturers of America (PhRMA)[156] have established educational policies, guidelines or guidances, which allow communication between industry and the Continuing Medical Education (CME) providers, with the proviso that the final decisions and control rest with the accredited provider. Recently, the Office of Inspector General (OIG) issued a guidance that prohibits the pharmaceutical industry from direct communication with CME providers and calls for an intermediary organization to develop CME programs.[157] The following factors are provided in the OIG Guidance: Does the arrangement skew clinical decision-making? Is the information complete, accurate, not misleading? Does the arrangement have the potential to be a "disguised discount" or result in inappropriate over or underutilization? Does the arrangement raise patient safety, quality, or care concerns?[157] Importantly, for pharmacists providing DI as industry clinical education consultants or medical liasons, as of January 15, 2005, the Accreditation Council for Pharmacy Education (ACPE) decided to stop accrediting pharmaceutical and biomedical manufacturers.[158] However, only 10 states actually require all of a pharmacist's continuing education activities to be accredited by the ACPE.[159]

The PhRMA Code, which became effective in July 2002, is the most specific and stringent and deals with various interactions between industry and health care professionals, such as informational presentations, professional meetings, consultant activities, scholarships and educational funds, and educational and practice-related items.[160] Scholarships for pharmacists, students, and residents to attend selected educational conferences may be provided. Salient features of the PhRMA Code are found in Table 12–4 and at <<http://www.phrma. org/ publications/policy//2004-01-19.391.pdf>>.

The FDA Guidance seeks to draw a distinction between educational activities that the FDA considers nonpromotional and those it considers promotional. The distinction is important, especially with regard to off-label uses, which can be an important component of educational activities. The FDA's factors to determine independence of the educational activity are found in Table 12–5.[161]

Some health care institutions have established their own best practices approach to developing ethical guidelines for pharmaceutical industry support. The practice involves a process similar to weighing the risks and benefits of a particular medication or therapeutic intervention, whereby each proposal for support can be viewed as having potential value, which may or may not outweigh any potential drawbacks inherent in the involvement of funding from a for-profit company. A four person committee assesses proposals based on the apparent balance between these factors and a set of guidelines developed by the institution.[162]

In general, most policies and procedures prohibit acceptance of commercial support of educational activities if such acceptance would appear to (1) create an atmosphere limiting

TABLE 12–4. PHRMA CODE ON INTERACTIONS WITH HEALTH CARE PROFESSIONALS

Gifts
 Generally prohibited
 Exceptions—$100 or less that benefits patients (e.g., branded promotional gifts for office or practice) or nominal value (e.g., pads, pens, BUT NOT golf balls) or medical textbooks or anatomical models
Meals
 Modest meals accompanying informational presentations
Entertainment
 Generally prohibited
 Exception—entertainment at meetings with bona fide consultants
Spouses
 Never appropriate for lodging, travel, meals, entertainment
Consultants
 Must be bona fide via written contract, appropriate venue, selection criteria related to purpose of service, must exclude spouses
Financial sponsorship of educational conferences
 Support should be provided to conference sponsor, not individual pharmacist
 Sponsor should control selection of content, faculty, educational materials, venue
 Faculty, but not attendees or spouses—may be paid/reimbursed for time, travel, and lodging
 Exception—companies may pay for travel/lodging for students to attend educational conferences; educational institutional must select individual students
Informational presentations
 Should be modest by local standards
 Should occur in a venue and manner conducive to informational communication
 Should provide scientific or educational value

TABLE 12–5. FACTORS USED BY THE FDA TO DETERMINE INDEPENDENCE

Control of content and selection of faculty: Is there scripting or other actions designed to influence the content by the supporting company?

Disclosures: Does it include: company funding the program, relationship between provider(s) and presenters to the supporting company, off-label discussion?

The focus of the program: Does the title accurately represent the presentation; is there fair-balanced educational discussion?

Relationship between provider and supporting company: Is there a legal, business, or other relationship between the parties?

Provider involved in sales or marketing: Are provider employees also doing marketing or promotional programs?

Provider's demonstrated failure to meet standards: Does the provider have a history of biased programs?

Multiple presentations: Do they serve public health interests?

Audience selection: Is the audience generated by sales or marketing departments to influence marketing goals?

Opportunities for discussion: Is there an opportunity for meaningful discussion?

Dissemination: Is the supporting company distributing additional information after the activity—unless requested by participant and then through an independent provider?

Ancillary promotional activities: Are promotional activities taking place in the educational meeting room?

Complaints: Are provider(s), faculty, or others complaining about the supporting company?

academic freedom and the free exchange of ideas and information, (2) introduce bias or otherwise threaten objectivity, (3) create a conflict of interest, or (4) be in conflict with the mission and profit status of the health care organization.[163]

RELATIONSHIP TO ANTIKICKBACK STATUTE

Particular arrangements between pharmacists and the pharmaceutical industry pose potential risks under the antikickback statute. The antikickback statute makes it a criminal offense to knowingly and willfully offer, pay, solicit, or receive any remuneration (in cash or in kind) to induce (or in exchange for) the purchasing, ordering, or recommending of any good or service reimbursable by any federal health care program.[164] Funding that is conditioned, in whole or in part, on the purchase of product implicates the statute, even if the educational or research purpose is legitimate. Several cases hold that intent is improper if one purpose, not the sole or even primary purpose, is to induce the purchase or recommendation of a company's goods or services.[165,166] When a grant is provided to a customer or potential customer, it may violate the antikickback statute if one purpose is to induce the customer to buy the company's product. Educational grants, for example, were at the heart of the $161 million Caremark settlement[167] and research grants were at the heart of the $450,000 Hoffmann La-Roche settlement.[157] Furthermore, to the extent the manufacturer has any influence over the substance of an educational program or the presenter, there is a risk that the educational program may be used for inappropriate marketing purposes.

In the area of DI, specific practices that may be problematic under the antikickback statute include gifts, use of pharmacist customers as consultants or members of speaker's bureaus, and questionable research grants. Problems under the antikickback statute could arise where the DI pharmacist participates in any of these activities and also advises on formulary choices or is a member of a formulary committee or is involved with purchasing decisions. If you recommend a product or service and you stand to make financial gain from it, and that service is paid for in part or in whole by the federal government, you may be violating the antikickback statute. Similarly, no gifts should be accepted if there are strings attached.

Educational activities or speakers can be funded by the pharmaceutical industry, whereas promotional marketing activities that purport to be of an educational purpose but serve no direct patient benefit are prohibited. Hiring a DI pharmacists under the guise of a consultant or advisor, or focus group participant or advisory board member, or even as a speaker at a meeting, could be considered payments for referrals. Similarly, compensating DI pharmacists as consultants, when all they do is attend conferences primarily in a passive capacity, is suspect. Other suspect activities include compensation for speaking, researching, listening to marketing pitches, or providing preceptor, shadowing or ghost-writing services.

However, where the pharmacist is compensated for actual, reasonable, and necessary services, the activities may be considered legitimate.

The antikickback statute prohibits involvement with research contracts that come through a pharmaceutical company's marketing department, research not reviewed by the manufacturer's science department, research that is unnecessarily duplicative or not needed for any purpose other than the generation of business, and postmarketing research used as a pretense for product promotion.[168] Manufacturers should use "Chinese walls" for marketing and grant-making activities to demonstrate that grants are bona fide and not improperly influenced by marketing considerations. The antikickback statute requires that grants be given in exchange for fair market value research consideration. This is often difficult to accomplish, since the precise costs and schedules of research activities are not knowable in advance and sometimes not conducive to being reduced to written agreements.

Conclusion

By now the reader has undoubtedly discovered that the liability aspects of DI include more than just negligence. Liability for off-label uses, consumer advertising, copyright infringement, liability issues unique to the Internet, privacy concerns, and industry support for educational activities are all connected to DI practice. The DI practitioner must at least have a working awareness of these areas. DI services provide a foundation for the provision of pharmaceutical care. To date, pharmacists providing DI have only speculated about and not actually faced malpractice lawsuits. Hopefully, this chapter has shed some light on how courts would react to malpractice suits against pharmacists for negligent provision of DI. However, legal precedents can be used by analogy; they cannot be relied on to predict the future. What can be done to avoid malpractice and other causes of action? First, be good at what you do. Second, have good relations with requestors and make sure they are aware of vagaries or information systems and sources. Third, make no outrageous claims about the accuracy and thoroughness of the information provided. Finally, carry your own malpractice insurance policy.

The future of DICs clearly lies in their ability to provide consultative DI services. While in the past most of the reported appellate decisions against pharmacists have involved routine dispensing errors, not mistakes in DI or other expanded practice, in the future this situation may change. Pharmacists should not be preoccupied with the risk of incurring liability, but should take the necessary steps to limit exposure and develop an appreciation of modern legal philosophy. Definitive guidelines need not emerge only through court decisions. It remains most important that DI be recognized as a liability-reducing factor for the institution and personnel who provide health care to patients.

Study Questions

1. What is negligence and what are the four elements of a negligence case?

2. Is a pharmacist liable if he or she does not provide a DI sheet or PPI?

3. Can a DI pharmacist be held liable for errors in online databases?

4. Describe methods to protect against malpractice.

5. Under what circumstances is written work protected by copyright?

6. What are the risk areas for industry support for scientific and educational activities and what factors may be used in assessing independence?

7. What is HIPAA and how does it relate to DI practice?

REFERENCES

1. Willig S. Legal considerations for the pharmacist undertaking new drug consultation responsibilities. Food Drug Cosmet Law J. 1970;25:444–52.
2. American Society of Health-System Pharmacists. ASHP supplemental standard and learning objectives for residency training in drug information practice. Practice standards of ASHP. 1995–1996. Bethesda (MD): American Society of Health-System Pharmacists; 1995.
3. Southwick AF. The law of hospital and health care administration. 2nd ed. Ann Arbor (MI): Health Administration Press; 1988.
4. Dobbs DB, Hayden PT. Torts and compensation. 3rd ed. St. Paul (MN): West Publishing; 1997. p. 336.
5. Baker K. OBRA '90 mandate and its impact on pharmacist's standard of care. Drake Law Rev. 1996;44:503–8.
6. Rosenberg v. equitable life insurance society of the United States, 595 N.E.2d 840 (NY 1992).
7. Keller v. Manhattan eye, ear & throat hospital, 563 N.Y.S.2d 686 (Sup. Ct. 1989).
8. Kashkin v. Mt. Sinai Medical Center, 538 N.Y.S.2d 686 (Sup. Ct. 1989).
9. Kelly WN, Krause EC, Krowinski WJ, Small TR, Drane JF. National survey of ethical issues presented to drug information centers. Am J Hosp Pharm. 1990;47:2245–50.
10. Doppelparker Case, OLG Karllsrule GRUR 1979 P267.
11. Perkins E. John Hopkins' tragedy: could librarians have prevented a death? Info Today [serial on the Internet]. 2001 Aug [cited 2004 Aug 2]: [about 2 p.] Available from: http://www.infotoday.com/newsbreaks/nb010806-1.htm
12. 805 S.W.2d 380 (Tenn. Ct. App. 1991).
13. 453 N.Y.S.2d 121 (1987).
14. 544 N.W.2d 727, 731 (Mich. Ct. App. 1991).
15. 191 A.D.2d 178, 594 N.Y.S.2d 195 (1993).
16. 579 N.E.2d 1255 (Ill. App. 1991) reversed by 605 N.E.2d 557 (Ill. 1992).

17. Brushwood DB, Belgado BS. Judicial policy and expanded duties for pharmacists. Am J Health Syst Pharm. 2002;59:455–7.

18. 780 So.2d 930 (Fla. App. 2001).

19. 1 S.W.3d 519 (Mo. App. 1999).

20. 737 N.E.2d 650 (Ill. App. 2000).

21. 30 S.W.3d 455 (Tex. App. 2000).

22. 827 F. Supp. 1522 (D.Nev. 1993).

23. 598 N.Y.S.2d 592 (App. Div. 1993).

24. Brushwood DB, Simonsmeier LM. Drug information for patients. J Leg Med. 1986;7:279.

25. Howe A. Are independent prescribing rights for pharmacists set to increase in 2004? Suppl Prescr Pract. 2004;1(2):5–6.

26. Canadian Society of Hospital Pharmacists [homepage on the Internet]. Information paper on pharmacist prescribing within a health care facility. Canada; 2001 Aug [cited 2005 Mar 2]: [about 17 p.]. Available from: http://www.cshp.ca/.

27. Abood RR, Brushwood DB. Pharmacy practice and the law. New York: Aspen Pub; 2001.

28. Berry M. The Canadian pharmacist's duty to counsel. Pharm Law Annu. 1992;19–75.

29. Hall M, Honey W. The evolving legal responsibility of the pharmacist. J Pharm Mark Manage. 1994;8:27–41.

30. Brushwood DB. The pharmacist's drug information responsibility after McKee v. American home products. Food Drug Cosmet Law J. 1993;48:377–410.

31. *In re* Michael A. Gabert, No. 92 PHM 21 (Wis. Pharmacy Examining Bd., Dec. 14, 1993).

32. Rees W, Rohde NF, Bolan R. Legal issues for an integrated information center. J Am Soc Inf Sci. 1991;42:132–6.

33. Restatement (Second) of Torts, Section 311, 1982.

34. Beaird S, Coley R, Blunt JR. Assessing the accuracy of drug information responses from drug information centers. Ann Pharmacother. 1994;28:707–11.

35. Calis KA, Anderson DW, Auth DA, Mays DA, Turcasso NM, Meyer CC, et al. Quality of pharmacotherapy consultations provided by drug information centers in the United States. Pharmacotherapy. 2000;20:830–6.

36. McDonagh AF, Lightner, DA. Attention to stereochemistry. Chem Engin News. 2003;Feb 3:2.

37. Gray JA. Strict liability for the dissemination of dangerous information? Law Lib J. 1990;82:497–517.

38. 694 F. Supp. 1216 (D. Md. 1988).

39. Bundesqe Richtsaf. Neue Juristische Wochenschrift (1970), 1973.

40. 110 Misc.2d 799, 442 N.Y.S.2d 945 (N.Y. Sup. 1981).

41. 938 F.2d 1033 (9th Cir. 1991).

42. 432 F. Supp. 990 (E.D.N.Y. 1977).

43. Prod. Liab. Rep (CCH), Section 8968 (S.D.N.Y. Feb. 20, 1981).

44. Brannigan VM, Dayhoff RE. Liability for personal injuries caused by defective medical computer programs. Am J Law Med. 1981;7:123–44.

45. Joyce EJ. Software bugs: a matter of life and liability. Datamation. 1987;May 15:88–92.

46. Gage D, McCormick J. Case 108—we did nothing wrong. Panama's Cancer Institute. Baseline. 2004;28:32–47.

47. Cuzamanes PT. Automation of medical records: the electronic superhighway and its ramifications for health care providers. J Pharm Law. 1997;6:19.

48. Brocklesby v. Jeppesen, 767 F.2d 1288 (9th Cir. 1985), cert. denied, 474 U.S. 1101 (1986).

49. 472 U.S. 749 (1985).

50. 137 Misc.2d 94, 520 N.Y.S.2d 334 (N.Y. Civ. Ct. 1987).

51. Amerson AB. Drug information centers: an overview. Drug Inf J. 1986;20:173–8.

52. 705 P.2d 1360 (Ariz. Ct. App. 1985).

53. Rumore MM, Rosenberg JM, Costa JG. The pharmacist and the law: legal aspects of providing drug information. Wellcome Trends Hosp Pharm. 1989;Dec:6–8.

54. Gough AR, Healey KM, Rupp SR. Poison control centers, from aspirin to PCBs and the scarlet runner beam: a study of legal anomaly and social necessity. Santa Clara L R. 1983;23:791–809.

55. Brushwood DB, Simonsmeier LM. Drug information for patients—duties of the manufacturer, pharmacist, physician, and hospital. J Leg Med. 1986;7:279–341.

56. 656 P.2d 483 (Wash. 1983).

57. Sigell LT, Bonofiglio JF, Siegel EG. The role of drug information centers with consumers. Drug Inf J. 1987;21:201–8.

58. Arnold RM, Nissen JC, Campbell NA. Ethical issues in a drug information center. Drug Intell Clin Pharm. 1987;21:1008–11.

59. Okasas RM. Hospital drug information centers: a new role in patient counseling. PharmaGuide to Hospital Med. 1988;2:1–4.

60. Gray JA. The health sciences librarian's exposure to malpractice liability because of negligent provision of information. Bull Med Libr Assoc. 1989;77:33–7.

61. Mintz AP. Information practice and malpractice. Libr J. 1985:38–43.

62. Fidelity Leasing Corp. v. Dun & Bradstreet, Inc., 494 F. Supp. 786 (E.D. Pa. 1980).

63. Food & Drug Administration [homepage on the Internet]. Center for Drug Evaluation and Research, Office of Medical Policy, Division of Drug Marketing, Advertising and Communications, Comparative Advertising, Fair Balance, and the Patient-Consumer; c2003 [cited 2005 Mar 2]. Available from: http://www.fda.gov

64. Food & Drug Administration. Guidance for industry: consumer-directed broadcast advertisements. Washington, DC:FDA; 1997 Aug 8.

65. 21 U.S.C. § 352(n).

66. 21 C.F.R. § 202.1(e).

67. Wilkes MS, Bell RA, Kravitz RL. Direct-to-consumer prescription drug advertising: trends, impact, and implications. Health Aff. 2000;19:110–28.

68. FDA officials describe agency actions on problematic drug promotion activity. BNA Pharm Law Ind Rep. 2003;1(35):1006.

69. Schwartz TM. Consumer-directed prescription drug advertising and the learned intermediary rule. Food Drug Cosmet Law J. 1991;46:829–37.

70. Physician's Desk Reference Health (PDRHealth) [database on the Internet]. Florence (KY): Thompson Health care; c2004 [cited 2005 Mar 2]. Available from: http://pdr.net.html

71. Lyles A. Direct marketing of pharmaceuticals to consumers. Annu Rev Public Health. 2002;23:73–91.

72. 161 N.J. 1, 734 A.2d 1245 (N.J. 1999).

73. Ferrelli JJ. Perez creates exceptions to learned intermediary doctrine. NJ L J. 1999.

74. Gebhart F. Here comes the judge. Drug Topics. 2005; Jan 24:26–32.

75. 122 S. Ct. 1497 (2002). No. 01-344.

76. Rumore MM. Direct-to-consumer advertising of prescription drugs: emerging legal and regulatory issues. Hosp Pharm. 2004;39:1058–68.

77. Prescription Access Litigation Project. Claritin® lawsuit [home page on the Internet] [cited 2005 Mar 2]. Available from: http://www.prescriptionaccesslitigation.org/Claritin.htm

78. Anderson v. SmithKline Beecham Corp., W.D. Wash. No. CV 03-2886-L, 2003 Sept 22.

79. Patsy BM, Furburg CD, Ray WA, Weiss NS. Potential for conflict of interest in the evaluation of suspected adverse drug reactions: cerivastin and risk for rhabdomyolysis. JAMA. 2004;292:2585–90.

80. FDC Act § 312.7.

81. 21 U.S.C. §§ 360.999, 403 (1998).

82. 21 C.F.R. § 99.101(a)(3)-(4).

83. Ward SM. WLF and the two-click rule: The first amendment inequity of the food and drug administration's regulation of off-label drug use information on the Internet. Food Drug Law J. 2001;56:41–56.

84. Kennedy D. The old file-drawer problem. Science. 2004;305:451.

85. The medical science liaison: examining the role. CME Briefing. 2002; July–Sept 3:5.

86. American Academy of Pediatrics. Policy Statement 2002;110-1. 2002; July 181–3.

87. Understanding the approval process for new cancer treatments. Bethesda (MD): National Cancer Institute [homepage on the Internet]; c.2004 [cited 2004 Mar 3]. Available from: http://www.nci.gov/clinicaltrials/learning/approval-process-for-cancer-drugs/page 5

88. Vivian JC. Off-label use of prescription drugs. US Pharm. 2003;28:5–8.

89. Beck JM, Azari ED. FDA, off-label use, and informed consent: debunking myths and misconceptions. Food Drug Law J. 1998;53:71–103.

90. 21 C.F.R. pt. 50.

91. N.Y. Pub. Health L. § 2805-d(1) (McKinney 1993).

92. Wood JM, Dorfman HL. Dot.com medicine labeling in an Internet age. Food Drug Law J. 2001;56:143–78.

93. Moberg MA, Wood JW, Dorfman HL. Surfing the Net in shallow waters: product liability concerns and advertising on the Internet. Food Drug Cosmet Law J. 1998; 53:213–24.

94. 21 U.S.C. §§ 351–354 (1994).

95. Adams SR. Information quality-liability and corrections. Online. 2003; Sept/Oct 16–22.

96. Kane B. Guidelines for the clinical use of electronic mail with patients. White paper. JAMIA. 1998;5:104–11.

97. Gulick PG. E-health and the future of medicine: the economic, legal, regulatory, cultural, and organizational obstacles. Alb L J Sci Tech. 2002;12:351–60.

98. Engstrom P. Can you afford not to travel the Internet? Med Econ. 1996;73:173–80.

99. Lopez, et al. v. Aziz, 852 S.W.2d 303, 304 (Tex. App. 1993).

100. Cubby v. Compuserve, 776 F. Supp. 135,140 (1990).

101. Stratton Oakmont Inc. and Daniel Porush v. Prodigy Services Co. & Others (NY Sup. Ct. 1995).

102. Medivision [homepage on the Internet]. New York; c2004 [cited 2004 Jul 15]. Available from: http://www.medivision.ch/rechtliche_infos-en.asp

103. Kalb PE, Bass IS. Government investigations in the pharmaceutical industry: off-label promotion, fraud and abuse, and false claims. Food Drug Cosmet Law J. 1998;53:63–70.

104. 42 U.S.C. § 1320a-7b(b)(1) (1994).

105. Huntington S. Emerging professional liability exposures for physicians on the Web. Presentation to the American Bar Association Health Law Section, 2001 June 8.

106. Warnecke M. Tested IP litigation storm of '04: Fair use principles prove their pluck. Patent, Trademark Copyright J. 2005;69(1707):369.

107. Ticketmaster Corp. v. Tickets.Com, Inc., 2003 U.S. Dist. LEXIS 6483 (CD Cal. 2003).

108. eBay, Inc. v. Bidder's Edge, Inc., 100 F. Supp. 2d 1058 (N.D. Cal. 2000).

109. 1998 U.S. Dist. LEXIS 17282 (E.D. Pa. 1998).

110. D. Minn., No. 02-1782 ADM/JGL, 2005 Jan 28.

111. Warnecke M. Effortless nature of Web surfing makes it unlikely consumers can avoid confusion. Patent, Trademark Copyright J. 2005;69(1707):363–4.

112. Millstein JS, Neuberger JD, Weingart JP. Doing business on the Internet. New York: Law Journal Press; 2004, §3.02[17][a][iii].

113. Futuredontics, Inc. v. Applied Anagramics, Inc., 1998 U.S. App. LEXIS 17012 (9th Cir. 1998).

114. 17 U.S.C. § 102.

115. Eldred v. Ashcroft, 239 F. 3d 373 (D.C. Cir. 2001).

116. 17 U.S.C. § 106.

117. 17 U.S.C. § 109(a).

118. 35 U.S.C. § 107.

119. College Entrance Examination Board v. Pataki, 889 F. Supp. 554, 568 (N.D.N.Y. 1995).

120. Epstein E, Zulieve AJ. The Fair Use doctrine: commercial misappropriation and market diversion. Isaacson Raymond [homepage on the Internet] [cited 2005 Feb 8]. Available from: http://www.isaacsonraymond.com/fair_use_doctrine.html

121. 471 U.S. 539 (1985).

122. Guidelines for classroom copying in not-for-profit educational institutions. H.R. Rep. No. 1476, 94th Cong., 1st Sess. § 68–70 (1976).

123. Latman A, Gorman R, Ginsberg JC. Copyright for the nineties. 3rd ed. Charlottesville (VA): Michie; 1989. p. 655–6.

124. Campbell v. Acuff-Rose Music, 510 U.S. 569, 578 (1994).

125. 420 U.S. 376 (1975).

126. Perlman R. Williams & Wilkins Co. v. United States: photocopying, copyright, and the judicial process, 1975 Sup. Ct. Rev. 1976;355.

127. 74 F. 3d 1512 (6th Cir. 1996).

128. 758 F. Supp. 1552 (SDNY 1991).

129. 2004 WL 1008314 (2d Cir., May 7, 2004).

130. Findlaw [homepage on the Internet]. Available from: http://laws.findlaw.com/us/000/00-201.html

131. Greenberg v. National Geographic, 201 U.S. App. LEXIS 4270 (11th Cir. 2001).

132. Inducing infringement of copyright act of 2004 (S. 2560).

133. Davidson A. Copyright office releases draft version of inducement bill. Tech Law J. Daily e-mail alert. 2004 Sept 3 [cited 2005 Feb 9]. Available from: http://www.techlawjournal.com/topstories/2004/20040903.asp.html

134. American Libraries Association [homepage on the Internet]; c 2004 [cited 2005 Feb 10]. Crews KD. New copyright law for distance education: The meaning and importance of the TEACH Act. Am Libr Assoc. Available from: http://www.copyright.iupui.edu/teach_summary.htm

135. Smedinghoff TJ, editor. Online Law. New York: Addison Wesley; 1996. p. 139.

136. 17 U.S.C. § 512.

137. ISPs are not directly liable for passively copying material for others. BNA's Patent, Trademark & Copyright J. 2004;68:190–2.

138. Scott MD. Scott on multimedia law. New York: Aspen Pub; 2003 Suppl. p. 4-80–86.

139. Pack R. Honest writers. Washington lawyer. 2004 Sept;21–6.

140. Health Insurance Portability and Accountability Act of 1996, Pub. L. No. 104-191, 110 Stat. 1936 (1996) (codified as amended in scattered sections of 18, 26, 29 and 42 U.S.C.A.); 42 U.S.C.A. § 1320d to 42 U.S.C.A. § 1320d-8.

141. 45 C.F.R. § 160.103.

142. 45 C.F.R. §§ 164.502(d)(2), 164.514(a) and (b).

143. Daniels JG. Health care privacy and HIPAA. In: Cronin KP, Weikers RN, editors. Data security and privacy law. Minneapolis (MN): West Group; 2002. p. 115–24.

144. Clause SL, Triller DM, Bornhorst CP. Conforming to HIPAA regulations and compilation of research data. Am J Health Syst Pharm. 2004;61:1025–31.

145. 45 C.F.R. § 164.512(i)(1)(i).

146. 45 C.F.R. § 164.512(b)(1)(iii).

147. 42 U.S.C.A. § 290dd-2.

148. Bishop S. Interactions with individuals other than the patient. Part 2: Caregivers, personnel representatives, and minors. Pharm Today [serial on the Internet]. 2003 July [about 5 p.] [cited 2004 Aug 2]. Available from: http://www.pharmacist,com/articles/h_hi_0013.cfm

149. Bishop S. Interactions with individuals other than the patient. Part 1: notice of privacy practices and medication counseling. Pharm Today [serial on the Internet]. 2003 July [about 6 p.] [cited 2004 Aug 2]. Available from: http://www.pharmacist.com/articles/h_hi_0012.cfm

150. Car J, Sheikh A. Email consultation in health care: 2-Acceptability and safe application. BMJ. 2004;329:439–42.

151. E-health privacy policies. Oakland, CA: California health care foundation. 2000.

152. Baker DB. Provider-patient e-mail: with benefits come risks. J Am Health Info Mgmt Assoc. 2003;74:22–9.

153. ANA Compendium of Legislative Activities, p. 9.

154. D. Mass, No. 00-11672-JLT, 2003 Nov 6.

155. 18 U.S.C. § 2510 et seq.

156. Pharmaceutical Research and Manufacturers of America Code on Interactions with Health care Professionals, 2002 July.

157. OIG Compliance Program for Pharmaceutical Industry, 2003 Apr.

158. Accreditation Council for Pharmacy Education [home page on the Internet]. Accreditation Standards and Criteria; c2005 Jan [cited 2005 Mar 3]. Available from: http://www.acpe-accredit.org/ceproviders/standards.asp

159. 2005 National Association of Boards of Pharmacy (NABP) Survey of Pharmacy Law. Mount Prospect (IL): NABP; 2005.

160. Cutting the strings on gifts and other questionable marketing practices: PhRMA takes a stand. CME Briefing. 2002; July–Sept:1–6.

161. FDA guidance for industry-supported scientific and educational activities, 1997.

162. Steiner JL, Norko M, Devine S, Grottole E, Vinoski J, Griffith EE. Best practices: developing ethical guidelines for pharmaceutical company support in an academic health center. Psychiatr Serv. 2003;54:1079–89.

163. Rosner F. Pharmaceutical industry support for continuing medical education programs: a review of current ethical guidelines. Mt Sinai J Med. 1995;62:427–30.

164. 42 U.S.C. § 1320a-7b(b).

165. U.S. v. Greber, 760 F.2d 68 (3d Cir. 1985).

166. U.S. v. LaHue, 261 F.3d 993 (10th Cir. 2001).

167. *In re* Caremark Int'l, Inc. Derivative Litig., 698 A. 2d 959 (1996).

168. Astrue MJ, Szabo DS. Pharmaceutical marketing and the anti-kickback statutes. Food Drug Cosmet Med Device Law Dig. 1993;10(2):57–60.

13

Chapter Thirteen

Ethical Aspects of Drug Information Practice

Linda K. Ohri

Objectives

After completing this chapter, the reader will be able to

- Interpret and make use of examples of ethics rules, principles, and theories.
- Explain characteristics that differentiate an ethical deliberation from other types of decision-making.
- Identify and assess examples of ethical dilemmas that may arise for pharmacists when providing drug information, in various practice settings and for various types of clients and circumstances.
- Utilize the described process of ethical analysis in order to propose and justify a specific decision or course of action in an example ethical dilemma.
- Describe structures that can prepare, guide, and support pharmacists faced with ethical dilemmas during the course of providing drug information.

What Is Ethics and What Is Not

The Ethics Course Content Committee of the American Association of Colleges of Pharmacy (AACP) described ethics as "the philosophical inquiry of the moral dimensions of human conduct".[1] They mentioned that Aristotle taught ethics as "an eminently practical discipline"...dealing... "with concrete judgments in situations in which action must be taken despite uncertainty." These authors indicated that the term ethical is often used synonymously with the term moral to describe an action or decision as "good" or "right." They further stated that ethics is not values clarification, it is not the study of moral development, and it is not the law.

Veatch stated that "an ethical, or moral, issue involves judgments between right and wrong human conduct or praiseworthy and blameworthy human character."[2] This author indicated that an ethical deliberation may be differentiated from other endeavors by three characteristics: (1) it is ultimate or fundamental, there is no higher standard against which to measure the rightness of the decision or action; (2) the issue is universal, the parties in disagreement do not consider it simply a difference of opinion or taste—each party believes there is a right or wrong answer—even if they're not sure what the answer is; and (3) the deliberation takes into account the welfare of all involved or affected by the judgment at hand. Those engaged in the practice of pharmacy typically rely on an intuitive sense of these characteristics: we have the feeling that the situation we are confronting is a big deal, and somehow anticipate that we should not address only personal preference in the matter at hand.

Law might be defined as rules of conduct imposed by society on its members. By contrast, professional ethics has been defined as "rules of conduct or standards by which a particular group in society regulates its actions and sets standards for its members."[3] Law involves written rules set by the whole society (or its representatives) that address responsibilities of that society's members. Professional ethics focuses on explicit or implicit rules and standards set by a professional subgroup of society, and addresses the responsibilities of only those who are members of that subgroup. Certain ethical standards of a given profession may be institutionalized as law by society as a whole. However, professional ethical standards (for example, "do no harm" or "preserve life") are often impossible to fully regulate by law. Meeting an ethical standard also goes beyond legal requirements; indeed, our ethical beliefs may on occasion command our civil disobedience. On the other hand, as will be discussed further below, law represents one aspect of the culture within which ethical decisions are made. In considering the cultural perspectives of a given dilemma, relevant legal requirements must be identified and considered when one seeks to make an ethical decision.

Ethical Dilemmas in Pharmacy Practice

This chapter will present case scenarios potentially representing ethical dilemmas. These scenarios may be utilized to demonstrate a specific method for analyzing ethical dilemmas confronted by the pharmacist providing drug information. The discussion will address ethical dilemmas encountered by generalist and specialist patient care pharmacists providing drug information, as well as examples drawn from the experiences of drug information specialists.

All pharmacists provide drug information and must address the ethical dilemmas that arise in the course of providing this service. Such dilemmas may arise in a wide variety of settings and circumstances where pharmacy is practiced, such as:

- The community pharmacist requested by a patient at the counter to critique another health care provider's recommendations or to provide information on a topic about which the pharmacist has moral conflict.
- The hospital practitioner asked to provide information that might be used to speed the ending of a terminal patient's life.
- The drug information specialist confronted by a physician, or an administrator, pressuring for a certain formulary recommendation that is possibly more cost-containment than evidence-based.
- The home health care pharmacist who is asked to positively present questionably substantiated information on the efficacy of a given therapy, in order to support insurance reimbursement for a truly needy patient.
- The pharmacist working in industry, who is asked to prepare two versions of a consumer product promotion piece: One meets U.S. regulatory requirements to describe key safety issues; the other version for use in a country without such legal requirements omits all safety information.
- The pharmacist practicing in any patient care setting, who experiences another episode (in a repetitious pattern) where his or her patient would benefit from specific drug information, but who finds workload demands to be an impossible barrier to providing more than the minimum, legally required information.

In the fifth edition of their foundational text *Principles of Biomedical Ethics*,[4] Beauchamp and Childress address the following aspects of the moral life: principles and rules, rights, character and virtues, and moral emotions. The responsibilities (based on principles and rules) and rights of the pharmacist, and other involved parties will be addressed briefly in this chapter as considerations that must be dealt with in the course of responding to a specific dilemma. While acknowledging their importance, this chapter will not address the roles of character, moral virtue, or emotions in ethical decision-making by pharmacists. One might say that they constitute the pharmacist's inherent moral perspective that will direct and support his or her decision-making. The interested reader is referred to the text referenced above for a fascinating discussion of these factors.

The remainder of this chapter is intended to prepare and assist the pharmacist providing drug information to analyze and address dilemmas, such as those listed above. The primary focus here will be on the pharmacist's identification, consideration, and balancing of pertinent ethical rules and principles as he or she seeks to make a right decision or take the best course of action.

Basics of Ethics Analysis

This section briefly presents relevant terminology and definitions used in the field of ethics, as well as an overview of a specific process of analysis that may be used in assessing ethical dilemmas. In the section following this one, specific case scenario demonstrations of this process for analysis will be presented.

DEFINITIONS USED IN THE FIELD OF ETHICS

Beauchamp and Childress[5] defined ethics as "a generic term for several ways of examining the moral life." These authors described a process of deliberation and justification that is necessary when confronting a moral dilemma. They stated, "When we deliberate ... we are considering which judgment is morally justified...." They indicated that, "Particular judgments are justified by moral rules, which in turn are justified by principles, which ultimately are defended by an ethical theory." These authors presented a hierarchical diagram that depicts this approach to analysis (Figure 13–1).

The authors referred to these hierarchical levels of analysis (particularly rules and principles) as action-guides, which are utilized to justify a particular judgment. They describe a rule of ethics as specific to context and relatively restricted in scope; for instance, the moral rule about confidentiality that specifically addresses a patient's right to consent prior to release of privileged information.[5] Principles are more broad and fundamental in scope; for example, the principle of respect for autonomy, which is the patient's right to decide on personal issues. They describe ethical theories as "integrated bodies of principles and rules ... that may include mediating rules that govern cases of conflicts." The prominent rules and principles guiding ethical decision-making by health care professionals can generally be placed within one of two broad ethical theories: consequentialist theory or deontological (derived from the Greek word deon, meaning duty) theory.[5] Multiple versions exist of each of these broad categories. Consequentialist theories describe actions or decisions as morally right or wrong based on their consequences, rather than on any intrinsic features

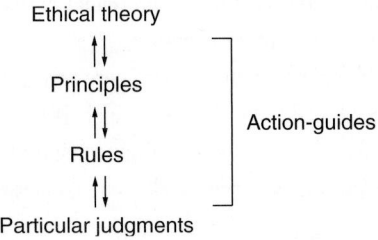

Figure 13–1

they may have. The two cardinal principles of consequentialist theory are beneficence (do that which promotes a good outcome) and nonmaleficence (do that which minimizes bad outcomes). Consequentialist theories focus on this one feature of an act, its consequences. For example, an informed consent ethical rule can be of value within consequentialist theory because consent generally results in improved compliance and outcome—good consequences. However, if informed consent was likely to result in a bad outcome, it would not be justifiable within consequentialist theory. A mediating rule utilized by many advocates of consequentialist theory is to hold nonmaleficence as more important, or more foundational, than beneficence.

Duty driven (deontological) theories look more to intrinsic qualities of an act or decision to assert its moral rightness or wrongness. Deontological theory considers other inherent features of an act, besides consequences, as also relevant and often of greater importance. For example, in various forms of deontological theory, the act is considered inherently wrong if it is dishonest or breaks confidentiality, or if it does not respect individual autonomy. Conflict between different rules are mediated by appealing to more foundational, underlying principles such as adherence to justice or to respect for persons.

Conscious recognition of the pertinent action-guides, and understanding mediating rules that operate within the pharmacist's preferred ethical theory or theories, can help pharmacists honestly and equitably analyze the ethical dilemma, and better comply with the required characteristics of ethical deliberation (see the beginning of this chapter).

OVERVIEW OF A SUGGESTED PROCESS OF ANALYSIS TO BE USED WHEN AN ETHICAL DILEMMA ARISES

In the article *Hospital Pharmacy: What is ethical?*, Veatch[2] indicated that often we reach a particular ethical decision without a great deal of conscious deliberation, through our moral intuition, and without subsequent challenge from any external party. However, on occasion, when pondering a certain ethical judgment, we are called on (internally or externally) to analyze and justify the basis for our conviction. He suggested that when this occurs, it is first important to understand the facts of the specific case. He then described progression through three additional process stages of reflection (on ethical rules, principles, and theories) by which we may identify, analyze, and present reasons for our judgment. In the same report, the author also emphasized the importance in one's reflection of taking into account the points of view of all parties. As stated earlier in this chapter, this is one of the key characteristics distinguishing an ethical deliberation. A survey of the text *Cross-Cultural Perspectives in Medical Ethics* (2nd ed.)[6] demonstrates that there are many commonalities, but also important differences across the ethical perspectives of different cultures. These cultural perspectives must also be considered if all parties' points of view are to be taken into account.

This section addresses the application of a proposed process of ethical analysis when identifying, analyzing, and resolving ethical dilemmas that may arise during pharmacists' provision of drug information. These steps of analysis are derived from the writings of Veatch, Beauchamp, and Childress, as well as other authors.[2,5-8] The process may be summarized as follows:

I. Identification of relevant background information.
   A. Factual details of the issue at hand.
   B. Consideration of who is affected by the ethical issue.
   C. Learn and respectfully address the cultural perspectives (including applicable legal requirements) for those affected by the dilemma.
II. Identification and justification of the relevant moral rules and principles (action-guides) pertinent to the case.
III. Deliberation, through the use of moral intuition and application of ethical theory, on how to rank/balance the rules and principles pertinent to the case in order to resolve the ethical dilemma.

Step I. Identification of Relevant Background Information

The first process step requires identification and evaluation of pertinent background information to insure that the facts of the specific case are understood. This first step deserves careful consideration and research. Once the facts of a case are known, the moral concerns may be resolved. This step has been divided into three parts: (A) Data gathering, (B) Consideration of the welfare of all affected parties, and (C) Respect for the cultural perspectives of these parties.

Pharmacists already use data gathering when they apply a "systematic approach" to answering any drug information question (see Chap. 2). When addressing a potential ethical dilemma, the pharmacist must learn about the factual details of the issue, who is directly involved, and whether there is conflict in factual understanding among the involved parties in the issue. For example, does the parent who calls to ask about the medication recently prescribed for her teenager already know that the teenager is taking a birth control pill prescribed by a gynecologist (rather than a dermatologist for acne) and simply wants to know the name of the product?

If the matter seems still to involve an ethical dimension once data gathering clarifies the facts, the next step is to consider the rights and responsibilities of all affected parties. As previously mentioned, this has been described as an essential component of any ethical deliberation.[2] The pharmacist, the direct client (patient), other indirect but individual clients (e.g., any existing or unborn children, or spouse), other health professionals (e.g., the patient's physician), other societal groups (e.g., other patients who might be harmed by an incompetent practitioner), and any higher power recognized by the pharmacist have rights and/or responsibilities that should be considered.

Finally, during first consideration of any potential ethical issue, the pharmacist should take into account the cultures of the affected parties.[7] In his reviews of the foundations of modern medical ethics theories, Veatch[6,8] described how the unique perspectives of Western, Chinese, Hindu, Jewish, Catholic, Protestant, and other cultural groups have affected the formulation of their dominant medical ethics traditions. Other cultural classifications might include socioeconomic status, political affiliation, age category, and racial or ethnic group. A report by Najjar et al.[9] demonstrates some important similarities (e.g., requests to assess physician's recommendations) and differences (e.g., requests to serve as a primary health care provider), compared to those reported at U.S. centers, in the types of ethical dilemmas that are identified by drug information specialists functioning within the cultural environment of Saudi Arabia.

In a very interesting case study, Carrese et al.[10] discussed the ethical obligations of medical professionals in caring for those of a different ethnic culture. In this case, a young Laotian mother had utilized a traditional Mien folk cure to treat her infant. The treatment involved placing several small burns on the child's abdomen to treat "gusia mun toe," an apparently transient, but very distressing, colic-like ailment. The cure resulted in several small scars, but no other obvious ill effects. The mother indicated that the cure worked. The physician recognized the value in supporting the positive impacts of the woman's attachment to her cultural support group. However, the physician was confronted with the dilemma of how to respond to this mother's revelation of a culturally-promoted treatment measure that was not scientifically supported and could be dangerous. Sometimes, culturally-based actions may conflict with the professional's goal to avoid harm and promote benefit. However, failing to consider a cultural perspective may also have harmful effects. An extended discussion of how differing cultural perspectives affect ethical decision-making is beyond the scope of this chapter. However, the pharmacist should strive to be aware of and respect the cultural perspectives of the affected parties when contemplating an ethical dilemma. The interested reader is encouraged to refer to the resources cited here and above for further discussion of cultural factors in ethical analysis.[6,8]

One final issue should be addressed relative to cultural considerations. The legal requirements of the society within which an ethical dilemma occurs are part of the culture and must be identified. A specific ethical decision will not always exactly conform to the existing legal requirements of society. The ultimate nature of ethical deliberations may result in decisions that are more demanding than the legal requirements and, unfortunately, may even occasionally involve perceived or true conflict with specific legal requirements. This may involve, for instance, a decision not to divulge confidential communications between a professional and client, which may or may not be acceptable within the law. In another case, the pharmacist may decide not to provide information related to abortion or capital punishment, even though these activities are acceptable within the law. Obviously, legal requirements cannot be ignored or dismissed lightly when making a specific ethical decision.

Step II: Use of Rules and Principles (Action-Guides) to Assist in Analysis of an Ethical Dilemma

If the dilemma persists, once the available background information has been identified and considered, the process of full ethical deliberation should proceed. Veatch suggests that the involved party/parties can proceed as far as necessary through successive stages of general moral reflection assessing at the level of moral rules and then at the level of ethical principles, within their accepted ethical theory.[2] These might be described as the action-guides referred to by Beauchamp and Childress.[5] This second process step of analysis will look at moral rules that may apply to the specific case, as well as at more general pertinent ethical principles. Definitions are provided at the end of this section for a number of ethical rules and principles that are considered particularly relevant to decision-making by pharmacists.

It should be noted that specific action-guides may be considered a rule within one ethical theory and a principle within another. For example, veracity (truth telling) as mentioned above, may be considered by some ethicists to be a specific moral rule and by others to be a general principle, depending on which ethical theory is followed. For the practitioner immediately involved in analyzing a specific ethical dilemma, defining the relevant action-guides as rules or principles is important only to the extent that this helps in assessing which are more fundamental to the issue at hand. Therefore, in this chapter, both rules and principles will be included within the same process step of ethical analysis.

Examples of moral rules within biomedical ethics include: a confidentiality rule dictating that patient-entrusted information should not be disclosed or an informed consent rule that addresses the individual's right to information before agreeing to a specific medical procedure. Unfortunately, there is no definitive list universally defining all moral rules and, sometimes, multiple pertinent rules can be in conflict. Furthermore, there are acceptable exceptions to most moral rules. For instance, disregarding the informed consent rule might be justifiable in an acute situation to protect the life of the client, suffering may be necessary in order to achieve cure of serious disease, and many consider killing justified under certain circumstances. Therefore, there may not be a specific rule that resolves a particular ethical dilemma.

When such a circumstance arises, the pharmacist may begin a more general level of analysis by looking at the ethical principles that apply to the case. Sometimes, the involved parties can reach an acceptable resolution to an ethical dilemma once they recognize the more broad relevant ethical principles. In a given dilemma, the professional may decide that the primary principle is to respect the autonomy of the client and that this requires providing complete information that enables the client to make an informed decision. In another dilemma, if do no harm is considered the most fundamental ethical principle, decisions or acts that deny this principle would be considered unethical. It becomes immediately obvious, however, that relevant ethical principles such as these may also come into conflict. This problem can be demonstrated by the following example: The pharmacist may believe that full disclosure will result in noncompliance by the patient, with significant risk of resultant harm. The pharmacist therefore confronts two conflicting principles: "respecting client autonomy" versus the duty to "do no harm."

Step III: Ethical Theory as a Means to Clarify or Resolve Ethical Dilemmas

This third step of ethical analysis reveals how relevant moral rules and principles interact within the preferred ethical theory to address the given dilemma. When confronted with conflicting ethical rules or principles, the pharmacist may simply resolve the dilemma through his or her moral intuition of "the right thing to do"; even if unconscious, this reflects the individual's at least temporary affiliation to some theory of what constitutes "good versus bad" or "right versus wrong." Sometimes, the professional will find it valuable to more consciously deliberate on how various ethical theories suggest that the relevant rules and principles should be prioritized or balanced. According to Veatch,[2] this process step can lead to more rational and honest decision-making or action-taking. He suggests that these ultimate deliberations at the level of ethical theory will be affected by our most basic religious and/or philosophical commitments. It is important that the pharmacist recognizes and acknowledges the impact on decision-making of his or her own personal ethical perspective. Those dilemmas that cannot be fully resolved can at least be viewed with greater clarity.

Veatch[8] states that, "The components of a complete theory will answer such questions as what rules apply to specific ethical cases, what ethical principles stand behind the rules, how seriously the rules should be taken, and what constitutes the fundamental meaning and justification of the ethical principles." In this reference and another text, the author reviews the foundations of consequentialist, deontological, and other ethics theories particularly relevant to health professionals, including: the Hippocratic tradition; Judeo-Christian and other religious-based traditions; the philosophies of the modern secular West; and medical ethics theories outside the Anglo-American West, including Socialist, Islamic, Hindu, African, Chinese, and Japanese traditions.[6,8] Frequently, versions of the broad consequentialist and deontological theories are expressed in various ways across these traditions. Particular note should be given to the core of the various Hippocratic Oaths, since this has been the central ethical tradition of Western medicine: "Those who have stood in that (Hippocratic) tradition are committed to producing good for their patient and to protecting that patient from harm."[8] In Hippocratic tradition, there is also a special emphasis placed on the responsibility of the medical professional to the specific patient versus obligations to other less directly affected parties or to society in general. A contract theory of medical ethics has also been proposed, which describes an implicit (unwritten) contract between professionals and patients.[8] This modern theory is of special relevance to the pharmacist providing drug information as a service within an implicit pharmaceutical care contract.[8,11] First of all, this theory represents a shift in thinking for those pharmacists who might have considered their primary obligation to be to the prescriber rather than to the patient. Furthermore, this contract between patient and professional suggests an obligation for more substantive communication with patients and a higher level of caregiving than some pharmacists have previously felt obligated to offer. The reader is referred to foundational writings by Veatch, as well as those of Beauchamp and Childress, for a more in-depth discussion of various medical ethics theories.[5,6,8]

AN ANNOTATED LISTING OF RULES AND PRINCIPLES (ACTION-GUIDES) APPLIED IN MEDICAL ETHICS INQUIRY

The following rules and principles of ethical conduct will be described and subsequently used in the analysis of case scenarios provided in the next section. Their description will necessarily be brief. The reader is referred to other sources to read more about these rules and principles.[5,8]

1. *Nonmaleficence*—A basic principle of consequentialist theory; encompasses the duty to do no harm. This tenet has a long history as part of the Hippocratic tradition, where it has often been described in terms of the health care provider's duty to the individual patient. The principle is also cited as justification for actions benefiting all. Sometimes, application of the principle requires addressing conflicts between the needs of one and all.

2. *Beneficence*—Another basic principle of consequentialist theory that expresses the duty to promote good. Again, conflict can arise between what constitutes "good" for one individual versus the larger societal group. Good or bad consequences are also of importance within deontological theories, but are evaluated along with other principles that may be considered of equal or greater importance.

3. *Respecting the patient-professional relationship*—A moral rule, often referring to respect for the physician-patient relationship, but also applicable to other professional-patient relationships, as well. This rule has been mentioned in published reports of ethical dilemmas arising during the provision of drug information.[9,12–14] As expressed in Hippocratic traditions, this rule indicates that the physician's primary duty is to the patient and tends to give the physician, rather than the patient, control in the relationship. This rule is particularly noted in duty-driven (deontological) ethical theories that consider the professional's duty to the patient, but also supports consequentialist theory to the extent that good outcomes are enhanced.

4. *Respect for autonomy*—A principle described particularly within deontological theory. This principle is founded on a belief in the right of the individual to self-rule. It speaks to the individual's right to decide on issues that primarily affect self.

5. *Consent*—A moral rule related to the principle of autonomy which states that the client has a right to be informed and to freely choose a course of action; for example, informed consent to receive a therapy or procedure.

6. *Confidentiality*—A moral rule, also related to the principle of autonomy, which specifically addresses the individual client's right to give or refuse consent relative to release of privileged information.

7. *Privacy*—Another rule within the principle of autonomy, more generally relating to the right of the individual to control his or her own affairs without interference from or knowledge of outside parties. This rule has been addressed in deliberations on the rights of individuals with AIDS versus those of their potential contacts.

8. *Respect for persons*—A principle expressing duty to the welfare of the individual, particularly described within religion-based deontological theories. This principle may also be expressed within dignity of life or sanctity of human life principles. It has common elements with the respect for autonomy principle, but addresses more directly a belief in the inherent value of human life, independent of characteristics or abilities of the specific human being.

9. *Veracity*—This term addresses the obligation to truth telling or honesty. Veracity is considered an ethical principle within deontological theory. However, it is considered a useful rule within consequentialist theory, to the extent that it promotes good.

10. *Fidelity*—Another principle of moral duty in deontological theory that addresses the responsibility to be trustworthy and keep promises. This principle also relates to a duty of reciprocity—consideration of the other's point of view. Descriptions of pharmaceutical care have spoken of the need to develop an ethical covenant between pharmacist and client.[11] This covenant details the characteristics of a relationship requiring fidelity and reciprocity, in which each party takes on certain responsibilities and gives up certain rights in order to achieve specific good outcomes (consequentialist theory). Success of this contract depends in good measure on consideration by each party of the other's point of view.

11. *Justice*—This concept has been presented within various principles that relate to fairness and tendering what is due; providing that to which the individual is entitled. A number of justice theories have also been developed to connect and justify these various principles.[5]

These are certainly not the only relevant rules or principles, nor are they necessarily universally accepted definitions. However, these action-guides seem particularly pertinent to medical ethics inquiry. Furthermore, several of these rules and principles have been specifically discussed in published reports that describe ethical dilemmas encountered by drug information specialists.[12,13] Such dilemmas have also been described in situations where pharmacists are providing drug information directly to patients, either from a formal drug information center or during the process of providing patient care.

Demonstration of the Process for Analyzing Ethical Dilemmas

The following example demonstrates an ethical dilemma that might arise for a pharmacist providing drug information to consumers in the course of dispensing prescriptions. This case will be utilized to demonstrate the aforementioned process of analysis for the pharmacist encountering an ethical dilemma.

DEMONSTRATION OF CASE ANALYSIS

Case # 1

Ms. Jamison, a regular patient at your pharmacy, comes to the counter and asks to speak to the pharmacist on duty. When Dr. Bradley arrives at the counter, the patient asks if she can talk to her privately. Once they have stepped over to a private area, the patient tells the pharmacist that she has a question about the "morning after pill." She reveals that she has had unprotected sexual relations in the last 12 hours and is now concerned about becoming pregnant. She has heard that this agent is available by prescription and that it might even be obtained over-the-counter. She would like some information about this treatment and asks if she can buy it without prescription.

ANALYSIS

I. Identification of relevant background information.
  A. Factual details and circumstances of the issue at hand: The pharmacist is familiar with this patient and her family, and gains additional information through discussion with her.
    1. Ms. Jamison is 18 years of age, unmarried, lives at home, and is in her first year at a local liberal arts college. Her family belongs to the same Roman Catholic Church as the pharmacist.
    2. Ms. Jamison indicates that she has been dating the young man involved for awhile, but is not interested in a long-term relationship with him. When asked tactfully, Ms. Jamison indicates that she is opposed to abortion, but states quite vehemently, "This is just a birth control pill to prevent pregnancy before it starts."

3. Dr. Bradley is aware that the product being discussed is currently under consideration by the FDA for transfer to nonprescription status (as of the time of writing this text).

4. Dr. Bradley is also aware that there is considerable controversy over whether this agent works only as a contraceptive or whether it also acts as an abortifacent agent by preventing implantation of a fertilized ovum. She understands that the controversy particularly revolves around various arguments about when human life begins. Dr. Bradley feels considerable personal conflict about this controversy, based on her values regarding individual autonomy and her religious convictions, and about whether abortion is ever justifiable.

B. Identification of who is affected by the ethical issue: As the pharmacist reflects on this patient's inquiry, it is important to consider who might be impacted by her response to the patient's questions and any subsequent request for assistance.

1. Dr. Bradley, relative to her own desire to do "right," her desire to maintain a good relationship between herself and this patient, and her concern over her role in affecting this patient's and any offspring's future well-being.

2. Ms. Jamison, relative to any current and future life experience (as well as any emotional or spiritual impacts) that may result from the decisions made/actions taken around this issue.

3. Any infant that may or may not be born as a consequence of this sexual encounter.

4. The young man involved in this situation (although he may or may not be informed of whatever action taken).

5. The related families, significant others, and society in general, relative to the impacts of either pregnancy or no pregnancy for this woman.

C. Consideration for the cultural perspectives of those affected by the dilemma.

The pharmacist will consciously or unconsciously act within her own cultural and religious framework, and her understanding of her legal obligations. Awareness of her own perspective, as well as consideration of the cultural perspectives of others who may be affected, is important if she is to pursue a truly ethical course of action. To repeat Veatch's words differentiating ethical deliberations, "The deliberation takes into account the welfare of all involved or affected."[2] Each involved party's welfare is affected by his or her cultural perspective. Cultural, religious, and legal perspectives that the pharmacist must seek to consider in this case might include:

1. Her own personal moral beliefs about: (1) when life begins and about participating in actions that might lead to ending a specific life; (2) individual rights to autonomy and privacy; and (3) her moral beliefs about her obligation to respond to her patient's request for information.

2. Her patient's presumed (or stated) moral beliefs about when life begins and about potentially ending a specific life.

3. Legal requirements placed on the pharmacist in terms of responding to patient requests for information and/or service.
4. Dr. Bradley's employer may also have policies/procedures directing a general or specific course of action to be taken in response to patient requests for information or service. These rules represent another aspect of the culture within which the pharmacist practices.
5. The pharmacist may or may not also feel bound by known religious constraints of her and her patient's Roman Catholic faith.
6. Known cultural (including social and religious) perspectives of other affected parties, such as the woman's sexual partner and her parents.

II. Identification and justification of the relevant moral rules and principles (action-guides) pertinent to the case at hand.

It does not seem likely that the background information will fully dismiss the pharmacist's ethical concerns. If she feels morally confident that use of the requested therapy is morally justifiable, she may still feel an obligation to discuss controversial aspects of this product's proposed mechanisms of action with the patient, particularly since she is aware that the young woman belongs to a religious group that generally seems to condemn abortion (as well as artificial contraception, according to official doctrine). As Dr. Bradley ponders how to respond, she may find it helpful to consider the ethical rules and principles presented earlier in this chapter in order to clarify the dimensions of her concern. It is most useful to first identify all potentially pertinent action-guides, and seek an understanding of how fundamentally each applies to the situation,

Ethical action-guides (rules and principles) that seem pertinent to this inquiry include:

1. *Nonmaleficence/beneficence*—Intuitively, it seems relatively clear that harm could potentially result for at least some affected parties, whichever way the pharmacist acts. It also seems likely that preventing a pregnancy would be in the best interests of most concerned.
2. *Respecting the patient-professional relationship*—According to traditional interpretation of the Hippocratic Oath it would seem that Dr. Bradley's primary ethical obligation is to the welfare of her immediate patient, Ms. Jamison. However, current thought, and the ethical imperative to consider all affected parties, tends to value a narrowed interpretation of this rule as generally true but not paramount relative to wider societal and professional obligation.
3. *Respect for autonomy*—This principle is key in speaking to Ms. Jamison's right to decide, once appropriately informed, what she will do in this situation, as long as no laws are broken. However, this principle does not require that the pharmacist deny

whatever moral code she lives by. Furthermore, Ms. Jamison's rights might be considered limited in judgments by her obligations to and the rights of any child that might have been conceived through her sexual interaction.

4. *Consent*—A mediating moral rule that speaks to Ms. Jamison's right to be informed and to freely choose the course of action that she will take. This rule is considered an extremely important one, both legally and morally, within the principle of autonomy. The rule is limited by legal constraints relative to the product's current prescription or nonprescription status.

5. *Confidentiality*—Whatever the pharmacist decides relative to the issue at hand, this moral rule demands that Dr. Bradley respect this patient's right to privacy, relative to sharing the content of this discussion with anyone else without express permission of Ms. Jamison. This certainly extends to the patient's parents with whom Dr. Bradley is acquainted; the issue of confidentiality might be a bit more controversial if this patient was under 18 years of age.

6. *Privacy*—This rule related to the principle of autonomy speaks to Ms. Jamison's right to control her own affairs and to privacy while dealing with this issue. Conflict can again arise between the rights of one individual to privacy versus legitimate claims to interference for the sake of other individuals or society as a whole.

7. *Respect for persons*—This principle expresses the pharmacist's duty to Ms. Jamison's welfare; however, it presents conflicts with the duty Dr. Bradley may also feel to any child that may naturally result from these circumstances, or even (probably to a lesser degree) to other affected persons mentioned above. Within some religious moral traditions, this principle becomes even more demanding as a duty to respect the sanctity of human life.

8. *Veracity*—Addresses Dr. Bradley's responsibility to tell the truth (with acknowledgement of areas where clear knowledge does not exist) in answer to Ms. Jamison's questions, as the pharmacist understands it. This may be considered a basic principle of obligation within deontological theory, or a useful rule within consequentialist theory (to the extent that it promotes good).

9. *Fidelity/reciprocity*—A principle of obligation to an ethical covenant between Dr. Bradley and Ms. Jamison (within deontological theory) requires that Dr. Bradley fully answer Ms. Jamison's questions. However, to the extent that this covenant asks that each party take on certain responsibilities and give up certain rights in order to achieve specific good outcomes, the provision of certain information content may not be ethically required if Dr. Bradley believes it will cause harm. For instance, Dr. Bradley may not feel ethically bound to respond if she were morally opposed to Ms. Jamison utilizing specific information (identification of the product and its nonprescription status, if that is true) to purchase and use medication with negative consequences for any child that had been conceived. Obviously, a choice by the

pharmacist to withhold requested information may also have legal or job consequences. Referral to another pharmacist is another option within this professional
duty that may or may not be acceptable to all concerned.

10. *Justice*—This principle is considered of intrinsic value within certain deontological theories, and addresses Ms. Jamison's (and other affected parties') right to be given what
is due—entitlement to information may be considered justice in this case. Certainly,
Dr. Bradley's time and expertise might be legitimately considered due to her patient.

The reader may believe that other ethical rules or principles are pertinent to this case. If
so, they should also be considered as the analysis proceeds.

III. How should these rules and principles be ranked or balanced against each other in
order to resolve the ethical dilemma?

It is not likely that this step will be easily accomplished through simple use of moral
intuition, unless both Dr. Bradley and Ms. Jamison turn out to have similar beliefs about
when life begins, about what constitutes acceptable versus unacceptable forms of contraception, and about the moral acceptability of abortion at various stages of pregnancy.
Careful consideration of ethical theory can suggest which are the more fundamental
action-guides to be applied of those considered above. In this case, it will probably be
necessary to balance similarly weighted principles (depending on one's point of view)
against each other, clarifying which appears to be of greater weight in this case.

How Dr. Bradley ranks/prioritizes the rules and principles she considers most pertinent in this dilemma over how to respond to Ms. Jamison's inquiry will be strongly
impacted depending on the pharmacist's personal belief system and her commitments to
the other parties (including primarily Ms. Jamison and any child who might result from
the sexual encounter) potentially affected by this decision. The principle of autonomy,
particularly addressing Ms. Jamison's rights and acknowledging the incapability of the
fetus to achieve immediate autonomy, will seem paramount in some belief systems.
Others may focus most on respect for persons; whether this respect is focused on
Ms. Jamison or on the potential fetus will be strongly dependent on the decision-maker's
beliefs about when life begins. Furthermore, the decision will be affected by whether
those beliefs stem more from a theoretical construct of absolute respect for life as
paramount or a consequentialist perspective weighing good versus bad outcomes. A
deontologic (duty-driven) perspective coupled with a strong belief in the sanctity of life
is likely to result in an unwillingness to be a party to perceived destruction of human life.
If the respect for persons is focused on Ms. Jamison, or even if both Ms. Jamison and
the potential child are equally considered, and Dr. Bradley mainly focuses on weighing good versus bad consequences, she may agree that a pregnancy is a negative

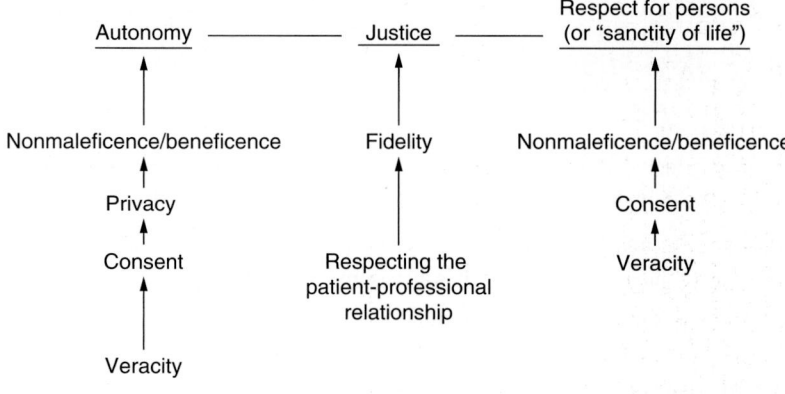

Figure 13–2

consequence and an unwanted child is better off not being born. On the other hand, she may consider that adoption is an alternative that could at least partially serve Ms. Jamison's needs, while aiming at a long-term good outcome for the potential child who would otherwise be destroyed. Perhaps, Dr. Bradley's sense of justice for all affected parties would become a deciding factor in such a deliberation. Ultimately, Dr. Bradley is called in this case to make an ethical judgment, resulting in provision of some accompanying service or refusal to provide service (Figure 13–2).

SUMMARY

Core to Dr. Bradley deciding on a course of action in this case is for her to clarify what she truly believes in regard to her immediate patient's right to autonomy/privacy versus the rights of other potentially affected parties. Her decision is likely to depend on when she believes that life begins, whether she believes that the product in question would prevent versus destroy life, as well as her own moral beliefs about the independent value of human life at various stages of fetal development.

It is well known that all will not agree on the ranking or balancing of the pertinent rules and principles in this case, nor will there be universal agreement about what constitutes the right resolution to the ethical dilemma presented. It is necessary to remember that an ethical issue has been defined as one where most agree that there is a right answer, but cannot always agree on what that answer is. The interested reader is referred to a publication by Cantor and Baum in the *New England Journal of Medicine* that further discusses ethical implications and conscientious objection related to this difficult issue.[15]

The reader is referred to Appendix 13–1 for discussions of further case scenarios, and identification of additional situations that might constitute ethical dilemmas for the pharmacist providing drug information.

Resources for Use by Pharmacists Seeking to Learn More About Medical Ethics

The first goal in learning more about medical ethics should be to learn to recognize opportunities for ethical deliberation when they confront us. Situations will arise where ethical judgments will be made that have moral consequences—with or without the conscious understanding of the parties involved. It is just as important that pharmacists are prepared to deal with these situations, as it is for them to learn how to address efficacy and safety concerns relative to drug therapies. This section of the chapter offers a survey of medical ethics resources that can assist pharmacists who personally desire to learn how to better recognize ethical situations and how to respond to them, or who will be teaching others in formal settings or informally in the workplace.

Formal coursework, inservices, or continuing education opportunities can teach skills that will aid pharmacists in handling ethical dilemmas related to work responsibilities. Thornton et al.[7] discussed what should be taught in basic ethics education that takes place within and outside the academic environment. Their review of important elements to be included in ethics education is worthwhile reading for anyone who may desire to participate in these teaching activities. They also refer the reader to other useful resources on the topic. In Davis's manual on patient-practitioner interactions, the author presents an easy to understand description of the stages of moral development, comparing two commonly identified models proposed by Piaget and by Kohlberg.[16] This information is valuable to assist in gaining insight into one's personal moral development, as well as that of others. This workbook, published by a physical therapist for the purpose of assisting in the professional socialization process, also offers a description of moral values associated with development as a professional. The author goes on to present a framework for resolving ethical dilemmas that has similar elements to those presented in this chapter; she also provides exercises that could be readily adapted for use in pharmacist education or inservices. Haddad et al.[1] have provided a comprehensive guideline on pharmacy ethics course content; this is also valuable reading for those wishing to address ethics topics in continuing education of the pharmacist. This guideline describes examples of educational methods including: case presentation and debate; scenario building, with identification and discussion of potential ethical issues; and role-playing activities. The authors indicate that such educational methods should involve group participation to conduct the analysis of sample cases for the ethical issue being discussed. Writing techniques, such as a "5-minute write" exercise prior to discussion can serve to focus the participant's ideas and facilitate the resultant discussion.[17] The guideline also provides an extensive bibliography of resource materials. Two other texts, one edited by Haddad[18] and the other by Veatch and Haddad[19], provide further discussion of teaching methods and many case examples of ethical dilemmas confronted by pharmacists. Pirl[3] described the use of role-playing assignments for pharmacy students. This article also listed case scenarios that could be used in continuing education programs for practitioners who are exploring ways to resolve ethical dilemmas arising in pharmacy practice. Smith et al.[20] have written a book on pharmacy ethics that also provides background discussion and case examples that relate to many target areas of pharmacy practice. This resource can be very useful for the pharmacy practitioner who wishes to address ethical issues in a particular area of practice.

Information technology is an integral part of the provision of drug information by pharmacists. Sometimes technology is utilized as a tool to access literature and other information sources utilized by the pharmacist responding to an inquiry. In other cases, the pharmacist may utilize the Internet to offer drug information to various target audiences, both professional and the lay public. Anderson and Goodman have authored a text *Ethics and Information Technology: A Case-based Approach to a Health Care System in Transition.*[21] This text addresses many ethical issues of pertinence to pharmacists, related both to web-based services and drug information. Case studies on topics such as provision or use of inaccurate information, conflicts of interest, issues of confidentiality and data sharing, and ethical standards that have been set for health websites are presented.

Poirier and Laux[22] have discussed redesign of a drug information resources course to meet the needs of nontraditional Pharm D students; this report describes addition of a course section where ethical issues associated with drug information questions received at the author's practice site were utilized to demonstrate how to deal with such situations. The authors utilized self-study, computer-assisted instruction, and recitations to teach the course. Published descriptions of ethical dilemmas arising during the provision of drug information may be utilized to build case discussions; these scenarios are helpful for educators of both traditional and nontraditional students, as well as for in-services aimed at practicing pharmacists.[9,14,23,24]

Structures That Support Ethical Decision-Making

Berger describes the need for an ethical covenant between the pharmacist and the patient who is being provided pharmaceutical care.[11] This term suggests an implicit contract between client and health care provider that broadly describes the relationship involved whenever a pharmacist provides drug information. Within this contract, the service recipient has a right to receive competently provided information as well as respectful treatment. He or she also has the obligation to provide background information needed by the pharmacist. Likewise, the provider pharmacist has the right to adequate background information (and respectful treatment as well), and the obligation to give competent, trustworthy, and caring service. Recognition of this implicit contract can occasionally suggest corrective action to resolve or avoid perceived ethical dilemmas. Such recognition is especially helpful when there has been a failure to adequately communicate, or there has been a lack of mutual respect in the interaction. Pharmacists also have a revised Code of Ethics for Pharmacists available to them since 1994, which may serve as a general guide to those obligations implicit to the patient-pharmacist relationship.[25,26] The text of this Code is provided in Appendix 13-2.

It is also important to establish organizational structures that guide and support the pharmacist providing drug information (in any setting), when he or she is faced with an ethical dilemma. Some formal structures, such as ethics committees[27,28] and other policy setting bodies, are generally available in larger hospitals. Formal attention to anticipatory planning activities on how to address ethical conflict situations is also needed within smaller institutions, the chain pharmacy setting, or in smaller organizations such as the independent community pharmacy. Furthermore, it is imperative that pharmacists participate in policy setting that may affect how they are expected to practice. Both the organization and the individual pharmacist have an obligation to plan in advance how they will handle situations where ethical conflict might arise, particularly relative to compliance with any policy affecting the employee's patient care obligations. A February 2004 Associated Press news story demonstrates this message very clearly (and was one source for the example case analysis presented earlier in this chapter).[29] The story describes an incident where a pharmacist on duty at a branch of the Eckerd pharmacy chain declined to fill a prescription written for an emergency contraception product for a rape victim. (Apparently all three pharmacists on duty refused to fill the prescription or to refer the patient to someone who would fill the prescription.) One pharmacist was fired for the action by Eckerd. His stated reason for declining the prescription was that he believed the product could cause an abortion if fertilization had already occurred, expressing his unwillingness to participate in such action. A spokesman for the Eckerd chain indicated that their employment manual was clear that their pharmacists could not decline to fill a prescription for moral or religious reasons. The pharmacist claimed that he was not aware of the policy until he was fired; his attorney protested that such a policy violated part of the Civil Rights Act. The attorney said that this Act "prohibits private companies from forcing employees to do something that violates their religious beliefs." In practice, pharmacists may have to deal with a specific ethical dilemma very rapidly and alone in order to decide or act in a timely manner. Policies and procedures to support the clinician in overall client interactions, and in ethical analysis and decision-making, can better prepare the pharmacist to address the real life dilemmas he or she will encounter. This case makes it clear that pharmacists must also be involved early (whatever their side in the issue) to make their voices heard during initial policy development, and must keep themselves informed about existing organizational policies in order to protect themselves and their patients. In the opinion of this author, after the fact controversy over unfamiliar policies does not serve the needs of pharmacists, patients, or organizations.

Organizations can assist professionals by sponsoring the creation of explicit policies addressing certain issues that have demonstrated a history of ethical controversy. For example, a written policy might state that pharmacists may refer questions (perhaps at a minimum back to the prescriber), where provision of an answer would violate their personal ethics. This could at least partially resolve a potential dilemma for the pharmacist who has been asked to provide information that involves ethical conflict. A policy that states pharmacists are not required to answer questions from a client who refuses to provide required background information could guide response in the dilemma of dealing with an unidentified client who wants to know how long amphetamine can be detected in the urine. Another policy might address adequate staffing requirements to ensure the community pharmacist of adequate time to perform counseling services. Of course, the legal and ethical rights of clients have to be recognized during development of such policies. This author believes that, as professionals, pharmacists should demand the right to a major role in organizational policy development that affects their practice, preferably with input from client/patient representatives. To be useful, organizational policies must be developed with attention to avoiding what constitutes infringement on the domain of personal ethics (such as a personal prohibition against euthanasia).

Finally, it is imperative that institutions engaged in the professional education of pharmacists provide foundational education in the area of ethics, and that organizations employing pharmacists continue this education through the use of various continuing education programs that foster increasing skills in application of ethical principles to practical decision-making.

Summary

All pharmacists will be called on to provide drug information. On occasion they will encounter ethical dilemmas regarding what information, if any, should be provided. It is important that the pharmacy professional approach such moments prepared to (often quickly) identify the pertinent facts, analyze relevant points of the situation, and rank or balance the pertinent ethical rules and principles that are involved. The individual pharmacist must recognize his or her rights and responsibilities relative to the client, to other involved individuals, to society as a whole and to any higher power to whom the pharmacist feels accountable. Organizations can assist the employee pharmacist by formal recognition of certain implicit and explicit policies. Furthermore, opportunities for deliberate study and rehearsal of important analytic steps are important to help pharmacists be prepared to address ethical dilemmas that arise when providing drug information.

Study Questions

A nurse (a member of the hospital's pain management team) on one of the medical-surgical units of your hospital calls with a question. She has a patient who she believes is being undertreated for pain. He is a young man who was admitted from the Emergency Room (ER) the previous evening after a motorcycle accident. He is a frequent patient in the ER, known to have a drug problem, with use of a variety of street products. She does not believe that he is in withdrawal, but does think he is getting inadequate pain medications for the severe bruises, scrapes, and a broken leg. However, the admitting physician (coincidentally, the rather testy Chair of the Pharmacy and Therapeutics Committee) is quite adamant that he will not enable the patient's drug habit, and maintains that perhaps living with some pain will encourage the patient to mend his ways. The nurse asks you to intervene with the physician to convince him that additional pain therapy is indicated, medically and ethically, for this patient.

1. Assess whether this drug information request constitutes a potential ethical dilemma, based on the three characteristics that differentiate such a situation.

2. What background information might you want to obtain to clarify this information request?

3. For pharmacists for whom this question constitutes an ethical dilemma, consider what moral rules and principles are likely to apply to this issue.

4. Assuming that some of these relevant action-guides conflict with others, describe further deliberations by which the pharmacist might prioritize or balance these conflicts in order to reach a decision on how to respond to the information request.

5. What organizational strategies might best prepare this pharmacist to most effectively respond to ethical dilemmas such as this one?

Refer to the article *Ethical dilemmas: Controversies in pain management* by Janet Brown to read the analysis of a similar case.[30]

REFERENCES

1. Haddad AM, Kaatz B, McCart G, McCarthy RL, Pink LA, Richardson J. Report of the ethics course content committee: curricular guidelines for pharmacy education. Am J Pharm Educ. 1993;57(Winter Suppl):34S–43S.

2. Veatch RM. Hospital pharmacy: what is ethical? (Primer). Am J Hosp Pharm. 1989;46:109–15.

3. Pirl MA. An ethics laboratory as an educational tool in a pharmacy law and ethics course. J Pharm Teach. 1990;1(3):51–68.

4. Beauchamp TLC, Childress JF. Principles of biomedical ethics, 5th ed. New York: Oxford University Press; 2001.

5. Beauchamp TLC, Childress JF. Principles of biomedical ethics, 4th ed. New York: Oxford University Press; 1994:15.

6. Veatch RM. Cross-cultural perspectives in medical ethics, 2nd ed. Sudbury (MA): Jones and Bartlett Publishers; 2000.

7. Thornton BC, Callahan D, Nelson JL. Bioethics education: expanding the circle of participants. Hastings Cent Rep. 1993;23(1):25–9.

8. Veatch RM. A theory of medical ethics. New York: Basic Books Publishers; 1981.

9. Najjar TA, Al-Arifi MN, Gubara OA, Dana MH. Ethical requests received by drug and poison information center in Saudi Arabia. J Soc Adm Pharm. 2000;17(4):234–7.

10. Carrese J, Brown K, Jameton A. Culture, healing, and professional obligations. Hastings Cent Rep. 1993;15–7.

11. Berger BA. Building an effective therapeutic alliance: competence, trustworthiness, and caring. Am J Hosp Pharm. 1993;50:2399–403.

12. Arnold RM, Nissen JC, Campbell NA. Ethical issues in a drug information center. Drug Intell Clin Pharm. 1987;21:1008–11.

13. Kelly WN, Krause EC, Krowsinski WJ, Small TR, Drane JF. National survey of ethical issues presented to drug information centers. Am J Hosp Pharm. 1990;47:2245–50.

14. Schools RM, Brushwood DB. The pharmacist's role in patient care. Hastings Cent Rep. 1991;12–7.

15. Cantor J, Baum K. The limits of conscientious objection: may pharmacists refuse to fill prescriptions for emergency contraception? N Engl J Med. 2004;351(19):2008–12.

16. Davis CM. Patient practitioner interaction: an experiential manual for developing the art of health care. Thorofare (NJ): SLACK; 1989.

17. Coach R. 5-minutes to monitor progress. Teaching Prof. 1991;5(9):1–2.

18. Haddad AM, editor. Teaching and learning strategies in pharmacy ethics, 2nd ed. Binghamton (NY): Pharmaceutical Products Press; 1997.

19. Veatch RM, Haddad A. Case studies in pharmacy ethics. New York: Oxford University Press; 1999.

20. Smith M, Strauss S, Baldwin HJ, Alberts KT. Pharmacy ethics. New York: Pharmaceutical Products Press; 1991.

21. Anderson JG, Goodman KW. Ethics and information technology: a case-based approach to a health care system in transition. New York: Springer-Verlag; 2002.

22. Poirier TI, Laux R. Redesign of a drug information resources course: responding to the needs of nontraditional PharmD Students. Am J Pharm Educ. 1997;61:306–9.

23. Arnold RM, Nissen JC, Campbell NA. Ethical issues in a drug information center. Drug Intell Clin Pharm. 1987;21:1008–11.

24. Kelly WN, Krause EC, Krowsinski WJ, Small TR, Drane JF. National survey of ethical issues presented to drug information centers. Am J Hosp Pharm. 1990;47:2245–50.

25. Vottero LD. Code of ethics for pharmacists. Am J Health Syst Pharm. 1995;52:2096, 2131.

26. Code of ethics adopted. Am Pharm. 1994;NS34(11):72.

27. Mappes TA, Zembaty JS, editors. Biomedical ethics, 3rd ed. New York: McGraw-Hill; 1991.

28. Mappes TA, Degrazia D, editors. Biomedical ethics, 5th ed. Boston (MA): McGraw-Hill; 2001.

29. Austin L. Emergency contraception denial raises moral, legal issues. Denton (TX): Associated Press State and Local Wire; 2004.

30. Brown J. Ethical dilemmas: controversies in pain management. Adv Nurse Pract. 1997;69–72.

14

Chapter Fourteen

Pharmacy and Therapeutics Committee

Patrick M. Malone • Mark A. Malesker • Paul J. Nelson •
Nancy L. Fagan

Objectives

After completing this chapter, the reader will be able to

- Describe the pharmacy and therapeutics (P&T) committee.
- Define the functions of the P&T committee.
- Describe attributes and structure of a P&T committee likely to promote its ability to function successfully.
- Describe where and how the P&T committee fits into the organizational structure of a health care institution or other groups.
- Describe how the pharmacy department participates in P&T committee activities.
- Describe and explain the concepts of drug formularies and drug formulary systems, and how pharmacy participates in their establishment and maintenance.
- Describe how P&T committee activities contribute to the quality improvement of medication use.
- Describe how to develop policies and procedures for the process of medication use.

Introduction

When considering how a pharmacist can have an impact on a patient's drug therapy, it is common to consider the individual practitioner dealing with a specific patient or, perhaps, a small group of patients. Certainly the clinician can have a deep impact this way, but it does have the disadvantage of dealing with a very limited number of patients. In order for pharmacists to efficiently impact a great number of patients, a different approach is necessary. Fortunately, one way pharmacists have that opportunity is through participation in the activities of a P&T committee or its equivalent, which generally oversees all aspects of drug therapy in an institution. Physicians and pharmacists have collaborated to implement cost-effective prescribing practices and assess clinical outcomes through educational initiatives, administrative programs to restrict ordering practices, use of formularies and prescribing guidelines, and financial incentives.[1] There are data to show that P&T committee actions are useful.[2,3]

Before proceeding, it must be stated that while this chapter deals with the P&T committee, which is usually the group responsible for overseeing all aspects of drug therapy in an institution, there is sometimes a similar body referred to as the formulary committee. This latter group deals strictly with determining which drugs are carried within an institution or organization, whereas, the P&T committee has numerous other tasks, covering all aspects of drug therapy (e.g., adverse drug reaction [ADR]/medication error monitoring, quality assurance, policy and procedure approval), although the exact group of functions may vary from place to place.[4] Some institutions use a formulary committee, since other bodies may perform the additional P&T committee tasks described later in this chapter. Also, some health care groups may use both committees, with one body addressing the issues for the group as a whole, while the other is located separately at various institutions to address issues specific to that location (e.g., only one institution in the group has an oncology unit, therefore, the committee for that individual institution will consider specific antineoplastic agents that are not of much use for the rest of the group). In this chapter, anything discussed regarding which drugs are available within an institution or group applies to both bodies, whereas, all other items are for the P&T committee only.

It should be noted that while P&T committees have normally been associated with institutional pharmacy, other organizations have increasingly used P&T-type committees in an attempt to improve drug therapy while lowering costs. Some places where such committees are seen include managed care organizations (MCOs),[5] insurance companies, pharmacy benefit management (PBMs) companies, unions, employers,[6] state Medicaid boards, state departments of public institutions,[7] Medicare,[8] long-term care facilities,[9] ambulatory clinics,[10] and even community pharmacies.[11] Much of this chapter will use examples from institutional pharmacy and managed care, simply because much of the published literature deals with those areas of practice and it is the most likely setting in which a pharmacist will be directly involved in P&T committee activities. However, the concepts covered are applicable to any P&T-type committee and comply with recommendations of the American Medical Association (AMA),[12,13] American Society of Health-System Pharmacists (ASHP),[14] the Joint Commission for the Accreditation of Health care Organizations (JCAHO),[15] and the Academy of Managed Care Pharmacy (AMCP).[16]

The role of the P&T committee has been continuously expanded over the years and now encompasses a great number of functions and activities that cover all aspects of overseeing drug therapy. As some of these are of sufficient size and importance, they are covered separately in other chapters (e.g., drug monographs and quality assurance). In addition, there are a number of areas (e.g., investigational drugs) in which P&T committees play a secondary role, and these too are covered in other chapters. This chapter will serve to provide a base to tie together discussion of all of these areas and a number of smaller functions or activities that will be covered as a portion of this chapter. The information is appropriate both for those just learning about the concepts and also for those individuals who are involved with P&T committee activities.

Organizational Background

The concept of a P&T committee represents a unique niche within the structure of the hospital. The current role of a hospital in western countries[17] began about 200 years ago, at a time when very few efficacious medications were available, although drug formularies had been developed during the Revolutionary War to list the drugs available.[18] The original hospital was a place to receive basic health care when a person had no extended family to provide the basic needs of good health. After infection control became a recognized concept and anesthesia for surgery evolved around 1900, the value of the modern hospital progressively became a recognized need for all segments of society. The origins for standards of how a hospital functioned subsequently developed during the first half of the twentieth century. This began with the early efforts of the American College of Surgeons in the United States to develop the first accreditation standards for hospitals. Later, the Joint Commission on Accreditation of Hospitals (JCAH), now known as JCAHO, evolved to centralize the basic requirements for the functional character of a U.S. hospital. The concept of the P&T committee originated and evolved to help hospitals meet various standards regarding drug therapy. The first P&T committee was formed at Bellevue Hospital in New York City in the mid-1930s.[18,19] While it dealt with true compounding formulas, it was originally founded to ensure quality and efficacy of those products, which is still a portion of the functions of P&T committees.

In keeping with the social origins of the hospital, the legally sanctioned or licensed privilege of being a professional health care provider evolved.[17] Both the physician and pharmacist were considered unique for the needs of society. Minimum standards evolved, including the accreditation of their training as a basis for being licensed. Originally, physicians and pharmacists functioned primarily as independent professionals. The nature of a physician's independence was legally defined to further support their obligations to a patient. Many states in the United States legally prohibited a physician from being employed by a corporation. Eventually, these laws were all repealed, but they had the effect of creating the basis for a medical staff as being a separate legal entity within a hospital. The medical staff reflected the legally evolving traditions of a physician, and indirectly the pharmacist, as being independent professionals committed only to the care of a patient without unnecessary outside influences. This evolution has had a major impact on the organizational structure of hospitals.

A typical hospital organization is shown in Figure 14–1. The board of directors divides the functions of its organization into two entities. First, the administration of the hospital operates as a typical business with a chief executive officer, chief operating officer, and so forth. Second, the board of directors authorizes that a medical staff be formed that reports separately to the board of directors. While the medical staff as a whole is ultimately in charge of all clinical aspects of care in the hospital, in most institutions this is unworkable without an administrative structure of some kind. Therefore, the medical staff may elect officers and either elect or appoint some body to oversee all aspects of patient care. In this example, the term medical executive committee is used for that body, although the name and exact function may vary. The medical staff functions to certify the credentials of its members, establish their scope of practice where appropriate, monitor the quality of health care provided by its members, and maintain the means to collaborate with the administration of the hospital.

In modern medicine, there are so many clinical areas to consider that it is unrealistic for one committee to adequately oversee all aspects of patient care, except in very small

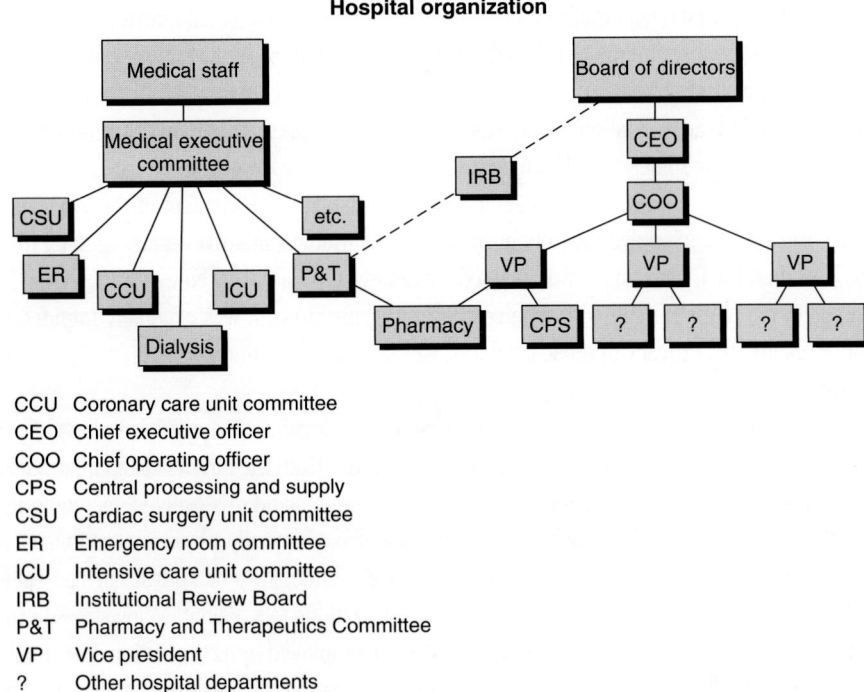

Hospital organization

CCU   Coronary care unit committee
CEO   Chief executive officer
COO   Chief operating officer
CPS   Central processing and supply
CSU   Cardiac surgery unit committee
ER   Emergency room committee
ICU   Intensive care unit committee
IRB   Institutional Review Board
P&T   Pharmacy and Therapeutics Committee
VP   Vice president
?   Other hospital departments

Figure 14–1. Hospital organization.

institutions. For this that reason, various subcommittees of the medical executive committee are usually necessary, as can be seen in Figure 14–1. As a means to coordinate the needs of the medical staff and the operation of the hospital pharmacy, the modern P&T committee developed. From the traditions established by JCAHO and ASHP, the P&T committee developed as a function of the medical staff's responsibilities. This committee or related committees may have other names, such as the drug and therapeutics committee in Australia,[20] but the functions are the same. While the P&T committee has been referred to in JCAHO accreditation standards in the past, it is no longer specifically required and may be replaced by some other committee or body,[15,21,22] although the P&T committee concept is supported by many national and professional organizations.[23] Given the continuing growth in the number, complexity, and expense of medications, both the importance and number of functions of the P&T committee have continued to increase. Policy and procedures to set up a P&T committee are described in Appendix 14–1, but the following will serve as a general description of P&T committees and their actions.

In some cases, the P&T committee may be part of a corporation of hospitals and medical centers, rather than just being for a specific institution. While the philosophy of operating one P&T committee within this corporate structure seems reasonable, this is not often accomplished without problems and decentralization of these efforts may be better.[24] Different patient populations, medication needs, cross hospital physician participation, meeting time, length and location of meetings, and differing clinical cultures within a specific institution are examples of barriers that may be present. The P&T model may need to be revised to work with these challenges.[25-30]

Although it is easy to assume from its name that the P&T committee is organizationally a part of the pharmacy department, such is not the case, as was mentioned above. Instead, it is usually a medical staff entity and, perhaps, only one or two pharmacists may actually be members of the committee (possibly *ex officio* members without voting privileges). Commonly, the pharmacy director or clinical coordinator, serving as the committee's secretary (e.g., taking minutes, collating, and arranging the agenda), may be the sole official pharmacy representative. Other pharmacists may also attend to act as consultants to the committee, often having great impact on the committee's decisions, even if they cannot officially vote. Fortunately, in larger hospitals, it appears that more pharmacists are now becoming members of the P&T committee.[31]

Typically, the voting members of an institutional P&T committee are limited to members of the medical staff. Membership is mostly physicians (preferably a wide variety of physicians from various areas of practice), but usually includes at least one pharmacist and often members from other areas of the hospital (e.g., nursing, administration, quality assurance, medical records, laboratory, and risk management).[32] A pharmacoeconomicist also can be extremely helpful. It may be best to try to keep down the number of physician members to encourage a smaller group to participate more fully, while taking care of addressing the wide variety of issues by calling in physicians to consult with the committee on an as-needed basis.[33] In some cases, the pharmacy department is asked to recommend physicians for the committee. If possible, pharmacy should suggest physicians that are noted for their commitment to rational drug therapy.[34] As an example, the Department of Defense has procedures for appointment of members, including nonphysician members, of the P&T committee that are available on the Internet.[35] Also, efforts should be made to ensure that the physician chosen to be chairman of the committee is an advocate of the pharmacy department. It is possible for the medical executive committee of the medical staff to pass a resolution to approve a policy broadening the voting members of the P&T committee (e.g., director of pharmacy or hospital vice president) or delegating the functions of the P&T committee to the hospital. In this latter arrangement, the medical staff would reserve the right to terminate the policy if the P&T committee fails to support the needs of the medical staff. If the P&T committee is a hospital committee, rather than medical staff committee, a pharmacist or nurse might more easily obtain voting privileges, given appropriate physician quorum requirements in the authorizing policy.

The P&T committee of MCOs and government bodies often have similar membership to that in institutional committees, however, there may need to be a requirement for at least some of the members to be independent practitioners (i.e., having no financial ties to the organization or group that sponsors the P&T committee).[36]

Once the general organizational setting of the P&T committee has been determined, the operating policy of the P&T committee requires careful attention to two key problems. The first key issue is obvious (e.g., to whom does the P&T committee report and to what degree can the decisions of the P&T committee be overturned by another segment of the organization). It is important to point out that the P&T committee may act only as an advisory body to the medical executive committee. Decisions of the P&T committee may not be considered final (and therefore not be implemented) until they are reviewed and approved by the medical executive committee. In this situation, a report is forwarded from the P&T committee after each meeting to the medical executive committee. In addition, an annual report of the P&T committee may be prepared for both internal review and review by the Medical Executive Committee. This annual report is time consuming in preparation, but is a very important means of tracking P&T activities and action over time.

The second key issue is that the P&T committee will likely be successful based on the leadership qualities of its members and the chairperson. The role of the chairperson includes developing the respect and involvement of all members.

PHARMACY BENEFIT MANAGEMENT (PBM) P&T COMMITTEE ORIGIN

The origin of the PBM organizations dates back to the late 1960s. Their primary focus was on claims administration for insurance companies. Later, it became a challenge for the insurance companies to efficiently manage the increase in drug coverage in the private sector when the prescription volume was high and the cost per claim was low.[37] The plastic drug benefit card began in the 1970s and changed the way many prescriptions were bought and paid for by the insurance company and employee. From then on, any employee with an ID card, using a pharmacy network, only had a small copayment.[37] In addition, administration costs for the third-party payer, whether it is the insurance company, health plan, or employer, were reduced, with the PBM creating pharmacy networks and mail service benefits. Pharmacy networks are a group of pharmacies that are under contract with the insurance company, health plan, and/or their contracted PBM partner to promote prescription services at a negotiated discounted fee.[38] Mail service is a program offered by the PBM, whereby pharmaceutical agents, both prescription and nonprescription, are offered through the mail at a discounted price compared to those offered at the independent and chain pharmacies.[38]

In the late 1980s came the introduction of real-time electronic claims processing. Not only was there two-way communication between the pharmacy and the PBM for claim processing, but also for clinical information as well. In the 1990s, the PBMs moved toward a greater emphasis on patient health by offering a variety of new services in addition to the claims processing. Since 2000, there has been an emphasis on consumer behavior modification, enhanced patient interventions, physician connectivity, clinical consulting, disease management, and retrospective drug utilization review (DUR; see Chap. 16 for further information) to name a few.[37]

One of the key functions of a PBM is to design, implement, and administer outpatient drug benefit programs for employers, MCOs, and other third-party payers. PBMs manage prescription drug benefits separate from other health care services (i.e., physician and hospital services).[38] Determining which medications are most cost effective, without compromising patient care, is one of the key elements for controlling the cost of a prescription drug benefit.[6] PBMs accomplish this by developing drug formularies.[6] Formularies define what medications are covered (i.e., paid for) and provide the main component of the pharmacy benefit. Specific PBM drug payment and management activities occur within this formulary structure, such as therapeutic interchange and disease management programs. Eighty to hundred percent of most PBM covered lives receive some type of formulary management service.[6,38] The use of drug formularies is in flux due to the advantages and disadvantages identified over the last decade or so, however, they are likely to be continued for at least the foreseeable future, particularly due to the proposed Medicare drug formulary requirements.[39]

Development and maintenance of drug formularies for third-party payers is an ongoing process. The formulary must be continuously updated to keep pace with new drugs, therapies, and prices; recent clinical research; changes in medical practice; and updated Food and Drug Administration (FDA) information.[40] PBMs use a panel of experts called the P&T committee to develop and manage their drug formularies. P&T committee members consist of physicians and pharmacists. Many times individuals with special clinical expertise are consulted when considering medications within a specific therapeutic class.[40] Meetings are usually held on a quarterly basis, and not only are drug formulary recommendations made, but this group also provides input into other clinical areas, such as development of disease management programs.[6,37-40]

Many PBMs establish their own P&T committee to evaluate the efficacy, safety, uniqueness, cost of therapeutic equivalent drugs, and other appropriate criteria. In addition, PBMs work with the health plan, employer, or insurance company P&T committee to develop drug formularies using the same evaluation process. In either case, if the P&T committee determines that one drug provides a clear medical benefit over the other, therapeutically equivalent drugs in that same therapeutic category, the drug is usually added to the formulary.[6] However, if there are drugs in the same therapeutic category that have very similar efficacy and safety profiles and no unique properties that would make it a better drug, then the net cost becomes a deciding factor as to which drug should be added to the formulary.[6] There has been some discussion as to whether drug costs are weighted too heavily, while drug efficacy and other clinical information is weighted too lightly when it comes to drug formulary decisions.[37,38] The committee leadership needs to recognize the potential for conflicts of interest between efficacy and economic interests of the PBM and to establish means of resolving conflicts that arise.

In the case of a health plan, employer, or insurance company's own P&T committee, the drug formulary recommendations made by the PBM P&T committee are presented and reviewed by the organization's P&T committee. The PBM recommendations regarding drug formulary recommendations can be either accepted or denied by the organization's P&T committee and the organization's own decision made regarding formulary inclusion.

PHARMACY SUPPORT OF THE P&T COMMITTEE

Although it is not uncommon for pharmacists to downplay or misunderstand the importance of P&T committee support in comparison to other clinical activities, such support is vital for pharmacy to impact patient care. P&T committee support and participation can have far-reaching effects on the overall quality of drug therapy in an institution and must be given a great deal of attention. While such attention is time consuming,[41] it can be of value to the pharmacy since this is an opportunity to present recommendations to a decision-making body and P&T committees often accept pharmacy recommendations;[42,43] therefore, pharmacy departments can have a great and far-reaching impact on drug therapy through this mechanism.

Some pharmacists who participate in P&T committee activities feel they are serving their function by just providing information requested by physicians and considering drugs for formulary approval only following physician requests. This can rapidly deteriorate into crisis management, where the pharmacy department reacts to problems, fighting each fire as it occurs. It is much better for a pharmacy to be proactive,[44,45] seeking to address issues (e.g., changes in drugs carried on the formulary, new policies and procedures, quality assurance activities, and so forth) before they become problems. JCAHO accreditation requirements include annual evaluation of all drugs and/or drug classes.[15] Through prospective actions with the P&T committee it is possible for the pharmacy to better get physician support for all of their clinical activities.

In the specific instance of P&T committee support, one or more pharmacists must be identified to conduct the necessary planning. This may consist of a pharmacy-based steering committee and might include administrators, purchasing agents, or clinicians, and, particularly, drug information specialists. These people must develop and regularly evaluate data sources to anticipate physicians' needs[46] (see Table 14–1). For example, it is necessary to find out what drugs have recently been FDA-approved in order to identify drugs for possible formulary inclusion. FDA approval often comes about 3 months before commercial availability and is published on the FDA website (<<http://www.accessdata.fda.gov/scripts/cder/drugsatfda/index.cfm>>). Therefore, there is time for the drug to be considered for formulary addition before the first orders arrive from the nursing units, which necessitates a review of some sort under JCAHO standards.[15] In a case where it is not possible to consider a drug before it is commercially available, it has been suggested by some that drugs rated "P" (priority) by the FDA be made available to physicians until the drug can be fully considered (the FDA classification codes are found on Table 14–2 through Table 14–5, with the priority vs. standard explanation found on Table 14–4).[47] This latter procedure may be effective, but considering the drug before commercial availability is preferable, because if the ultimate P&T committee decision is to leave the drug off the drug formulary, there may be difficulties in getting physicians to stop use of the product. It is also a good idea to track older drugs. For example, the use of nonformulary drugs may be tracked within the hospital.[48,49] If patterns of increased use are noted, it is best to identify a reason for that use. If the use is inappropriate, the physician(s) should be contacted and given information about alternative formulary

TABLE 14–1. AREAS WHERE PHARMACISTS SHOULD BE SUPPORTING A PHARMACY AND THERAPEUTICS COMMITTEE

Planning future agendas (including medications, policies and procedures, quality assurance, and other subjects to be addressed)

Gathering data to create drug monographs and other necessary documents

Evaluating medications for formulary adoption or deletion

Preparing and conducting quality assurance programs (including drug usage evaluation and monitoring of adverse effects and medication errors)

Preparing policies and procedures

Communicating information from the P&T committee to other areas of the institution

Creating hard copy and electronic versions of the formulary

TABLE 14–2. FDA CLASSIFICATION BY CHEMICAL TYPE*

Type	Definition
1	New molecular entity not marketed in the United States
2	New salt, ester, or other noncovalent derivative of another drug marketed in the United States
3	New formulation or dosage form of an active ingredient marketed in the United States
4	New combination of drugs already marketed in the United States
5	New manufacturer of a drug product already marketed by another company
6	New indication for a product already marketed
7	Drug that is already legally marketed without an approved NDA
	First application since 1962 for a drug marketed prior to 1938
	First application for DESI (Drug Efficacy Study Implementation)-related products that were first marketed between 1938 and 1962 without an NDA
	First application for DESI-related products first marketed after 1962 without NDAs. In this case, the indications may be the same or different from the legally marketed product

NDA–New Drug Application.
*Efficacy supplements approved in fiscal year 2004 [home page on the Internet]. Washington: Food and Drug Administration; [updated 2004 Sept 30; cited 2004 Nov 11]. Available at <<http://www.fda.gov/cder/rdmt/ESFY04AP.htm>>.

agents. In some cases, new information may be available showing a new advantage or use for an old agent, which can lead to its reconsideration for formulary adoption. Related to this is the necessity to regularly consider the material being promoted by the drug company representatives. It is worth mentioning that some hospitals will restrict drug representative access to the institution or restrict the drugs that may be promoted by those representatives to only

TABLE 14–3. EFFECTIVENESS SUPPLEMENTAL CODE DEFINITIONS*

Type	Definition
N (Chemical Type 6)	NDA Type 6—new indication
SE1	New indication or significant modification of an existing indication. Includes removal of a major limitation to use
SE2	New dosage regimen, including an increase or decrease of daily dose, or change in administration frequency
SE3	New route of administration
SE4	Comparative efficacy or pharmacokinetic claim naming another drug
SE5	Change in any section other than INDICATIONS AND USAGE that would significantly alter the patient population being treated (e.g., addition of pediatric dosing information)
SE6	Switch from prescription to over-the-counter (OTC)
SE7	Complete the traditional part of a product originally receiving accelerated approval
SE8	Incorporates other information based on at least one adequate and well-controlled clinical trial

*Efficacy supplements approved in fiscal year 2004 [home page on the Internet]. Washington: Food and Drug Administration; [updated 2004 Sept 30; cited 2004 Nov 11]. Available at <<http://www.fda.gov/cder/rdmt/ESFY04AP.htm>>.

TABLE 14–4. FDA CLASSIFICATIONS BY THERAPEUTIC POTENTIAL*

Type	Definition
P	Priority handling by FDA—before 1992 this was two categories: A: Major therapeutic gain B: Moderate therapeutic gain
S	Standard handling by FDA—before 1992 this was referred to as class C, which indicated the product offered only a minor or no therapeutic gain
O	Orphan Drug

*Efficacy supplements approved in fiscal year 2004 [home page on the Internet]. Washington: Food and Drug Administration; [updated 2004 Sept 30; cited 2004 Nov 11]. Available at <<http://www.fda.gov/cder/rdmt/ESFY04AP.htm>>.

items approved for use in the hospital in order to prevent this problem. There may also be new indications or other information that will increase demand for nonformulary items. If there are sufficient changes noted in the use(s) of a particular class of drugs, it is useful to review the class as a whole to decide which drug(s) are to be retained on the formulary. JCAHO now requires annual review of all medications,[10-15] which is useful because there may be new information not otherwise noted that necessitates changes in formulary items in a particular class, both additions and deletions. However, these situations that have been noted above may necessitate moving up the review. Other items, such as trends in reported ADRs in the institution or published data for new products with little information in the literature on first approval may also be useful in determining products for P&T committee consideration or reconsideration.[50] Although there must be a mechanism by which physicians can request that drugs be added to the formulary, all of the above methods and others can help the pharmacy anticipate physician needs, allowing time for information gathering, evaluation of products, and P&T committee consideration before the need becomes too urgent to permit proper consideration.

To guide clinicians into considering the logic of requesting the addition of items to the drug formulary, a specific request form may be useful. Items that a physician may be

TABLE 14–5. FDA SUPPLEMENTARY DESIGNATORS*

Type	Definition
AA	Drug used for acquired immunodeficiency syndrome (AIDS) or complications of that disease
E	Drug developed or evaluated under special procedures for a life-threatening or severely debilitating illness
F	Drug under review for fraud policy; validity of data submitted being assessed
G	Drug originally given Type F designation, once its data are found to be reliable
N	Product with nonprescription marketing for some indication
V	Orphan Drug

*Efficacy supplements approved in fiscal year 2004 [home page on the Internet]. Washington: Food and Drug Administration; [updated 2004 Sept 30; cited 2004 Nov 11]. Available at <<http://www.fda.gov/cder/rdmt/ESFY04AP.htm>>.

TABLE 14–6. ITEMS THAT MAY BE ON A REQUEST FOR FORMULARY CONSIDERATION FORM

Date and time of request

Name of product (e.g., generic, trade, and chemical)

Source of product (e.g., manufacturer and distributor)

Specific information about drug product (e.g., class of drug, mechanism, adverse effects, and clinical studies)

Anticipated use of drug (e.g., what type of patient and how often)

Comparable drugs already on the formulary

Why the product is needed

What drugs could be removed from the formulary

What restrictions, policies, cautions, and so forth are necessary

How the drug fits into any clinical guidelines

Action requested (e.g., addition, deletion, and restriction)

required to fill out or attach to the form can be seen listed on Table 14–6.[51] An example form is seen in Appendix 14–2.

The P&T committee should be kept advised by the above-mentioned pharmacy-based steering committee of future plans, so that it can be aware that a rational planning process is governing its agenda. Also, it is a good idea for one or more representative(s) of this steering committee to meet with the pharmacy director, chairman of the P&T committee, and a representative of the hospital administration on a regular basis to assist with planning and ensure their concerns are addressed. This meeting could be held shortly before the P&T committee actually meets to present preliminary formulary evaluations, drug usage evaluation (DUE) material, and policy and procedure documents for an initial review, allowing modifications addressing physician and administration concerns to be made before formal committee review and action. During this meeting, plans for future months can be made or adjusted as the circumstances dictate. Other appropriate physicians or groups should also be consulted in order to assure that their concerns are addressed. For example, if changes to the cephalosporins carried on the drug formulary or their permitted uses (e.g., restrictions to particular uses or prescribing groups) are considered, the infectious disease specialists should be contacted to provide input. Note: This does not mean that recommendations are changed to account for physician preferences, but that their options and concerns are specifically addressed in the evaluation.

Regarding to quality assurance activities, the pharmacy department should obtain data to guide the selection of upcoming quality assurance programs. This will be covered in greater detail in Chap. 16.

The pharmacy should also investigate what medications may need specific policies and procedures developed to guide their use and monitoring. This may be done when the drug is first being evaluated for formulary addition or later if problems (e.g., increased ADR reports, medication errors, and overuse) are noted. For example, concerns about a new thrombolytic agent leading to increased morbidity and mortality through improper use might prompt the P&T committee to approve specific protocols for the use of the agent. Policy and procedure documents are covered later in the chapter.

Finally, it is extremely important for the P&T committee to make sure that physicians are informed about the actions taken. Often the pharmacy is heavily involved in providing this information to physicians. While a great deal of effort is placed on communication within the committee itself, it is also necessary to keep the entire medical staff informed. This may be accomplished through medical department meeting presentations, newsletters and websites (refer to Chap. 11), or other mechanisms.

AD HOC COMMITTEES

A P&T committee may find it necessary to create ad hoc committees to address various issues, depending on their complexity and size. Some of the common committees are discussed below. Institutions may or may not use these committees (sometimes referred to as subcommittees) and their exact use varies from place to place, depending on their needs or desires.[4]

Adverse Reactions

A comprehensive ADR monitoring and reporting program is an essential component of the P&T committee (see Chap. 17 for further information about ADRs and how they are handled). A subcommittee may be helpful to review the entire ADR data for trends and any necessary actions that need to be taken. The P&T committee will usually report the ADR data on a monthly or quarterly basis. Following approval of this report, the P&T committee is responsible for the dissemination of information to the medical staff and other health professionals in the institution. This includes recommending processes to cut the rate of preventable ADRs. This subcommittee may be combined with the medication errors subcommittee.

Antimicrobials/Infectious Disease

Antibiotics can represent the largest category of formulary medications.[52] Frequent category review and revision is necessary and complex.[53] Cunha has defined five factors to consider when reviewing antimicrobial agents for formulary inclusion: microbiologic activity,[54] pharmacokinetics and pharmacodynamics profiles,[55] resistance patterns,[56,57] adverse effects,[58] and cost to the institution.[59]

The P&T committee or a subcommittee of the P&T may be responsible for developing appropriate antibiotic selection and use in both inpatient and outpatient settings.[60,61] Some institutions may rely on input from the infection control committee regarding antibiotic formulary management and appropriate utilization. Multidisciplinary antibiotic use committees have limited inappropriate prescribing of antimicrobials and increased the medical staff's knowledge on appropriate antibiotic use.[59,62,63]

Medical Devices

The P&T committee or a subcommittee may be responsible for the approval of some medical devices within an institution. This subcommittee is often multidisciplinary and is given the opportunity to review medical devices before purchases are made or contracts are signed. The committee is also responsible for reviewing the safety information associated with these devices because adverse medical device events are an important patient safety issue.

Medication Errors

A medication error or medication misadventure subcommittee should be multidisciplinary in nature. This subcommittee will review medication misadventures and medication errors that occur within the institution or health care system. The role of the subcommittee is to provide guidance and recommendations to the P&T committee. For example, they may suggest the implementation of a set of policies and procedures for use of a particular agent or drug class. A report will commonly be presented to the P&T committee on a quarterly or semiannual basis (see Chap. 17 for further information about medication errors and how they are handled).

Quality Assurance of Medication Use

A subcommittee of the P&T committee may be placed in charge of planning and overseeing the plan for quality assurance regarding drug therapy. Details about this activity are found in Chap. 16.

P&T COMMITTEE MEETING

Before beginning the description of a typical P&T committee meeting, it is important to note that a smoothly functioning P&T committee has certain needs. The committee will need the support of its parent organization. A room for the meetings should be carefully selected (see Appendix 14–3). The agenda for the meeting should be prepared in advance by the committee's secretary and sent to the members. Most often, as mentioned previously, an informal meeting of the supporting pharmacists and others is required between P&T committee meetings to plan the activities necessary to support the agenda. The chair of the committee may also attend such planning meetings to ensure that issues are addressed before the meeting. Formulary reviews represent a special concern when sending out an agenda, since they may trigger the outside influences of dedicated pharmaceutical marketing efforts if companies learn from committee members that their products or their competitor's products are being evaluated. Efforts must be made to make sure the committee is not distracted by outside influences, such as the pharmaceutical industry and advertisements. This consideration should be reflected in the selection of members and it may be necessary to avoid sending out some materials ahead of time, to lessen the chance of them being obtained by pharmaceutical company representatives. Also, if it is possible to prevent pharmaceutical representatives from knowing the membership of the committee, many of these problems may be avoided. If materials are sent out, it may be found that sending minutes from the previous P&T committee meeting is not always appropriate, since it may be difficult to adequately describe the full basis of a decision in a set of minutes. As a result, the minutes might be open to inappropriate projection regarding the basis for the P&T committee decision process. Some institutions simply make the minutes a pure recording of the decisions, eliminating any information about the discussion to avoid this problem. A sample set of minutes is seen in Appendix 14–4. Along with sending an agenda to members, a reminder phone call, fax, and/or e-mail may be useful to facilitate attendance. Each P&T committee meeting will require extensive preparation by the pharmacists involved in its affairs. Specifically, management of the formulary requires extensive background research and the preparation of written reports for any addition or deletion. Similarly, quality-related functions require time-consuming review of patient records. Finally, the P&T committee functions will be peripherally related to other affairs of the parent organization, e.g., the standard order set preparation by other segments of a hospital. This requires special attention in order to prevent the use of nonformulary products. These items will be discussed in greater detail in the next section. Finally, the chairperson should be skilled at guiding an efficient meeting (see Appendix 14–5). In respect of the time commitment for members, meetings should always start and end at the scheduled times.

P&T Committee Functions

Typically, P&T committee functions include determining what drugs are available, who can prescribe specific drugs, policies and procedures regarding drug use (including pharmacy policies and procedures, standard order sets, and clinical guidelines—see Chap. 9 for the latter), quality assurance activities (e.g., DUR/DUE/medication usage evaluation–see Chap. 16), ADRs/medication errors (see Chap. 17), dealing with product shortages, and education in drug use.[15,64] Many of those functions are quality assurance-type activities, because they are designed to improve the quality of drug therapy.[65] Because the functions may improve drug therapy quality, they may actually provide some legal protection for an institution, as long as the reason for decisions is not strictly based on financial considerations.[66] P&T committee functions can also include investigational drug studies; however, that is often delegated to the Institutional Review Board (IRB) that oversees all investigational activities in the hospital (see Chap. 18). In addition, some P&T committee functions may be delegated to subcommittees (e.g., quality assurance, antibiotic, and medication errors subcommittees);[67] however, this can be cumbersome and is often avoided, except in larger institutions.

According to the JCAHO, the medical staff, pharmacy, nursing, administration, and others are to cooperate with each other in carrying out the previously mentioned functions.[15] Although the medical staff normally takes overseeing drug therapy very seriously and expects to approve all activities of the P&T committee, it is common for the pharmacy department to do much of the preparation work for the committee. Although it is tempting to say the reason pharmacies are charged with all of the work is that they are the drug experts, which is often true, it is probably more realistic that the reason is that pharmacists are paid to do this as part of their salary, whereas, physicians often do not obtain any direct monetary compensation for this committee's preparatory work, although such compensation may be considered by an institution to encourage more physician participation.

FORMULARY MANAGEMENT

Drug Formulary

Wherever a drug formulary system is in place, there is usually a drug formulary published, as a hard copy book and/or in electronic format (e.g., website). In its simplest form, the drug formulary contains a list of drugs that are available under that formulary system, which reflects the clinical judgment of the medical staff.[68] This list will be arranged alphabetically and/or by therapeutic class (American Hospital Formulary Service [AHFS] classification usually), and usually contains information on the dosage forms, strengths, names (e.g., generic, trade, and chemical), and ingredients of combination products. Many drug formulary publications contain a great deal more material related to the drugs, including a summary of indications, side effects, dosing, use restrictions, and other clinical information.[69] An example of a web-based drug formulary may be seen at <<http://www.intmed.mcw.edu/drug.html>>.

A related term, the formulary system, can be thought of as a method for developing the list, and sometimes even as a philosophy.[70] In theory, a well-designed drug formulary can guide clinicians to prescribe the safest and most effective agents for treating a particular medical problem.[71] Some people argue that the formulary system itself does not work because it is not properly implemented and recommend replacing it with counterdetailing by pharmacists or computers at the time a prescription order is written.[72] However, whether or not that is true has yet to be determined. The most well-known article indicating that formularies may ultimately result in higher patient costs was written by Horn et al.[73] While this may be one of the best articles on the topic and the author has defended criticism of the article,[74] there are nevertheless various deficiencies in the study that make it uncertain whether it was truly the drug formulary or other factors that lead to increased costs.[75-78] Horn and associates[79] also published a similar study conducted in the ambulatory environment, which appears to have similar results and deficiencies. In the case of national drug formularies, there has been a positive[80] effect on prescribing habits shown in Canada. Further research is needed before a definite conclusion may be reached on the effectiveness of formulary management.[81] For now, a well-constructed formulary is still believed to improve patient care while decreasing costs.

The goal of the formulary system is to provide a decision-making process leading to the selection of medications necessary for the treatment of any disease states likely to be seen in that institution. These formulary medications should be the most efficacious and cost-effective agents with the fewest side effects.[15] Other factors should also be taken into consideration, such as the variety of dosage forms available for the medication, estimated use, convenience, dosing schedule, compliance, abuse potential, physician demand, ease of preparation, and storage requirements.[82] Typically, only two or, perhaps, three drugs from any drug class are added to the formulary. Some people would argue that only one agent is necessary from any class; however, some individuals will not respond and/or tolerate certain agents, so at least one secondary agent is usually desirable. Therapeutic redundancy must be minimized, however, by excluding superfluous or inferior preparations. This should improve the quality of prescribing and also lead to improved cost effectiveness, both by eliminating less cost-effective agents that do not improve patient care and by assisting patients to become well faster.

Whether an institution has a very strict formulary with a minimum number of items or a less-restricted formulary that excludes items that are significantly inferior is sometimes a matter of philosophy. The former will cut down the pharmacy department's inventory and often save money through avoidance of highly priced products, but may only be practical in closed health maintenance organizations (HMOs) where the same formulary is used in both the inpatient and ambulatory environments. In cases where physicians are free to prescribe whatever products they prefer in the ambulatory environment, they have been shown to have difficulty in remembering what products are contained on the formularies of third-party payers.[83] Therefore, the increased time necessary for pharmacists to contact physicians for order changes may lead to the disruption of patient care. As a result, a less restricted formulary may be more practical. As an example, a patient is admitted to the hospital on a nonformulary medication. While there would be other satisfactory medications in the same therapeutic category on the formulary, it may be best to simply allow use of the nonformulary product, rather than adding another complicating factor to the patient's hospital treatment by attempting to change therapy. Pharmacist and physician time would also be saved.

Even in cases where an institution has a strict and enforced drug formulary, it should be noted that there are occasions when it is necessary to prescribe a drug that is not on the drug formulary. This might be due to a patient with a rare illness, a patient who does not respond or has intolerable side effects to the formulary drugs, a patient stabilized on a nonformulary medication where it would be difficult or dangerous to change, a conflict between the institutional formulary and the patient's insurance company formulary,[84] or some other valid reason. A mechanism must be in place to promptly obtain the particular drug when it is shown to be necessary (the National Committee for Quality Assurance [NCQA] requires such a mechanism for HMOs,[85] as does JCAHO for other hospitals,[15] but it must try to prevent physicians ordering nonformulary drugs "because I said so!"). Some institutions require specific requests forms to be filled out (see example in Appendix 14–2), sometimes with a cosignature from the physician's department head, or at least require a consultation between a pharmacist and the physician before the drug is obtained. Also, patients may be charged more for the nonformulary medications. In some HMOs and insurance company plans, the physicians or pharmacies may be financially penalized for use or overuse of nonformulary medications.[86] Whatever mechanism is used, it is important to make it easy to obtain necessary nonformulary medications, but difficult to obtain unnecessary medications, otherwise the benefits of the formulary system may be negated.[48] Also, it is necessary to track which nonformulary drugs are being used regularly and why that is happening because it may be worthwhile to add some of those agents to the drug formulary.[87]

Some physicians feel that a drug formulary serves only to keep costs down, at the expense of good patient care.[88] These physicians must be reassured that there is evidence to support that a good formulary does keep expenses down[89] without negatively affecting care,[90] although in some cases the costs are merely transferred to other hospital expenses.[91,92] One study demonstrated that a well-controlled formulary or therapeutic substitution (substituting a different medication that is effective for the disease being treated for the one ordered by the physician) results in 10.7% lower drug costs per patient day, and both a well-controlled formulary and therapeutic substitution together could cause 13.4% lower drug costs per day.[93] Some physicians do not like formularies because they consider them to be a limitation to their authority.[88] It is necessary to keep in mind that when physicians become a part of a medical staff or sign up to participate in some managed care group they are given "privileges" not "rights." The privileges generally do include limitations on what medications they can prescribe, and when and how they can prescribe them. If a drug formulary system is run well there is little reason to feel there are inadequate drugs available; however, it does take some effort for the physician to learn to use the drugs available rather than the drugs they normally prescribe. An effort must be made to help physicians in this regard and to reassure them that every effort is being made to ensure the best drugs are available for the patients. Additionally, all changes to the drug formulary must be quickly and effectively communicated to the physicians to avoid confusion. A lack of such communication can negate some of the benefits of the formulary and lead to poor physician/pharmacist relations.[91] Also, it is important for physicians to be aware that it is the medical staff that makes these decisions, in order to avoid pharmacy being perceived as the "policeman" who is waiting to jump on the unsuspecting physician.[94] In the future, physicians will enter prescription orders into the computer, which can quickly inform the physician of formulary drug choices and guide therapeutic decisions. Currently, however, pharmacists may have to tactfully contact the physician about nonformulary drugs in order to make a formulary system work.

Similarly, pharmacies filling prescriptions for an HMO must be kept informed of the formulary status of drugs. One suggestion is to have a help desk to answer pharmacist questions and to provide information.[95]

Oftentimes, the drug formularies will have a number of other sections that may include information about the P&T committee and pharmacy department, policy and procedure information (e.g., how to obtain nonformulary drugs, how to request a drug be placed on the formulary), laboratory test information, dietary supplement charts, pharmacokinetics information, approved abbreviations, sodium content, nomograms, dosage equivalency charts, apothecary/ metric equivalents, drug-food interactions, skin test directions, cost data, antimicrobial therapy charts, and any other brief clinical information tables felt to be necessary. Use of linking in websites can make such information much more readily available and usable, since users can hop back and forth between these tables and the drug list. MCOs may need to include the procedure they use to limit choice of drugs by physicians, pharmacists, and patients.[96,97]

In institutional pharmacies, a hard-copy book has normally been published once a year. Often it was published in a pocket size format that could be carried in lab coats by physicians, pharmacists, and nurses. There may also have been a larger loose-leaf binder published that could be updated regularly throughout the year. Such a book is no longer justified.[98] It is now becoming more common for this reference to be available electronically. The electronic form can be made more widely available and can be kept continually up to date by making changes, as necessary, at one central location (an example can be found at <http://www.intmed.mcw.edu/drug/antibiotics.html>>). Also, the electronic formulary coupled with physician order entry may lead to the most efficient and effective way to encourage or enforce the use of formulary items,[99-101] although there is some evidence that electronic messages may be ignored by physicians.[102] Also, other information can be included to improve drug therapy. For example, this may include a requirement for a consultation by a specialist or pharmacokinetic monitoring. For outpatient drug formulary books this may include quantity level limits and requirements for prior authorizations.

The publication of a hard copy drug formulary can be a very time-consuming process. If at all possible it is best if the pharmacy can download the information about drug products carried in the institution from their computer system or a separate database management program to a word processing or other suitable program.[103] This list can then be manipulated to a more readable and understandable format without a big problem in transcription errors, and the other clinical information can easily be placed into the document (particularly if it is just being updated from a previous year). Almost any high-end word processing program or desktop publishing program can be used to do this, producing a printer ready copy that can be more inexpensively reproduced, in both time and dollars, than a typeset copy. Later, use of colored paper and an edge index can make use of the final product easier. Even with the availability of computer technology, the production of a drug formulary is a very time-intensive effort, requiring a few weeks to several months of work. Fortunately, technical and clerical personnel can do much of the work. One or more pharmacists, however, should carefully proof all material to ensure it is correct. Often this task will be divided up so that somebody involved with purchasing will check the drug list, an administrator will review the policies and procedures, and a clinician will update the clinical information. Even if an electronic drug formulary is produced, rather than the hard copy, this checking of the material is necessary on a regular basis.

Pharmacies can also use commercial vendors who will take their drug lists and prepare a professional looking formulary (hard copy and/or electronic). These commercial formularies can also include condensed monograph information (e.g., indications, dosing, side effects, and so forth), which can be of value to the prescriber.

Preferably, the pharmacy can use the information on their computer system to create a formulary that is constantly up to date. The information can be accessed as part of the prescription order software and/or it may be interfaced with web software. The latter makes it possible to embed other information easily, but may take further work by the pharmacist. In any case, this information should be available to the physician and other health care professionals wherever necessary—potentially even by wireless connection. As a side note, many institutions do not want information about their formularies readily available to individuals not directly associated with the institution (e.g., pharmaceutical manufacturers), but this should not be a problem using Virtual Private Network (VPN) software and firewalls to secure the data—allowing access to only qualified individuals.

PBMs, in conjunction with an organization, may publish a patient pocket formulary in addition to the formulary published for physicians and provided online for pharmacies. These patient pocket formularies may contain the top therapeutic categories and other information as well. Within these categories are the key drugs in that specific therapeutic class as well as the designated preferred products and the associated patient cost index. Patients are encouraged to take these pocket formularies on their physician visits as a means of ensuring formulary compliance when discussing therapeutic options. Physicians may also have the capability of prescribing online, whereby the physician enters the prescription in an electronic device and instant messaging occurs alerting the physician to potential drug interactions or formulary status of the prescription, allowing the physician to change the prescription immediately and eliminating the need for a pharmacist to call.[38,104]

In addition to pocket formularies, one method whereby the pharmacist educates the physician about formulary drugs is academic detailing. Through mailings, phone conversations, and personal visits the pharmacist discusses with the physician his or her prescribing patterns and, using evidence-based medical literature, supports the rational for preferred formulary product selection and clinically appropriate, cost-effective prescribing without compromising quality.[38]

Evaluating Drugs for Formulary Inclusion

The establishment and maintenance of a drug formulary requires that drugs or drug classes be objectively assessed based on scientific information (e.g., efficacy, adverse effects, cost, contribution to some critical treatment pathway,[105] and other appropriate items), not anecdotal physician experience.[70,106] Medication selection and procurement were specifically added to the JCAHO accreditation process under medication management in the 2004 standards.[107] There is an emphasis in the literature that P&T committee activities should be a result of evidence-based decisions.[108] Regarding the formulary process, JCAHO standard MM.2.10 calls for written criteria for addition or deletion of medications.[15] Any health care practitioner who is involved with ordering, dispensing, administering, and monitoring medications needs to be involved with the development of the criteria.[107] A process must also be in place to monitor patient responses to a new medication. All formulary medications are to be reviewed at least annually based on safety and efficacy information. This means that in addition to new formulary additions, all categories of the AHFS therapeutic classification should be reviewed at least yearly.

According to JCAHO, the criteria used for approving addition of a drug to a formulary need to minimally include the following:[107]

- Indications for use
- Effectiveness
- Risks (e.g., adverse effects, drug interactions, and potential for medication errors[109])
- Cost

A procedure for preparing the written evaluation of drug products is found in the next chapter, however, this section will go further into how the P&T committee should use that information and other items to do the actual evaluation.

When a P&T committee considers a drug for formulary adoption, it is quite common for the discussion to include statements such as "In my clinical experience...," which leads the discussion into rather subjective areas. It must be kept in mind that physicians are most likely to request drugs if they have met with the pharmaceutical company representative or received money from the drug company (e.g., speaking fees and travel funds to a meeting).[102,110] Valid formulary decisions should be based on objective evidence, particularly clinical studies,[111] rather than a few cases of "clinical experience" by a physician attending a meeting. Efforts must be made to guide discussions to scientific information when it wanders into vague subjective areas.[112] In some cases this is rather difficult because many new drugs have limited published information when they are first commercially available. The information that is available is generally placebo-controlled studies that are funded by the manufacturer. In situations such as this, the decision on formulary addition may need to be postponed until adequate information is available. Sometimes the decision cannot wait, as is the case with many managed care companies, who need to review a drug before a patient picks up the drug from the pharmacy so that appropriate coverage determination can be made, or in hospitals in response to the new JCAHO accreditation standards.[107] Then the P&T committee's decision-making process needs to be structured in a manner that is very objective and data driven, and takes into account the lack of data. In these cases, a committee may make a decision and then place the product on a 6-month follow-up for an additional review, after which time additional prescribing and patient use data or clinical trial data may be available.

While there is a temptation to think that anything new is better, which is an attitude that is certainly pushed by drug company representatives with new products to sell, it cannot be assumed and must be proven. In some cases, experts have determined that the new products pose no significant advantages to the patients to justify the costs.[113–115] The rate at which the new chemical entities are approved by the FDA has been declining from what it has been in the past,[116] although there was a slight increase in 2003.[117] Often, manufacturers are trying to get products approved and on the market that may be in a different strength or dosage form, single isomer of a product, a new indication for a product, or even an extended release version of a product (sometimes several different extended release versions).[118] All of the products potentially need to be given consideration by a P&T committee. However, with a lack of published trials and, in many cases, objective and reliable data, the P&T committee faces the challenge of creating a sound drug formulary that represents the needs of an organization or patient population in an objective manner that encompasses current clinical practice, established guidelines of patient care, and a thorough risk-benefit analysis of the drug product.[23] Some places have even tried computerized methods to make more objective decisions;[119,120] however, there does not seem to be any data demonstrating the superiority of such a method. Similarly, there are processes called System of Objectified Judgment Analysis (SOJA), which uses a computer program to score different aspects of drugs in the same class to determine the best product,[121,122] and multi-attribute utility technology.[123]

Other Aspects of Formulary Evaluation

Also, it is necessary to determine whether people involved in the discussion and decision about a drug's formulary status have some conflict of interest (i.e., would receive some direct or indirect compensation from having a drug available, e.g., stock in a company, honoraria for speaking, consulting fees, and gifts or grants from a company[124,125]) and avoid that biasing factor. Perhaps a conflict of interest policy, requiring regular disclosure of any possible conflicts, needs to be established.[23,126,127] An example form to gather information about conflicts of interest is found in Appendix 14–6. In certain cases, regular voting P&T committee members may have to abstain from the vote if they disclose a possible conflict of interest or the committee may vote to determine whether the conflict is considered to be significant enough to prevent voting by the individual in question.

Patent expiration is a common question that should be considered for all products or drug classes undergoing formulary review, since the introduction of generic products after that date may lead to decreasing prices. Patent expiration information can be found at <<www.fda.gov/cder/ob/default.htm>>.

The JCAHO Medication Management Standards for 2004 are focused on medication safety. The definition of a medication goes beyond prescription products and the FDA classification as drugs. Also considered medications in the 2004 standards are herbal/alternative therapies, vitamins, nutraceuticals, OTC products, vaccines, diagnostic and contrast agents, radioactive agents, respiratory treatments, parenteral nutrition, blood derivatives, intravenous (IV) solutions, anesthetic gases, sample medications, and anything else deemed by the FDA to be a drug.[107] The pharmacist is required to review the appropriateness of all medication orders before a medication is dispensed.[15,107,128]

While it is now necessary to evaluate herbal or other alternative medicine products,[129-131] some institutions may instead handle them as nonformulary requests or investigational drugs.[132] Although alternative and herbal medications seem somewhat unusual to the P&T committee, they can still be treated much the same way as any drug product, perhaps with additional evaluation of the purity and composition of the products (see Dietary Supplement Medical Literature section of Chap. 7 for additional details regarding how to evaluate for these products).[133] Some pharmacies also have other policies and procedures,[134] perhaps some that are highly restrictive,[135] including requiring pharmacists to verify labeled product ingredients.[136]

In addition to considering the cost of drug products in the institution, it is necessary to consider the cost to the patient, once he or she returns home. If a product is so expensive that an uninsured or underinsured patient cannot afford it in the ambulatory environment, it may not be good to place the patient on that drug in the hospital. However, in some cases pharmaceutical companies may offer assistance to this type of patient. More information about such assistance programs can be found in Appendix 14–7.

Open versus Closed Formularies

When setting up a drug formulary there are several things to consider. First is whether there will be an open or closed formulary.[137] The open (or voluntary) formulary essentially means any drug on the market is available, and some would argue that the term open formulary is really an oxymoron.[112] One exception to this definition is that the NCQA states that an open formulary for a MCO can be a list of recommended drugs, as long as there are no requirements concerning its use.[138] A closed (or restricted) formulary means that only a limited number of agents are available. This is certainly preferable, because such agents should be chosen by objective evidence in the scientific literature that supports the superiority of the agents over other similar drugs and because closed formularies can result in cost savings.[139] Closed formularies are becoming much more common in HMOs.[140,141] In some instances of closed formularies, patients may have access to these nonformulary or nonpreferred drug products by paying a substantially higher co-payment, by paying the difference between the formulary and nonformulary products in addition to the co-payment, or by paying for the nonformulary drug in its entirety unless there is a prior authorization to allow this drug.[37]

Issues may arise with a closed or restricted formulary in that it may be too restrictive for those patients who cannot afford the drug, even though the drug is still available in a closed formulary. A growing health policy concern is the ability to successfully appeal for coverage of a nonformulary product. Newer breakthrough medications and biotechnology products are making their way onto the market. Although clinically valuable, they are very expensive. In addition, PBMs have managed or preferred formularies. In a managed or preferred formulary, interventions may be used to encourage physicians to use the preferred products. Some of these interventions for physicians include academic detailing, prior authorizations, and coverage rules. For pharmacies this may mean a higher dispensing fee for formulary compliance. For the patient this may mean higher co-payments if the formulary or preferred product is not used.

Unlike hospitals, PBMs along with their clients (i.e., health plans) place their formulary and nonformulary medications into tiers with an associated co-payment with each tier. This tier co-payment structure came about in response to the rising cost of prescription drugs. The first tier is generally reserved for generic drug products. This tier usually has the lowest co-payment (e.g., $10.00). The second tier is usually reserved for those name brand drugs that are formulary (e.g., $15.00). This tier has a higher co-payment than the first tier due to the added cost of the brand-name drug. The third tier is reserved for those drug products that are nonformulary brand names. This co-payment is significantly higher than the other two tiers (e.g., $30). However, some third-tier co-payments may be calculated as a proportion of the drug cost, even as much as one-third as a form of co-insurance, or require paying for the drug in its entirety. The reason for the co-payment structure is to encourage the patient to use the most clinically appropriate, cost-effective drug without compromising quality care.[37]

The closed formulary can also be broken down into what is referred to as positive or negative formularies. This is the method by which the formulary is developed. A positive formulary effectively starts with a blank sheet of paper and specifically adds agents. While this is probably the best method to limit the number of drugs available, it is often not very popular when first implementing the formulary because every agent must be considered. That means the physicians must even make specific decisions on whether they should add such things as acetaminophen and amoxicillin to the formulary. Therefore, in hospitals just establishing a formulary, it is often more popular and easier to use a negative formulary system. This essentially starts with the current hospital drug stock, with each drug class being evaluated to eliminate agents that are not necessary.[142] The first steps in this process may be as simple as eliminating multiple salts/esters of the same drug. Then classes of drugs with multiple similar products could be addressed (e.g., analgesics, antacids, laxatives, vitamins, and topical steroids). While in some ways this process is easier, it is also likely to result in a much bigger formulary, since the decision will be made as to what drugs are definitely not needed, rather than which drugs the institution definitely needs. However, the specific institution's situation will need to be assessed before the method of determining the formulary items can be decided on. Overall, the goal is to provide the optimal agents; it is easy to end up with too many duplicative agents; however, having a greater number of agents to choose from can lead to better patient care in some areas.[143,144]

Therapeutic Interchange

The AMA[12,137] defines therapeutic interchange as "authorized exchange of therapeutic alternatives in accordance with previously established and approved written guidelines or protocols within a formulary system." An example would be the use of cefazolin in specific doses whenever any other first-generation injectable cephalosporin is ordered. Therapeutic interchange is used in nearly 90% of U.S. hospitals[145] for reasons that include cost savings,[146,147] improved patient outcomes, decreased adverse effects, decreased inventory, fewer medication errors,[148] or other benefits. Therapeutic interchange has been shown to decrease costs without adversely affecting patient outcomes.[45,149] There is even reason to believe that when therapeutic interchange is properly performed, and not entirely based on financial considerations, it may produce lower legal liability on an institution,[66] although there are no published legal cases regarding therapeutic interchange to demonstrate either increased or decreased legal liability.[150] The concept of therapeutic interchange through collaborative interactions with interdisciplinary teams to develop protocols and comprehensive therapeutic assessments has been described. Several medication classes may be the target of therapeutic interchange and an aggressive IV to PO conversion may be part of this process.[151] The most common classes of drugs for therapeutic interchange are, in order: H_2 antagonists, proton pump inhibitors, antacids, quinolones, potassium supplements, cephalosporins, and hydroxymethylglutaryl-coenzyme A reductase inhibitors.[145] Some drugs classes, such as low-molecular weight heparins, that at first glance may appear to be possible places for therapeutic interchange to take place, may be found to be unacceptable after a closer inspection.[152]

Therapeutic interchange is considered acceptable to the AMA, unlike therapeutic substitution, which they define as the "act of dispensing a therapeutic alternative for the drug product prescribed without prior authorization of the prescriber" (note: prior authorization may be a blanket authorization, not a specific authorization for each case[153]).[154] Therapeutic interchange has also been found to be acceptable by other organizations, including the American College of Clinical Pharmacy (ACCP), American College of Physicians (ACP) (they require immediate prior consent by the physician),[155] ASHP, American Pharmacists Association (APhA), American Association of Colleges of Pharmacy (ACCP), AMCP,[156] and the American Society of Consultant Pharmacists (ASCP).[157,158] The American College of Clinical Pharmacy spells out the concept of therapeutic interchange in great detail and suggests that it not only be conducted under the auspices of a P&T-type committee, but also that it specifically include DUE, a set method for informing the physicians and other staff that interchange is taking place (should be well planned and thorough[159]), and a mechanism under which the therapeutic interchange policies may be overridden in specific cases. Evaluations for therapeutic interchange should also consider medical, legal, and financial evaluations.[152] Other practical aspects, such as communication forms, policies and procedures, medical staff bylaw changes, and other items may need to be addressed by the institution.[160] Electronic means to provide authorization for interchange may be seen more in the future.[161] Outside of an institution (e.g., ambulatory environment), therapeutic interchange may not be as easy to implement due to practical procedure methods and because patients are not as closely monitored; however, it may still be possible.[162,163] In the ambulatory situation, the AMA states that therapeutic interchange recommendations must be approved by the majority of physicians affected and must otherwise follow similar standards to that described for inpatient settings.[137]

The consideration of certain therapeutic agents for interchange may result in strong differences of opinion among medical staff members regarding their appropriate use. The process for evaluating any product, especially those having deeply held physician opinions, should be followed, along with efforts being made by committee members to actively approach appropriate influential individuals before a crisis occurs. Through anticipatory, structured negotiation, it is more likely that rational and balanced decisions will be made. Also, it is necessary to take into consideration whether a short-term interchange of products, while the patient is in a hospital, may cause confusion or other difficulties when the patient returns to the outpatient environment and may be restarted on the original agent.[164] Working with the physicians to resolve this issue is a necessity for long-term care of patients.

Generic substitution is also considered by the P&T committee in some cases, but many pharmacies consider generic substitution to be one of their responsibilities and do not take such decisions to the P&T committee for approval. The one exception may be drugs with narrow therapeutic indexes (e.g., anticonvulsants), where a P&T committee may determine a list of products where generic substitution is not allowed,[165] although the FDA insists that such precautions are unnecessary.[166] In relation to generic substitution, it must be mentioned that pharmacies must determine quality suppliers. The ASHP has guidelines for this function.[167] Also, states may have a variety of laws governing generic substitution. They may also publish so-called positive and negative formularies, which differ in definition from those terms used elsewhere in this chapter in that they are lists of drugs that may or may not be substituted for one another, respectively.[150]

In some instances, physicians may prefer that no generic substitution or therapeutic substitution occur on a written order or prescription by indicating "Dispense as Written" on that document. This can occur in the inpatient setting as well as the outpatient setting. Depending on the state, dispense as written is synonymous with the following: no substitution, do not substitute, medically necessary, brand necessary/medically necessary, no drug product selection, brand medically necessary, substitution prohibited without permission of physician or patient, or no substitution/brand necessary.

In most states, the law provides that pharmacists can use a generic version of any medication on a prescription or medication order if the physician has not precluded that action by indicating dispense as written. In the outpatient setting, in general, if a patient wants a generic medication, they should be sure that their pharmacist knows of their desire.

In some benefit plans, if the physician requests a brand name medication when a generic equivalent is available, the patient member may be responsible to pay the difference in cost in addition to the generic co-payment. In some instances, members may not be required to pay this cost difference, if their physician documents that the brand name medication is necessary.

Nonformulary Usage

Many institutions track the drug use patterns of prescribers, as was mentioned previously in describing the tracking of nonformulary drug products. Annually, a listing of nonformulary products and expenses should be made available to the P&T committee. It is helpful if the pharmacy director can report the total cost of nonformulary items as a percent of the total budget, particularly since the cost can exceed the cost of carrying the nonformulary product on the formulary.[168] Ideally, a report of the number involved and costs of nonformulary orders will be made available to each prescriber. This process is helpful in improving the appropriate use of medications and has also been linked to the prescriber credentialing process.[169]

Unlabeled Uses

While some third-party payers may attempt to limit the use of drugs to only FDA-approved label indications, this may unnecessarily restrict use of products for indications that may have significant literature support. This should not be supported.[170] However, as will be discussed in more detail in the next chapter, it is sometimes necessary for institutions to specifically restrict drugs to specific uses when they may be used inappropriately. While at first glance this seems to be the same, in reality, such restrictions may be totally unrelated to approved labeling. In this situation, it may be found that products are permitted to be used for unlabeled indications where there is adequate literature support and, conversely, may not be permitted to be used, at least without special approval within the institution, for FDA-labeled indications when there may be more appropriate drugs available.

New Product Introductions

When new drug products are added to the formulary, it is best to prepare physicians, nurses, and others.[102] To begin with, it is necessary to inform affected individuals that the drug will be available as of a specific date. That could be immediately or at some time in the near future. There are various reasons for a delay. For example, a drug may have been approved by both the FDA and the P&T committee, but the company may not have yet made it commercially available because they have not yet produced a sufficient supply or they are not yet ready to start their marketing efforts. In some cases it is necessary for specific equipment to be obtained and installed. Such was the case a number of years ago when Fluosol®-DA was made available for a limited period of time. This parenteral product required very specialized preparation method involving a warm water bath and percolating a mixture of gases through an IV bag under sterile conditions. Few, if any, pharmacies had the necessary equipment at the time of introduction and it would have taken some time to get the equipment, set it up, and train pharmacists and technicians in its use, requiring a delay in making the product available in an institution. Most commonly, the reason for the delay is likely to be the time it takes to inform all individuals likely to be involved in the prescribing, preparing, and administering of the drug that the drug will be available and to educate them in the proper use, including applicable policies and procedures. These education efforts may be provided through newsletters, websites, portals, e-mail, memos, educational programs, RSS (Really Simple Syndication) aggregators, or other methods. The method chosen should generally be a standard method used within the institution and should be appropriate for the specific medication product introduction. In cases where a product is particularly complicated, dangerous, or prone to misuse, several methods of instruction, perhaps along with prescribing restrictions, should probably be employed. Further information about newsletters and websites is found in the Chap. 11.

POLICIES AND PROCEDURES

Occasionally, policies and procedures must be developed to support the rational use of medications. While the pharmacy department may decide they need to have their own policies and procedures for internal functions that is not the focus of this discussion.[171] Instead, policies and procedures for the use of medications in an institution, clinic, and so forth will be discussed, since that is often provided through a P&T committee.

The JCAHO has specifically stated that they expect policies and procedures for the following types of orders:[107]

- As needed (prn) medications
- Standing order medications
- Hold medications
- Automatic stop
- Resume medications
- Dosage adjustment
- Dosage taper
- Compounded or admixed drugs
- Medication-related devices
- Investigational medications
- Herbal/natural medications
- Discharge medications
- Self-administered medications

Some examples of policies and procedures can be found on the Internet at <http://www.hosp.uky.edu/pharmacy/departpolicy/departmentalpolicies.html>> and <<http://www.utmb.edu/rxhome/Policies_Frames.htm>>.

To begin this discussion, the definitions for policies and procedures should be considered.[172] A policy is a broad general statement that describes the goals and purposes of the document. The procedures are specific actions to be taken. In some ways, policies and procedures may resemble a cookbook-type approach, in that a set of steps to be accomplished are described in order. Taken together, these policies and procedures may be a logical, step-by-step explanation of why and where a product may be used, how to use it, and who is to follow the policy (i.e., there may be different portions of the document addressed to pharmacists, technicians, nurses, and physicians),[173] along with a brief introductory statement describing why the process is necessary.

Before developing a specific policy and procedure, the first step should be deciding whether it is necessary at all. In other words, is there a good reason for the existence of that particular policy and procedure and is it likely to be used? This can be looked at as a risk-benefit decision. For example, is there sufficient risk that a particular medication will be used incorrectly (e.g., prepared wrong, administered wrong, and used for an inappropriate indication) to make it worthwhile to develop a policy and procedure? Generally, the answer will be "no," but in a certain number of cases, policies and procedures may be necessary. Examples of where a policy and procedure may be necessary include thrombolytic agents (where the drug can cause serious or fatal effects if used improperly), antibiotics (where it is found that expensive, broad-spectrum antibiotics are being used where amoxicillin should suffice), injectable drugs (where specific individuals who will administer the medication and the process will be defined),[174] and even for drugs where reimbursement may be a problem.

Once a decision is reached to develop the policy and procedure, a logical and orderly course should be followed. It is undesirable to wait until after problems occur before deciding that policies and procedures are necessary. This process should follow the drug formulary process, where a mechanism is set up to help determine that a policy and procedure is necessary. In many cases, a policy and procedure for use of drugs likely to be misused may be developed in conjunction with its consideration for addition to the drug formulary.

As in any process, it is first necessary to decide who will be coordinating the effort and the likely endpoint. That person, or designee, will then need to investigate various sources for background material necessary to develop the policy and procedure. This might include doing a literature search, talking to experts in the field, talking to other institutions that have already developed policies on the same topic, reviewing published professional (e.g., <<http://www.ashp.org/bestpractices/index.cfm>>) or clinical guidelines (e.g., <<http://www.guideline.gov>>), and checking out the institution's requirements for developing policies and procedures. If the policy and procedure is for a hospital group, other institutions in the group must also be involved. In particular, it is necessary for the person developing the policy and procedure to have good communications with those to be affected. After all, if the final product is looked at as being more trouble than it is worth, it is not likely to be followed.

Where the policy and procedure fits in relation to other institutional policies and procedures will also have to be evaluated. Finally, a document should be written, reviewed, and revised, using many of the skills outlined in the Chap. 11.

As part of the process of preparing the policy, it is important to be clear as to when it is applicable and where there may be exceptions. For example, institutions have policies for the automatic stop of specific medications (e.g., stopping an antibiotic after 7 days). There needs to be careful consideration of only applying that policy in cases where it will be likely to improve drug therapy. There also needs to be a mechanism to make sure that such an automatic stop, which may be programmed into the computer system, may not cause harm to particular patients[175] (e.g., patients with osteomyelitis receiving antibiotics for an extended period of time).

Once the policy and procedure is finished, it will need to be approved by the same mechanism that drug formulary changes go through (i.e., P&T committee, medical executive committee, and so forth). The approval and/or effective date for the policy and procedure should be recorded on the document itself to ensure it is not confused with earlier or later documents. A plan for implementing the policy and procedure will need to be developed. Forms may need to be prepared and distributed. Copies of the policy and procedure will have to be distributed to those affected (preferably on the computer network), and educational programs will need to be planned and given. At that point, the policy and procedure can be implemented, perhaps in conjunction with the first appearance of a particular agent on the drug formulary. That is not the end of the process, however. At some point, the policy and procedure should be evaluated to determine if it is being properly followed and having the desired effect as a part of a quality assurance plan. A method to enforce compliance with the policies and procedures is required and it is necessary for legal reasons to demonstrate that this enforcement method is used.[173] Also, the policy and procedure will need to be reviewed, revised (if necessary), and reapproved on a regular basis (probably once a year). As part of that process, the actual need for the policy and procedure should be reconsidered. The policy and procedure should be eliminated if no longer needed. One way to determine whether the policy and procedures are consulted is if they are on a web server, where the number of times the specific page is opened is recorded. Superseded copies (i.e., previous versions) of the policies and procedures should be kept on file for background and for legal purposes.

It is also necessary to have policies and procedures for the operation of the P&T committee itself (see Appendix 14–1 for policies and procedures for setting up a P&T committee). Some examples of other policies and procedures that may need to be developed include how new drugs are requested for addition to the formulary, how nonformulary drugs can be used, what procedure is used to evaluate new drugs,[107] the composition of the committee, and other committee functions (e.g., conflict of interest). These have been discussed elsewhere in the chapter and will not be dealt with further at this point.

Clinical Guidelines

P&T committees may be involved with the development, alteration (to fit local circumstances), and/or approval of evidence-based clinical guidelines. The reader is directed to Chap. 9 to obtain further information.

Standard Order Set Development

Many physicians, both in their offices and in institutions (e.g., hospital and nursing home), make use of something called standard orders. This usually consists of some sort of form, preprinted hardcopy, or electronic checklist, which lists various orders that are often written for specific patients under certain circumstances. This can include medications, laboratory tests, x-rays, other diagnostic tests, diet restrictions, preoperative preparation, and many other things. For example, there may be a specific set of orders for all patients a physician admits to the hospital in general or for a specific diagnosis, or a set of orders for a patient who is scheduled to undergo a specific procedure, such as an operation. Standing orders are commonly used for some medications, such as total parenteral nutrition solutions and oncology agents, where the order can be complex and confusing, perhaps resulting in potential medication errors. The physicians using the standing orders can simply indicate which of the items they wish their patients to receive and provide various necessary details, such as dose or duration. The use of standing orders can be a very good practice, since they act much like checklists do for pilots or astronauts—saving time and ensuring that important items are not inadvertently missed or misused. This can be particularly important in the use of drugs that can be dangerous or ineffective if not properly used, such as chemotherapeutic regimens in oncology patients. However, the disadvantage is that the standing orders do take time to establish and maintain, and may not keep up with actual practice standards, therefore, contributing to the perpetuation of outmoded or inappropriate practices. While many P&T committees do not address standing orders directly, leaving them to the individuals or groups that use them, it is something that still needs to be considered for several reasons.

First, P&T committees are responsible for overseeing all things related to medication use in an institution. Second, the standing orders may contain medications that may be removed from the formulary for various reasons. This requires the P&T committee to make a special effort to communicate with those individuals or groups with standing orders that contain drugs that may be eliminated from the formulary. This communication should begin prior to recommendation for removal of a product from the formulary, in order to find out the reason for the use of the product and the acceptability of available substitutes. By maintaining copies of standing orders, the pharmacy department can help facilitate this process. Also, once it has been decided that a particular product on standing orders is to be removed from the formulary, that decision must be quickly communicated to the affected individuals and groups, with enough time allocated before the removal becoming effective for the standing orders to be updated and the new ones be put into use. This process may be delayed by the frequency of meetings of the groups affected, the time it takes to have new standing order sheets either printed or put on the computer system, and the necessity to adequately train personnel in the use of the replacement products. In all likelihood, it may take several months after a decision by the P&T committee before the changes can be put into affect. Finally, P&T committees may find that products on standing orders may be used in ways that are not supported by the medical literature and/or hospital policy, which means that they need to make sure the physicians or groups that use those orders make necessary changes.

Optimally, individuals or groups using standard orders should be required to review and reapprove their use on a regular basis (probably at least once a year). It may also be necessary to have standing orders go through an institutional standing orders committee. In any case, the JCAHO requires a specific policy and procedure for how institutions handle standing orders.[107] Any changes should be reported to both the affected groups (e.g., nursing units, pharmacy, and information technology) and to the P&T committee in cases where the standing orders include drugs. All printed sets of the standing orders must include their revision date, to make sure that that old copies are not inadvertently used. Old copies of the orders must be maintained for medicolegal purposes, with the length of time for keeping such records to be determined by the institution's legal counsel.

Credentialing and Privileges

Health care institutions are required by various groups to verify that physicians and other health care professionals have the credentials to practice.[176] This can include degrees, licenses, training, and experience. Based on the credentials, professionals may be given privileges to practice within that institution and perform certain activities.[177] Please note that this term is privilege, not right. For example, while all physicians may have the same license, only those trained in surgery may be allowed to do more than very minor surgical procedures (e.g., suturing lacerations and removing minor skin growths). There may be even more specific rules, such as those preventing a chest surgeon from performing neurosurgery. These privileges can also extend to drugs. For example, it may be decided within the P&T committee that only oncologists have privileges to prescribe most antineoplastic agents. This type of policy and procedure is the basis for some restrictions that may be placed when a drug is considered for formulary addition. In addition to restrictions placed within an institution, restrictions may be enforced from outside the institution. For example, the use of dofetilide (Tikosyn®) requires the credentialing of both the prescriber and hospital by the company, see <<http://www.tikosyn.com/>> for details.

It also must be mentioned that policies and procedures may be in place within an institution to require pharmacists to perform certain operations, whether that is the preparation of particular agents or performing specific clinical functions (e.g., pharmacokinetics and warfarin dosing).[176] Institutions may have a method by which pharmacists are credentialed to perform such services.

Quality Improvement within the P&T Committee—Internal Audit

A variety of topics regarding the quality of medication use are normally part of the activities of a P&T committee. Many of these activities are covered in Chap. 16, however, the items described in the following sections may be considered to be specific to the P&T committee.

MEDICATION QUALITY ASSURANCE

In addition to determining which medications are available and providing direction in their use, it is necessary that the quality of use is regularly measured in whatever areas are felt to be necessary, including medication use evaluation (MUE), drug use evaluation (DUE), and other similar activities. The P&T committee will likely be involved in this, although coordination of such efforts, including preparing an annual plan of quality assurance activities, may be through other groups, such as a quality assurance committee. The initial plan may be developed by pharmacists but multidisciplinary feedback is essential before the focused areas of evaluation are finalized. Ideally, all practice areas of the medical staff are given opportunity for input into these focused evaluations. The project list should be continually reviewed and allow for special urgent projects when necessary. If a project is not completed during the year, it may be reconsidered for the next year. DUE criteria should be selected that can be used for continuous improvements that meet JCAHO accreditation requirements. DUE activities may be used to identify ADRs, contain cost, and expand clinical pharmacy activities.[178] Even if the P&T committee does not direct quality assurance efforts, they must be kept informed of the information gathered and the medication-related quality improvement efforts that are being instituted. This way the P&T committee can be supportive of such efforts directly (e.g., making changes to the drug formulary or policies and procedures to improve medication use) or less directly (e.g., providing statements supporting such activities). Quality assurance is a large topic and further information is available in Chap. 16.

ADVERSE DRUG REACTIONS

The P&T committee has a responsibility to review adverse reaction data in an institution to identify trends. One tool they can employ is to monitor the use of medications, sometimes referred to as tracer drugs, to treat the symptoms and side effects of other medications.[179] For example, the monitoring of epinephrine, flumazenil, phytonadione, or protamine to try to detect allergic responses, benzodiazepine overdoses, warfarin overdoses, or heparin overdoses, respectively. The topic of ADRs is covered more in the Chap. 17.

MEDICATION ERROR INCIDENTS

Data collected regarding medication errors may be reported to the P&T committee and, probably, for investigational drugs, to the IRB. A systematic method to collect data about medication errors must be set up within an institution, perhaps using internal incident report forms employed by the institution to track all unusual occurrences regarding patients. All incidents are reviewed by severity (none, minimal, moderate, major, death) and by process (prescribing, transcription, dispensing, administration, other). A multidisciplinary review of all incidents should take place and trends in the specific quality indicators should be shared with the entire professional staff. High-alert medications (narcotics, patient-controlled analgesia, insulin, anticoagulants, electrolytes, neuromuscular blockers, thrombolytics, and chemotherapy) should be benchmarked and followed to identify trends to improve the medication management system and ultimately enhance patient safety.

Another monitoring consideration is related to errors with medical devices and may also be monitored by these committees. A recent study completed in a 520-bed tertiary teaching institution demonstrated that more intensive surveillance methods yielded higher rates of medical device problems as compared to voluntary reporting.[180]

The topic of medication errors is covered in more detail in Chap. 17.

ILLEGIBLE HANDWRITING, TRANSCRIPTION, AND ABBREVIATIONS

It is important to work with the medical staff and all other health professionals regarding illegible handwriting and transcription errors. Typically, a task force assigned by the P&T committee is given the charge of evaluating and trending illegible handwriting, followed by developing process improvement measures. A report can be made to the P&T on an ongoing or quarterly basis. An education process must be in place for those individuals who consistently demonstrate poor handwriting. Hands-on reminders have been helpful or, in some extreme cases, handwriting school is recommended. In addition, institutions have adapted the 2004 JCAHO unapproved abbreviation list.[15] Unacceptable abbreviations may have an intended meaning but often are potentially misinterpreted and can lead to serious complications. In many institutions, the nurse or pharmacist must clarify the order with the prescriber when an unapproved abbreviation is written. In some cases, the only effective prevention of this problem has been when the medical staff has determined, probably through the P&T committee, that orders contained unapproved abbreviations are invalid and must be rewritten by the physician.[181] The addition to the formulary of look-alike, sound-alike medications is discouraged.[182–185] Increasingly, institutions are implementing computerized physician order entry (CPOE), which eliminates the problem of illegible handwriting and decimal point errors, thus reducing medication errors,[186] although implementation costs are considerable and some institutions may currently feel that it is not yet worth the effort and expense.[187]

TIMELINESS

The time for medication orders to be filled and sent to the floor may be tracked by the P&T committee. One area of importance is the response time sequence for a stat (immediate) order. The time should be evaluated from the time the order was written, to when the order was filled, to when the patient receives the medication. There are many obstacles in the order process and getting the medication to the patient. Each institution should have a standard expectation of the turnaround time for stat orders and a policy that will assure that the medication is dispensed and administered promptly. Benchmarking should be done to make sure the policy is followed.

Although not quite as imperative, the timeliness of ordinary order fulfillment must also be evaluated for appropriateness.

COUNTERFEIT DRUG PRODUCTS

Counterfeit drugs can be considered to be those that do not contain the ingredients claimed on the labeling, perhaps having no active ingredients, incorrect dose, or even other drugs.[188] Counterfeit drugs appear to be an increasing problem, although the actual incidence is unknown.[189] The ASHP announced in February 2004 that it will partner with the FDA in a program to keep pharmacists informed about entrance of counterfeit drug products into the nation's drug supply. The ASHP plans to provide rapid alerts to hospital pharmacy departments about counterfeit drug incidents.[190] Also, there are methods being developed or implemented that will help to ensure the "pedigree" of products, particularly those imported from foreign countries, to help avoid counterfeit products. This may include the use of radio frequency identification (RFID) tags to help track products.[191]

The FDA website may be consulted at <<http://www.fda.gov/medwatch/SAFETY/2004/safety04.htm>> for a list of counterfeit products that are updated weekly. Because of the potential problems associated with counterfeit drug products, the P&T committee must be kept informed of any situations that affect the institution, as should the medical staff as a whole.[189] This topic also may be handled with medication errors, since it leads to such errors.

SAFETY ALERT

A variety of other safety-related items are also important to P&T committees, including recalls, black box warnings, and product shortages, which will be covered in the following subsections. The items covered in this section can also be considered related to ADRs and medication errors, since some portions fit under those categories.

Recalls

The pharmacy department constantly reviews medication products recalled by the manufacturer or the FDA due to a safety issue.[192] This information is provided to the pharmacy by the wholesaler and the manufacturer. If a product lot number involved in the recall is found in the pharmacy inventory, that product should be removed from the inventory immediately and recalled from other areas of the institution that may stock it.[107] In the outpatient environment, a recall from consumers may be necessary. A report of medications that have been pulled from the pharmacy inventory should be made available to the P&T committee and the committee may need to decide whether or not to identify patients who may have been affected by the safety issue. Further actions would be based on these findings. The P&T committee chair should be contacted when a patient has significant consequences in relation to a product recall. When a product recall requires the removal of a product treating a disease with limited alternative treatments from the pharmacy inventory, therapeutic alternatives must be made known to the prescribers.[10]

Black Box Warnings

The safety of medications is under constant evaluation and the safety of new agents cannot be known until the product has been on the market for a period of time.[193] Some newly reported serious adverse effects result in black box warnings being inserted in the product labeling, due to requirements of the FDA, which necessitates action up to the withdrawal of the medication from the market. The reason for this name is that the warning is set off from the rest of the information in the package insert by a thick black box that is drawn around it. It is the responsibility of the P&T committee to review safety data for every medication on the formulary. Many P&T committees have a standing agenda item to review all new black box warnings or newly released FDA safety alerts for medications. The P&T committee needs to review the safety data and make any formulary, policy and procedure, and/or other changes as required. The black box safety data of formulary products need to be disseminated to the medical staff, including any special restrictions or actions taken on a specific product.

PRODUCT SHORTAGES

Product shortages should be continuously monitored by the pharmacy department in an organized fashion; this is a JCAHO requirement.[107,192] There is a trend of more frequent medication shortages in recent years.[194] In some cases, evaluation of information may show that acceptable alternative products or treatments may be interchanged for products affected by a shortage. The appropriate health care professionals (e.g., physicians, drug information service, pharmacy director, and buyer) need to be immediately notified of product shortages that may have an affect on therapeutic outcomes, along with plans or recommendations on how to address the situation.[195] In some instances the chief of the medical staff and even the ethics committee may need to be consulted when policies need to be put into place to ration drug supplies. The shortage of intravenous immunoglobulin (IVIG) in the 1990s necessitated a complete medical staff and pharmacy department agreement for appropriate patient selection for treatment.[196] This shortage required product rationing with the available supply. Unfortunately no therapeutic alternatives were available for the IVIG shortage. Methods of alerting medical staff of shortages include personal communication, the use of posters or message boards in key areas of the hospital (e.g., medical staff lounge, dictation area, parking garage, and high traffic areas), e-mail, computer notification during physician order entry, and the use of newsletters or faxes. A guideline is available from the ASHP to aid in determining how to handle a variety of types of shortages.[192]

In today's health care environment, it is essential to keep medication shortages as a standard agenda item for each P&T meeting. Products with limited availability and products that are not available need to be evaluated constantly. Formulary alternatives for these product shortages then need to be communicated to the medical staff.

Communication within an Organization

INVESTIGATIONAL REVIEW BOARD ACTIONS

While P&T committees are generally responsible for overseeing all aspects of medication use in a hospital, they often turn the major responsibility for overseeing investigational drug use over to an IRB. The IRB should provide a regular overview of its actions to the P&T committee for review, but oftentimes this is all that is done. Further information about IRBs can be found in Chap. 18.

COST, BUDGET, AND FORECASTING

How does the P&T committee actively balance its quality promoting activities as well as the economic requirements of its parent organization? For an individual hospital, this is probably an easier task as long as the economic pressures on the hospital's margin are manageable. As previously mentioned, a closed formulary can result in lowered costs within an institution.[139] However, the P&T committee decisions will be more difficult for the PBM function of a health insurance company or HMO. In the latter situation, the pressures of cost containment, the contents of an insurance plan's Certificate of Benefits, and the applicable payer regulations represent formidable obstacles for building broad support for the decisions of a PBM's P&T committee. In comparison to institutional formularies, PBMs have instituted tier-based formularies that encourage the use of more cost-effective agents to control prescription costs and improve therapy.[197,198] In spite of the economic influences on the P&T committee functions of a PBM, there is no end to opportunities for quality improvement by a PBM since there is no other organization that has the ability to access outpatient medication use to the same extent. Regardless of the organizational setting, the requirements for quality as a basis for decisions should be the chief focus of a P&T committee. Obviously, this is a potentially moving target because of the need to achieve a balance between the ethical standards involved in health care. The vested interests of the parent organization, patient's needs and expectations, the professional activities of physicians, pharmacists and nurses, the pharmaceutical companies, and the requirements of society may be very difficult to reconcile.

National drug expenditure projection data, and the factors likely to influence drug costs for a particular year, can be reviewed by the P&T committee on a yearly basis. Also, it is necessary to keep hospital administrators informed of drug costs.[199] An understanding of current trends is essential for formulary management.[116,200,201]

LIAISON WITH OTHER ELEMENTS OF THE ORGANIZATION

Within any organization, it is often found that the root of problems is communications or, perhaps more often, lack thereof. Unfortunately, the solution is not simply an increase in communication efforts in general. Instead, the need is for increasing appropriate communication, along with decreasing inappropriate communication. Some specific things have to be kept in mind.

First, make sure that everyone involved in any way in drug therapy receives some communication about medication-related matters. Often, this may simply be a list of new drugs available being given to practitioners, along with any policies and procedures. Newsletters and educational presentations may also be valuable, depending on the circumstances.

Second, be sure the amount of material is not overwhelming, otherwise it will be ignored. A news program on television a number of years ago described a situation that the military found regarding its pilots in Vietnam. They had a tape from the cockpit of an aircraft that had been shot down. Those listening to the tape could clearly hear the warning alarm letting the pilot know that a radar missile was locked on his aircraft and posing an imminent danger, however, it was also clear that the pilot did not even realize that warning was happening because of everything else going on. He mentally "tuned out" the warning and was shot down as a result. It became clear to those training pilots that it was necessary to limit the amount of information to whatever is most important, so that those items were noticed. This is also important in communicating P&T committee materials.

In addition, it is important to keep certain materials confidential for various reasons. In the case of quality assurance materials, keeping materials suitably confidential may protect that data from legal discovery in court (see Chap. 12 and consult attorneys for specifics). Also, some P&T committees keep the agenda and handouts confidential by not sending them to committee members in advance and by collecting the materials at the end of the meeting in order to destroy them. By doing so, they can often avoid pressure put on the committee by pharmaceutical company representatives, who may be trying to have their products included on the formulary, while having their competitor's products excluded. The disadvantage, of course, is that committee members are not able to prepare for a meeting in advance. In relationship to this, it is often a good idea to make sure the pharmaceutical company representatives do not know who members of the committee are and who is preparing the evaluation of a particular product, since that can lead to the evaluator being pressured to sway his or her opinion about a particular product.

Finally, an annual report of the P&T committee may be prepared for both internal review and review by the medical executive committee. This annual report is time consuming in preparation but is a very important means of tracking P&T activities and actions over time.

Overall, it is necessary for the chairman and secretary of the P&T committee to work in cooperation with other appropriate individuals and groups to make sure that essential information is provided wherever needed, while minimizing the amount of extraneous material.

Conclusion

The pharmacy department can have a major impact on the quality of drug therapy in an institution through participation in P&T committee functions and activities described in this chapter, many of which are related to the management of information or are commonly performed by drug information practitioners. While there are many "right" ways that may be used in addition to those outlined above, those described can be successfully used to improve drug therapy.

Acknowledgments

The authors would like to acknowledge the suggestions of George W. Benecke, MBA, RP and Christopher Holewinski, Pharm.D. in the preparation of this chapter.

Study Questions

1. What is the P&T committee, what are its functions, and how does the committee relate to a pharmacy department?

2. How should a pharmacy/pharmacist be involved in supporting a P&T committee?

3. Define drug formulary and formulary system. How do those items relate to one another?

4. Define open versus closed formularies, including the specific types of closed formularies.

5. How does a P&T committee improve the quality of medication use in a hospital?

6. Define policy. Define procedure.

7. What are the steps in preparing a policy and procedure?

8. Name and briefly explain four policies and procedures that may be implemented by a P&T committee.

9. How does an institutional P&T committee differ from one in a PBM?

10. Who must a P&T committee communicate with? What should they communicate and how should they communicate?

REFERENCES

1. Shulkin DJ. Enhancing the role of physicians in the cost-effective use of pharmaceuticals. Hosp Formul. 1994;29:262–73.
2. Nair KV, Ascione FJ. Evaluation of P&T committee performance: an exploratory study. Hosp Formul. 2001;3:136–46.
3. Zellmer WA. Dr. Avorn's wake-up call to pharmacy. Am J Health Syst Pharm. 2004;61:2010.
4. Nair KV, Coombs JH, Ascione FJ. Assessing the structure, activities, and functioning of P&T committees: a multisite case study. P&T. 2000;25(10):516–28.
5. Redman RL, Mays DA. Data analysis. Drug information services in the managed care setting. Drug Benefit Trends. 1997;9:28–40.

6. Sroka CJ. CRS report for Congress: pharmacy benefit managers. Washington, DC: Library of Congress; 2000 Nov 29.

7. Gourley DR, Halbert MR, Hartmann KM, Malone PM. Development and implementation of a P&T committee for state institutions. Hosp Formul. 1981;16(2):143–4, 149–51, 154–5.

8. McCutcheon T. Medicare prescription drug benefit model guidelines. Washington, DC: United States Pharmacopeial Convention; 2004.

9. Stefanacci RG. The expanding role of P&T committees in long-term care. P&T. 2003;28:720–3.

10. Feldman L. Pharmacists' role in the pharmacy and therapeutics committee. Pharm Times. 2004 Feb:26.

11. Jenkins A. Formulary development by community pharmacists. Pharmaceutical J. 1996;256: 861–3.

12. AMA Board of Trustees. Drug formularies and therapeutic interchange. Recommendations adopted at the American Medical Association (AMA) House of Delegates Interim Meeting 1993. Chicago (IL): American Medical Association; 1993.

13. H-125.991 drug formularies and therapeutic interchange. Chicago (IL): American Medical Association; 2000 [cited 2004 Mar 9]. 2 p. Available from: http://www.ama-assn.org/apps/pf_new/pf_online? f_n=browse&doc=policyfiles/HnE/H-125.991.HTM

14. Formulary management (medication-use policy development). Bethesda: American Society of Health-System Pharmacists; 2004 [cited 2004 Mar 9]. 1 p. Available from: http://www.ashp.org/ bestpractices/formulary.cfm?cfid=497523&CFToken=39106216

15. CAMH comprehensive accreditation manual for hospitals: the official handbook. Oakbrook Terrace (IL): Joint Commission on Accreditation of Health care Organizations; 2004.

16. Format for formulary submissions. Version 2.1. Alexandria (VA): Academy of Managed Care Pharmacy; 2005.

17. Raffel MW, Barsukiewicz CK. The US health system: origins and functions. Albany (NY): Delmar; 2002.

18. Balu S, O'Connor P, Vogenberg FR. Contemporary issues affecting P&T committees. Part 1: The evolution. P&T. 2004;29:709–11.

19. Millano C. Bellevue Hospital: the birthplace of formulary medicine? Pharm Pract News. 2004;31:14.

20. Plumridge RJ, Stoelwinder JU, Rucker TD. Drug and therapeutics committees: the relationships among structure, function, and effectiveness. Hosp Pharm. 1993;28:492–3, 496–8, 508.

21. Doherty EC. The JCAHO agenda for change: what changes in pharmacy and P&T activities do you need to prepare for in 1994. Hosp Formul. 1994;29:54–68.

22. The Joint Commission on Accreditation of Health care Organizations. 1995 comprehensive accreditation manual for hospitals. Oakbrook Terrace (IL): Joint Commission on Accreditation of Health care Organizations; 1994.

23. Academy of Managed Care Pharmacy. Principles of a sound drug formulary system. 2000 [cited 2004 Mar 18]. Available from: http://www.amcp.org/data/nav_content/drugformulary%2Epdf

24. Eavy GR, Swinkey NJ, Rehan A. Decentralizing the P&T committee: rationale and successes. Formulary. 2000;35:752–69.

25. Mubarak-Shaban H, Billups SJ. The pharmacy and therapeutics committee within a hospital corporation: challenges and solution. P&T. 1998;23(6):309–10, 332.

26. Herbert WJ, Mahaney LM. Consolidating P&T committees in an integrated health care system. Formulary. 1996;31:497–504.

27. Cano SB. Formularies in integrated health systems: Fallon health care system. Am J Health Syst Pharm. 1996;53:270–3.

28. Rizos AL, Levy E, Furnier J, Crowley K. Formularies in integrated health systems: sharp health care. Am J Health Syst Pharm. 1996;53:274–8.

29. Barkley GL, Krol G, Anandan JV, Isopi M. An integrated health care system's attempt to create a unified formulary. Formulary. 1997;32:60–74.

30. Jarry PD, Fish L. Insights on outpatient formulary management in a vertically integrated health care system. Formulary. 1997;32:500–14.

31. Mannebach MA, Ascione FJ, Gaither CA, Bagozzi RP, Cohen IA, Ryan ML. Activities, functions, and structure of pharmacy and therapeutics committees in large teaching hospitals. Am J Health Syst Pharm. 1999;56:622–8.

32. Balu S, O'Connor P, Vogenberg FR. Contemporary issues affecting P&T committees. Part 2: Beyond managed care. P&T. 2004;29:780–3.

33. Teagarden JR. How many members should be on a P&T committee. P&T Society. 2003 Fall.

34. Miller WA. Making the pharmacy and therapeutics committee more effective. Curr Concepts Hosp Pharm Manage. 1986;Summer:10–15.

35. Christopherson GA. Policy for implementation of the DoD pharmacy and therapeutics committee [Internet]. Washington: 1998 Mar 23 [cited 2004 Jan 23]. 4 p. Available from: http://www.tricare.osd.mil/policy/fy98/dptc9825.html

36. Barlas S. Role of P&T committees in Medicare: how much authority, accountability? P&T. 2004;29:678.

37. The ABCs of PBMs. A discussion featuring Peter D. Fox, Ph.D, Terry S. Latanich, Chris O'Flinn, J.D. LLM, and Phonzie Brown. Washington, DC: The George Washington University. National Health Policy Forum. Issue Brief No. 749; 1999 Oct 27.

38. Lipton HL, Kreling DH, Collins T, Hertz KC. Pharmacy benefit management companies: dimensions of performance. Annu Rev Public Health. 1999;20:361–401.

39. Teagarden JR. Perspectives on prescription drug benefit formularies. Hosp Pharm. 2004;39:1102–25.

40. PricewaterhouseCoopers. The value of pharmacy benefit management and the national cost impact of proposed PBM legislation. Pharmaceutical Care Management Association; 2004 July.

41. Butler CD, Manchester R. The P&T committee: descriptive survey of activities and time requirements. Hosp Formul. 1986;21:89–98.

42. Chi J. When R.Ph.s talk P&T committees listen. Hosp Pharm Rep. 1994;8(5):1, 7–8.

43. Gannon K. More power to you. Pharmacists flex their muscles and exert greater influence on P&T committees. Hosp Pharm Rep. 1998;12(2):18–20.

44. Chase P, Bell J, Smith P, Fallik A. Redesign of the P&T committee around continuous quality improvement principles. P&T. 1995;20(10):25–26, 29–30, 32, 34, 37–8, 40.

45. Croft CL, Crane VS. Redesign of P&T committee functions and processes: a model. Formulary. 1998;33:1105–22.

46. Crane VS, Gonzalez ER, Hull BL. How to develop a proactive formulary system. Hosp Formul. 1994;29:700–10.

47. Poirier TI, Vorbach M, Bache T. Linking a policy on nonformulary drugs to the FDA's therapeutic-potential classification system. Am J Hosp Pharm. 1994;51:2277–8.

48. Green JA, Chawla AK, Fong PA. Evaluating a restrictive formulary system by assessing nonformulary-drug requests. Am J Hosp Pharm. 1985;42:1537–41.

49. Hailemeskel B, Kelvas M. Nonformulary drug requests as a guide in formulary system management. Am J Health Syst Pharm. 1999;56:818, 820.

50. Adding drugs to the formulary: your work is never done. Hosp Pharm. 1999;34(7):828.

51. Shea BF, Churchill WW, Powell SH, Cooley TW, Maguire JH. P&T committee overview: Brigham and Women's Hospital. Pharm Pract Manag Q. 1998;17(4):76–83.

52. Cunha BA. Principles of antibiotic formulary selection for P&T committees. P&T. 2003;28(6):396.

53. Empey KM, Rapp RP, Evans ME. The effect of an antimicrobial formulary change on hospital resistance patterns. Pharmacotherapy. 2002;22(1):81–7.

54. Cunha BA. Principles of antibiotic formulary selection for P&T committees. Part 1: Antimicrobial activity. P&T. 2003;28(6):397–9.

55. Cunha BA. Principles of antibiotic formulary selection for P&T committees. Part 2: Pharmacokinetics and pharmacodynamics. P&T. 2003;28(7):468–70.

56. Cunha BA. Principles of antibiotic formulary selection for P&T committees. Part 3: Antibiotic resistance. P&T. 2003;28(8):524–7.

57. Polk RE. Antimicrobial formularies: can they minimize antimicrobial resistance? Am J Health Syst Pharm. 2003;60(Suppl 1):S16–S19.

58. Cunha BA. Principles of antibiotic formulary selection for P&T committees. Part 3: Antimicrobial side effects. P&T. 2003;28(9):594–6.

59. Cunha BA. Principles of antibiotic formulary selection for P&T committees. Part 5: The cost of antimicrobial therapy. P&T. 2003;28:662–5.

60. Motz JC. Influence of the P&T committee on antibiotic selection in a staff model HMO. P&T. 1998;23(8):411–8.

61. DiLiegro N, Groves AJ, Caspi A. Cost savings from an antimicrobial-monitoring program. P&T. 1998;23(8):419–24.

62. Carlson JA. Antimicrobial formulary management: meeting the challenge in a health maintenance organization. Pharmacotherapy. 1991;11(1 pt 2):32S–35S.

63. Quintiliani R, Quercia RA. How to create a therapeutics committee that is scientifically and economically sound. Formulary. 2003;38:594–602.

64. ASHP statement on the pharmacy and therapeutics committee. Am J Hosp Pharm. 1992;49:2008–9.

65. Chase P, Bell J, Smith P, Fallik A. Redesign of the P&T committee around continuous quality improvement principles. P&T. 1995;20(1):25–6, 29–30, 32, 34, 37–8, 40.

66. Brushwood DB. Legal issues surrounding therapeutic interchange in institutional settings: an update. Formulary. 2001;36:796–804.

67. Mutnick AH, Ross MB. Formulary management at a tertiary care teaching hospital. Pharm Pract Manag Q. 1997;17(1):63–87.

68. ASHP statement on the formulary system. Am J Hosp Pharm. 1983;35:326–8.

69. ASHP technical assistance bulletin on drug formularies. Am J Hosp Pharm. 1991;48:791–3.

70. ASHP guidelines on formulary system management. Am J Hosp Pharm. 1992;49:648–52.

71. Rucker TD, Schiff G. Drug formularies: myths-in-formation. Med Care. 1990;28:928–42.

72. Chi J. Hospital consultant foresees dim future for drug formularies. Drug Topics. 1999 April 19:67.

73. Horn SD, Sharkey PD, Tracy DM, Horn C, James B, Goodwin F. Intended and unintended consequences of HMO cost-containment strategies: results from the managed care outcomes project. Am J Manag Care. 1996;2:253–64.

74. Horn SD. Unintended consequences of drug formularies. Am J Health Syst Pharm. 1996;53:2204–6.

75. Goldberg RB. Managing the pharmacy benefit: the formulary system. J Manag Care Pharm. 1997;3(5):565–73.

76. Formulary effectiveness: many questions, but few clear answers. Consult Pharm. 1996;11(7):635.

77. Curtiss FR. Drug formularies provide a path to best care. Am J Health Syst Pharm. 1996;53:2201–3.

78. Formularies and generics drive up health resource use, study suggests. Am J Health Syst Pharm. 1996;53:971–5.

79. Horn SD, Sharkey PD, Phillips-Harris C. Formulary limitations and the elderly: results from the managed care outcomes project. Am J Manag Care. 1998;4:1105–13.

80. Marra F, Patrick DM, White R, Ng H, Bowie WR, Hutchinson JM. Effect of formulary policy decisions on antimicrobial drug utilization in British Columbia. J Antimicrob Chemother. 2005;55: 95–101.

81. Hepler CD. Where is the evidence for formulary effectiveness. Am J Health Syst Pharm. 1997;54:95.

82. Kelly WN, Rucker TD. Considerations in deciding which drugs should be in a formulary. J Pharm Pract. 1994;VII(2):51 – 7.

83. Shih Y-C T, Sleath BL. Health care provider knowledge of drug formulary status in ambulatory care settings. Am J Health Syst Pharm. 2004;61:2657–63.

84. Muirhead G. When formularies collide. Hospitals vs. health plans. Hosp Pharm Rep. 1994;8(10):1, 8.

85. 1999 accreditation standards address public concerns, says NCQA. Am J Health Syst Pharm. 1998;55:2221, 2225.

86. Bruzek RJ, Dullinger D. Drug formulary: the cornerstone of a managed pharmacy program. J Pharm Pract. 1992;V(2):75–81.

87. North GLT. Handling nonformulary requests for returning or transfer patients. Am J Hosp Pharm. 1994;51:2360, 2364.

88. Davis FA. Formularies: a dangerous concept for patients. Priv Pract. 1991 Sept:11– 17.

89. Palmer MA, Hartman SK, Gervais S. Introducing a formulary system in long-term care facilities: initial experience. Consult Pharm. 1994;9:307–14.

90. Shulkin DJ. Enhancing the role of physicians in the cost-effective use of pharmaceuticals. Hosp Formul. 1994;29:262 – 73.

91. Pearce MJ, Begg EJ. A review of limited lists and formularies. Are they cost-effective? Pharmacoeconomics. 1992;1:191–202.

92. Sloan FA, Gordon GS, Cocks DL. Hospital drug formularies and use of hospital services. Med Care. 1993;31:851–67.

93. Hazlet TK, Hu T-W. Association between formulary strategies and hospital drug expenditures. Am J Hosp Pharm. 1992;49:2207–10.

94. Pickette S, Hanish L. Dealing with demands for nonformulary drugs. Am J Hosp Pharm. 1992;49: 2920, 2923.

95. Corliss DA. Computer-assisted help desk for handling drug benefits. Am J Health Syst Pharm. 1977;54:1941–42, 1945.

96. NCQA draft accreditation standards for 2000 address formularies. Am J Health Syst Pharm. 1998;55:1266–7.

97. Format for formulary submissions. Version 2.1. Academy of Managed Care Pharmacy [modified 2005 Apr 1; cited 2005 Nov 15]. Available from: http://www.fmcpnet.org/data/resource/Format~Version_2_/~Final_Final.pdf

98. Le AG, Generali JA. From printed formularies to online formularies. Hosp Pharm. 2004;38:1003.

99. Navarro RP. Electronic formulary control. Med Interface. 1997;10(8):74–6.

100. Drug czars, electronic formulary systems increase formulary compliance. Formulary. 1997;32: 171–2.

101. Ukens C. Hospital finds computer carrot can save drug dollars. Hosp Pharm Rep. 1994;8(6):20.

102. Computerized drug cost information fails to sway physician prescribing. Am J Health Syst Pharm. 1999;56:1183–4.

103. Sateren LA, Sudds TW, Tyler LS. Computer-based system for maintaining and printing a hospital formulary. Am J Hosp Pharm. 1987;44:1367–70.

104. E-prescribing applications help physicians with Vioxx recall. Pharm Pract News. 2004;31(11):67.

105. McCaffrey S, Nightingale CH. How to develop critical paths and prepare for other formulary management changes. Hosp Formul. 1994;29:628–35.

106. Current formulary decision-making strategies and new factors influencing the process. Formulary. 1995;30:462–70.

107. Rich DS. New JCAHO medication management standards for 2004. Am J Health Syst Pharm. 2004;61:1349–58.

108. Neumann PJ. Evidence-based and value-based formulary guidelines. 2004;23(1):124–34.

109. Murri NA, Somani S. Implementation of safety-focused pharmacy and therapeutics monographs: a new University HealthSystem Consortium template designed to minimize medication misadventures. Hosp Pharm. 2004;39:654–60.

110. Chren M-M, Landefeld CS. Physicians' behavior and their interactions with drug companies. JAMA. 1994;271:684–9.

111. Haslé-Pham E, Arnould B, Späth H-M, Follet A, Duru G, Marquis P. Role of clinical, patient-reported outcome and medico-economic studies in the public hospital drug formulary decision-making process: results of a European survey. Health Policy. 2005;71:205–12.

112. Rucker TD, Schiff G. Drug formularies: myths-in-formation. Med Care. 1990;28:928–42.

113. Asmus MJ, Hendeles L. Levalbuterol nebulizer solution: is it worth five times the cost of albuterol? Pharmacotherapy. 2000;20:123–9.

114. Desloratadine (Clarinex). Med Lett. 2002;44(W1126B):27–9.

115. Escitalopram (Lexapro) for depression. Med Lett. 2002;44(W1140A):83–4.

116. Hoffman JM, Shah ND, Vermeulen LC, Hunkler RJ, Hontz KM. Projecting future drug expenditures—2004. Am J Health Syst Pharm. 2004;61:145–58.

117. FDA sees rebound in approval of innovative drugs in 2003 [Internet]. New York: Science Daily; 2004 Jan 19 [cited 2004 Apr 22]. 4 p. Available from: http://www.sciencedaily.com/releases/2004/01/040116074839.htm

118. Most medications approved in the 1990s not new, but modified versions of older drugs, report states [Internet]. Menlo Park (CA): kaisernetwork.org; 2002 May 29 [cited 2004 Apr 22]. Available from: http://www.kaisernetwork.org/daily_reports/print_report.cfm?DR_ID-11414&dr_cat=3

119. Senthilkumaran K, Shatz SM, Kalies RF. Computer-based support system for formulary decisions. Am J Hosp Pharm. 1987;44:1362–6.

120. Computer tool lets P&T members assess Tx classes with their own weightings, product ratings. Formulary. 2000;35:603.

121. Janknegt R, Steenhoek A. The system of objectified judgement analysis (SOJA). A tool in rational drug selection for formulary inclusion. Drugs. 1997;53(4):550–62.

122. Janknegt R, van den Broek PJ, Kulberg BJ, Stobberingh E. Glycopeptides: drug selection by means of the SOJA method. Eur Hosp Pharm. 1997;3(4):127–35.

123. Zachry WM III, Skrepnek GH. Applying multiattribute utility technology to the formulary evaluation process. Formulary. 2002;37:199–206.

124. Berghelli JA. Conflict of interest policy approved. P&T. 1995;20:497.

125. Alpert JS. Doctors and the drug industry: how can we handle potential conflicts of interest? Am J Med. 2005;118:88–100.

126. Palmer MA. Developing a conflict-of-interest policy for the pharmacy and therapeutics committee. Am J Hosp Pharm. 1987;44:2012–4.

127. Fredrick DS, Maddock JR, Graman PS. Hashing out a policy on conflicts of interest for a P&T committee. Am J Health Syst Pharm. 1995;52:2791–2.

128. JCAHO unveils medication-management standards. Am J Health Syst Pharm. 2003;60:1400–1.

129. Cardinale V. Alternative medicine: the law, the marketplace, the formulary. Hosp Pharm Rep. 1999;13(7):15.

130. Is alternative medicine poised for hospital formularies. Drug Util Rev. 1999;15(5):65–8.

131. Brubaker ML. Setting up the herbal formulary system for an alternative medicine clinic. Am J Health Syst Pharm. 1998;55:435–6.

132. Beal FC. Herbals and homeopathic remedies as formulary items. Am J Health Syst Pharm. 1998;55:1266–7.

133. Johnson ST, Wordell CJ. Homeopathic and herbal medicine: considerations for formulary evaluation. Formulary. 1997;32:1166–73.

134. Malesker MA, Meyer RT, Kuhlenengel LJ, Galt MA, Nelson PJ. Development of an alternative medication use policy [abstract]. ASHP Midyear Clinical Meeting. 1998;33(Dec):P-406R.

135. Walker PC. Evolution of a policy disallowing the use of alternative therapies in a health system. Am J Health Syst Pharm. 2000;57:1984–90.

136. Ansani NT, Ciliberto NC, Freedy T. Hospital policies regarding herbal medicines. Am J Health Syst Pharm. 2003;60:367–70.

137. H-125.911 Drug formularies and therapeutic interchange [Internet]. Chicago (IL): American Medical Association [cited 2004 Apr 23]. Available from: http://www.ama-assn.org/apps/pf_new/pf_online?f_n=browse&doc=policyfiles/HnE/H-125.991.HTM

138. NCQA draft accreditation standards for 2000 address formularies. Am J Health Syst Pharm. 1999;56:846.

139. Chiefari DM. Effect of a closed formulary on average prescription cost in a community health center. Drug Benefit Trends. 2001;13:44–5, 52.

140. Survey reveals continued HMO shift toward closed and partially closed formularies. Formulary. 1997;32:781–2.

141. Survey finds HMOs, PBMs still moving to restricted formularies, quickly advancing in informatics. Formulary. 1998;33:622, 625.

142. Abramowitz PW. Controlling financial variables—changing prescribing patterns. Am J Hosp Pharm. 1984;41:503–15.

143. Open formularies improve oncology outcomes in capitated care system. Formulary. 1996;31:878, 881.

144. TennCare formulary restrictions hurt patient care, survey says. Formulary. 1996;31(6):443.

145. Schachtner JM, Guharoy R, Medicis JJ, Newman N, Speizer R. Prevalence and cost savings of therapeutic interchange among U.S. hospitals. Am J Health Syst Pharm. 2002;59:529–33.

146. Bowman GK, Moleski R, Mangi RJ. Measuring the impact of a formulary decision: conversion to one quinolone agent. Formulary. 1996;31:906–14.

147. Chase SL, Peterson AM, Wordell CJ. Therapeutic-interchange program for oral histamine H_2-receptor antagonists. Am J Health Syst Pharm. 1998;55:1382–6.

148. Stoysich A, Massoomi F. Automatic interchange of the ACE inhibitors: decision-making process and initial results. Formulary. 2002;37:41–44.

149. Frighetto L, Nickoloff D, Jewesson P. Antibiotic therapeutic interchange program: six years of experience. Hosp Formul. 1995;30:92–105.

150. Vivian JC. Legal aspects of therapeutic interchange. 2004 Aug 15 [cited 2004 Oct 22];[6 screens]. Available from: http://www.uspharmacist.com/index.asp?show=article&page=8_1129.htm

151. Janifer AN, Chatelain F, Goldwater SH, Mikovich G. Reengineering hospital pharmacy through therapeutic equivalency interchange while maintaining clinical outcomes. P&T. 1998;23(2):78–82, 85–8, 90–2.

152. Merli GJ, Vanscoy GJ, Rihn TL, Groce JB III, McCormick W. Applying scientific criteria to therapeutic interchange: a balanced analysis of low-molecular-weight heparins. J Thromb Thrombolysis. 2001;11(3):247–59.

153. Reich P. Therapeutic drug interchange. Med Interface. 1996;9(5):14.

154. H-125.995 Therapeutic and pharmaceutical alternatives by pharmacists [Internet]. Chicago (IL): American Medical Association [cited 2004 Apr 23]. Available from: http://www.ama-assn.org/apps/pf_new/pf_online?f_n=browse&doc=policyfiles/HnE/H-125.995.HTM

155. American College of Physicians. Therapeutic substitution and formulary systems. Ann Intern Med. 1990;113:160–3.

156. AMCP position statement on therapeutic interchange. 1997 Sept 13 [cited 2000 Feb 4]:[1 screen]. Available from: http://www.amcp.org/public/legislative/position/therapeutic.html

157. American College of Clinical Pharmacy. Guidelines for therapeutic interchange. Pharmacotherapy. 1993;13(2):252–6.

158. Massoomi F. Formulary management: antibiotics and therapeutic interchange. Pharm Pract Manag Q. 1996;16(3):11–8.

159. Heiner CR. Communicating about therapeutic interchange. Am J Health Syst Pharm. 1996;53:2568–70.

160. Rosen A, Kay BG, Halecky D. Implementing a therapeutic interchange program in an institutional setting. P&T. 1995;20:711–7.

161. Kielty M. Improving the prior-authorization process to the satisfaction of customers. Am J Health Syst Pharm. 1999;56:1499–1501.

162. Carroll NV. Formularies and therapeutic interchange: the health care setting makes a difference. Am J Health Syst Pharm. 1999;56:467–72.

163. Nelson KM. Improving ambulatory care through therapeutic interchange. Am J Health Syst Pharm. 1999;56:1307.

164. D'Amore M, Masters P, Maroun C. Impact of an automatic therapeutic interchange program on discharge medication selection. Hosp Pharm. 2003;38:942–6.

165. Banahan BF III, Bonnarens JK, Bentley JP. Generic substitution of NTI drugs: issues for Formulary Committee consideration. Formulary. 1998;33:1082–96.

166. FDA comments on activities in states concerning narrow-therapeutic-index drugs. Am J Health Syst Pharm. 1998;55:686–7.

167. ASHP guidelines for selecting pharmaceutical manufacturers and suppliers. Am J Hosp Pharm. 1991;48:523–4.

168. Sweet BV, Stevenson JG. Pharmacy costs associated with nonformulary drug requests. Am J Health Syst Pharm. 2001;58:1746–52.

169. Tse CST, Roecker W, Benitez M, Musabji M. How to tie a drug therapy improvement program to physician credentialing. Hosp Formul. 1994;29:646–56.

170. ASHP statement on the use of medications for unlabeled uses. Am J Hosp Pharm. 1992;49:2006–8.

171. Steinberg SK. The development of a hospital pharmacy policy and procedure manual. Can J Hosp Pharm. 1980;XXXIII(6):194–5, 211.

172. Ginnow WK, King CM Jr. Revision and reorganization of a hospital pharmacy and procedure manual. Am J Hosp Pharm. 1978;35:698–704.

173. Van Dusen V, Pray WS. Issues in implementation and enforcement of hospital pharmacy policies and procedures. Hosp Pharm. 2001;36(4):398–403.

174. Piecoro JJ, Jr. Development of an institutional I.V. drug delivery policy. Am J Hosp Pharm. 1987;44:2557–9.

175. Grissinger M. Eliminating problem-prone, automatic stop-order policies. P&T. 2004;29:344.

176. Galt KA. Credentialing and privileging for pharmacists. Am J Health Syst Pharm. 2004;61:661–70.

177. Galt KA. Privileging, quality improvement and accountability. Am J Health Syst Pharm. 2004;1:659.

178. Sass CM. Drug usage evaluation. J Pharm Pract. 1994;7(2):74–8.

179. Orsini MJ, Funk Orsini PA, Thorn DB, Gallina JN. An ADR surveillance program: increasing quality, number of incidence reports. Formulary. 1995;30:454–61.

180. Samore MH, Evans RS, Lassen A, Gould P, Lloyd J, Gardner RM, et al. Surveillance of medical device-related hazards and adverse events in hospitalized patients. JAMA. 2004;291:325–34.

181. Traynor K. Enforcement outdoes education at eliminating unsafe abbreviations. Am J Health Syst Pharm. 2004;61:1314, 1317, 1322.

182. Baker De. Sound-alike and look-alike drug errors. Hosp Pharm. 2002;37:225.

183. Vaida AJ, Peterson J. Common sound-alike, look-alike products. Pharm Times. 2002;68:22–3.

184. Starr CH. When drug names spell trouble. Drug Topics. 2000;144:49–50, 53–4, 57–8.

185. Cohen M. Medication error update. Consult Pharm. 1997;12:1328–9.

186. Soulliard D, Hong M, Saubermann L. Development of a pharmacy-managed medication dictionary in a newly implemented computerized prescriber order-entry system. Am J Health Syst Pharm. 2004;61:617–22.

187. First Consulting Group. Computerized physician order entry: costs, benefits and challenges. A case study approach. Long Beach: First Consulting Group; 2003.

188. FDA's counterfeit drug tasks force interim report. Washington, DC: U.S. Department of Health and Human Services, 2003 Oct [cited 2004 Mar 8]. Available from: http://www.fda.gov/oc/initiatives/counterfeit/report/interim_report.html

189. Generali JA. Counterfeit drugs: a growing concern. Hosp Pharm. 2003;38:724.

190. Young D. FDA urges adoption of anticounterfeit technologies by 2007 [Internet]. Bethesda (MD): American Society of Health-System Pharmacists, 2004 Feb 19 [cited 2004 Mar 8]. Available from: http://www.ashp.org/news/ShowArticle.cfm?cfid=497458&CFToken=73579785&id=4194

191. Redwanski J, Seamon MJ. Impact of counterfeit drugs on the formulary decision-making process. Formulary. 2004;39:577–9, 583.

192 ASHP guidelines on managing drug product shortages. Am J Health Syst Pharm. 2001;58:1445–50.

193. Lasser KE, Allen PD, Woolhandler SJ, Himmelstein DU, Wolfe SM, Bor DH. Timing of new black box warnings and withdrawals for prescription medications. JAMA. 2002;287:2215–20.

194. Fox ER, Tyler LS. Managing drug shortages: seven years' experience at one health system. Am J Health Syst Pharm. 2003;60:245–53.

195. Leady MA, Adams AL, Stumpf JL, sweet BV. Drug shortages: an approach to managing the latest crisis. Hosp Pharm. 2003;38:748–52.

196. Schrand LM, Troester TS, Ballas ZK, Mutnick AH, Ross MB. Preparing for drug shortages: one teaching hospital's approach to the IVIG shortage. Formulary. 2001;36:52–9.

197. Huskamp HA, Deverka PA, Epstein AM, Epstein RS, McGuigan KA, Frank RG. The effect of incentive-based formularies on prescription-drug utilization and spending. N Engl J Med. 2003;349:2224–32.

198. Thomas CP. Incentive-based formularies. N Engl J Med. 2003;349:2186–8.

199. Crane VS, Hull BL, Hatwig CA, Teresi M, Croft CL. Presenting drug cost information to a board of directors: a case example. Formulary. 2001;36:857–64.

200. Shah ND, Vermeulen LC, Santell JP, Hunkler RJ, Hontz K. Projecting future drug expenditures—2002. Am J Health Syst Pharm. 2002;59:131–42.

201. Shah ND, Hoffman JM, Vermeulen LC, Hunkler RJ, Hontz K. Projecting future drug expenditures—2003. Am J Health Syst Pharm. 2003;60:137–49.

Chapter Fifteen

Drug Evaluation Monographs

Patrick M. Malone • Mark A. Malesker •
Nancy L. Fagan • Paul J. Nelson • Linda K. Ohri

Objectives

After completing this chapter, the reader will be able to

- Describe and perform an evaluation of a drug product for a drug formulary.
- List the sections included in a drug evaluation monograph.
- Describe the overall highlights included in a monograph summary.
- Describe the recommendations and restrictions that are made in a monograph.
- Describe the purpose and format of a drug class review.

Introduction

The establishment and maintenance of a drug formulary requires that drugs or drug classes be objectively assessed based on scientific information (e.g., efficacy, safety, uniqueness, cost, and other appropriate items), not anecdotal physician experience. The way to decide which drug is best for formulary addition is to rationally evaluate all aspects of the drug in relation to similar agents. In particular, it is necessary to consider need, effectiveness, risk, and cost (overall, including monitoring costs, discounts, rebates, and so forth)—often in that order. Some other issues that are evaluated include: dosage forms, packaging, requirements of accrediting or quality assurance bodies, physician preferences, regulatory issues, patient/nursing convenience, advertising, and consumer expectations.[1] It is expected that in the future there will be more emphasis on evaluating clinical outcomes, continuous quality assurance information, comparative efficacies, pharmacogenomics, and quality of life.[2] Even such a factor as the public image of the institution may have an impact on the decision to add a drug to the formulary. An in-depth drug evaluation monograph can be prepared to assist in this process as described below. The drug evaluation monograph provides a structured method to review the major features of a drug product. Once a monograph is prepared, it can easily be used as a structured template or overview of a drug product. That allows for easy comparison or contrast to other products that may be used for the same indication or that are in the same product class. Commercially prepared monographs can also be obtained from several sources that can be used "as is" or with modifications to suit the needs of the institution. If this latter method is used, be aware that the quality of the commercial monographs may vary, even from the same publisher, and they may need extensive updating. Often, writing a new drug evaluation monograph may be easier than improving a commercial monograph. When a pharmacy and therapeutics (P&T) committee desires to review an entire class of drugs, the drug category review is often another method used. Drug class reviews are often more lengthy than a single product drug evaluation monograph; however, they can also use a similar structure and format. Hospitals, health-systems, and managed care organizations review an entire class of drugs on a scheduled basis, which must be at least annually, according to accreditation standards.[3] This allows an organization the opportunity to reevaluate the formulary status of products in light of new publications or trials, new products that have entered the market, or oftentimes reevaluate a drug class for possible deletion of particular products from the class. Samples of drug class reviews prepared by the Veterans Administration are available on the Internet at <<http://www.vapbm.org/PBM/reviews.htm>>. Whether or not the monograph is commercial or prepared by a member from within the organization, the material should reflect the local conditions or current prescribing practices and may be sent to P&T committee members at a reasonable time before the meeting in order to allow full consideration of the information. In order to prevent drug company representatives or others from obtaining the material, however, some institutions only distribute this material for review during the meeting and then require the materials to be returned at the end of the meeting. Some institutions even number each monograph with a unique numbering system to assist in tracking the return of P&T committee documents.

Although there are recommendations concerning monograph contents,[1,4] information that may be valuable and specific to an institution, and necessary for an objective review of the product, is commonly missing.[5] An outline of a sample monograph is found in Appendix 15–1. Each of the sections of this monograph will be discussed below. An example of some of the information found in the various parts of a monograph is seen in Appendix 15–2. This sample monograph meets or exceeds the recommendations of the American Society of Health-System Pharmacists (ASHP),[4] and should serve as a good example for most circumstances. Guidelines published by the Academy of Managed Care Pharmacy (AMCP)[1,6] and the Joint Commission for Accreditation of Hospital Organizations (JCAHO)[3] are also noted and discussed for situational applicability. The AMCP format is actually the standard recommended by an organization for drug companies to submit data to managed care organizations. It is designed to restrict the marketing impact of the company in providing information and, while it has applicability as to how an institution may evaluate a drug, it also has restrictions as to the amount of information that it can cover in some areas that may make it undesirable in some cases. However, it may be very worthwhile for institutions or other organizations to request this information from the drug company, preferably, well in advance of the time it is needed. Please note, in some cases this request may require signing a nondisclosure agreement, since it may contain proprietary information.[1]

Overall, the precise monograph should be tailored to the institution, organization, patient population, clinic, and so forth. Several sections not recommended by ASHP have been added to increase the utility of the monograph for other sites of practice, including ambulatory clinics, pediatric institutions, long-term care facilities, managed care or pharmacy benefit managers, or even Medicare or Medicaid formularies. Also, in some cases, the information has been divided into multiple sections or subsections to increase clarity. This format can also be used to evaluate whole classes of drugs. In most cases, a specific drug is compared to others in the same class. The only difference in a class review is that one drug is not receiving the greatest attention; all drugs are being compared with equal attention. Comparative charts and tables are often more prevalent in drug class reviews, as they can serve as a concise method to provide an overview of comparative features for the products in a particular drug class.

Specific formats, differing somewhat from the one presented here, may be required by organizations or governments. For example, Australia (<<http://www.tga.gov.au/pmeds/argpm.htm>>),[7] Ontario, Canada (<<http://www.health.gov.on.ca/english/providers/pub/drugs/dsguide/dsguide_mn.html>>),[8] the United Kingdom (<<http://www.nice.org.uk/pdf/TAP.pdf>>),[9] and the European Medicines Agency (<<http://www.emea.eu.int/htms/human/d70ar/d70ar.htm>>)[10] have very specific published guidelines that need to be followed for a drug product to be considered for their formularies. Where appropriate, features of these formats have been incorporated into the description presented in this chapter. While the format described in this chapter does provide much of the information in those government standards, with the exception of details about product manufacturing and specific pricing for the particular country, the order and amount of information is often different and the reader is referred to those standards for details.

Before discussing details about monograph preparation, it should be emphasized that the drug monograph is a powerful tool for the pharmacy to guide the rational development of a drug formulary. Although the pharmacy department or an individual pharmacist may have few, if any, votes in the ultimate adoption of a formulary agent, the monograph guides the evaluation process and is likely to be a major factor in the final decision. While monograph preparation can be very time consuming, it is extremely important and should be given proper attention. The structured evaluation process of a drug monograph, in many cases, is the only time a full, fair, and balanced review of a drug may be presented to a practitioner. Pharmacists have a unique role in the preparation of a monograph in that they view the drug product from a whole and macroeconomic view—all aspects of the drug product are objectively reviewed in a monograph, whereas, oftentimes when a physician is presented information about a new drug product, they may be basing their use or nonuse of the product on a single study, package insert data, pharmaceutical representative information, or some other microeconomic view of a drug product that may or may not represent the full utility of the drug product.[11]

In addition to FDA-regulated drug products, pharmacists need to be aware of complementary/alternative medicine use, along with the responsibilities and implications that it has for pharmacy services. These products can only be marketed as dietary substances, since the FDA does not regulate herbal products, so manufacturers and distributors cannot make specific health claims. Although there may be minimal scientific evidence regarding efficacy and safety of these products, pharmacists must provide information relating to all therapeutic agents patients are receiving, preparing a drug monograph for the P&T committee, much the same as for any FDA-approved product. This can also follow the format described in this chapter.[12]

The following sections describe the parts of the drug monograph, as shown in the appendices.

SUMMARY PAGE

The first page of the monograph is essentially a summary of the most important information concerning the drug, and includes a specific recommendation of the action to be taken on the product. Some P&T committees only review this first sheet; however, the remainder of the document should be prepared in order to completely evaluate a drug product and to provide a record of all that was taken into consideration. The summary and recommendation could be placed at the end of the monograph, but it is probably best to keep it on the front to make it easier to refer to during the meeting.

The format of the summary page usually begins with general institutional information. Following the name header, specific introductory information about the product is included. The generic name, trade name, and manufacturer are self-explanatory, but the classification may require some explanation. This is meant to give the readers a very quick way of classifying the agent in their head. It includes the prescription/controlled substance status, American Hospital Formulary Service (AHFS) classification, and FDA classification. It may also contain other classification schemes used by particular organizations, such as the Veteran's Administration (see <<http://www.vapbm.org/natform/vaclass.htm>>). Managed care organizations may use more detail drug product identification schemes, such as those established by First DataBank (<<http://www.firstdatabank.com>>).

The AHFS classification can be found in the *AHFS Drug Information* reference book, published by the ASHP. This classification can help the reader determine where this new agent falls in therapy. Most of the time new drugs will be evaluated for possible formulary addition before they are actually placed in that book, so it will be necessary to consult the

TABLE 15–1. FDA CLASSIFICATION BY CHEMICAL TYPE[62]

Type	Definition
1	New molecular entity not marketed in United States
2	New salt, ester, or other noncovalent derivative of another drug marketed in United States
3	New formulation or dosage form of a active ingredient marketed in United States
4	New combination of drugs already marketed in United States
5	New manufacturer of a drug product already marketed by another company
6	New indication for a product already marketed
7	Drug that is already legally marketed without an approved NDA
	• First application since 1962 for a drug marketed prior to 1938
	• First application for Drug Efficacy Study Implementation (DESI)-related products that were first marketed between 1938 and 1962 without an NDA
	• First application for DESI related products first marketed after 1962 without NDAs. In this case, the indications may be the same or different from the legally marketed product

therapeutic classification table in the front of the *AHFS Drug Information* reference book or online at <<http:// www.ashp.org/ahfs/classes.cfm?cfid=3356571&CFToken=16885847>> to decide where the product fits. The classification of similar products listed in *AHFS Drug Information* can also be checked before deciding where to categorize the new product.

The FDA classification is given to nonbiologic products during the review process and is finalized when the new drug application (NDA) is approved. This classification gives some idea of the importance of the product. The classification consists of Chemical Type classification (see Tables 15–1 and 15–2) and Therapeutic Rating classification (see Table 15–3). An

TABLE 15–2. EFFECTIVENESS SUPPLEMENTAL CODE DEFINITIONS[63]

Type	Definition
N (Chemical Type 6)	NDA type 6-new indication
SE1	New indication or significant modification of an existing indication. Includes removal of a major limitation to use
SE2	New dosage regimen, including an increase or decrease of daily dose, or change in administration frequency
SE3	New route of administration
SE4	Comparative efficacy or pharmacokinetic claim naming another drug
SE5	Change in any section other than INDICATIONS AND USAGE that would significantly alter the patient population being treated (e.g., addition of pediatric dosing information)
SE6	Switch from prescription to over-the-counter (OTC)
SE7	Complete the traditional part of a product originally receiving accelerated approval
SE8	Incorporates other information based on at least one adequate and well-controlled clinical trial

TABLE 15–3. FDA CLASSIFICATION BY THERAPEUTIC POTENTIAL[62]

Type	Definition
P	Priority handling by the FDA—before 1992 this was two categories: A—major therapeutic gain; B—moderate therapeutic gain
S	Standard handling by the FDA—before 1992 this was referred to as class C, which indicated the product offered only a minor or no therapeutic gain
O	Orphan drug

FDA classification of 1P (or 1A prior to 1992) would indicate a drug that was given a priority review status by the FDA. This means that the product offered a therapeutic advance over existing products in the market, may be for a new disease state, or may represent a new drug class. The FDA generally reviews these products in an expedited manner, often not requiring as many clinical trials or a lower number of patients enrolled in the trials before the drug is approved to be on the market. In contrast, a classification of 3S (or 3C prior to 1992) is probably a "me-too" product, meaning that it is an additional product in a class of medications that is already on the market and is similar in many ways to the other products already marketed. These products are generally reviewed by the FDA in a standard review manner and do not receive an expedited review process. A supplementary designation (see Table 15–4) may be added to the two-character designation previously discussed. For example, a new AIDS drug might be classified 1P, AA. Knowing and understanding the FDA classification status of a product can assist a reviewer in preparing the drug evaluation monograph in several ways. First, if the reviewer knows that the product they are reviewing has an FDA classification status of 1P, the reviewer will often have to compare the product to a drug outside of the class of the product they are reviewing. For example, if a new class of antibiotics was developed called ketolides, the reviewer will not have any other drugs in the class to compare the product to, and therefore he or she may need to search for studies or review articles of products that fall in other classes of antibiotics, such as the macrolides. Oftentimes in cases in which cancer chemotherapy medications are approved for a treatment that was previously treated by

TABLE 15–4. SUPPLEMENTARY DESIGNATORS[63]

Type	Definition
AA	Drug used for acquired immunodeficiency syndrome (AIDS) or complications of that disease
E	Drug developed or evaluated under special procedures for a life-threatening or severely debilitating illness
F	Drug under review for fraud policy; validity of data submitted being assessed
G	Drug originally given type F designation, once its data are found to be reliable
N	Product with nonprescription marketing for some indication
V	Orphan drug

nondrug therapy, a surgical procedure or radiation therapy may be the best comparator for the product. In the cases of products that are given an FDA classification status of 3S, the reviewer generally will be able to prepare a head-to-head comparison of the product to another product that is in the same drug class. For example, if a new hydroxymethylglutaryl-CoA (HMG-CoA) reductase inhibitor was approved by the FDA, the reviewer would normally want to the compare the product to other HMG-CoA reductase inhibitors. Usually, when 3S or standard review products enter the market, if there are already a number of similar products available in the market, the manufacturer will conduct head-to-head trials with the product that was introduced first in the class. This product is generally then referred to as the comparator or "gold standard" product. The reviewer will want to discuss the comparator product and any other similar agents in the class. This can assist the decision makers in the P&T committee in reviewing the new product if they are already familiar with other products in the class.

Additional product introductory information may include the product's patent exclusivity date and/or the product's patent expiration date. This information can generally be located on the FDA's website at <<http://www.accessdata.fda.gov/scripts/cder/drugsatfda/index.cfm>>. A particular institution may request additional or specific information that maybe be relevant to include in the introductory information. It is also common to provide a list of similar agents.

The summary itself is a brief overview of the important aspects of the drug product. If there are similar products or different drugs used for the same indication, it is important to state how the drug being reviewed compares to those products. If a comparison between the agent in question and some other treatment is possible, that comparison must make up the bulk of the section, just as the comparison must be a prominent feature in every other section of the document. The summary will include information on the efficacy, safety (e.g., adverse effects and drug interactions[13]), uniqueness, cost, and other factors, such as the likelihood patients would be more compliant with one agent or another[14,15] or how the therapy fits into published clinical guidelines. Information should be limited in this section to those items where a drug has a definite advantage/disadvantage or, if products are similar, where there would be concern about the possibility of a clinically significant difference. Items that are not clinically significant and not likely to be of concern should be left out of the summary to avoid distractions. In cases where the new drug under evaluation is indicated for a disease that has normally received nondrug treatment (e.g., surgery, radiation, and physical therapy), the drug should be compared to that standard treatment. It is worth pointing out that the summary should be just that—a summary of the material presented in the body of the document. Like a conclusion of a journal article, this is not the place to put new material or, for that matter, to provide citations; both of those items belong in the body.

Finally, a definite recommendation must be made based on need, therapeutics (including outcome data and the use of evidence-based clinical guidelines), side effects, cost (full pharmacoeconomic analysis, if possible), and other items specific to the particular agent (e.g., dosage forms, convenience, dosage interval, inclusion on the formulary of third party payers, hospital antibiotic resistance patterns, and potential for causing medication errors[16]), usually in that order.[17,18] When making formulary recommendation as it pertains to third party payers, consideration should also be given to the placement of the formulary agent into a multi-tiered copayment system where the copayment varies according to the cost of the drug and/or formulary status. The member is required to pay these varying amounts of copayment out-of-pocket at the time the prescription is filled. If the drug is a generic, the placement is at the first tier which has the lowest copayment. If the drug is a brand name drug preferred by the health plan, it is usually placed in the second tier with a higher copayment. All other brand name, nonpreferred drugs are usually placed in the third tier with the highest copayment. Drugs in the third tier, the nonpreferred agents, usually have therapeutic alternatives in either the first or second tier. Members are encouraged to talk to their physicians about switching to the more cost-effective, therapeutic alternative drugs in the lower tiers.[19,20] Tier designation or formulary status may change, based on the discretion of the health plan and/or pharmacy benefits management (PBM), in the absence of significant new clinical evidence.[21] Quality-of-life information and patient preferences should be considered, if possible. Recommendations for third party payers may also include a step therapy approach, quantity limits on the prescription, prior authorization, and coverage rule criteria in order for the drug to be covered. Third party payers may require some drugs to have a prior authorization before being dispensed. Prior authorization is usually required for those drugs that are high cost and/or are likely to be used inappropriately. Examples include appetite suppressants and growth hormones. Prior authorization requires that predetermined guidelines must be met by the member before the drug can be covered by the third party payer. As an example, the member may be required to try an older, less expensive drug first. If this drug proves to be ineffective or the patient is unable to tolerate the therapy, then the third party payer may cover a newer, more expensive therapeutically equivalent drug.[22]

Recommendations should be specific to the circumstances in the institution, hospital system, third party payer plan, and/or other organization in which it is being considered. Recommendations to conduct drug use evaluation on the drug (see Chap. 16), clinical guidelines to be followed (see Chap. 19), how physicians are to be educated about the new drug and other items may also be necessary. Education may range from a simple newsletter or web page, to a specific educational program and certification required before a physician can prescribe a drug product.[23]

Some people strongly object to the presence of specific recommendations being placed in the document. This may be because they do not feel it is appropriate for them to make these decisions; however, this should not be a concern if adequate research was done in preparing the evaluation. Sometimes, they have a philosophy that an unbiased decision should be reached only through a group consensus after discussing the matter in the P&T committee meeting; however, that too should not be a concern. For one thing, the person preparing the document, who also obtains input from other appropriate individuals, is in the best situation to advance a logical recommendation. Second, without a recommendation, the discussion does not have a foundation to begin with—allowing the discussion to wander aimlessly to some conclusion that may not make optimal sense. Third, the lack of a specific recommendation allows emotion and "noise" to overcome logic and science. The provision of a specific recommendation is one of the best opportunities for pharmacists to have a deep and wide-ranging impact on patient care, and should not be neglected.

The recommendation must be supported by objective evidence (presented in the summary). Subjective factors that are likely to be significant from the point of view of all involved parties i.e, physicians, pharmacists, nurses, and patients should also be considered. Decision analysis can be used to show the best drug at the least cost (effectively pharmacoeconomic analysis—see Chap. 8 for details).[24–27] Other factors may also be considered and given weight to indicate importance (e.g., multiattribute utility theory[28]). These methods may be commonly seen in HMOs.[29] They look at the possible decisions and their likely outcome, allowing a decision to be made that is likely to lead to the most desirable outcome. Meta-analysis may also find a place in the decision-making process[30]; however, it seems unlikely that most individuals evaluating products for formulary addition would have the skill or time to use that method. Tentative recommendations should be discussed with appropriate physicians and any clinical pharmacists specializing in that area of therapy before the recommendation is finalized. For example, if a cardiac medication is being evaluated, one or more cardiologists should be consulted to identify their concerns and desires. That does not mean the recommendation should necessarily be changed to what a physician wants. If the objective evidence supports the original recommendation, that is the one that should be made; however, it is necessary to demonstrate that the physicians' concerns were addressed.

Overall, the items most likely to be added to the formulary include those that are unique, that serve the specific population, that are most cost-effective and, unfortunately, those with the biggest marketing drive by the marketer. Multiple ingredient products or products that are the extended release or other variations on the patent of a product are least likely to be added in the institutional setting.[31]

The recommendation should be whatever logical conclusion is supported by the objective evidence and the needs of the health care system, including health care staff needs, distribution concerns, drug administration, and drug availability. Whenever possible, at least in the case of recommendations prepared for an institutional pharmacy, it is best to follow the ASHP guidelines for recommendations, which would place the drug into one or a combination of the following groups.[4]

- Added for uncontrolled use by the entire medical staff
- Added for monitored use—No restrictions placed on use, but the drug will be monitored via a quality assurance study (e.g., drug usage evaluation and medication usage

evaluation) to determine appropriateness of use. This is a tie-in to the institution's quality assurance/drug usage evaluation process.[32] Please note: this category does not mean that the patient is monitored, since that is necessary for every drug. It means that the quality and appropriateness of how the drug is used is monitored.

- Added with restrictions—The drug is added to the drug formulary, but there are restrictions on who may prescribe it and/or how it may be used (e.g., specific indications, certain physicians or physician groups, and certain policies to be followed).
- Conditional—Available for use by the entire medical staff for a finite period of time.
- Not added/deleted from formulary.

Note, there may be different recommendations presented for specific strengths, forms, sizes, and so forth of a drug being reviewed; however, being that specific sometimes does not result in any real benefit and may only make things more complicated to manage, with little improvement in drug therapy or decrease in costs.[33]

Most drugs should be added for uncontrolled use or, at the other extreme, not be added, simply because the three other categories cause greater work for the pharmacy or other departments. As a side point, if a recommendation to not add the drug to the formulary is approved, it is often good to require a time period before the drug can be considered again (typically 6 months) to prevent heavy political action pushing through approval of a less than desirable drug, just because the P&T committee gets tired of having it requested every month. Monitored use is occasionally needed if there is concern that a drug might be used in some inappropriate manner or has a great risk for adverse events. A limited drug usage evaluation would be conducted until it is evident that the drug is being appropriately used or not causing adverse events. One example where monitored use might be considered is an expensive biotechnology product that only has one or two approved indications, but multiple investigational uses, where it could be inappropriately prescribed without an investigational protocol. Also, a very toxic product might be monitored to see if adverse effects are appropriately addressed by the prescriber. As electronic drug usage evaluation becomes standard, monitoring may be used to a greater extent, but is seldom justified in systems requiring the pharmacist to manually collect data. Conditional addition to the formulary is a recommendation of last resort, simply because it is much easier to keep a drug off the formulary rather than try to delete an inappropriate drug that is being used by physicians. This type of approval might be used when it is very difficult to clearly determine whether an agent will benefit the institution, if available data are limited at the time of the P&T meeting. If conditional approval is given, it is absolutely necessary to specify when the P&T committee will reconsider whether the drug should be retained on the formulary.

The added with restrictions choice deserves more explanation. Occasionally there are drugs that should be added to a drug formulary, but are dangerous,[34] or prone to misuse or overuse. This could include agents such as antineoplastics, thrombolytics, and third or fourth generation cephalosporins.[35] In such cases, it may be desirable to limit the use of the drugs in some manner.[36] For example, the antineoplastics might be limited to prescriptions from oncologists or a defined group that might include a few physicians who are not oncologists (e.g., rheumatologists using methotrexate). Specific antibiotics might be limited to either infectious disease physicians or to specific, culture-proven diagnoses. Often antibiotics may be restricted to a specific length of therapy, after which a new order must be written or the original order will automatically be discontinued. Other restrictions could include specific floors/areas of the institution or that the physician must receive counter-detailing by the pharmacist before the drug is dispensed.[37] Relatively new methods of restriction involve formularies for managed care organizations, where there may be a cap or limitation on the price, quantity, or on how many times a patient may receive a drug (e.g., one time use for nicotine patches to quit smoking); how much a patient may receive at one time (e.g., 3-month ambulatory supply); a medication may be subject to prior authorization or precertification before the drug can be made available to a patient; there may be step therapy or medications which have to be tried and failed before a specific agent may be available for coverage for a patient; or whether the practitioners (e.g., physicians and pharmacists) may receive financial or other incentives to cut back on the use of specific products.[38] Whenever possible, these types of restrictions should be based on objective data, such as the FDA recommended maximum dose limitations or prescribing contraindication that can be obtained from drug usage evaluation.

Some physicians will object to restrictions, but remember that the physicians are given "privileges" to prescribe drugs and not "rights." Usually, this is not much of a problem because good physicians realize there is a reason for the restrictions. The real problem, however, is the desire to use this category much too often in an attempt to ensure proper use of all drugs. While restrictions can be effective in changing usage of specific formulary agents,[39] every time a restricted drug is prescribed, more time and effort by the pharmacy, managed care organization and, perhaps, the physician is required to ensure compliance with restrictions. At the very least, a policy and procedure, and probably appropriate forms or computer restriction methods, will need to be developed or adapted and be presented as part of the drug recommendation to the P&T committee. A cost-benefit analysis may also need to be conducted to ensure that the restriction is valid, meaning that it really does assist in curbing inappropriate prescribing or use of an agent. A drug use evaluation may also be performed to assess the usefulness of the restriction. If the results of the drug usage evaluation suggest an acceptable level of appropriate use, the P&T committee may need to reconsider the restriction placed on the product or the restriction could be costing the institution more to administer and monitor than it is saving or avoiding. Therefore, unless the computer system can eliminate much of the effort, there needs to be great restraint used when deciding to recommend that a drug be added to the drug formulary with restrictions. Oftentimes, adding with monitoring may be a viable alternative. A relatively new twist to the "restrictions" or "monitoring" types of approval is the use of critical or clinical pathways.[40,41] In this case, a drug may be approved for use in a particular manner for the treatment of a particular disease. These critical pathways may be established for several target populations or target diseases, where additional guidance of patient treatments can result in significant improvement in patient care and/or significant decreases in costs. Because a great deal of time is necessary to develop and manage these critical pathways, they will most likely only be seen in a few areas of any institution at any given time. The recommendation should state that if the drug is to be used as part of some clinical guidelines or disease state management (DSM) program.[42] The reader is referred to Chap. 9 for further information. In managed care organizations, critical pathways may be incorporated into the use parameters of a drug through prior authorization or precertification criteria. These are specific criteria that must be met, based on clinical guidelines, current medical practices, and product prescribing information before a product is deemed "medically necessary" for use.

While the decision to add or delete a drug from the formulary is seldom black or white, a general rule of thumb may be helpful. If the drug is less expensive or the same price as others, and more efficacious or safer—add it to the formulary. If the drug is more expensive without added benefit, such as increased safety or effectiveness—do not add to the formulary (or delete it from the formulary if it is already on it). The problem comes when the drug is more expensive and also has more benefits. In that case, the careful analysis of the literature and weighing of the institution's needs must be carried out. This is the gray area that has no right answer, but the most appropriate decision must be found. This latter decision may also involve "conditional" or "monitored" use.

Whenever a recommendation is made to add a new agent, consideration should be given to the possibility of removing agents that will no longer be necessary or, in the case of a PBM company, moving the agent to a different classification for reimbursement. This whole process can be used as a way of removing extraneous agents on the formulary; however, removal of agents can be difficult if the products are frequently prescribed. (Note: it is often worthwhile to annually review a list of products that have seen little or no use in the previous year in an attempt to remove these products from the formulary.) Whether removing agents individually, or through a review of an entire therapeutic class, there needs to be adequate information presented to the P&T committee to show the product is no longer necessary. The reasons for removal may include superior agent(s) on the formulary, safety, low or no use, and high cost.[43] A timetable for deleting these agents from the formulary must then be developed and the physicians must be informed when the agent will no longer be available. In 2004, the JCAHO, in their medication management standards, stated that as a requirement for accreditation, health care organizations should review medications that are available for dispensing or administration on at least an annual basis for safety and efficacy information.[3] Many managed care organizations accomplish this via the use of the drug class review on a scheduled basis. The drug classes may be placed on a schedule for review in which all classes are reviewed over the course of the year. No matter what system an institution chooses to use to delete or review agents, the use should be monitored and follow-up is necessary to ensure the formulary deletions proceed smoothly.[44] Communication of these deletions can generally appear in newsletters or, if one is aware of a particular physician who is the only one utilizing a product, personal contact may be best to communicate the change as well as to provide information to the prescriber of alternative products.

Finally, therapeutic interchange must be considered.[45] If this concept is acceptable to the institution, and legal in the state, it may be appropriate that the new drug be used to substitute for a less desirable agent, or vice versa. Please refer to Chap. 14 for further information on this subject.

All of the material on recommendations presented above may be confusing. However, to state it simply, the most logical decision to benefit the patient and the institution should be recommended to the P&T committee.

BODY OF THE MONOGRAPH

Many parts of the body of the monograph are self-explanatory from their names and will not be discussed further. Some specific points, however, do need to be made about the body. First, the body may not always be reviewed by the P&T committee and, even if presented, it may be covered only briefly. The body needs to be written as a means to compile the information for reference and further information. Importantly, it serves as a way of bringing all of the information together in a logical order for preparation of the summary. Some P&T committees will want to review the data presented in the body of the monograph, but all need to know that the clinical data were reviewed adequately. Other times, an abbreviated monograph may be presented to the P&T committee and the full monograph is presented to the chairman.

Second, efforts must be made to ensure that the drug in question has been adequately compared to other therapies (whether drug, surgical, radiation, or something else). The person preparing a monograph must go through each section and ask "Have comparisons been made between this drug and the appropriate alternative therapy?" If not, there should either be a good reason for the lack of comparison or some explanation must be put in the section. Sometimes, there will be no published comparison with other drugs or therapies. For example, when anistreplase was first marketed there were only comparisons to streptokinase available, but physicians wanted to know how the drug compared to alteplase. In that case, information comparing both drugs to streptokinase was used to discern how the drugs would compare to each other. Scientifically, this leaves much to be desired, but sometimes there is no choice in the matter. Other indirect methods of comparison may also be necessary. If at all possible, studies directly comparing the drug being evaluated to the standard of therapy should be used. Also, if there are outcome studies data, that can be very important to put in the evaluation, including such hard to quantify items as quality of life.[46]

Third, every item should be addressed, even if only to state that information was not available or that it is not applicable (absorption of IV drugs, for example). This follows the rule that "if it was not written down, it was not done," or in this case was not reviewed.

Finally, the source of the information should be mentioned—any important statement of fact must be referenced, or must be suspected of being inaccurate. The package insert (now often available from <<http://www.accessdata.fda.gov/scripts/cder/drugsatfda/index.cfm>> for newly approved products) will serve as a basis for some of the information, particularly to define what is the FDA-approved information, but other references must be used to fill in the gaps and to back up that information. Other information can be obtained from the manufacturer, as stated in the Format for Formulary Submissions, Version 2.1 by the AMCP[1] (an example letter requesting such information is available as a part of that document), but the person preparing the monograph should also personally do an adequate literature search.

The Pharmacologic Data section is often one of the briefest. A simple one-paragraph explanation of the proposed mechanism of action and how it differs from the comparator agent(s) usually will suffice for the drug in question. More may be needed if the agent is being compared to a drug with an entirely different mechanism of action (e.g., comparing a new angiotensin converting enzyme [ACE] inhibitor to a calcium channel blocking agent). If the agent under consideration is an antibiotic, the spectrum of activity should be discussed, which will be much longer.

The therapeutic indications section normally requires the most work. This section may be broken into three main subsections. The first is a brief coverage of what indications the drug has been used to treat. It is necessary to clearly indicate which uses are FDA-approved, non-FDA approved but reasonably supported and likely to be seen, and those that are early in investigation. Non-FDA-approved indications or possible uses may be difficult to find for new drugs; however, a literature search may be conducted to determine if any abstracts or case reports have been published for uses that were not approved by the FDA. It is important to note these non-FDA-approved uses as they may be helpful in determining possible restrictions to place on the drug in the recommendations section of the monograph. Also, they can be vital when evaluating medications in a pediatric institution or various other subpopulations. Often, non-FDA-approved uses, if found to have therapeutic benefit, will be studied further and manufacturers will submit a request to the FDA to add indications for their product. So, their consideration is important when considering possible future use of the product. They can have an impact on use of an agent for an institution. If at the time the reviewer is researching the product and no off-label uses are noted, it is appropriate to note that fact in the evaluation.[47]

The second subsection will explain how the product and any comparison products fit into any published clinical guidelines. This should include methods for treatment of the condition, both pharmacologic and nonpharmacologic treatment approaches. An excellent source of these guidelines is the National Guidelines Clearinghouse (<<http://www.guideline.gov/>>).

The reader may also consult Chap. 9 for further information. The use of clinical guidelines is important for a P&T committee's consideration. The inclusion of clinical guidelines allows the reader to see the product's anticipated place in therapy. If the product will be a new first-line agent, an agent should often be available for second- or third-line therapy after other agents have failed. The product's place in therapy for a particular disease or indication can play an important role in budgetary decisions when determining the usage potential of a particular product. A pharmacy department may want to increase their budget in anticipation of a new drug that will see a lot of usage for a particular condition. For example, if a new vaccine was developed to help reduce or prevent Alzheimer's disease, a nursing home or long-term care pharmacy provider may want to increase their medication budget to allow for a larger supply of the product to be on hand. However, if a product is for an indication that occurs in less than 1% of a specific gender of a particular ethnic group, the recommendation for the product may be to not add it to the formulary.

The third subsection will be abstracts of clinical studies supporting the various uses (see Chap. 11 for further information on how to prepare an abstract of a study). In the rare case where a product only has one use, data from several studies on that use should be reviewed in the monograph. If there are multiple uses, one well-conducted study for each FDA-approved or likely to be seen indication are usually reviewed; more can be added, but may be redundant and provide no added benefit. If there are several similar studies, one may be covered in depth with a statement at the end of the paragraph that the use is supported by other studies, giving their citations. If one well-conducted study for a use cannot be found, several less desirable studies may be needed to provide sufficient information. Whenever possible, clinical comparison studies should be used. When reviewing newly approved drugs, it is not unusual to find that no comparison studies have been published. In that case, a simple efficacy study should be used. In some cases, it may be necessary to use a meta-analysis, simply because the disease state is rare and a typical clinical study cannot be performed. In cases where no human trials are available, unless there are extenuating circumstances, the drug should generally not be added to a drug formulary until sufficient published information is available. An example of extenuating circumstances would be when a new drug is available for a previously untreatable illness. In that case, the philosophy of anything is better than nothing may apply.

The information should be presented in a manner that is similar to the description of abstracts given in the appendices to Chap. 11, making sure all information is covered. When reviewing the clinical study, the person writing the drug evaluation monograph should point out strengths and weaknesses of the studies, along with applicability of the information to the patients that are covered by the drug formulary. This evaluation may be vital in the arriving at the final recommendation.

A new item to consider in this section is pharmacogenomics. If the genetic makeup of patients is a factor in how the medication is to be used, such clinical study information should be presented in this section. In addition, where appropriate, pharmacogenomic information should be presented in other appropriate sections, such as pharmacokinetics, adverse effects, summary, and so forth

In cases of pediatric drug use, studies may focus on adult literature and the data for pediatric literature may be available in abstracts or poster presentations only. The situation may be the same in other areas where there may not be a great deal of information on the use of the product under review. For these cases, a summary of evidence table, such as the one in Table 15–5, may be beneficial to include in the product review, which should cover material whether it is positive or negative. This provides a concise overview of all the available literature, as well as a rating system for the weight of evidence that is available for a particular indication in the pediatric population. It also contains a comparative summary, in a tabular formation, of the literature and evidence available in the adult population. In cases in which published clinical trials are not available, the summary of evidence table serves to provide the P&T committee with an overview of the data available.

Other information may also be covered in the therapeutics section, including quality-of-life studies.

The Bioavailability/Pharmacokinetics section is similar to what would be found in most publications, but the information may be difficult to find for some new drugs. In some cases, a new dosage form may be considered in a drug evaluation. For example, when a drug is released in IV form, its use may be entirely different from the oral form, so the P&T committee might separately consider it. A change in route, however, does not necessarily mean that elimination is significantly different in the same patient population. Therefore, oral data may be more useful than no information. Whenever possible, a table comparing the drug in question to other products may be helpful.

The Dosage Form section is a good place to point out the limitations in dosage forms available for some drugs. For example, perhaps the drug in question is available only as an oral solid, but the agent it is compared to is available in oral solid, oral liquid, and injectable forms which could be an advantage. This section can also be used to discuss unusual preparation directions or pointing out which product would be easier, quicker, and less expensive to prepare. Additionally, this section should state if the product has any limitations on access (i.e., the product is only available from a registry or available to select facilities), distribution, supply limitations, or possible anticipated shortages.[48] Medication management standards[3] released in 2004 by the JCAHO also emphasize the importance of the handling of medications that have a high-risk for serious injury if misused. The dosage form section should also address special provisions for the procurement, storage, ordering, dispensing, and monitoring of these high-risk agents. Medication error problems in this area are related to professional practice procedures describing product labeling and packaging, nomenclature, compounding and dispensing, education, administration, monitoring and use. Specific recommendations are available regarding antineoplastic agents that address health care professionals, organizations, and patients.[49]

TABLE 15–5. SUMMARY OF EVIDENCE TABLE

Summary of evidence Place drug name here:		
Literature Type	**Comments**	**Weight of Evidence**[*]
Pediatric evidence		
Efficacy		
Controlled trials		
Published reports		
Abstract		
Uncontrolled trials		
Published reports		
Abstract		
Experience reports		
Published reports		
Abstracts		
Local specialists' experience		
Safety		
Published		
Abstract		
Local specialists' experience		
PK/Dosing		
Published		
Abstract		
Adult evidence		
Efficacy		
Evaluative reviews		
Controlled trials		
Other		
Summary comments		

ABBREVIATIONS: Ra, randomized; DB, double-blind; PC, placebo-controlled; F/U, follow-up studies.
[*]Levels of evidence: good, fair, poor, and none.

TABLE 15–6. EXAMPLE SUMMARY OF EVIDENCE TABLE

Summary of evidence Zonisamide (Zonegran®):		
Literature Type	**Comments**	**Weight of Evidence**[*]
Pediatric evidence		
Efficacy		
Controlled trials		
Published reports	Two trials; total n = 333 subjects; generalized and partial; intellectual disability and/or refractory	Good documentation of efficacy
Abstract		
Uncontrolled trials		
Published reports	One review/study and 2 study reports on use for infantile spasms; total n = ~109	Good documentation for efficacy; poor for safety
Abstract	(Much of the pediatric literature is from Japan, with limited availability in English language) Fourteen prospective, open-label Japanese trials involving 1237 subjects were reviewed in an *Epilepsia* abstract. Direct study review available for some trials.	Poor documentation Response (↓ by > 50%): Generalized: 47%, 152/325 Partial: 63%, 578/912
Experience reports		
Published reports	Two reports; total n = 4 infants with infantile spasms	Good documentation for these cases
Abstracts	Eight abstracts; total n = 135; most were pediatric	Poor documentation of varied experience from multiple independent groups
Local specialists' experience	Not available	
Safety		
Published	Ten case/case series reports published, with extensive description of adverse events	Good documentation of ADR experience reports
Abstract	Two U.S. summaries of Japanese safety experience; 1st 4 data sources, n = 2574; 2nd 14 studies, n = 1237. Likely overlap between 2 reports	Poor documentation; rather extensive experience
Local specialists' experience	Not available	
PK/Dosing		
Published	Two reports; total n = 194; children and adults	Good documentation; limited data

TABLE 15-6. EXAMPLE SUMMARY OF EVIDENCE TABLE (*Continued*)

Summary of evidence Zonisamide (Zonegran®):		
Literature Type	**Comments**	**Weight of Evidence***
Abstract	~Six reports; children and/or adults; drug interaction effects on pharmacokinetics (PKs)	Poor documentation of limited data
Adult evidence		
Efficacy		
Evaluative reviews	Cochrane review of adjunctive use for refractory partial epilepsy in 3 Ra studies; total n = 499; 12 weeks duration An assessment of Japanese experience was compared against clinical guidelines for antiepileptic drugs (AED) use (established by the League Against Epilepsy); International n = 1008 (ped n = 403)	Reviewer conclusions: Effective as adjunctive tx for refractory partial seizures. Authors concluded that zonisamide was effective against both partial and refractory generalized seizures.
Controlled trials	Deferred review; FDA-approved for adjunctive therapy of partial seizures in adults	Good documentation, based on FDA approval
Other		
Summary comments	Extensive, independent pediatric reports of efficacy in a variety of seizure types, both published and abstracts; demonstrated benefit in refractory seizure types, including infantile spasms; substantial published experience literature on a variety of adverse events, generally documenting reversibility with dosage adjustment or discontinuation. Limitations in evaluation: multiple publications representing the same subjects	

ABBREVIATIONS: Ra, randomized; DB, double-blind; PC, placebo-controlled; F/U, follow-up studies.
*Levels of evidence: good, fair, poor, and none.

A problem often develops in presenting the information in the Known Adverse Effects/Toxicities section. Quite simply, some drugs have so many adverse effects listed that pages could be written. What should be done is to concentrate on the serious and/or common adverse effects for both the specific drug and the drug class. Whenever possible, incidence and severity should be included. An incidence comparison table listing the agent under consideration and other similar agents may be an efficient and informative method to show the material. If there are many rare, minor adverse effects, a statement to that effect can be listed at the end of the discussion. Conversely, other agents may have very little information available on adverse effects, simply because they are too new. In that case, it may be necessary to discuss adverse effects common to that class of agent, making it clear that they have not yet been seen with the new drug, but are possible. The new agent should be compared to other agents used for the same indication to determine whether there are any advantages. Keep in mind that these tables can be somewhat deceiving because older agents may have 20 years of side effect reports, whereas, a number of adverse effects of the new agent may not yet be discovered.

The JCAHO now requires patient safety information to be addressed in all monographs.[3] In response, P&T committees are implementing safety focused drug monographs, which include information regarding medication errors.[50] In response to the public's concern about drug safety, the FDA has created a special advisory board to advise them.[51]

The Patient Monitoring Guidelines and Patient Information sections listed are items not suggested by ASHP. These sections were added for use in the ambulatory environment, although they can be quite informative in any practice area. The Patient Information section complies with the Omnibus Budget Reconciliation Act (OBRA) '90 standards for prospective Drug Utilization Review (DUR).

The final section to be discussed is the cost comparison, where the product being reviewed is compared in price to other similar products. Typically, three or four medications (possibly including both trade name and generic products) are compared, although sometimes it is necessary to compare a dozen or more products or dosage forms. Preferably, a pharma-coeconomic analysis should be prepared[52] (see Chap. 8), because the seemingly more expensive agent may turn out to be less expensive, overall, as it decreases the length of hospi-talization, degree of monitoring, or number of adverse events that would otherwise occur.[53] Sometimes it may even be necessary to provide a spreadsheet, which may be used during the meeting using a computer projector, to show what effect changes in assumptions may have on the economic analysis. In the case of reports prepared in the method of the AMCP guidelines, the information in this section may provide detailed abstracts of pharmacoeconomic studies, in a manner similar to that seen for clinical studies in the Therapeutics section.[1]

Often, a full pharmacoeconomic review is not practical because of lack of time or expertise, although most large hospitals do report doing a formal economic analysis of some kind for each drug reviewed for possible formulary addition.[54] With particularly expensive products, a com-prehensive pharmacoeconomic analysis becomes much more necessary.[55,56] Even when a full pharmacoeconomic analysis is not practical, any pertinent information that could be used in a full analysis should be included. After all, it sometimes can be determined that the most expen-sive (per dose) drug product may actually be much cheaper in the long run because of increased or faster efficacy, decreased incidence of adverse effects, or lower monitoring costs.

In some cases, a simple price comparison can be prepared using just the cost of the drugs and the frequency of administration. Such a price comparison must consider that the patient may be getting medications both within an institution and after returning home, because insti-tutional pharmacies may get considerable discounts. Therefore, both the institution's cost for the medication and the average wholesale price (AWP) price should be considered. Some medications are extremely inexpensive to the institution, making it tempting to include those agents on the formulary instead of similar therapeutic agents; however, if the AWP price is quite high, the patient may not be able to afford the product in the community, which could quickly lead to readmission into the hospital when the patient's disease is no longer being treated. In those cases, it may not be a good item to carry on the formulary. Also, the differences in package sizes and frequency of administration must be considered. In most cases, products can be compared on the cost of a typical day's therapy at a relatively normal dose; however, in some cases, a different approach may be necessary. For example, an antineoplastic agent may need to be compared with other agents based on a per cycle or per cost of therapeutic regimen basis. Another example that resulted in unusual cost comparisons in the past was Norplant® (an implantable contraceptive agent that was effective for 5 years). The cost of both the drug and the implantation procedure needed to be compared to a 5-year supply of other contraceptive agents. In cases like this, over a period of years, it may be necessary to include calculations of inflation or other factors likely to change over the time period.[57] Other costs should also be considered when possible, such as drug preparation costs, administration costs, laboratory tests, monitoring requirements, and changes of length of stay/therapy—after all, it is not a savings overall if costs are simply shifted from the pharmacy (i.e., drug price) to the laboratory (i.e., monitoring costs).[58] Some pharmacies even include such items as the cost to order and hold the drug, and the cost of preparing the evaluation of the drug for the P&T committee.[59] Also, it is becoming more common to take into account some more difficult to assess items, such as the probability and cost of therapeutic failure in comparison to other similar agents, impact of specific drug therapy on other health care costs (a drug may be cheaper, but require an increase in the cost of other non-drug therapy for the patient), and the cost of adverse drug effects.[60] Because these items may depend on the characteristics of the patients (e.g., age, socioeconomic status, and education level), the figures used are necessarily going to be uncertain. In some cases, however, they will be very important in the final formulary decisions; a drug that at first glance seems more expensive, may be found to actually cost the institution less in the end.[61] Also, it is necessary to consider nondrug therapy (e.g., surgery, radiation therapy, and physical therapy) in the comparison, when they are legitimate alternatives to drug therapy. Overall, the goal is to ensure that the comparison makes sense and takes into consideration all of the relevant economic factors. While some people think that cost is emphasized too much in formulary decisions, it is still an extremely important item. Some drugs cost thousands of dollars per dose, and that can quickly deplete a pharmacy department's budget and significantly affect the economic status of an institution.

Conclusion

Preparation of a drug evaluation monograph requires a great amount of time and effort, using many of the skills discussed throughout this text to obtain, evaluate, collate, and provide information. However, the value of having all of the issues evaluated and discussed can be invaluable in providing quality care.

REFERENCES

1. Format for formulary submissions, version 2.1. Alexandria (VA): Academy of Managed Care Pharmacy; 2005.
2. Wade WE, Spruill WJ, Taylor AT, Longe RL, Hawkins DW. The expanding role of pharmacy and therapeutics committees. The 1990s and beyond. PharmacoEconomics. 1996;10(2):123–8.
3. Comprehensive accreditation manual for hospitals: the official handbook. Chicago (IL): Joint Commission on Accreditation of Health care Organizations; 2004.
4. ASHP technical assistance bulletin on the evaluation of drugs for formularies. Am J Hosp Pharm. 1991;48:791–3.
5. Majercik PL, May JR, Longe RL, Johnson MH. Evaluation of pharmacy and therapeutics committee drug evaluation reports. Am J Hosp Pharm. 1985;42:1073–6.
6. AMCP position statement on therapeutic interchange. 1997 Sept 13. [cited 2000 Feb 4]: [1 screen]. Available from: http://www.amcp.org/public/legislative/position/therapeutic.html
7. Australian regulatory guidelines for prescription medicines. Woden, Australia: Australian Government, Department of Health and Ageing, Therapeutic Goods Administration; 2004.
8. Ontario guidelines for drug submission and evaluation. Toronto: Ministry of Health and Long-Term Care; 2000.
9. Guide to the technology appraisal process. London: National Institute for Clinical Excellence; 2004.
10. CHMP D70 assessment report templates [homepage on the Internet]. London: European Medicines Agency; 2004 [updated 2004 Sept; cited 2004 Nov 11]. Available from: http://www.emea.eu.int/index/indexh1.htm
11. Groves KE, Fanagan PS, MacKinnon NJ. Why physicians start or stop prescribing a drug: literature review and formulary implications. Formulary. 2002;37(4):186–8, 190–4.
12. Cohen KR, Cerone P, Ruggiero R. Complementary/alternative medicine use: responsibilities and implications for pharmacy services. P&T. 2002;27(9):440–6.
13. Chan L-N. Consider potential for drug interactions during formulary review. Am J Health Syst Pharm. 2000;57:391.
14. Feldman JA, DeTullio PL. Medication noncompliance: an issue to consider in the drug selection process. Hosp Formul. 1994;29:204–11.
15. Sesin GP. Therapeutic decision-making: a model for formulary evaluation. Drug Intell Clin Pharm. 1986;20:581–3.
16. Cohen MR. Adding drugs to the formulary: your work is never done. Hosp Pharm. 1999;34:828.
17. Hedblom EC. Pharmacoeconomic and outcomes data in the managed care formulary decision-making process. P&T. 1995;20:462–4, 468, 471–3.
18. Klink B. Formulary influences. Drug Top. 1998;142(20):72.
19. Abourjaily P, Kross J, Gouveia WA. Initiatives to control drug costs associated with an independent physician association. Am J Health Syst Pharm. 2003;60:269–72.
20. Gleason PP, Gunderson BW, Gericke KR. Are incentive-based formularies inversely associated with drug utilization in managed care? Ann Pharmacother. 2005;39:339–45.
21. Reissman D. Issues in drug benefit management. Drug Benefit Trends. 2004; Dec:598–99.
22. Sroka CJ. CRS report for Congress: pharmacy benefit mangers. Washington, DC: Library of Congress; 2000.

23. Dedrick S, Kessler JM. Formulary evaluation teams: Duke University Medical Center's approach to P&T committee reorganization. Formulary. 1999;34:47–51.

24. Kresel JJ, Hutchings HC, MacKay DN, Weinstein MC, Read JL, Taylor-Halvorsen K, et al. Application of decision analysis to drug selection for formulary addition. Hosp Formul. 1987;22:658–76.

25. Szymusiak-Mutnick B, Mutnick AH. Application of decision analysis in antibiotic formulary choices. J Pharm Technol. 1994;10:23–6.

26. Basskin L. How to use decision analysis to solve pharmacoeconomic problems. Formulary. 1997;32:619–28.

27. Kessler JM. Decision analysis in the formulary process. Am J Health Syst Pharm. 1997;54 (Suppl 1):S5–S8.

28. Schumacher GE. Multiattribute evaluation in formulary decision-making as applied to calcium-channel blockers. Am J Hosp Pharm. 1991;48:301–8.

29. Barner JC, Thomas J III. Tools, information sources, and methods used in deciding on drug availability in HMOs. Am J Health Syst Pharm. 1998;55:50–6.

30. Gibaldi M. Meta-analysis. A review of its place in therapeutic decision-making. Drugs. 1993;46:805–18.

31. Gannon K. Uniqueness of a drug key to formulary inclusion. Hosp Pharm Rep. 1996;10:27.

32. Chase P, Bell J, Smith P, Fallik A. Redesign of the P&T committee around continuous quality improvement principles. P&T. 1995;20(1):25–6, 29–30, 32, 34, 37–8, 40.

33. Ain KB, Pucino F, Csako G, Wesley RA, Drass JA, Clark C. Effects of restricting levothyroxine dosage strength availability. Pharmacotherapy. 1996;16(6):1103–10.

34. Limit potential dangers by restricting problem drugs on formulary. Drug Util Rev. 1997;13(4):49–51.

35. Anassi EO, Ericsson C, Lal L, McCants E, Stewart K, Moseley C. Using a pharmaceutical restriction program to control antibiotic use. Formulary. 1995;30:711–4.

36. Berndt EM. Drug expenditures. A medical center's experience with antibiotic cost-saving measures. Drug Benefit Trends. 1997;9:32–6.

37. McCloskey WW, Johnson PN, Jeffrey LP. Cephalosporin-use restrictions in teaching hospitals. Am J Hosp Pharm. 1984;41:2359–62.

38. Goldberg RB. Managing the pharmacy benefit: the formulary system. J Manag Care Pharm. 1997;3(5):565–73.

39. Hayman JN, Sbravati EC. Controlling cephalosporin and aminoglycoside costs through pharmacy and therapeutics committee restrictions. Am J Hosp Pharm. 1985;42:1343–7.

40. McCaffrey S, Nightingale CH. The evolving health care marketplace. How to develop critical paths and prepare for other formulary management changes. Hosp Formul. 1994;29:628–35.

41. Dana WJ, McWhinney B. Managing high cost and biotech drugs: two institutions' perspectives. Hosp Formul. 1994;29:638–45.

42. Armstrong EP. Disease state management and its influence on health systems today. Drug Benefit Trends. 1996;8:18–20, 25, 29.

43. Kelly WN, Rucker TD. Considerations in deciding which drugs should be in a formulary. J Pharm Pract. 1994;VII(2):51–7.

44. Lemay AP, Salzer LB, Visconti JA, Latiolais CJ. Strategies for deleting popular drugs from a hospital formulary. Am J Hosp Pharm. 1981;38:506–10.

45. Boesch D. Formularies and therapeutic substitution: gaining ground in long-term care. Consult Pharm. 1994;9:284–97.

46. Lewis BE, Fish L. Drug approvals. Formulary decisions in managed care: the role of quality of life. Drug Benefit Trends. 1997;9:41–7.

47. ASHP statement on the use of medications for unlabeled uses. Am J Hosp Pharm. 1992;49:2006–8.

48. Leady MA, Adams AL, Stumpf JL, Sweet BV. Drug shortages: an approach to managing the latest crisis. Hosp Pharm. 2003;38:748–52.

49. ASHP guidelines on preventing medication errors with antineoplastic agents. Am J Health Syst Pharm. 2002;59:1648–68.

50. Murri NA, Somani S, University HealthSystem Consortium Pharmacy Council Medication Management/Quality Improvement Committee. Implementation of safety-focused pharmacy and therapeutics monographs: a new University HealthSystem Consortium template designed to minimize medication misadventures. Hosp Pharm. 2004;39(7):653–60.

51. Harris G. FDA to create advisory board on drug safety. NY Times. 2005 Feb 16. [cited 2005 Feb 16]: [about 3 p.]. Available from: http://query.nytimes.com/gst/abstract.html?res=F40916FF385E0C758DDDAB0894DD404482&incamp=archive:search

52. Sanchez LA. Pharmacoeconomics and formulary decision-making. PharmacoEconomics. 1996;9(Suppl 1):16–25.

53. Heiligenstein JH. Reformulating our formularies to reflect real-world outcomes. Drug Benefit Trends. 1996;8:35, 42.

54. Mannebach MA, Ascione FJ, Gaither CA, Bagozzi RP, Cohen IA, Ryan ML. Activities, functions, and structure of pharmacy and therapeutics committees in large teaching hospitals. Am J Health Syst Pharm. 1999;56:622–8.

55. Shepard MD, Salzman RD. The formulary decision-making process in a health maintenance organisation setting. PharmacoEconomics. 1994;5:29–38.

56. Johnson JA, Bootman JL. Pharmacoeconomic analysis in formulary decisions: an international perspective. Am J Hosp Pharm. 1994;51:2593–98.

57. Basskin L. Discounting in pharmacoeconomic analyses: when and how to do it. Formulary. 1996;31:1217–27.

58. Macklin R. Understanding formularies. Drug Store News Pharmacist. 1995;5:82–8.

59. Myers CE, Pierpaoli P, Smith MA. Measurement of formulary inclusion costs. Hosp Formul. 1981;16:951–3, 957–8, 967–8, 970–1, 975–6.

60. Crane VS, Gonzalez ER, Hull BL. How to develop a proactive formulary system. Hosp Formul. 1994;29:700–10.

61. Heiligenstein JH. Reformulating our formularies to reflect real-world outcomes. Drug Benefit Trends. 1996;8:35, 42.

62. CDER drug and biologic approvals for calendar year 2004 [homepage on the Internet]. Washington: Food and Drug Administration; [updated 2004 Sept 30; cited 2004 Nov 11]. Available from: http://www.fda.gov/cder/rdmt/ndaaps04cy.htm

63. Efficacy supplements approved in fiscal year 2004 [homepage on the Internet]. Washington, DC: Food and Drug Administration [updated 2004 Sept 30; cited 2004 Nov 11]. Available from: http://www.fda.gov/cder/rdmt/ESFY04AP.htm

16

Chapter Sixteen

Quality Improvement and the Medication Use Process

Mark A. Ninno • Sharon Davis Ninno

Objectives

After completing this chapter, the reader will be able to

- Explain the evolution of quality management in industry and health care.
- Describe the processes used to assess and improve quality.
- Define the role of the pharmacist in modern health care quality improvement initiatives.
- Explain quality in health care as outlined by the Joint Commission on the Accreditation of Health Care Organizations (JCAHO).
- Define ORYX® and its role in health system accreditation.
- Discuss the role of National Committee for Quality Assurance (NCQA) as it pertains to quality measures in managed health care.
- Describe the role of medication use evaluation (MUE) as a component of an organization's quality improvement program.
- Outline the general process of MUE.
- Describe the role of pharmacists and other health professionals in the MUE process.
- Discuss quality improvement techniques applied in drug information practice.

Quality Improvement

Probably no initiative has had a bigger impact on the delivery of health care in the United States during the past decade than the emphasis being placed on quality. For many years, it was accepted that the quality of the American health care system was second to none and the consumer public was rather passive in their belief that the standard of health care in the

United States was exceptionally high.[1,2] However, quantification of this perceived level of quality is difficult as the standard of care varies from state to state, institution to institution, practitioner to practitioner, and even patient to patient. Increasing competition in the health care market place, decreasing dollars with which to treat patients, and greater access to the availability of medical information through media outlets and the Internet, has served to increase the public's awareness about the need to be more actively involved in the management of their health. As a result, there is an increasing demand for quality health care services at more affordable costs.[3] This demand is coming from all sectors of the community including health care providers, institutions, third-party payers, the government, and most importantly, the consumer public. More and more consumers are seeking information to compare health care providers and payers, and are "shopping" for health care services. Similarly, employers are seeking the best health care coverage for their employees while trying to reduce the costs associated with expanding medical technology. Balanced against all of this is an effort to ensure that all individuals, regardless of payer status, receive the same level and quality of health care, which has resulted in an unprecedented focus by governmental, consumer, and private health care organizations to quantify and regulate the quality of health care in the United States.

For the profession of pharmacy, the new focus on quality of health care comes as both a great opportunity and challenge. While in the past, the assessment of quality was the domain of only a few pharmacy practitioners, today it has become an integral part of every pharmacy practice setting.[4] The use of quality management techniques in assessing therapy and influencing outcomes blends well with pharmacy's initiative to shed its traditional role in medication dispensing and become more involved in the provision of patient-focused care; however, determining "what is quality" and how it is measured has provided many hurdles in achieving this goal. Complicating matters are the numerous national, state, local, and private organizations, and regulatory bodies, that each defines quality in their own terms. As a result, a survey that asks the question: "what is quality health care?" may be greeted with as many different responses as responders.

DEFINING QUALITY

The term quality has meant different things to different groups for as long as the term has been defined. Compounding the confusion in defining quality has been the multitude of terms used to express the process of assessing quality in providing a product or service. Terms such as quality control, quality assurance, quality improvement, continuous quality improvement (CQI), total quality management (TQM), and performance improvement have all been used, sometimes interchangeably, to define the process of determining and improving quality. In its most basic definition, quality is "a degree or grade of excellence" and can be applied to goods, services, processes, or even people.[5] Measures of quality can be applied to any service or good, but is most often associated with a physical product such as an automobile, computer, appliances, or other products. Often the association of quality is made with the service of a product and not the product itself (e.g., we may not be as aware of the quality in the construction of a dishwasher as we are of the dishwasher repair service). More often, quality is associated with intangible items, such as friendliness or timeliness (e.g., we may not be as aware of the quality of the construction of the dishwasher or the repair service as we are of the friendliness of the repairman).

Quality measures have been used for years in the industrial sector. Some quality assurance programs can be traced back to J.C. Penney and Company in 1913.[6] Walter Shewart is often viewed as the founding father of the American quality improvement initiative. Shewart and others at Bell Laboratories during World War II used quality improvement techniques in its zero-defect program.[7,8] Shewart, a statistician, recognized that quality could be best improved by preventing the defects that can be expected with any process. In order to prevent defects, one had to first identify them through a continuous analysis of data produced by the process. By continually reviewing these data, variations and defects can be anticipated and prevented, thus improving quality.[1,8] Shewart developed the simple model of *plan, do, check, and act* (PDCA); a model frequently employed in quality management today. This view of quality control as a statistical process is at the heart of modern quality management initiatives. The first real use of quality assurance techniques in large-scale industry can be traced back to the Japanese in the 1950s.[7,8] In an effort to rebuild their economy after World War II, the Japanese began to compete in markets traditionally dominated by the United States and Western Europe, such as automobile manufacturing. The Japanese had a limited infrastructure and few resources with which to begin manufacturing goods. Gaining insight from early quality pioneers, such as Deming and Juran, the Japanese employed quality improvement techniques to manufacturing. The Japanese recognized that to be competitive they needed to prevent defects because they did not have the resources to correct them after they had occurred, as was the practice in American manufacturing.[8] Early Japanese automobiles had a notorious reputation for being inferior in design and construction, and were held with little regard in the marketplace. Utilizing quality management techniques outlined by Shewart and others, the Japanese soon began to revolutionize the automotive industry with higher quality cars at competitive prices, much to the chagrin of many U.S. automobile manufacturers. Application of similar quality techniques ultimately lead to Japanese dominance in other industrial fields and, to some degree, to the revitalization of the U.S. automobile industry.[7]

Having access to quality management techniques has not always proven to be the key to successful quality improvement. Many U.S. industries started to adopt quality assurance techniques when faced with stiff competition from abroad.[2,7] Unfortunately, many of these quality programs focused on measures of productivity and financial profitability without much regard to the final product or customer satisfaction. In this environment, individuals involved in the production of a good or service focused on identifying and changing the work habits of problematic departments or workers in an effort to improve quality. This practice is known as quality assurance or quality control and differs in practice from quality improvement. In most situations, quality assurance is retroactive, seeking to identify problems and those responsible for allowing problems to occur.[1,9] Additionally, quality assurance tends to focus only on the quality of a particular component within the process, but not the entire process. For example, individuals building the engine of a car may focus only on the quality of the engine production, but not be involved with those responsible for bolting the engine to the chassis. While it may have resulted in a top quality engine, it does little good when the engine falls out of the car! Unfortunately, many quality assurance programs took on an accusatory and punitive aspect for those individuals or departments that did not meet the established expectation of quality.[1] This shortsighted view of quality lead to the demise, or near demise, of many facets of the American industrial sector.

In more recent years, the focus has been shifted away from quality assurance and quality control to embrace a different discipline in the search for quality—TQM. TQM takes a more investigative approach to identifying barriers to quality in the processes of providing goods or services.[1,8,9] TQM works under the basic principle that individuals are committed to quality; however, the processes under which they operate may not be conducive for allowing them to achieve that level of quality. In TQM, all participants are involved in the search for more efficient and cost-effective ways to improve the quality of services, products, and processes. TQM is a statistical, data-driven process that strives to improve quality by limiting variation in the processes involved in providing a good or service.[1] This contrasts with quality assurance, in which the assessment of quality and the plan to improve quality were managed by a limited few and focused on standards that may or may not be driven by data. A table comparing and contrasting the differences in approach and methodology between TQM and quality assurance is provided in Appendix 16–1.

CQI is the term given to the methodologies used in the process of TQM. By using a systematic approach to identify internal and external factors that influence processes and functions, CQI seeks to remove the subjectivity from the assessment of quality and provide an ongoing mechanism for improving quality. CQI uses tools such as brainstorming, Pareto charts, scatter diagrams, fishbone diagrams, run charts, control charts, and other statistical and investigational tools to provide insight into which barriers are decreasing quality (or which processes are improving quality), and to what extent those barriers exist.[9] Examples of these tools are provided in Appendix 16–2.

The shift in the global workplace from quality assurance to TQM has revolutionized many industries. Many companies now embrace these practices very zealously and have incorporated these techniques into their daily routine. While this change has come more quickly to some industries, health care is just now beginning to embrace these philosophies. Accrediting organizations such as the JCAHO and the NCQA have been instrumental in bringing these philosophies to the forefront of contemporary health care. Despite this, many obstacles remain in place as health care seeks to improve quality. In the following sections of this chapter, changes and barriers to quality in health care as well as the expectations of quality set forth by some of the national health care accrediting bodies are reviewed. TQM, as it pertains to the medication use process, and steps to implement a medication quality program are outlined.

Beyond Total Quality Management: Six Sigma Quality

Over the past decade, a new approach to quality, based on the principles of TQM, has emerged and been embraced by many manufacturing and service industries. This principle is called Six Sigma quality and incorporates many of the tools used in TQM. Six Sigma quality derives its name from the statistical term sigma; a measure of deviation from a desired value. Six Sigma is a data-driven, statistical process designed to eliminate defects and improve quality to a level of near perfection (99.99966% defect-free or six sigma). To better understand Six Sigma, it is of value to review an example familiar to most pharmacists; filling an automated medication dispensing machine.[10]

For any given process, there exists opportunities for quality or defects in that process. In this example, each time the automated dispensing unit is filled, it can either be filled correctly or incorrectly. Thus, there is a chance for a defect with each opportunity. If the pharmacy fills the automated dispensing units 1 million times each year and does so at a level of accuracy of 99% (i.e., % yield) then it can be expected that there will be 8800 defects per million opportunities (DPMO). That is to say, in 1 million attempts to fill the dispensing unit, the unit will be filled incorrectly 8800 times. A pharmacy functioning at this level would be achieving approximately four sigma quality for the process of filling automated dispensing machines. Let us say that the same pharmacy desired to achieve Six Sigma quality in the same process. In order to accomplish this goal, the pharmacy would need to produce only 3.4 defects (incorrect fills) per 1 million opportunities (99.99966% defect-free yield). A pharmacy that performs this function at a three sigma level (93.32% defect-free yield) can expect 66800 DPMO. As demonstrated by this example, performing a process at 90 to 99% yield will still leave the potential for a significant number of defects. Most pharmacy managers would be pleased with 99% accuracy in any process; however, in the case of filling an automated dispensing machine, being 99% accurate still will produce 8800 defects, each potentially leading to a dangerous medication misadventure. Six Sigma calculators are available online to assist in determining the yield and DPMO for any given process, as well as provide additional information and explanation of the Six Sigma process (<<www.isixsigma.com>>).

Beyond determining the percent yield and DPMO for a process, the Six Sigma discipline also utilizes a variety of tools and strategies to improve quality. Many of these strategies are similar to those employed in TQM and are based on the PDCA model. Six Sigma employs the strategies of DMAIC (define, measure, analyze, improve, control) and DMADV (define, measure, analyze, design, verify) to improve or incorporate quality into a process or function.[10] The former (DMAIC) is used when improving an existing process that is performing below a desired standard; the latter process is employed when developing a new process. The approach taken with these processes is very similar. A working group of all parties involved in the process (e.g., multidisciplinary group of pharmacists, nurses, and physicians) meet to define the process (e.g., how are automated dispensing units filled? by whom? when?), measure the number of opportunities for that process (e.g., how many times is the automated dispensing unit filled? how many times is it filled incorrectly?), analyze the data (e.g., what is the current percent yield of accuracy and DPMO), improve the process (e.g., reduce pharmacy technician workload or provide double-check method), and control or verify (e.g., determine if the changes improved accuracy). Many of the tools used in TQM and outlined in Appendix 16–2 (e.g., Pareto charts, flow charts, and fishbone diagrams) are employed by the working group to better define the process, the nature and cause of the defects, and the most successful methods for improving performance. While Six Sigma quality practices are being employed in an increasing number of industries, its application in the health care industry is relatively new and not well established. For Six Sigma techniques to be fully effective in the health care industry, industry leaders will need to develop the resources and personnel specifically trained in the techniques of Six Sigma quality.

QUALITY IN HEALTH CARE

In the industrial setting, assuring quality has often focused on materials, people, and processes to achieve a common goal of a quality product.[8] The measure of quality is usually associated with the final product and is often very tangible (e.g., car has no defects, functions, and has a low repair record). Health care is not different in that quality also focuses on materials, people, and processes; however, the end product or service is often much more difficult to quantify than a physical product.[11] Differences in diseases, treatments, facilities, and health providers, all impact the level of quality. More importantly, differences in patients, their expectations, and their response to a given therapy significantly influence the perception of quality. Unlike the industrial sector, health care is also hampered by the complexity of its health systems and payer structure. While an automobile manufacturer may recognize the need to improve quality and can call on all of its employees to contribute to obtain the desired goal, health care has many autonomous practitioners seeking to meet the expectation of quality of numerous institutions, governmental agencies, third-party payers, and patients.

Problems associated with quality in health care fall into one of three categories: overuse, underuse, and misuse.[12] Overuse occurs when a service is provided, but is not needed, and thus the risk of harm from that service outweighs the potential benefit. Underuse results when a needed service is unavailable or not provided. Misuse occurs when the correct service is provided so poorly that the full benefit is not seen. In the past, health care addressed these problems through quality assurance techniques. Traditionally, a committee or group would identify a standard that was thought to reflect quality (e.g., infection rate after surgery, cart fill errors, and readmission rates) and would establish an acceptable threshold for performance of that standard. A review of the performance of a particular group or individual would be compared against the standard and some corrective action taken if variations existed. Often, such programs had a limited effect on quality and were perceived as punitive or judgmental. In an effort to avoid the drawbacks of quality assurance techniques, many health care practices are employing the principles of TQM. However, utilizing these techniques is difficult work and is still facing many barriers in the health care setting.

Many health practitioners take an isolated view of their role in providing care and do not consider how their actions and processes affect others involved in the care of the patient. For example, the pharmacy may only focus on decreasing the number of missing doses by getting the right drug into the right medication drawer; whereas, it may be more appropriate to assist nursing in improving the documentation on the medication administration record to achieve the same goal. Additionally, a physician may view the delay of medication delivery as a quality issue among pharmacy and nursing, and not address the role that his or her illegible handwriting contributes to the process. This compartmentalized (or departmentalized) view is a barrier to quality in many health care systems and has unfortunately become entrenched in many practices.[9] The classic battle between pharmacy and nursing over missing doses is an excellent example of a systems breakdown. While it is easier to blame nursing for misplacing the dose or pharmacy for not sending the dose, it is more effective to apply the principles of TQM and systematically identify those process problems that contribute to poor quality (i.e., missing dose). The role of the pharmacist in TQM process is varied and determined by their role within the department and the institution. Most importantly, pharmacists must be willing to work within multidisciplinary groups and serve as leaders in identifying barriers to quality within pharmacy processes as well as in other processes that impact patient care.

The process of quality improvement must involve all practitioners involved in the aspect of care under assessment.[8,13] Within health care organizations, quality improvement functions are often coordinated through the pharmacy and therapeutics (P&T) committee or other similar multidisciplinary groups. The approach to quality improvement varies among organizations and is often specific to the opportunities for improvement identified. The section discussing MUE outlines an example of how quality improvement activities can be conducted. Regardless of the process involved, there are some aspects of multidisciplinary group dynamics that are important to consider.

Working within multidisciplinary groups can pose significant challenges. Busy schedules, politics, and poor communication and planning can contribute to dysfunction. Often, physicians or other health practitioners are left out of quality improvement initiatives for a variety of reasons. Perceptions of aloofness or disinterest, fear of reprisal or admission of guilt, or previous conflicts may result in the exclusion of individuals or groups that are essential to the quality improvement process. Likewise, it is important when interfacing with a group charged with resolving quality issues that one goes about the process with an open mind. Understand where your current practices may provide a barrier to others and how you can change those practices without creating barriers for yourself. All groups or individuals involved in the process should be included as early as possible, preferably from the beginning.[14] One of the single greatest barriers to effective quality improvement is the addition of a new group or individuals once work has begun. This not only delays the process, but is likely to leave that group feeling slighted and likely to be less cooperative.

Leadership is one of the most important aspects of a successful quality management initiative.[14] Most people can recall a committee that has seemingly met forever, always covering the same ground, and seldom reaching closure on any issues. Strong leadership is essential to help keep working groups focused on the task at hand. It is important to establish which systems are contributing to the majority of problems and address only those that will have the biggest impact. It is of little benefit to expend a great deal of time and resources on a process that contributes little to the resolution of the problem. Establishing clear goals, a timeline for completing tasks, and routine follow-up on progress will facilitate involvement and assist in bringing closure and documenting results. Although strong leadership is needed to facilitate any large working group, such as a committee or quality improvement team, the leadership of that group should not override the group's ideas or present an accusatory or punitive image.[1,8,12,14] It is important that all involved with quality initiative feel free to speak their minds and contribute to the process. The approach to developing and implementing a successful quality management program is varied and complex; however, some time-tested approaches, such as FOCUS-PDCA, SMART, and the Ten-step method, can be employed. Appendix 16–3 defines and outlines the key components of these quality management tools.

The application of quality management techniques in health care is not very different than in other industries. Strong leadership, an open mind, willingness to put past differences or processes behind, and, most importantly, a willingness to improve the existing system are required to assure that quality goals are met. Often, it is most beneficial to examine programs or processes that work well and determine what makes them successful. Flow charts are useful in describing a process and can illustrate how a system is designed to work well. An example of a flow chart appears in Appendix 16–2. Applying these successes to processes that need improvement (e.g., problematic or high-risk processes) will often result in additional successes while making the most efficient use of time and resources. Determining the expectation of quality can often be the largest challenge facing a quality improvement initiative.

For this reason, many national organizations and accrediting bodies have set forth to establish benchmarks for quality in health care. This will be discussed in the next section.

QUALITY AND JCAHO

Undoubtedly, the single most influential group directing quality improvement in the health system setting is the JCAHO, (<<http://www.jcaho.org>>). Established in 1951 as the Joint Commission on the Accreditation of Hospitals, the JCAHO has been a leader in assessing and promoting quality in the health care setting.[15] The JCAHO currently oversees the accreditation of more than 5000 hospitals and 15,000 health care organizations including laboratories, home-care organizations, long-term care organizations, behavioral health organizations, and integrated health systems.[15] Accreditation by the JCAHO is an important component in maintaining eligibility for reimbursement from Medicare and Medicaid and often serves as a means for comparison to similar health systems. The importance of the JCAHO accreditation to many health systems is so great that a significant amount of resources are committed on an ongoing basis to meet their standards.

Prior to the early 1990s, the JCAHO took a fairly standard stance on quality in the health care setting. The JCAHO standards were divided into departmental areas, outlining the roles of those departments and the quality measures that should be expected from activities governed by those departments.[15] This departmental approach to quality focused more on function than outcome and did not meet the needs of modern health systems that were looking to improve quality and contain costs. As a result, the JCAHO initiated its *Agenda for Change* in 1986, shifting the focus of quality away from departments and departmental roles to process-oriented quality.[16] For example, there were no longer standards for pharmacy or specific mention of P&T committees, drug use evaluation (DUE), or formulary management in the current standards. However, traditional activities that pharmacy had been closely associated with were now contained in other standards.[15] This initiative was designed to remove the responsibility of a particular activity away from a particular group or department, and increase the responsibility of all practitioners within the system for all aspects of patient care. The *Agenda for Change* reflected the shift from quality assurance to TQM and CQI.

In 1999, the JCAHO continued the evolution of their accreditation services toward CQI by reexamining the entire accreditation process. This reevaluation culminated with the launch of *Shared Visions—New Pathways* in January 2004. Shared Visions represents a radical restructuring of the JCAHO accreditation process and involves all components including application, standards, survey methodology, scoring, and follow-up. The goal of the restructuring is to move the accreditation process from a score-driven survey that is conducted once every 3 years to a continuous, systematic, quality-focused process. As such, many of the standards used in previous accreditation manuals still exist; however, they have been reorganized and more clearly defined. Additionally, many of the old methodologies for the survey process and scoring have been abandoned, and new methodologies and requirements implemented. While these changes may initially produce a significant degree of stress and anxiety for health system administrators and staff, the goal of these changes is to improve the consistency, objectivity, and quality of the accreditation process and hopefully improve the quality of health care. While this chapter will attempt to summarize the changes in the JCAHO accreditation process, many of the changes are detailed and beyond the scope of this reference. As such, the reader is advised to consult the appropriate JCAHO Accreditation Manual or the JCAHO website (<<www.jcaho.org>>) for additional information.

The sweeping natures of the JCAHO's reforms are best understood if divided into the various components of the accreditation process. As such, a description of the changes as they apply to the JCAHO standards, application process, the on-site survey process, performance measurement, periodic performance review (PPR), quality reports, and scoring will be discussed.

STANDARDS

The heart of the JCAHO accreditation process is the standards. Like all other components of the accreditation process, and perhaps to a larger degree, the standards for 2004 have been significantly restructured and heavily scrutinized. While many of the standards remain unchanged from previous years, their definition, organization, interpretation, and scoring have been significantly altered. As the first phase of the Shared Visions initiative, the JCAHO created a multidisciplinary Standards Review Taskforce to reevaluate all of the standards for ambulatory care, behavioral health care, home care, hospital, laboratory, and long-term care programs. This task force was comprised of many leaders in health care, including quality directors, nurses, physicians, pharmacists, risk managers, CEOs, COOs, and the Joint Commission staff. The task force was charged with many goals relating to the standards including eliminating redundant requirements between the standards for different programs, improving the clarity of the standards, focusing standards on patient safety and quality of care, and reducing paperwork and documentation to name just a few. As a result of this review, the most notable change is the creation of two new chapters of standards. The chapter entitled Provision of Care, Treatment and Services encompasses many of the standards previously listed in the Assessment, Care of Patients, Education, and Continuum of Care chapters. More significantly for pharmacists, an entire new chapter entitled Medication Management has been included. This chapter includes many of the medication-related standards previously included in the Care of Patients chapter, but has been expanded and clarified with a clear focus on patient safety and quality of care as it relates to the management of medications.

Because the JCAHO understands that not all barriers to quality are shared among health systems and that there is no one way to affect changes in quality, there are few specific mandates to be found in the revised standards. Unlike previous version of the standards, the

JCAHO has made a greater effort to clarify the intent of the each standard and eliminate some of the variation in interpreting the standards. Nonetheless, the specific system for defining, assessing, and documenting quality is still left to be established by each institution or health system. As in the past, the revised JCAHO accreditation standards are divided into three main sections, further subdivided into chapters relating to aspects of organizational activity.[17] Within these chapters, the specific standards are detailed. The sections and chapters as well as a description of the goals of each chapter are provided below.

PATIENT-FOCUSED CARE

- *Ethics, Rights and Responsibilities (RI)*: This chapter outlines the institution's role in recognizing the patient's rights and special needs. Included are standards that outline the provision of care while maintaining the dignity and autonomy of the patient, and involving family and other caregivers.
- *Provision of Care, Treatment, and Services (PC)*: The chapter, covering provision of care, outlines how the delivery of care should be coordinated from inpatient to outpatient, and is based on assessments of risk and benefit of continuing care or providing additional care.
- *Medication Management (MM)*: This chapter is the most important for most health system-based pharmacists. It addresses all aspects of the provision of, through the use of, pharmaceuticals including procurement, storage, ordering and transcribing, preparing and dispensing, administration, and monitoring.
- *Surveillance, Prevention, and Control of Infection (IC)*: This chapter specifically addresses the standards for reducing the occurrence of hospital-acquired infections.

ORGANIZATION-FOCUSED FUNCTIONS

- *Improving Organization Performance (PI)*: This chapter outlines the performance-improvement goals that the health system should strive to achieve. In recent years, this chapter has focused more on patient safety and reducing system failures.
- *Leadership (LD)*: This chapter outlines the institutional leadership's responsibilities to ensure that the organization strives to improve its services and has the appropriate resources (people, equipment, and processes) to affect those improvements.
- *Management of the Environment of Care (EC)*: The standards in this chapter largely address the safety and functionality of the work place with a focus on producing an environment that is safe for the employee and the patient.
- *Management of Human Resources (HR)*: Standards in this chapter address the qualifications and competencies of the employees and others who provide services to the health system.

- *Management of Information* (*IM*): This chapter addresses the use, storage, and distribution of information. While the chapter addresses many aspects of modern health care computerized technology, most of the standards contained in this chapter apply equally as well to paper documentation.

STRUCTURES WITH FUNCTIONS

- *Medical Staff* (*MS*): This chapter specifically conveys that the medical staff has an essential role in the oversight of the provision and quality of care, and is designed to ensure that decisions about patient care are made by clinicians on the patients' behalf, rather than business personnel.
- *Nursing* (*NR*): This chapter covers the role of nursing leadership in the provision of care, including nursing practice standards.

MEDICATION MANAGEMENT STANDARDS

Because of the impact that the creation of the Medication Management standards will likely have on pharmacists and pharmacy practice, it is worth exploring these standards in greater detail. Currently, there are 21 standards within the Medication Management chapter. These standards cover all aspects of medication management from the initial selection of agents to be included on the formulary, through patient administration and monitoring for clinical effects and adverse events. It is important to note that the JCAHO has established a definition of medication as it relates to the standards. This definition of medications includes not only traditional pharmaceutical agents (i.e., prescription and over-the-counter medications), but herbal remedies, vitamins, nutraceuticals, vaccines, diagnostic/radiologic agents, blood derivatives, intravenous solutions, and parenteral nutrition. Not included in this definition are enteral nutrition products, oxygen, or other medical gases.

The implication of this definition is that all of the Medication Management standards apply to these agents, including aspects such as procurement, ordering, dispensing, administration, and monitoring. As such, it will be crucial for health systems to include these agents in existing policies governing medications or to create separate policies for these agents. As with traditional pharmaceutical agents, it will be the JCAHO's expectation that quality improvement initiatives will include all medications routinely used at the institution. This may pose a challenge for some organizations as it relates to the use of herbal remedies and nutraceuticals where clinical evidence is still somewhat sparse.

For each standard, the JCAHO provides a definition and a list of elements of performance (EP). The EPs are those functions against which the organization must conduct a self-assessment and, ultimately, will be gauged by the Joint Commission at the time of the on-site survey.[18] The EPs are divided into three categories: A, B, and C. By way of definition, Medication

Management standard MM 1.10 will be used as an example. This standard is defined as "patient-specific information is readily accessible to those involved in the medication management system." Category A EPs are those related to structural requirements, such as policies or procedures. These EPs either exist or do not exist within the institution and are scored as such. A Category A EP for standard MM 1.10 is that "A written policy describes the minimum amount of information about the patient that is to be available to those involved in medication management." Category B EPs also have a structural component, but contain some qualitative aspect in addition, usually with several components. Scores within these EPs can be either compliant or noncompliant. A Category B EP would include additional qualitative information. In this case, it would include the type(s) of patient information that should be readily accessible (i.e., the patient's age, sex, current diagnosis, current medications, relevant laboratory values, allergies and sensitivities, weight and height, pregnancy and lactation status, and any other information the organization may require). Category C EPs are scored based on the number of times the organization is not compliant with the EP. A Category C EP for this standard would be "The information is accessible when needed." Each time the JCAHO finds instances where the information is *not* accessible when needed, they would score against this element. For this example, one can summarize the EPs as "does your organization have a policy for the availability of patient information?" (Category A); "does that policy contain the correct components?" (Category B); and "does your organization adhere to the policy?" (Category C). Additional information about the EPs and their associated scoring can be found at the JCAHO website (<<www.jcaho.org>>).

The Role of the JCAHO's Standards in Institutional Quality Improvement

The JCAHO utilizes the standards and scoring methods outlined above to conduct their triennial on-site survey. This survey, in conjunction with the PPR, is used to establish benchmarks of performance for a specific institution and is an integral step in the evolution of the JCAHO accreditation as it relates to quality improvement. PPR is a process by which the institution submits performance data to the JCAHO on an ongoing basis to establish internal benchmarks of the institution's compliance with the JCAHO standards and National Patient Safety Goals. Historically, the JCAHO conducted surveys of institutions on a triennial basis, with very little follow-up occurring between survey periods. The result was a lack of CQI as most institutions focused on achieving a high score during the on-site survey. Although the JCAHO will continue to conduct triennial on-site surveys, the PPR will provide a mechanism for assessing the institution's compliance with the standards and improving areas of noncompliance at a midpoint in the accreditation cycle. The benchmarks established as part of PPR are not only intended to be used by the institution as an internal measure of their performance, but also as an external measure as they relate to similar institutions. This benchmarking process assists the institution in establishing goals and, through the routine collection and submission of performance data to the JCAHO, move toward improving services.

ORYX Core Measures

In 1997, the JCAHO developed a system by which to assess the level of performance improvement a health system has achieved and to compare that to a national benchmark. This initiative is known as ORYX® and it has been called the "next evolution in accreditation." The ORYX® initiative was introduced by the JCAHO to mandate the use of performance measurement tools to monitor outcomes and to integrate these data into the accreditation process.[19] The goal of ORYX® is to establish a data-driven survey that compliments the accreditation process, allowing institutions to use their own performance data in comparison to national benchmarks to ultimately improve care.

In 1997, the JCAHO mandated that all hospitals and home care organizations that were currently being accredited by the JCAHO identify, by the end of 1998, the performance measurement system they would use to report performance-improvement data.[19,20] A performance measurement system is an automated database that is used to assist an institution or organization in collecting and disseminating performance-improvement data. Not only must the performance measurement system allow the institution to conduct internal evaluation and comparison of performance, but must also be available to compare the performance against other institutions. All performance measurement systems must first be approved by the JCAHO prior to the institution using that system for accreditation purposes. The JCAHO had contracted with more than 60 different vendors of performance measurement systems, including the JCAHO's own Indicator Monitoring System (IMS). Each institution being surveyed must select core measures for assessment of performance. These measures may include areas of performance, such as the number of surgical infections or the management of myocardial infarction patients. For hospitals, the core measures selected were to reflect the types of health care services it provided. Performance measurement systems provide a format by which organizations can collect and report data and compare their performance to similar organizations. On July 1, 2002, accredited hospitals were required to begin collecting data on two standardized core measures from the four sets of measures approved by the JCAHO: acute myocardial infarction, heart failure, community-acquired pneumonia, and pregnancy and related conditions. For each measure selected, the institution must demonstrate the ability to reliably collect, analyze, and interpret data and design performance-improvement systems to address any issues identified through the process. Examples of the measures of myocardial infarction performance include the time to treat the patient from entry into the hospital and the appropriateness of pharmacologic agents used for treatment. The institution must be able to consistently and uniformly collect and analyze the data. While the JCAHO does not provide specific instructions on how an institution is to address any deficiencies it may find through this process, it expects that multidisciplinary groups will employ the principles of TQM to improve performance on this measure.

Beginning in 2004, the JCAHO mandated that hospitals begin gathering data on a third core measure. The expanded core measurement requirements allow hospitals to satisfy

JCAHO requirement to participate in the Quality Initiative: A Public Resource on Hospital Performance. The quality initiative is led by several large national organizations including the American Hospital Association, the Federation of American Hospitals, and the Association of American Medical Colleges, and has the support of the JCAHO and the Centers for Medicare and Medicaid Services. This initiative is designed to collect and compare performance-related measures among the participating institutions and to provide the public with meaningful performance-based information. As such, the public will be able to make more informed decisions about the quality of health care provided by a given institution and create a competitive environment that will foster additional performance improvement. In addition to the currently approved core measures, JCAHO is developing additional hospital core measures including surgical infection prevention, ICU care, pain management, and asthma care for children. Also, JCAHO has plans to develop core measures for other accredited programs including home care, behavioral health, and long-term care.

Initially, the JCAHO was flexible in allowing institutions to use a wide variety of quality measurement tools to satisfy the needs of ORYX®. Quality management initiatives such as the Maryland Hospital Association's Quality Indicator Project and others met the requirements for quality data collection outlined by the JCAHO.[21] The Maryland Hospital Association's Quality Indicator Project is a statewide system developed to measure and compare outcomes data in acute care hospitals. Many of the measures in this system have been previously mentioned (e.g., perioperative mortality and Caesarian section rates). However, the multitude of different quality measurement tools and indicators now being employed has made the development of a national benchmarking database nearly impossible. To this end, the JCAHO has developed core indicators to collect data on specific aspects of care related to specific disease states (e.g., patients with congestive heart failure and low left ventricular ejection fraction prescribed an angiotensin-converting enzyme inhibitor at discharge) or health system activities (e.g., timing of prophylactic antibiotic administration during surgery). Use of these indicators would increase the number of institutions collecting data on a particular indicator. In turn, this would increase the data pool size and be used to develop national benchmarks. More detailed information about the specific core measures can be obtained from the JCAHO (<<www.jcaho.org>>).

QUALITY AND MANAGED CARE

The increasing role of managed care in the United States has created the need to assess the quality of care provided by these organizations. Depending on who is providing the analysis, Health Maintenance Organizations (HMOs) either represent the best or worst quality that health care has to offer.[22] The focus of quality improvement as it relates to managed care has not always been on the quality of the care provided and the related patient outcomes, but rather a function of financial considerations (e.g., co-pays and the extent to which services are covered) and the provider network (i.e., which physicians or institutions participate in the plan). That is to say, quality managed care providers were those that offered the best co-pays or greatest flexibility for physician selection and not necessarily those that provided the best care to their patients. As a result, selecting a quality-managed care provider, whether as an employer or an individual, can be confusing at the very least.

As the number of individuals enrolled in managed health plans continued to grow throughout the 1980s and 1990s, several staff- and group-model HMOs recognized the need to collect and report quality measurement data among managed care providers.[23-25] To this end, the NCQA was formed in 1990.[23] The NCQA (<<http://www.ncqa.org/>>) is a nonprofit organization dedicated to assessing and reporting on the quality of managed care plans. The NCQA assesses the quality of managed care in three different ways. The first is to survey and accredit managed care organizations much like the JCAHO accredits hospitals.[23] The NCQA also manages the Health Plan Employer Data and Information Sets (HEDIS) performance measures for the managed care community. The HEDIS is a series of performance measures that allows consumers of managed care to compare managed care organizations. Lastly, the NCQA conducts national member satisfaction surveys. The mission of the NCQA is "to provide information that enables purchasers and consumers of managed health care to distinguish among plans based on quality, thereby allowing them to make more informed health care decisions."[23] Since its first survey in 1991, the NCQA has been refining its performance measurement and survey/accreditation process and has grown steadily. Approximately 50% of the HMOs in the United States are currently accredited by the NCQA accreditation process, since it is not a requirement for their operation, and many more use the HEDIS measurement indicators.

Accreditation from the NCQA is a vigorous and voluntary process that includes both on-site and off-site surveys. The NCQA compares managed care organizations by use of the HEDIS performance measures. These measures cover several domains or aspects of care provided by the managed care provider and within these domains there are over 60 NCQA standards that must be met.[23] The standards within each domain more specifically identify therapeutic or service issues or activities that will be measured for performance. The current HEDIS performance domains are the following:

- *Effectiveness of Care*: This domain includes such measures as childhood immunizations, breast cancer screening, and beta-blocker treatment after myocardial infarction to name only a few.
- *Access/Availability of Care*: This domain includes measures such as adult's access to preventative/ambulatory health services, prenatal and postpartum care, and claim timeliness.
- *Satisfaction with the Experience of Care*: This includes standardized customer satisfaction surveys conducted by the NCQA.

- *Health Plan Stability*: Addresses aspects of managed care such as practitioner turnover and years in business.
- *Use of Services*: These measures evaluate how managed care resources are utilized, including such examples as frequency of ongoing prenatal care, well-child visits, inpatient utilization, and mental health utilization.
- *Health Plan Descriptive Information*: These measures evaluate the quantitative or qualitative features of the plan, such as board certification, total enrollment, cultural diversity of membership, and others.

The HEDIS measures are used to compare managed health care plans.[23-25] Since its inception in 1992, the HEDIS has been regularly updated to include new advancements in medical practice and changes in the standard of care. Data from the HEDIS are included into the NCQA's Quality Compass, a large, national database of NCQA accreditation and HEDIS data. These data are made available to the consumer public for use as a comparison between managed care providers. The intent of the HEDIS was to allow consumers, either individuals or corporate purchasers of health care plans, to compare the performance of a managed care organization on many aspects of the service they provide including everything from quality of care to access of care. For example, using HEDIS data, consumers could compare the frequency and availability of mammograms provided by the managed care organization or the number of patients who have had a myocardial infarction who were treated with appropriate pharmacotherapy. In recent years, however, the number of managed care providers opting to allow the NCQA to release their HEDIS data to the public has decreased.[26,27] A review of HEDIS data has shown that the level of quality is lower among those managed care providers that elect not to release their HEDIS data than for those managed care plans that do.[22,26-28] It has been speculated that without other incentives to participate, poorer performing managed care organizations have little reason to want their HEDIS data disclosed. This change in the willingness to make the HEDIS data publicly available has concerned some in the industry who feel this may be the only system for measuring the quality of managed care providers. The managed care plans who have restricted access to their data point out that the HEDIS system does not take into account the poor quality of documentation that often occurs in physician-based practices.

For 2005, the latest release of HEDIS includes new specific drug use performance measures.[23] New measures include disease-modifying antirheumatic drug (DMARD) therapy in rheumatoid arthritis and persistence of beta-blocker therapy after a heart attack. Other new measures including physical activity in older adults, glaucoma screening in older adults, and the use of imaging studies for low back pain are also included. Likewise, some measures are no longer used, including utilization of maternity services measures and the management of menopause survey. In general, none of the measures address the impact or role of pharmacy in improving performance related to these measures; however, the pharmacist's role in meeting the HEDIS requirements should include development of performance criteria, assessment and analysis of data, and involvement in institutional performance-improvement initiatives.

The ultimate impact of the NCQA and the HEDIS performance-monitoring program has yet to be determined; however, it is reasonable to assume that as the number of patients receiving their health care through managed care providers increases and competitive market forces demand higher quality service for the dollar, accreditation and benchmarking data such as HEDIS will become increasingly important in the selection process for care providers, provided, of course, that such information is routinely available to the consumer public.

Drug Regimen Review and Drug Use Review

The next section of this chapter discusses MUE and will include examples of quality improvement activities occurring as part of the MUE process. Although MUE is generally conducted in organized health systems, two other processes with similar names, drug regimen review (DRR) and drug use review (DUR), focus on therapy provided within nursing facilities and for outpatients. DRR is a requirement of the Health Care Financing Administration (HCFA), mandating pharmacist review of drug regimens for patients in nursing facilities. The intent of the regulation requiring DRR is to assure that the drug therapy provided for each resident is reviewed monthly and that pharmacists are making appropriate recommendations to health care professionals to improve drug therapy. This requirement was implemented in 1974 through Medicare (Title XVIII) and Medicaid (Title XIX) regulations and was expanded in 1987 to include intermediate care nursing facilities.[29,30]

The Medicare Catastrophic Coverage Act of 1988 required an assessment of medication prescribing in outpatient settings. It was rescinded in early 1990. The Medicaid Anti-Discriminatory Drug Price and Patient Benefit Restoration Act (Pryor II), enacted in 1990, includes similar requirements. This bill mandates prospective and retrospective assessment of medication prescribing and utilization, and requires that each state establish educational outreach programs for outpatient pharmacy services. The intent of this provision is to assure that prescription drugs are "appropriate, medically necessary, and not likely to result in adverse medical results." This legislation requires that drug utilization review (DUR) programs be designed to educate physicians and pharmacists in identifying and reducing the frequency and patterns of fraud, abuse, gross overuse, or inappropriate or medically unnecessary care. Claims data are used as the primary source of information. Although the Act did not specify the mechanism for education of health care professionals, the intent was that an assessment of prescribing patterns and patient medication compliance be used to reduce unnecessary or inappropriate medication use. Over time, the term DUR had also been adopted to describe an early version of what was referred to as DUE and that has now evolved into a broader process referred to as MUE. These latter processes are largely employed in acute care settings and, unlike DUR, compare actual medication use to evidence-based standards adopted by the specific organization. These processes are further compared and contrasted within the following section. Long-term care facilities meeting the DRR requirements of the Department of Health and Human Services are exempt from the provision requiring DUR.[29–33]

MEDICATION USE EVALUATION

MUE is the component of a health care organization's quality improvement program that should examine all aspects of medication use and most often requires direct involvement of pharmacists.[34,35] MUE uses definitions of safe and effective use of medications to assess the quality of medication use within the organization. These definitions are usually described as criteria and are endorsed by the organization within which they are to be applied. The manner in which medications are used, administered, and monitored within the organization is compared to the criteria to determine if actual practice matches the best (or at least acceptable) practice as stated with the criteria. Endorsement is usually provided by a multidisciplinary group that includes medical staff. The goal of MUE is to provide all patients with the most rational, safe, and effective drug therapy through the assessment and improvement of specific medication use processes. MUE may focus on a specific medication (e.g., alteplase), a class of medications (e.g., thrombolytics), medications used in the management of a specific disease state or clinical setting (e.g., thrombolytics in acute myocardial infarction), medications related to a clinical event (e.g., drug therapy within the first 24 hours for patients admitted with acute myocardial infarction including aspirin, beta-blockers, thrombolytics, and so forth), a specific component of the medication use process (e.g., time from admission to administration of thrombolytic), or can be based on specific outcomes (e.g., vessel patency following thrombolytic administration). MUE is not designed to address "if-then" questions (such as if one dose is used instead of another will outcomes be effected) but simply determines if the actual use of a medication is consistent with the standards established within the criteria. This important function is required by the JCAHO performance-improvement standards. Unfortunately, the standards related to MUE remain among the most challenging for many institutions. Lack of resources or authority, politics, difficulty in identifying issues (e.g., high-use, high-risk, or problematic medications or processes) or in acting on data to improve performance, and cumbersome or ineffective reporting structure or processes can all contribute to ineffective MUE programs.

THE MEDICATION USE PROCESS

In 1989, a multidisciplinary task force was organized by the JCAHO to describe the medication use process as a component of their effort to develop tools to assess medication use.

The original definition of the medication use process included prescribing, dispensing, administration, monitoring, and systems and management control (see Table 16–1). This description serves as the basis for contemporary MUE. [36,37] Medication acquisition, storage, distribution, and disposal may also be assessed if pertinent.

It is important to note that this description outlines a process more multidisciplinary than the categories might imply. For example, while the prescribing category may imply a physician function, pharmacists are often involved as they assist in drug selection and individualization of the therapeutic regimen.

MEDICATION USE EVALUATION AND THE JCAHO

The terminology used to describe MUE has changed over time and can be confusing. MUE, DUE, DUR, and AUR (antibiotic use review) are often used interchangeably, but are different in their approach and application. This section will attempt to provide some background as to how these terms developed and changed over time. Table 16–2 summarizes several key events in the development of MUE as it relates to the JCAHO and governmental activities in the United States.[29,30,38,39]

Table 16–3 compares several of the acronyms applied to the evaluation of medications. The process has evolved from a retrospective evaluation of prescribing to a thorough assessment of how a medication is used and its effects monitored within patient care provided throughout an organization. The focus has expanded from simply identifying issues to seeking systematic resolution to the issues identified and assessing the impact of these efforts to assure that the use of the medication has improved. One of the first calls for a process to evaluate the use of

TABLE 16–1. DESCRIPTION OF THE MEDICATION USE PROCESS

Prescribing	Assessing the need for/selecting the correct drug
	Individualizing the therapeutic regimen
	Designing the desired therapeutic response
Dispensing	Reviewing the order for correctness of dosing and indication for use
	Processing the order
	Compounding/preparing the drug
	Dispensing the drug in a timely manner
Administering	Administering the right medication to the right patient
	Administering the medication when indicated
	Informing the patient about the medication
	Including the patient in administration
Monitoring	Monitoring and documenting the patient's response
	Identifying and reporting adverse drug reactions
	Reevaluating the drug selection, drug regimen, frequency, and duration
Systems/management control	Collaborating and communicating among caregivers
	Reviewing and managing the patient's complete therapeutic drug regimen

TABLE 16–2. SUMMARY TIMELINE: THE EVOLUTION OF MEDICATION USE EVALUATION

1969	Task Force on Prescription Drugs (Department of Health, Education, and Welfare—DHEW) Report calls for development of programs to monitor drug use
1974	HCFA regulation mandate pharmacists' monthly review of medication for all residents of skilled nursing facilities, this was later (1987) expanded to include residents of intermediate care nursing facilities
1978	Antibiotic utilization review standards included in Accreditation Manual for Hospitals
1980	Quality Assurance Standard included in Accreditation Manual for Hospitals
1986	Drug Usage Evaluation Standard included in Accreditation Manual for Hospitals Agenda for Change initiated
1987	Omnibus Budget Reconciliation Act (OBRA): required states to develop retrospective and prospective DUR programs
1994	Medication Use Evaluation Standard included in Accreditation Manual for Hospitals
1996	Indicator Monitoring System (IMS) initiated
1997	Medication Use Evaluation Standard included in PI.3.2.2 and TX.3.9 in the Accreditation Manual for Hospitals

medications appeared in the final reports of the Task Force on Prescription Drugs (United Stated Department of Health, Education, and Welfare).[38] This 1969 report called for development of programs to monitor medication use. A retrospective evaluation process referred to as DUR was suggested.

The Joint Commission on Accreditation of Hospitals (JCAH), as the JCAHO was known at the time, required antibiotic utilization review (AUR) beginning in 1978. This assessment

TABLE 16–3. ACRONYMS ASSOCIATED WITH THE EVALUATION OF MEDICATION USE

Term	Origin	Description
Drug use review (DUR)	1969 Task Force on Prescription Drugs[37]	Retrospective evaluation to monitor medication use patterns. Usually quantitative and limited to trending
	1990 Medicaid Anti-Discriminatory Drug Price and Patient Benefit Restoration Act (Pryor II)	Usually retrospective evaluation based on claims data. Results used to direct education and to reduce fraud, abuse, overuse, and inappropriate or unnecessary care
Antibiotic use review (AUR)	1978 JCAHO Standards	Retrospective evaluation of antibiotic use. Usually quantitative and limited to identifying patterns of use
Drug use evaluation (DUE)	1986 JCAHO Standards	Expansion of AUR to all drugs. Concurrent evaluation of prescribing and outcome only. Multidisciplinary involvement
Medication use evaluation (MUE)	1992 JCAHO Standards	Expansion of DUE to include all medications (e.g., vaccines and biotechnology medications) Evaluation expanded to include all aspects of medication use: prescribing, dispensing, administering, monitoring, and outcome

was largely retrospective, quantitative, and evaluated trends in antibiotic use. The JCAHO standards evolved to include other medications in the mid-1980s. The number and specific type of evaluation was not specified and patterns of drug use (vs. a qualitative evaluation of individual cases) were often the focus. The term DUR was also used during this time period to describe retrospective review of other drugs and should not be confused with the current use of DUR as discussed in the Quality and Managed Care section. The requirement was expanded to include all drug therapy and the terminology was changed to DUE in 1986. The 1986 standards implied that concurrent evaluation of drug use was required. The responsibility for this function was shared by the medical, pharmacy, nursing, and other staff (as appropriate) and was assigned to the medical staff as a P&T committee activity. The activity was to be ongoing, planned, systematic, and criteria based using current knowledge and experience. Data from these activities were also to be used in the process of medical staff reappointment and recredentialing within the organization.[39,40]

An initiative called the *Agenda for Change* was adopted by the JCAHO in 1986. [16,41] It was intended to improve standards by focusing on key functions of quality of care, to monitor the performance of health care organizations using indicators, to improve the relevance and quality of the survey process, and to enhance the accuracy and value of JCAHO accreditation. The revised process was to focus on actual performance versus the capability to perform well. Within this initiative, the JCAHO endorsed the concept of CQI and included CQI within its standards beginning in 1994. As part of this process, the *Accreditation Manual for Hospitals* (AMH) was significantly modified and much of the definition of expectations related to organization performance was deleted. Multidisciplinary involvement in the evaluation of medication use was emphasized. Eventually, the standards were moved from the Medical Staff chapter of the AMH to the Care of Patients and Performance Improvement chapters. In 1992, the terminology was also changed from Drug Use Evaluation to Medication Use Evaluation to reflect that all medications (including vaccines, biotechnology derivatives, and so forth) and all medication-related functions are included in the standard. This change broadened the scope to reflect the JCAHO's expanded reach into nonacute care settings and clarified that the process did not focus on illicit drug use. This terminology is also consistent with the medication use process as delineated by a group of practitioners who were developing medication use indicators as described in the *Agenda for Change*. Previously, the evaluation of medication use typically focused on only the prescribing and outcome components of the process. With this change, dispensing and administration were specifically included. MUE standards first appeared in the 1992 edition of the AMH and were required of all institutions beginning in 1994.

Current standards focus on quality improvement but no longer require that a specific approach be used.[17] The organization is allowed to select, based on its characteristics and structure, a performance-improvement approach (e.g., FOCUS-PDCA, SMART, and the Ten-step method) that best meets its needs and that of its patients. Appendix 16–3 briefly describes these approaches. Standards state that MUE should be a systematic, multidisciplinary process focusing on continual improvement in the medication use process and patient outcomes. The use of data for reappointment/recredentialing is still required but the emphasis is on CQI.

Priorities should be established based on:

> Effect on performance and improved patient outcomes.
> Selected high-volume, high-risk, or problem-prone processes.
> Resources and organizational priorities.

Evaluation of the use of high-cost medications is often a priority within organizations hoping to optimize use of available financial resources. However, in the past, many organizations based their topic selection solely based on cost-saving initiatives rather than on improving the quality of medication use. As a result, this category, when stated as a sole rationale for topic selection, is no longer considered to be consistent with the goals of MUE. Currently, high-cost medications continue to be a focus of evaluation, but organizations are careful to justify the evaluation based on other criteria, such as the use of the medication being problem prone or its importance in determining patient outcome.

The pharmacist plays a key role within the multidisciplinary MUE process. Although not always involved in specific initiatives, all pharmacists should actively identify opportunities for improvement in processes.[3,42] Although many pharmacists within the organization will have some role in the MUE process, those responsible for coordination and implementation of MUE initiatives are often those with drug information or quality improvement responsibilities, as well as those with specialized knowledge or experience in the component of medication use under assessment. Many of these pharmacists are self-taught using continuing education opportunities or the literature.[43] The American Society of Health-System Pharmacists (ASHP, <<http://www.ashp.org>>) has developed guidelines for pharmacists' participation in DUE and MUE.[35,44] These guidelines can serve as a resource to those developing or revising a MUE program or for practitioners new to the process.

The Medication Use Evaluation Process

Figure 16–1 outlines the process of MUE. This figure is an adaptation of the Ten-step process described by the JCAH in 1989.[45,46] The next section will follow the major steps of the process and provide examples of what occurs within each step.

Responsibility for the Medication Use Evaluation Function

The Ten-step process begins with the organization defining which group or groups will participate in and be responsible for the evaluation of medication use. These groups are the ones overseeing the process, since it has to be assumed that everyone will have to provide effort toward actually performing or implementing quality assurance activities. Although the JCAHO standards no longer assign the responsibility for MUE to the P&T committee, nor do

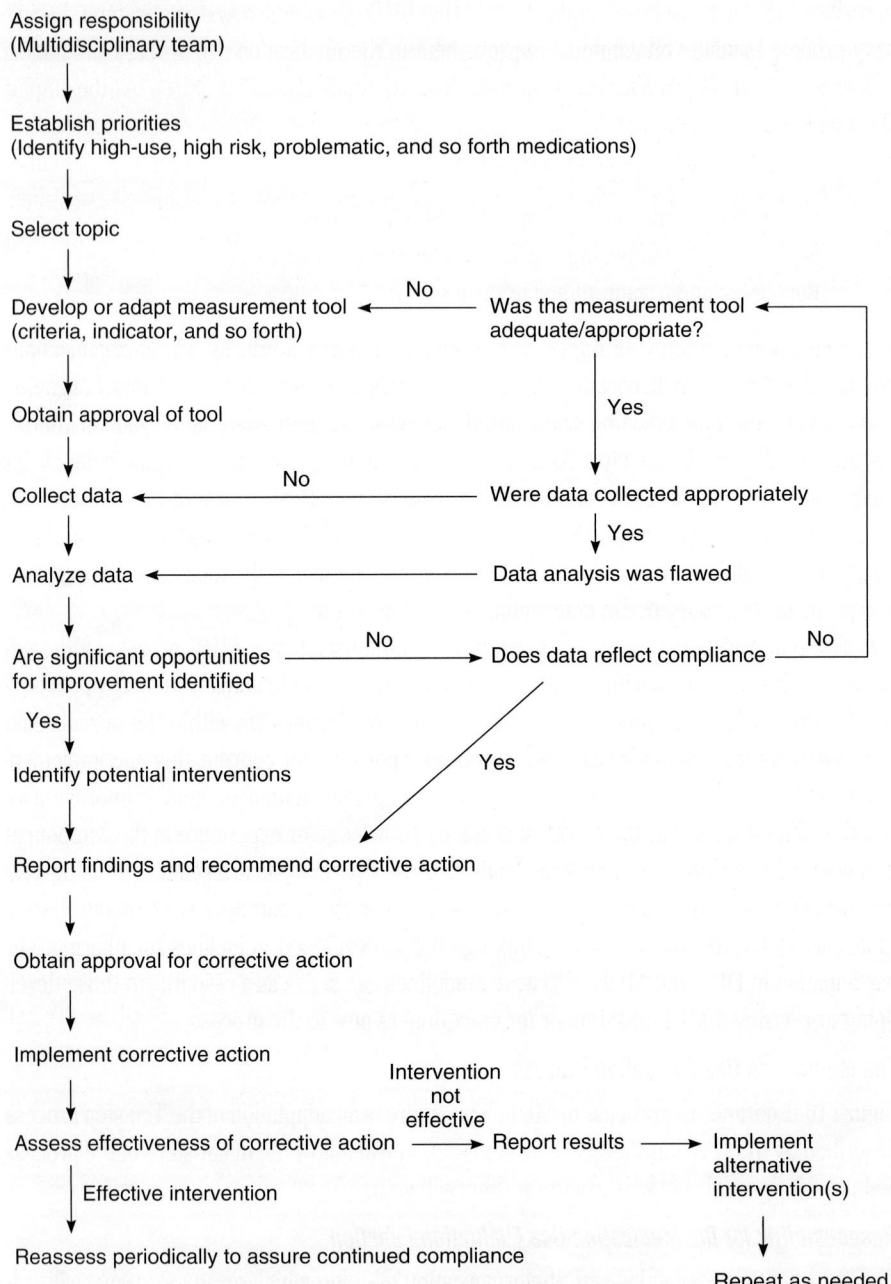

Figure 16–1. Medication use evaluation process.

they require a P&T committee at all, the function is well suited to this group as well as to a performance/quality improvement committee. Some organizations have formed a MUE subcommittee to the P&T group, while others have distributed the responsibility for MUE along patient population or product lines. A patient safety committee may also play a role in identification of topics, evaluation of findings, and implementation of corrective actions. The entire committee may participate in evaluations or working groups consisting of committee members and nonmembers may be appointed to address specific issues. The size, scope, and makeup of the health care organization and its approach to quality improvement should determine the approach to be used. The participants in the group charged with overseeing MUE must have a clear understanding that the purpose is that of improving the quality of the medication use process and that each member is expected to actively participate.[14] Newly formed groups may benefit from an overview of the organization's overall approach to quality improvement and how MUE contributes to overall goals.

Topic Selection

Topic selection should be based on the mission and scope of care of the organization and should focus on high-volume, high-risk, or problem-prone medication-related processes. Topics may also focus on institutional priorities (e.g., initiation of new clinical programs or services). Several sources of information are commonly used to identify these agents and issues. They include medication error reports, adverse drug reactions (ADRs), advances in patient care modalities that involve changes in optimal pharmacotherapy, disease- or diagnosis-based length of stay or cost outliers within an organization, purchasing reports indicating a significant increase in the use of an agent (without a related shift in patient population), medications that are a key component of a process or procedure (e.g., thrombolytics and glycoprotein 2b3a receptor inhibitors), and so forth. Many organizations emphasize antibiotics within their MUE programs. It is essential that the topics selected reflect the overall scope of medication use throughout the organization, including inpatients, outpatients, emergency care, short-stay settings, and so on.

The inclusion of specific requirements within the JCAHO's Medication Management standards related to identification and monitoring of medications described as high risk or high alert within the organization provides another mechanism to target specific medications for additional assessment. High-risk or high-alert medications are those that are most likely to result in adverse outcomes if used inappropriately or if errors are made.

Ideally, the group charged with MUE should establish an annual plan that will establish goals for new topics to be assessed and provide for follow-up on previous evaluations. Priorities should be reevaluated and the scope and breadth of recent evaluations should be assessed relative to the scope of care provided within the organization. For example, if recent MUE efforts focused primarily on issues related to antibiotic use, the plan for the upcoming year should deemphasize assessment of this class in favor of a more balanced topic selection.

The planning process can identify follow-up assessments (used to assess and document that previous efforts were successful in improving performance) that remain to be performed. The failure to perform and document these follow-up evaluations is problematic in many organizations, but is a key component of the quality improvement process. Development of an annual plan also allows an opportunity to discontinue activities that are no longer useful, such as an ongoing assessment that has demonstrated sustained improvement and can now be replaced by periodic rechecks to assure continued compliance.

Criteria, Standards, and Indicators

Criteria are statements of the activity to be measured and standards define the performance expectations. For example, criteria for the management of patients with pneumonia might state that "the first dose of antibiotic must be administered within 2 hours." The standard for this criteria statement would be set at 100% if there were no acceptable exceptions to this timeframe (see Table 16–4 and Appendix 16–4). Criteria should be based on current best, or at least accepted, practice or available organization-based clinical care plans, appropriate for the target patient population(s), and be supported by current literature. Ideally, a multidisciplinary group develops the criteria. The membership of this group (e.g., prescribers, nurses, pharmacists, respiratory therapists, social workers, clinical laboratory and information systems personnel, and discharge planners) should be determined by the nature of the process under evaluation. A flow diagram (see Appendix 16–2) outlining the process is often useful. Based on this diagram, additional disciplines should be invited to participate in the evaluation process as appropriate. Respiratory therapists, discharge coordinators, and social workers are a few of the disciplines not routinely represented as core members of medication-related committees. Inclusion of all involved disciplines initially will also facilitate implementation of corrective actions. However, criteria are most often developed by one or two of the involved disciplines and are subsequently approved by a multidisciplinary group with representation from all applicable practice groups (e.g., prescribers, pharmacists, and nurses). Explicit (objective) criteria are preferred in that they are clear cut, based on specific measurable parameters, and are better suited for automation. Implicit (subjective) criteria require that a judgment be made and require appropriate clinical

TABLE 16–4. EXAMPLES OF IMPLICIT AND EXPLICIT CRITERIA STATEMENTS

Implicit Criteria Statements	Explicit Criteria Statements
Blood work ordered	Pretreatment WBC with differential ordered and completed within 48 hours prior to the initiation of therapy
Renal function assessed routinely	Serum creatinine evaluated every 3 days
Neutropenic patients	Patients with WBC < 1000/mm^3

WBC = white blood count.

expertise to be effective. Table 16–4 compares implicit and explicit criteria statements. It is imperative that the appropriate oversight group approves the criteria prior to initiation of data collection.

Criteria should be phrased in yes/no or true/false (along with *not applicable* as appropriate) formats and should avoid interpretation on the part of data collectors. They should assess important aspects in the use of the medication or therapy under evaluation and focus on aspects most closely related to outcomes of the care provided. Definition of outcome should also be established within the criteria based on the scope of care provided within the organization. For example, in a truly acute care setting, the outcome assessment of antibiotic management of pneumonia may be limited to a decrease in clinical signs and symptoms indicating a response to therapy and the ability to be discharged on an oral antibiotic(s). However, in an integrated system that includes both acute and ambulatory or long-term care, outcome could be assessed at the conclusion of therapy.

It is helpful to consider how opportunities for improvement identified via a criteria statement could be addressed. If the corrective action would involve participation of a group not represented in the development process, it may be wise to include them in the development and assessment process. Table 16–5 outlines several questions to test the validity of criteria or indicators.[47,48]

Criteria are available from a variety of published sources.[49–59] Many group purchasing organizations and other networks have systems to facilitate sharing of MUE materials (e.g., criteria and data collection forms) and methods of comparing results with those from similar organizations. The advantages to using predeveloped criteria include prior expert review and

TABLE 16–5. TESTS OF THE VALIDITY OF CRITERIA OR INDICATORS

Face validity	Are they important to patient outcome?
	Do they assess a problematic area?
	Do they have some utility in improving patient care?
	Do they reflect system-wide performance?
	Are they appropriately based on current practice standards and literature?
External validity	Have they been thoroughly reviewed by practitioners with expertise in the use of the medication?
	Are they applicable within organization?
	Has the review process clarified and improved the criteria/indicators without weakening their intent?
Feasibility of data collection and retrieval	Are they clear and not subject to interpretation?
	Are data available?
	How many cases will need to be evaluated in order to provide adequate data?
	How difficult or complex will the data collection process be?
	What benefits will be gained vs. the effort associated with data collection?
	Will data collection methods be consistent?

assessment and time savings. However, criteria developed outside the organization must be adapted to the practice setting and patient population as appropriate and must be approved by the designated multidisciplinary group prior to data collection. For example, criteria intended for use in a general adult population may not be appropriate for geriatric patients without modification. Also, criteria may include uses of a medication not applicable to certain settings or aspects of use that are not a priority for assessment within the organization. For example, criteria for the use of benzodiazepines, including use in conscious sedation in a setting where conscious sedation is not performed or criteria related to the use of antibiotic to treat an infection when the concerns prompting the evaluation relate solely to perioperative use. Criteria may also be derived from guidelines for use developed or adopted within the organization. For example, the P&T committee may agree to add a medication to the formulary for specific indications and require that the use of the agent and patient outcomes be concurrently evaluated based on these guidelines.

Performance indicators can also be used within the MUE process. An indicator is a quantitative measure of an aspect of patient care that is used as a screening tool to detect potential problems in quality.[50,60] (Table 16–6 provides some examples of indicators.) While criteria are very focused and assess specific important components of medication use, indicators measure symptoms of a medication use system that could indicate that something is not working well. Indicators are not direct measures of quality, they simply serve as a tool to identify potentially problematic aspects of care that require more detailed assessment in order to identify the cause. Indicators can be used to monitor rate-based events (e.g., how often something does or does not occur, such as preoperative antibiotic administration within 2 hours of the first surgical incision) or sentinel events (events that occur rarely but are significant in impact, such as an adverse drug event that results in the patient's death). Indicators can assess structure, process, or outcome. Structure refers to the resources, tools, and other established attributes of the setting in which care is provided. Process refers to the activities that take place in giving and receiving care. Outcome denotes the effects of care on the health status of the patient or population. Indicators can be used as a mechanism to monitor the overall medication use

---

TABLE 16–6. EXAMPLES OF INDICATORS

Examples of indicators

  Patients >65 years old in whom creatinine clearance (CrCl) has been estimated

  Patients undergoing surgery who receive prophylactic antibiotics >2 hours before the first incision

  Frequency of pharmacy stock outages

  Frequency of discrepancies in automatic dispensing units

  Patients with a diagnosis of acute myocardial infarction that are prescribed daily aspirin therapy at discharge

  Patients with a diagnosis of congestive heart failure receiving an angiotensin-converting enzyme inhibitor

  Patients discharged on >x number of prescription medications

system, either to screen for potential problems (e.g., to assess if a more comprehensive evaluation such as a MUE is needed), or to provide an ongoing monitor to assure that performance improvement is sustained following the completion of an evaluation or intervention.[35] For example, the first indicator listed in Table 16–6 involves the estimation of creatinine clearance in patients older than 65 years of age. If an estimation of a patient's renal function is performed (e.g., if a creatinine clearance is calculated or measured) and is available to caregivers, it can be used by caregivers to adjust therapy accordingly. The availability of an estimated creatinine clearance in the medical record of patients over the age of 65 suggests that the organization is systematically taking steps to adjust drug therapy in this population based on organ function. Of course, it cannot be certain that the information is used appropriately or even if it is used at all, but as an indicator, it does provide a useful screen related to patient-specific dosage adjustments. The lack of this information related to renal function in elderly patients may indicate that the organization is not routinely making these assessments as part of their medication use system. Organizations using this indicator have taken a variety of steps to make this information available as part of the routine medication use process. Some organizations have assigned the responsibility to the clinical laboratory with estimated creatinine clearances appearing within laboratory reports. Others have assigned the responsibility to pharmacy with some organizations automating calculations and screening within the dispensing information system and others requiring that pharmacists document calculations in the medical record.

Standards are used to define optimal performance and are usually set at 0% (should never happen) or 100% (should always happen). Thresholds specifying an acceptable level of compliance or performance are usually set higher than 0% or lower than 100% based on acceptable variation, standards of practice, or benchmarks.[61] Thresholds should not be used to avoid intervention, but are sometimes used instead of standards to allow limited noncompliance with the criteria when the clinical impact of noncompliance is felt to be of low risk. Thresholds are useful when the group overseeing the MUE process is most interested in addressing performance that is clearly unacceptable, while allowing some variation from best practice. Control limits define the limits of allowable or expected variation in performance (often two to three times the standard deviation from the mean initially) and may be used to assess the results on ongoing monitoring. As long as performance remains between the upper and lower control limits, action is not necessary to address the variations that occur over time. However, performance above or below the control limits is referred to as special variation and prompts assessment as to what factor(s) resulted in the special variation and should result in actions being taken to address the impact of these factors over time. For example, within an organization training medical residents, the number of pharmacists' interventions, as documented on a control chart, might spike upward around July 1st corresponding to the start date for the new residents. While the organization may have limited opportunity to stagger starting dates, specific aspects of their orientation process could be enhanced to improve initial performance. As actions are taken to address factors resulting in special variations and the overall variability is reduced, control limits should narrow.[50] An example of a control chart with limits appears in Appendix 16–2.

Performance, as demonstrated by data collected in the quality assurance process, not meeting the defined standard or threshold or falling outside the control limits indicates that intervention to improve performance is necessary. In some cases, performance outside the defined parameters may, on review, be acceptable to the oversight group. This usually results from expectations being set too high (e.g., that the rate of adverse effects with any agent will be 0%) or when the criteria fail to include the appropriate exceptions. When this occurs, the multidisciplinary oversight group must agree that the level of performance is acceptable and that intervention is not necessary. These decisions must be clearly documented in meeting minutes or summaries of results. If this is not done, regulatory bodies may infer that the organization chose to ignore the findings of the evaluation, thus failing to meet the quality improvement requirements.

Data Collection

Prior to the initiation of data collection, the multidisciplinary oversight group must approve the topic selection, criteria, patient selection process, sample size, sampling method (e.g., all consecutive patients, intermittent sampling, and random sampling), evaluation timeframe, data collection method, and standards of performance.[35] It may be appropriate to distribute the approved criteria as an educational tool prior to data collection. Although this may address some quality issues prior to data collection and result in less dramatic results, it may support the ultimate goal of improving care and do so in a more expedient manner. In this situation, if there is a need to document the overall impact of a MUE effort, collection of baseline performance data even as criteria are being finalized and approved can provide a more accurate representation of "before" and "after." If at any point, problems are identified in the criteria or indicators or with any component of the evaluation, the issue should be brought back to the oversight group and modifications made as appropriate.

The timing of data collection can be influenced by seasonal variations in the types of care provided (e.g., increased frequency of pneumonia in the winter months), systems issues (e.g., construction, implementation of new computer systems and initiation of new services), and personnel issues (e.g., the influx of new health professional graduates and medical housestaff that occurs during the summer months and staff absences during vacation or flu seasons). The timeframe for data collection, both in duration and time of year, should also be considered in the planning process. For example, an assessment of care provided to patients with pneumonia is usually best performed during the winter months when this diagnosis is more frequent, while an assessment of the management of near-drowning may be more appropriate during the summer months. The longer the data collection period, the more likely various fluctuations in quality of care will be identified.

Retrospective data collection was used primarily in the era of AUR and DUR. This method involved reviewing the patient's medical record after discharge. It allowed data collection to be scheduled when convenient or when staff was available, but was totally dependent on documentation in the medical record. If an opportunity for improvement was identified, there was no opportunity to improve that particular patient's care—it would only help future patients.

Concurrent data collection occurs while the patient is still actively receiving the medication, but after the first dose is dispensed or administered. Data sources other than the medical record are available (e.g., staff or patient interviews) and there is an opportunity to improve patient care. Based on more complete information, results may be more complete as well as more accurate.[62] However, the need for data collection is constant and must occur within a specific timeframe, which is not always convenient. This often results in an increased number of personnel being involved in the data collection process and increased inconsistency.

Prospective evaluation occurs before the patient receives the first dose of medication and is initiated whenever an order for the medication is generated. Simple prospective evaluations can be at least partially automated and are likely to become more common. An example of this is a computerized medication system that generates a warning to the pharmacist or prescriber if the dose of a drug is outside the normal limits based on a patient's organ function. Clinical judgment must also be applied in many of these settings.

In systems with computerized prescriber order entry, the system itself can drive prescribing to comply with guidelines and standards by limiting prescribing options or directing users to specific therapy. In some cases, the system can report instances where prescribers attempt to prescribe a medication outside established limits. These limits are usually developed by the P&T committee, optimally as the agent is being considered for addition to the formulary, and fall into three general categories: diagnosis, prescriber, and medication specific. Diagnosis-based limits may define the allowable indications for use or may drive the use of an agent under a specific protocol approved by the committee. Prescriber limits may restrict the use to an agent to a specific subset of prescribers (e.g., infectious disease or critical care specialists). Medication-specific limits can designate approved dosage regimens (e.g., disallow sublingual administration of nifedipine), frequency of administration (e.g., once-daily dosing of ceftriaxone), and duration of therapy (no more than x doses or days of therapy).

Prospective evaluations that are not automated are the most cumbersome to implement because the evaluation must occur promptly every time an order is initiated to avoid therapy delays. They require that personnel be available to collect data and report results at all times and force immediate interaction between practitioners. This approach offers the greatest opportunity for intervention and education, but also increases the risk for potentially negative interactions (e.g., ranting and raving) with prescribers and other health professionals, and can result in therapy delays. Furthermore, it is essential that the interventions made as part of the prospective evaluation are documented in order to evaluate workload, effectiveness of the interventions, and that outcomes are assessed in some manner.

Limiting the number of data collectors or automating data collection is valuable in maintaining consistency. When multiple data collectors are involved, it becomes even more important to have clear, explicit criteria not subject to interpretation.

The selection of patients or cases for inclusion in the evaluation should be determined and approved by the oversight group prior to data collection. It is essential that the selection be unbiased, consistent, and representative of the care provided. Sample size should be based on size of the patient population. It has been suggested that for frequently occurring events, a sample of at least 5% of cases be used, and for events occurring less frequently, a minimum of 30 cases be assessed.[63]

The term *target drug program* is often used to refer to programs that evaluate the use of a medication or group of medications on an ongoing basis. Within these programs, interventions are usually made at the time of discovery based on established criteria or guidelines. It is important that these interventions are documented by practitioners, and are periodically assessed by the multidisciplinary oversight group in order to determine the continued need for and appropriateness of the program.

Confidentiality is a key component of all quality improvement initiatives, including MUE.[14] It is important that the entire MUE program is identified as a performance-improvement activity. This helps to assure that the information collected as part of the program is legally "protected" and/or not "discoverable." Although regulations vary from state to state (check with attorneys in your area), in most cases this means that a plaintiff's lawyer pursuant to a case cannot request MUE information, nor can this information be available for review to identify potential plaintiffs. Within the program, individual patients and practitioners should usually be identified in some manner other than their actual name in order to assure anonymous review, although it is necessary that identification data be available in cases where additional actions necessitate its use (e.g., checking charts for details and implementing corrective actions that involve discussing actions with practitioners who do something outside of the criteria). Many institutions use medical record numbers and codes assigned to individual prescribers within reports. It is also important not to inadvertently identify a practitioner. For example, if the results of an evaluation are reported by practitioner specialty (e.g., pediatrics and pediatric infectious disease) and there are only one or two practitioners in certain subspecialties, you have in essence identified the practitioner for the small subspecialty area.

Ultimately, practitioner-specific reports should be generated in most cases, as the JCAHO requires that information related to medication use be considered in the reappointment/recredentialing of medical staff. Following peer-review, the practitioner's name may be revealed only to those responsible for the reappointment/recredentialing functions. Medical department chairpersons usually carry out this function. An example of a practitioner-specific report appears in Appendix 16–5.

Data Analysis

The multidisciplinary oversight group should conduct the analysis of results. Reports should compare actual performance with expectations defined by the standards (or thresholds or control limits) established and approved prior to data collection. Performance not meeting standards (or threshold or control limits) may be considered opportunities for improvement. Alternatively, the oversight group may determine that the standards were too rigorous, that unforeseen exceptions were encountered, and/or that actual performance falls within current acceptable standards of practice. Specific corrective actions should be recommended for all identified opportunities for improvement (e.g., for all criteria statements for which the standard of performance was not met) whenever possible. The need for and nature of follow-up should also be assessed based on the frequency, prevalence, and/or severity of the issue. For example, if an evaluation of the management of pneumonia identified no issues with drug selection, but did identify an unacceptable delay in time to first dose of antibiotic (e.g., greater than 2 hours after admission), the follow-up evaluation could focus on the time to first dose and not assess antibiotic selection. Furthermore, if this issue was identified in patients admitted to a particular unit, then the follow-up could focus on assessing and documenting improvement in only that unit.

Often, a multidisciplinary group does not perform the actual data analysis. In this situation, the findings and actions must be reviewed and approved by the appropriate multidisciplinary group prior to initiation of any corrective action or distribution of the results.

Computer software programs (e.g., relational databases and spreadsheets) can be very helpful in collecting data, managing data, and reporting results.[35,64–66] Handheld devices, bar code technology, proprietary software products, and computer systems used within the organization's clinical departments can be employed as tools to assist in patient identification, data collection and analysis, and documentation.[64–67]

The report to the oversight group should contain the rationale for the topic selection, team members involved in the evaluation, a description of the patient population evaluated, any selection criteria used, a copy of the criteria/indicators, discussion of the results, identification of likely causes for opportunities identified, and recommendations for corrective action and follow-up evaluation. An example is provided in Appendix 16–6. In most settings, delineation of results on a practitioner-specific basis is not appropriate at this level. The exception would be if the practice of only a small subset of practitioners consistently fell outside the criteria. In this situation, some sort of code (e.g., physician A or physician 28) should be used instead of their actual name.

Interventions and Corrective Actions

The key to quality improvement is improving the process and, ultimately, the results, not blaming an individual or group of individuals. Steps to improve performance or avoid similar outcomes in the future fall into three categories: educational, restrictive interventions, and process changes. Educational interventions are most appropriate when knowledge deficits contribute to performance outside the criteria. They are most effective when they are directed personally, take place soon after the problem occurs, the educator is a peer or superior of the person being educated, and when the education is well supported in the literature or by practice standards.[68] One-on-one or group discussion of results, letters, newsletters, computerized order entry educational screens, protocols or guidelines, and presentation via quality improvement channels are examples of educational approaches.[69,70] Generally, educational interventions incorporated into ongoing processes (e.g., education screens in computer order entry systems) are more effective while one-time efforts (e.g., newsletters) may not have a sustained effect. In most situations, educational interventions are the most palatable.[71]

Restrictive approaches may involve special ordering procedures, compliance with guidelines for use, consultation with a specialty service, or formulary restrictions. The impact of restrictive interventions often reverses when the restrictions are removed.[72] Restrictive interventions are perhaps most effective when used to establish appropriate practice patterns when an agent is first made available for use within the organization (see Chap. 14).

Process changes incorporate the correction into routine practice. This approach may involve changes in policy or procedures, implementation of new services, acquisition of new equipment, changes in staffing, or generation of regular notifications, and so forth, when practice does not appear to meet standards.

Follow-up

Follow-up evaluation should occur within a reasonable timeframe after completion of the initial evaluation and completion of the corrective action. Follow-up is designed to assess the effectiveness of the intervention. The same criteria, standards, and sample should be used for the follow-up assessment as in the initial evaluation. Exceptions to this rule should be made if there was a problem with the initial criteria, standards, and sample; the standard of practice changes in the interim; or there is an opportunity to focus on a subset of the original data elements or patient population. For example, if issues were only found in the administration component of the use of a medication (and not in the prescribing, dispensing, or monitoring components) or only in a specific age group, follow-up evaluation could focus on these issues or populations rather than repeating the broader assessment performed initially.

MUE has been criticized as being heavy handed, non-patient-focused, and for not addressing the issue of accountability for provision of care based on a unique body of knowledge.[3] If the approach termed MUE is utilized in its true spirit, many of these challenges are addressed. MUE is a truly multidisciplinary, process-oriented approach to evaluate the quality of medication use. The process goes beyond numbers and percentages to identify opportunities for improvement and, more importantly, to improve the quality of care.

Quality in Drug Information

Quality standards for drug information practice have not been established to date and quality assessment techniques used in drug information practice vary greatly among practice sites.[73-76] Several studies have found inconsistencies in the quality of drug information practice and have called for increased emphasis on quality and the development of practice standards.[77-79] Most drug information services conduct some form of quality assessment based on the scope of service provided by that center and preestablished levels of acceptable performance. Quality assessment is usually conducted on the responses provided to drug information requests, medical literature search, and evaluation processes, availability, accuracy, and timeliness of drug information resources, and the quality of materials produced by the drug information center staff (e.g., monographs, newsletters, and continuing education programs). Although some quality assessment processes are conducted concurrently, most assessments are done retrospectively, often by randomly sampling of drug information requests, monographs, and so forth. Furthermore, assessments may be performed via peer-review or may be performed by the director of the service. Currently, no standards have been developed for this process.

Assessment of the quality of responses to drug information inquiries may include components such as timeliness, completeness and appropriateness of response, and the method of communication of the response. Additionally, aspects such as documentation of search terms, references utilized, and the availability of appropriate background or patient-specific information may also be assessed. This assessment may be carried out internally based on standards of practice at the site. This usually offers the advantage of peer-review by practitioners skilled in these functions. Another method is to poll those using the service about the quality of service and response received. This approach is hampered because consumers of the response are rarely able to assess the quality or appropriateness of the search strategy utilized to formulate the response they received in lieu of performing the search themselves or being present while the search is performed. An example assessment tool appears in Appendix 16-7. Questions that are often asked in the process of assessing drug information responses include the following:

- Is the response correct and appropriate to the situation presented?
- Is the response provided promptly?
- Does the response completely address the question posed?
- Is the response communicated appropriately?
- Are search terms and references appropriately documented?
- Is the response clear, concise, and appropriate for the clinical situation?
- If follow-up was appropriate, was it provided?

The search process itself can be assessed by evaluation of the appropriate depth and breadth of resources used, the timeliness of the resources accessed, and the search strategy. This process can also assess documentation issues, the application of literature evaluation skills to the information, and resources used by the practitioner completing the search.

Drug information practitioners are often responsible for assessing and recommending drug information resources available within the organization. These resources may include printed references such as handbooks, textbooks, or educational materials, or electronic resources such as large search engines or Internet websites. This process should assess whether the appropriate information resources are available based on the scope of care provided and expertise of the practitioners and whether the resources contain accurate and timely information that can be applied in clinical situations. Available primary, secondary, and tertiary resources should be evaluated based on established standards. The explosion of medical information on the Internet has created new challenges in evaluating drug and medical information resources. Because there are currently no regulations of content of Internet sites, caution must be used when utilizing these resources to support clinical decision-making. With the number of websites expanding faster than most practitioners can assess their content and editorial policies (if any), it has become increasingly difficult for drug information practitioners to stay abreast of those sites that offer legitimate and validated information compared to those offering only conjecture and opinion. Information obtained from other sources including manufacturer's drug information services should also be assessed (see Chaps. 6 and 7 on assessing information).

A final component of quality relates to material produced by the drug information service. This includes newsletters, drug monographs, and guidelines developed by the service. Most drug information specialists measure quality related to the accuracy, timeliness, and clinical applicability of such documents. Unfortunately, more time is often spent assessing quality of grammar and writing style than is often devoted to clinical content and interpretation. Once again, Chaps. 6 and 7 provide further information on assessing the quality of the material itself.

Conclusion

The focus of quality in health care has increased significantly in the past decade and has become a major initiative among governmental agencies and accreditation organizations. Within organizations, the emphasis has shifted from departmental efforts to multidisciplinary efforts related to key processes reflecting the move to CQI. Within this context, the role of the pharmacist in quality improvement functions related to the medication use process has expanded. A practical working knowledge of TQM principles is essential for pharmacists to contribute to and lead initiatives to improve patient care.

Study Questions

1. Describe the differences between TQM and quality assurance.

2. List at least four statistical tools used in TQM to identify barriers to quality and to improve processes.

3. Describe the role of the pharmacist in TQM programs.

4. As asked by the JCAHO, what two questions define the "Dimensions of Performance"?

5. Give two examples of clinical measures that might be used to meet ORYX® requirements.

6. List two specific drug measures included in the HEDIS 2000 quality measures.

7. Compare and contrast DRR, DUR, and MUE based on current definitions.

8. Compare and contrast retrospective, concurrent, and prospective data collection in terms of timing relative to the provision of care, personnel requirements, and accessibility of important information.

9. Give one example of each of the following: educational intervention, restrictive intervention, and process intervention.

10. List three criteria or indicators that could be used to assess the use of a problematic medication within your practice.

11. Give one example of how each of the following could be used at your practice site to assist in a quality improvement effort: a flowchart, a Pareto chart, and a control chart.

REFERENCES

1. Goldstone J. The role of quality assurance versus continuous quality improvement. J Vasc Surg. 1998;28(2):378–80.
2. Decker MD. The application of continuous quality improvement to health care. Infect Control Hosp Epidemiol. 1992;13(4):226–9.
3. Enright SM, Flagstad MS. Quality and outcome: pharmacy's professional imperative. Am J Hosp Pharm. 1991;48:1908–11.

4. Zellmer WA. Symposium: opportunity for pharmacy leadership in integrated health care systems. Am J Health Syst Pharm. 1996;53(4):3S–4S.

5. Costello RB, editor. The American Heritage College Dictionary. Boston (MA): Houghton, Mifflin Company; 1997.

6. Jablonski JR. Implementing TQM. Competing in the nineties through total quality management. 2nd ed. Albuquerque (NM): Technical Management Consortium; 1992.

7. Decker MD. Continuous quality improvement. Infect Control Hosp Epidemiol. 1992;13(2):165–9.

8. Chambers DW. TQM: the essential concepts. J Am Coll Dent. 1998;65(2):6–13.

9. Dorodny VS. Quality and caring: a fad or a religion? Hosp Pharm. 1997;32(3):316, 320, 325–6.

10. iSixSigma.com [homepage on the Internet]. Bainbridge Island (WA): iSixSigma LCC; c2000-03 [cited 2004 Aug 18]. Available from: http://www.isixsigma.com/.

11. Relman AS. Assessment and accountability. The third revolution in medical care. N Engl J Med. 1988;319(18):1220–2.

12. Chassin MR. Quality improvement nearing the 21st century: prospects and perils. Am J Med Qual. 1996;11(1):S4–S7.

13. Cohen MR. Cooperative approaches to medication error management. Top Hosp Pharm Manage. 1991;11(1):53–65.

14. Tremblay J. Creating an appropriate climate for drug use review. Am J Hosp Pharm. 1981;38(2):212–5.

15. O'Malley C. Quality measurement for health systems: accreditation and report cards. Am J Health Syst Pharm. 1997;54:1528–35.

16. Ente BH. The Joint Commission's agenda for change. Curr Concept Hosp Pharm Manage. 1989; (Summer):7–14.

17. Joint Commission on the Accreditation of Health care Organizations. Accreditation manual for hospitals. Chicago (IL): Joint Commission on Accreditation of Health care Organizations; 2004.

18. The launch of shared visions-new pathways. Jt Comm Perspect. 2004;24:1–27.

19. Joint Commission to require performance data. Am J Health Syst Pharm. 1997;54:743.

20. Andrusko-Furphy KT. Oryx and performance measurement in home care. Am J Health Syst Pharm. 1998;55:2299–301.

21. Kazandjian VA, Lawthers J, Cernak CM, Pipesh FC. Relating outcomes to care: The Maryland Hospital Association's Quality Indicator Project (QI Project®). Jt Comm J Qual Improv. 1993;19(11):530–8.

22. Himmelstein DU, Woolhandler S, Hellander I, Wolfe SM. Quality of care in investor-owned vs. not-for-profit HMOs. JAMA. 1999;282(2):159–63.

23. ncqa.org [homepage on the Internet]. Washington, DC: National Committee for Quality Assurance; c2000-04 [cited 2004 Aug 18]. Available from: http://www.ncqa.org/.

24. Cortterell CC. Pharmacy and the proposed quality measures for managed care plans. Am J Health Syst Pharm. 1996;53:2619–22.

25. Spoeri RK, Ullman R. Measuring and reporting managed care performance: lessons learned and new initiatives. Ann Intern Med. 1997;127(8 pt 2):726–32.

26. Managed care shows moderate gains, reluctance to share performance data in 1998, says NCQA. Am J Health Syst Pharm. 1998;55:2351–2.

27. Spragins EE. What are they hiding? HMOs are getting more secretive about quality. Newsweek. 1999;133(9):74.

28. McCormick D, Himmelstein DU, Woolhandler S, Wolfe SM, Bor DH. Relationship between low quality of care scores and HMO's subsequent public disclosure of quality of care scores. JAMA. 2002;288:1484–90.

29. Omnibus Budget Reconciliation Act of 1987. Section 843.60, Level A requirement; Pharmacy services. 54 FR1989:5359–69.

30. Omnibus Budget Reconciliation Act of 1990. Section 1903(I)10(B)(g) Drug Use Review and (A) Prospective Drug Review.

31. Navarro RP. DUR applications in managed care. Med Interface. 1995;8(3):67–8.

32. Briesacher D, DuChane J. Drug utilization review in the managed care environment. Med Interface. 1995;8(3):72–8.

33. Feinberg JL. Meeting the mandate for quality assurance through drug-use evaluation. Consult Pharm. 1991;6:611–20.

34. Stolar MH. Drug use review: operational definitions. Am J Hosp Pharm. 1978;35:76–8.

35. ASHP guidelines on medication-use evaluation. American Society of Health System Pharmacists. Am J Health Syst Pharm. 1996;53(16):1953–5.

36. Nadzam DM. Development of medication-use indicators by the Joint Commission on Accreditation of Health care Organizations. Am J Hosp Pharm. 1991;48:1925–30.

37. Cousins DD. Medication use: a systems approach to reducing errors. Chicago (IL): Joint Commission on Accreditation of Health care Organizations; 1998.

38. DHEW Task force on prescription drugs: final report. Washington, DC: US Department of Health, Education, and Welfare; 1969.

39. Gutshall EL, Davidson HE, Ninno SD, editors. Medication usage evaluation: primer. 3rd ed. Norfolk (VA): Insight Therapeutics, LLC; 1999.

40. Todd MW, Keith TD, Foster MT. Development and implementation of a comprehensive, criteria-based drug-use review program. Am J Hosp Pharm. 1987;44:529–35.

41. New accreditation process model for 1994 and beyond. Am J Hosp Pharm. 1993;50:1111–2, 1121.

42. Flagstad MS, Williams RB. Assuming responsibility for improving quality. Am J Hosp Pharm. 1991;48:1898.

43. Terry AK, Draugalis JR, Bootman JL. Drug-use evaluation programs in short-term-care general hospitals. Am J Hosp Pharm. 1993;50:940–4.

44. ASHP guidelines on the pharmacist's role in drug use evaluation. Am J Hosp Pharm. 1988;45:385–6.

45. The Joint Commission on Accreditation of Hospitals. 1990 AMH. Accreditation manual for hospitals. Chicago (IL): Joint Commission on Accreditation of Hospitals; 1989.

46. Covington TR, Alexander VL. Drug use evaluation: the fundamentals. Indianapolis (IN): Eli Lilly; 1991.

47. Schaff RL, Schumock GT, Nadzam DM. Development of the Joint Commission's indicators for monitoring the medication use system. Hosp Pharm. 1991;26:326–9, 350.

48. Bernstein SJ, Hilborne LH. Clinical indicators: the road to quality care? Jt Comm J Qual Improv. 1993;19(11):501–9.

49. American Society of Consultant Pharmacists. Drug regimen review: a process guide for pharmacists. 2nd ed. Arlington (VA): American Society of Consultant Pharmacists; 1992.

50. Angaran DM. Selecting, developing, and evaluating indicators. Am J Hosp Pharm. 1991;48:1931–7.

51. Beers MH, Ouslander JG, Rollingher I, Reuben DB, Brooks J, Beck JC. Explicit criteria for determining inappropriate medication use in nursing home residents. Arch Intern Med. 1991;151:1825–32.

52. Criteria for drug use evaluation. Vol 1. Bethesda (MD): American Society of Hospital Pharmacists; 1989.

53. Criteria for drug use evaluation. Vol 2. Bethesda (MD): American Society of Hospital Pharmacists; 1990.

54. Criteria for drug use evaluation. Vol 3. Bethesda (MD): American Society of Hospital Pharmacists; 1992.

55. Gutshall EL, Davidson HE, Ninno SD, editors. Drug usage evaluation: a screening criteria manual for use in concurrent drug usage evaluation. 2nd ed. Norfolk (VA): Insight Therapeutics, LLC; 1999.

56. Knapp DA. Development of criteria for drug utilization review. Clin Pharmacol Ther. 1991;50 (pt 2):600–3.

57. American Psychiatric Association. Manual of psychiatric quality assurance. A report of the American Psychiatric Association Committee on quality assurance. Washington, DC: American Psychiatric Association; 1992.

58. Model drug use review criteria. Year one of HCFA project, model for developing strategies for outpatient drug use review, Center on Drugs and Public Policy, University of Maryland at Baltimore, Baltimore (MD). 1991 Feb.

59. Screening criteria for outpatient drug use review. Final report of HCFA project, model for developing methodological strategies for outpatient drug use review, Center on Drugs and Public Policy, University of Maryland at Baltimore, Baltimore (MD). 1992 Dec.

60. Melby MJ. A mid-sized hospital's experience in indicator data collection. Am J Hosp Pharm. 1991;48:1937–40.

61. Threshold vs. standards. QRC Advis. 1988;5(2).

62. Makela EH, Davis SK, Piveral K, Miller WA, Pleasants RA, Gadsden RH, Sr, et al. Effect of data collection method on results of serum digoxin concentration audit. Am J Hosp Pharm. 1988;45:126–30.

63. What is an adequate sample? QRC Advis. 1985;1(Aug);4–5.

64. Grasela TH, Walawander CA, Kennedy, Jolson HM. Capability of hospital computer systems in performing drug-use evaluations and adverse event monitoring. Am J Hosp Pharm. 1993;50:1889–95.

65. Zarowitz BJ, Petitta A, Mlynarek M, Touchette M, Peters M, Long P, et al. Bar-code technology applied to drug-use evaluation. Am J Hosp Pharm. 1993;50:935–9.

66. Burnakis TG. Facilitating drug-use evaluation with spreadsheet software. Am J Hosp Pharm. 1989;46:84–8.

67. Libby D, Grove C, Adams M. Collaborative use of informatics among hospitals to benchmark medication use processes. Jt Comm J Qual Improv. 1997;23:626–52.

68. Soumerai SB, McLaughlin TJ, Avorn J. Improving drug prescribing in primary care: a critical analysis of the experimental literature. Milbank Q. 1989;67:268–317.

69. Avorn J, Soumeri SB, Taylor W. Reduction of incorrect antibiotic prescribing through a structured educational order form. Arch Intern Med. 1991;151:1825–32.

70. Kowalsky SF, Echols RM, Peck F. Preprinted order sheet to enhance antibiotic prescribing and surveillance. Am J Hosp Pharm. 1982;39:1528–9.

71. Pierson JF, Alexander MR, Kirking DM, Solomon DK. Physician's attitudes toward drug-use evaluation interventions. Am J Hosp Pharm. 1990;47:388–90.

72. Himmelberg CJ, Pleasants RA, Weber DJ, Kessler JM, Samsa GP, Spivey JM, et al. Use of antimicrobial drugs in adults before and after removal of a restriction policy. Am J Hosp Pharm. 1991;48:1220–7.

73. Restino MS, Knodel LC. Drug information quality assurance program used to appraise students' performance. Am J Hosp Pharm. 1992;49(6):1425–9.

74. Wheeler-Usher DH, Hermann FF, Wanke LA. Problems encountered in using written criteria to assess drug information responses. Am J Hosp Pharm. 1990;47(4):795–7.

75. Moody ML. Revising a drug information center quality assurance program to conform to Joint Commission standards. Am J Hosp Pharm. 1990;47(4):792–4.

76. Smith CH, Sylvia LM. External quality assurance committee for drug information services. Am J Hosp Pharm. 1990;47(4):787–91.

77. Halbert MR, Kelly WN, Miller DE. Drug Information Centers: lack of generic equivalence. Drug Intell Clin Pharm. 1977;11:728–35.

78. Beaird SL, Coley RM, Blunt JR. Assessing the accuracy of drug information responses from drug information centers. Ann Pharmacother. 1994;28(6):707–11.

79. Calis KA, Anderson DW, Auth DA, Mays DA, Turcasso NM, Meyer CC, et al. Quality of pharmacotherapy consultations provided by drug information centers in the United States. Pharmacotherapy. 2002;20:830–6.

17

Chapter Seventeen

Medication Misadventures: Adverse Drug Reactions and Medication Errors

Philip J. Gregory

Objectives

After completing this chapter, the reader will be able to

- Define medication misadventures, adverse drug events, adverse drug reactions, and medication errors.
- Classify adverse drug reactions based on type and severity.
- Explain methods for determining probability and causality of an adverse drug reaction.
- Describe reporting systems for adverse drug reactions.
- Describe steps to develop an adverse drug reaction reporting program.
- Classify medication errors based on type and severity.
- Differentiate between slips and mistakes as they pertain to medication errors.
- Describe factors affecting cognitive function that lead to medication errors.
- Describe reporting systems for medication errors.
- Describe strategies health care practitioners and health systems can implement to reduce medication errors.

Pharmacists play a pivotal role in the medication use process. Throughout this process there is potential for unexpected adverse events, including errors in prescribing, dispensing, and administering medications, idiosyncratic reactions, and other adverse effects. These events can all be described as medication misadventures.[1] Pharmacists need to understand the potential for various medication misadventures and be prepared to recognize and prevent such occurrences and minimize adverse outcomes.

The terminology surrounding medication misadventures is often confusing. Medication misadventure is a very broad term. It refers to any iatrogenic hazard or incident associated with medications. A medication misadventure may or may not cause an injury to a patient. All adverse drug events (ADEs), adverse drug reactions (ADRs), and medication errors fall under the umbrella of medication misadventures. An ADE is the next broadest term. It refers to any injury caused by a medicine. An ADE refers to all ADRs, including allergic or idiosyncratic reactions, as well as medication errors that result in harm to a patient.[1-5] ADRs and medication errors are the most specific terms. ADRs refer to any unexpected, unintended, undesired, or excessive response to a medicine. Drug-drug interactions can also fall into the category of ADRs. A medication error is any preventable event that has the potential to lead to inappropriate medication use or patient harm.[1] Figure 17–1 shows one way of classifying these terms.

Medication misadventures are now an issue of national priority in the United States.[2-4] The mid to late 1990s served as a wake-up call. Several important studies documented the staggering economic burden of these events.[5-9] A landmark study in 1995 estimated that ADE-related costs were $76.6 billion annually in ambulatory patients alone.[6] Drug expenditures in ambulatory patients at that time were $80 billion per year. This means that for every $1 spent for a drug, almost $1 was also being spent due to a drug-related problem. These costs exceed the total costs of managing patients with diabetes or cardiovascular diseases.[7] A 2000 update to these figures indicates that the problem is not improving. In fact, costs related to ADEs seem to have more than doubled to $177.4 billion.[8]

About a third of these events are thought to be preventable.[5] Several agencies and professional organizations across the country are now contributing efforts to minimize these events (Table 17–1).

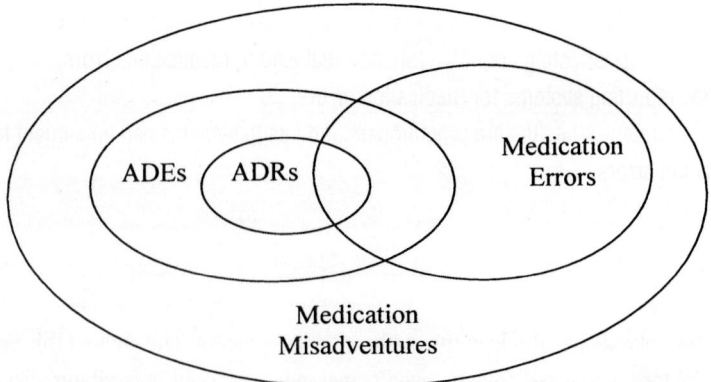

Figure 17–1. Relationship Among Medication Misadventures, Adverse Drug Events, Medication Errors, and Adverse Drug Reactions. Adapted from *American Society of Health-System Pharmacists. Suggested definitions and relationships among medication misadventures, medication errors, adverse drug events, and adverse drug reactions. Am J Health-Syst Pharm 1998;55:165–6.*

TABLE 17–1. ORGANIZATIONS INVOLVED IN PREVENTING ADVERSE DRUG EVENTS

Food and Drug Administration (FDA)	www.fda.gov
Joint Commission on Accreditation of Healthcare Organizations (JCAHO)	www.jcaho.org
World Health Organization (WHO)	www.who.int
Institute for Safe Medication Practices (ISMP)	www.ismp.org
The United States Pharmacopoeia (USP)	www.usp.org
American Society of Health-System Pharmacists (ASHP)	www.ashp.org

Efforts to minimize medication misadventures depend heavily on individual health care practitioners, including pharmacists, physicians, and nurses. Multiple studies have highlighted the impact individual pharmacists can have on minimizing medication misadventures and improving outcomes.[9–12] In one of the most significant studies, published in the *Journal of the American Medical Association*, pharmacists participating in hospital rounds in an intensive care unit decreased prescribing errors by 66% and saved an estimated $270,000 per year.[10]

Adverse Drug Reactions

All medications, including the excipients of a product, are capable of producing adverse effects.[13] Some of these are idiosyncratic and are unpredictable. But many are predictable, based on understanding of their pharmacology, and, therefore, they can be anticipated and prevented. It's estimated that 30 to 60% of ADRs are preventable.[14,15]

ADRs are estimated to account for about 3 to 15% of all hospital admissions and lead to an increase in morbidity and mortality.[7,14,16,17] Almost 16% of nursing home patients are hospitalized annually due to ADRs.[14] About 20% of the ambulatory population receiving medications experiences ADRs.[18] These outpatient events do not always result in hospitalization. The incidence of ADRs for patients in the hospital might be as high as 28%. These percentages are likely to be somewhat conservative because many ADRs go undetected, unreported, and untreated.[18] Many patients and health care professionals are not always adequately informed about medications and their potential for adverse events and, therefore, when an ADR occurs, it might not always be recognized.

Many countries, including the United States, have developed systems to encourage the reporting of adverse events. In addition, the Joint Commission on Accreditation of Healthcare Organizations (JCAHO) require hospitals to have a mechanism in place to monitor ADRs.[19] Many hospitals have developed extensive programs that provide a foundation for monitoring and reporting adverse reactions, including a warning system to prevent further problems. Sharing information about ADRs between health care practitioners and organizations is vital to the success of these programs. In addition, networking of ADR information can help provide a useful database to use for recognition or prevention of future ADRs.

DEFINITIONS

One of the first steps in establishing an ADR program is to define what the institution or facility categorizes as ADRs. There are many definitions for ADRs that have been described in the literature. Institutions, as well as clinicians, have used different definitions depending on their practice needs.

The WHO defines an ADR as "any noxious or unintended response to a drug that occurs at doses usually used for prophylaxis, diagnosis, or therapy of disease or for the modification of psychological function."[20]

The FDA definition of an ADR is any adverse event associated with the use of a drug in humans, whether or not considered drug related, including the following: adverse event occurring in the course of the use of a drug product in professional practice; an adverse event occurring from drug overdose, whether accidental or intentional; an adverse event occurring from drug abuse; an adverse event occurring from drug withdrawal; and any significant failure of expected pharmacologic action.[20] This definition is fairly broad and includes overdose situations, as well as areas involving abuse.

The FDA goes on to define an unexpected drug reaction. These unexpected ADRs are what should be reported, because they are new and not previously described in product labeling. This includes an ADR that may be symptomatically or pathophysiologically related to an ADR listed in the labeling, but may differ from the labeled ADR because of greater severity or specificity (e.g., abnormal liver function vs. hepatic necrosis). An ADR may also be due to a drug interaction, defined as a pharmacologic response that cannot be explained by the action of a simple drug, but is due to two or more drugs acting simultaneously.[20]

The use of "unexpected" in the language does limit the number of ADRs that the FDA expects health care professionals to report. This definition focuses on reporting the unusual, uncommon, or newly identified ADRs. Although the common or usual ADRs are relevant and important, they do not provide the FDA with additional information.

Karch and Lasagna[21] define a drug, an adverse event, and a patient drug exposure as the following:

- *Drug*: A chemical substance or product available for an intended diagnostic, prophylactic, or therapeutic purpose.
- *ADRs*: Any response to a drug which is noxious and unintended and which occurs at doses used in man for prophylaxis, diagnosis or therapy, excluding therapeutic failures.
- *Patient drug exposure*: A single patient receiving at least one dose of a given drug.

Many hospital programs use this definition because it excludes accidental poisonings, as well as problems with drugs of abuse.

CAUSALITY AND PROBABILITY OF ADVERSE DRUG REACTIONS

One of the difficulties in defining an ADR is determining causality. Cause and effect is difficult to prove, in general, and ADRs are no exception. Many publications have dealt with this problem by developing definitions, algorithms, and questionnaires that try to determine the probability that a drug caused a specific reaction. To date, none of these attempts have been able to prove actual causality. These tools, however, can help determine the probability or likelihood that a particular drug caused an adverse event.

These algorithms and definitions use several key concepts.[22] Dechallenge and rechallenge are often used to assess causality. Dechallenge occurs when the drug is discontinued and the patient is then monitored to determine whether the ADR abates or decreases in intensity. Rechallenge occurs when the drug is discontinued and, after the ADR abates, the drug is readministered in an attempt to elicit the response again. Dechallenge and rechallenge are effective means for establishing a strong case that the drug was responsible for the ADR. Unfortunately in clinical practice, a rechallenge may not be practical or desirable since it could actually cause further harm to the patient. Patients who suffer a serious ADR will not be interested in experiencing the reaction again in the name of science. On the other hand, a dechallenge is almost always done, especially in the case of a severe ADR, as it is often essential for improving patient care.

Another important factor to consider is the temporal relationship between drug administration and the event. Does the timeframe for development of the ADR make sense based on the actions of the drug? If there is literature on the ADR, does it describe a temporal relationship between the drug and the event? The medical literature and package inserts can be helpful in noting if a drug has been known to cause a certain type of reaction within a certain timeframe. But for rare or new ADRs, the medical literature is not likely to be helpful.

Naranjo and associates[22] developed the following definitions to assist in determining the probability of an ADR.

- Definite ADR is a reaction which: (1) follows a reasonable temporal sequence from administration of the drug, or in which the drug level has been established in body fluids or tissue; (2) follows a known response pattern to the suspected drug; and (3) is confirmed by dechallenge; and (4) could not be reasonably explained by the known characteristics of the patient's clinical state.
- Conditional ADR is a reaction which: (1) follows a reasonable temporal sequence from administration of the drug; (2) does not follow a known response pattern to the suspected drug; and (3) could not be reasonably explained by the known characteristics of the patient's clinical state.
- Doubtful ADR is any reaction, which does not meet the criteria above.

Several algorithms have been published that try to incorporate information about an ADR into a more scientific form. These algorithms determine the likelihood that the drug was responsible for the reaction and establish a rational and scientific approach to what previously required strictly clinical judgment. All of the algorithms are time-consuming and the results can vary according to the interpretation of multiple observers. In 1979, Kramer and coworkers[23] published a questionnaire composed of 56 yes or no questions (Appendix 17–1). This questionnaire includes sections about the patient's previous experience with the drug or related drugs, alternative etiologies, timing of events, drug concentrations, dechallenge, and rechallenge. Responses to each question are given a weighted value and these values are totaled. The total value then belongs to one of four categories: unlikely, possible, probable, or definite. One of the problems with this method is that clinicians can disagree on the weighted values because the user must make subjective judgments for some of the questions. Hutchinson and colleagues[24] evaluated the reproducibility and validity of the Kramer questionnaire. The authors concluded that although the questionnaire was cumbersome to use, the method described by Kramer was superior to clinical judgment alone. Another problem inherent with this questionnaire is that an unexpected ADR may not score well because of lack of literature or previous experience with the ADR. If the reaction is not universally accepted or in the most recent edition of the *Physicians' Desk Reference*, the reaction would score a zero in this section. Overall, however, the questionnaire provides professionals with the opportunity to use a standardized tool.

Naranjo and colleagues developed an alternative algorithm (Appendix 17–2). Today, it is probably the most commonly used tool to assess ADR causality.[14] This algorithm has 10 simple questions. The questions involve the following areas: the temporal relationship, the pattern of response, dechallenge or administration of an antagonist, rechallenge, alternative causes, placebo response, drug level in the body fluids or tissue, dose-response relationship, previous patient experience with the drug, and confirmation by any other objective evidence. The answer to each question is then assigned a score. The score is then totaled and placed into a category from definite to doubtful. The Naranjo algorithm also places emphasis on rechallenge and dechallenge, which may pose some problems in evaluating ADRs using this method. In the initial published report of this algorithm, Naranjo and colleagues[22] tested the reproducibility and validity of the algorithm. Like the study by Kramer and associates,[23] this algorithm was found to be a valid means of assessing ADRs.

In 1982, Jones and coworkers[25] published an algorithm that allows health care practitioners to answer a series of yes or no questions to determine if a true ADR occurred (Appendix 17–3). This type of format is similar to other published algorithms. The Jones algorithm is shorter and quicker to complete compared to Kramer's questionnaire.

All of the algorithms possess a certain degree of observer variability. However, all can be used to help determine whether an adverse event was precipitated by a certain drug or drug-drug combination. Michel and Knodel[26] compared the three algorithms by Kramer, Jones, and Naranjo. The study found that the Naranjo algorithm was simpler and less time-consuming, and compared favorably to the 56 questions asked by Kramer. The study found a higher correlation between the Naranjo algorithm and the Kramer questionnaire. Although there was agreement between the Naranjo and Jones algorithms, the correlation was not as high as that seen between the Naranjo and Kramer algorithms. The authors stated that more data were needed to support the use of the algorithm developed by Jones.

A Bayesian approach to assessing adverse reactions has also been developed by Lane.[27] Using the Bayesian approach, relevant information is collected and a quantitative measure of the odds that a particular drug caused a particular event is calculated. The Bayesian approach has the potential to be an outstanding tool for predicting populations that may be at higher risk for ADRs. But at this point it is too complex and time-consuming for daily application in a clinical setting. Rather than taking a few minutes with other tools for assessing causality, performing Bayesian analysis could take weeks.

CLASSIFICATION

Definitions and algorithms have also been used to classify the probability and severity of ADRs. Classification systems, such as those developed by Naranjo, Kramer, and Jones, as previously described, have been used to establish probability of ADRs. Other classification systems ranked the severity of ADRs from minor to severe.

One such classification system was developed by Lasagna and Karch, and classifies severity of ADRs into minor, moderate, severe, and lethal as defined below.[25]

- *Minor:* No antidote, therapy, or prolongation of hospitalization is required.
- *Moderate:* Requires a change in drug therapy, specific treatment, or an increase in hospitalization by at least 1 day.
- *Severe:* Potentially life-threatening, causing permanent damage, or requiring intensive medical care.
- *Lethal:* Directly or indirectly contributes to the death of the patient.

The FDA classifies an ADR as serious when it results in death, is life-threatening, causes or prolongs hospitalization, causes a significant persistent disability, results in a congenital anomaly, or requires intervention to prevent permanent damage.[28]

When developing an ADR monitoring program, these various systems can be used to determine probability (cause and effect) and severity of ADRs, and help describe and quantify data.

MECHANISM OF ADVERSE DRUG REACTIONS

Karch and Lasagna also described various mechanisms for ADRs.[21] These mechanisms are related to the pharmacologic or pharmacodynamic aspects of drugs and can be used to classify the type of reaction that occurs.

- *Idiosyncrasy:* An uncharacteristic response of a patient to a drug, usually not occurring on administration.
- *Hypersensitivity:* A reaction, not explained by the pharmacologic effects of the drug, caused by altered reactivity of the patient and generally considered to be an allergic manifestation.
- *Intolerance:* A characteristic pharmacologic effect of a drug produced by an unusually small dose, so that the usual dose tends to induce a massive overaction.
- *Drug interaction:* An unusual pharmacologic response that could not be explained by the action of a single drug, but was caused by two or more drugs.
- *Pharmacologic:* A known, inherent pharmacologic effect of a drug, directly related to dose.

When implementing an ADR program, these classifications can help health care practitioners to organize and present data. Potential causative drugs involved in ADRs can be listed, allowing trends to be followed over time. These trends can be used to change prescribing habits or alert the institution to potential problems. In addition, the data may also suggest the severity of reactions that are occurring and which medications cause the most severe reactions.

REPORTING

Well-designed programs that monitor ADRs, as well as network information to the medical community, are essential. Surveillance of ADRs makes it possible to detect early signals of a developing problem.[29] This is why postmarketing surveillance of ADRs is so important. Postmarketing ADR reporting can cause changes in prescribing drugs as well as result in the withdrawal of various drugs from the market.

FDA REPORTING

The size of preapproval drug studies prohibits detection of all potential adverse reactions. Adverse reactions that occur only rarely (e.g., 1 out of a million) often will not be detected until after a drug is approved and used in millions of people. Therefore, the FDA relies on postmarketing information to establish a better understanding of adverse events. Historically, drugs have been approved by the FDA only to be withdrawn from the market due to postmarketing adverse events, either voluntarily by the manufacturer or because of mandate from the FDA. Pharmaceutical companies are required by the FDA to submit quarterly reports of all ADRs for the first 3 years that a drug is on the market as part of the postmarketing surveillance system.

The FDA was required to have a Spontaneous Reporting System (SRS) with the passage of the Kefauver-Harris Amendment of 1962. This program allows for an inexpensive monitoring system of ADRs for all drugs marketed in the United States.[30] The problem in the past has been the lack of reporting by the medical community. In a study of community-based physicians, only 57% were aware of the voluntary system of reporting.[31] In the past, the FDA utilized Form 1639 to allow anyone to report an adverse event through the SRS. However, in June 1993, the FDA switched to a new program called MedWatch: The FDA Medical Products Reporting Program.

With this new program, the FDA receives reports via mailings, phone calls, faxes, and the Internet. Between June 1993 and September 30, 1993, the FDA received 1717 voluntary reports from pharmacists, physicians, nurses, risk managers, dentists, and other health and nonhealth professionals. Pharmacists provided 53% of the reports. Of the 1717 reports, 65% were ADEs and 3% were ADRs to biologics.[32]

To report a problem to the FDA, consumers and health care professionals can call 1-800-FDA-1088, fax a report to 1-800-FDA-0178, or send via the Internet from <<www.fda.gov/medwatch>>. In addition, the MedWatch Form, also known as FDA Form 3500, can be completed and mailed to the FDA[32] (Appendix 17–4).

A unit of the FDA called the Central Triage Unit receives voluntary reports. This unit screens the reports and forward them to the appropriate FDA program within 24 hours of receiving the report. In addition, they mail a letter to the sender acknowledging the report's receipt. The report becomes part of a database used by the agency to identify signals or warnings that would require further study or regulatory action. Like the previous FDA program, MedWatch is still interested in serious adverse events, which they describe as death, life-threatening events, hospitalization, disability, congenital anomaly, or requiring intervention to prevent permanent impairment or damage. The MedWatch program asks people to report an event even if they are not certain that the product was the cause.[33]

The MedWatch program does not overcome lack of reporting due to a voluntary system. It is important to note that pharmaceutical manufacturers are required to report all adverse events to the FDA, whereas, individual health care practitioners only do so voluntarily. Various explanations can account for the failure of practitioners to participate in the FDA program. Hoffman[33] best describes the lack of ADR reporting by physicians as follows:

1. Failure to detect the reaction due to a low level of suspicion.
2. Fear of potential legal implications.
3. Lack of training about drug therapy.
4. Uncertainty about whether the drug causes the reaction.
5. Lack of clear responsibility for reporting.
6. Paper work and time involved.
7. No financial incentive to report.
8. Unaware of reporting procedure or little understanding of it.

9. Lack of readily available reporting forms.
10. Desire to publish the report.
11. Fear that a useful drug will be removed from the market or given a bad name.
12. Complacency and lethargy.
13. Guilty feelings because of patient harm.
14. Reaction not worth reporting.

Other explanations for the lack of reporting are that medical record personnel, who might be used to categorize and report data, are not familiar with ADRs and/or their method of documentation. Therefore, the pharmacist can provide a valuable service by participating in the MedWatch program.

DIETARY SUPPLEMENTS

Dietary supplements, including herbs, vitamins, minerals, and nutraceuticals, are regulated much differently than pharmaceuticals. The most striking difference is that these supplements can reach pharmacies and grocery store shelves without FDA approval and without any proof of safety or effectiveness. Manufacturers of these products are not required to monitor safety of their products through postmarketing surveillance and they are not required to share information about safety with the FDA. For example, if a pharmacist or a consumer reported a potential ADR to a dietary supplement manufacturer, that manufacturer is not obliged to forward such information to the FDA.

Despite these lax standards, dietary supplements can and do cause ADRs. Many of these products have powerful pharmacologic effects and therefore they can cause ADRs. The medical literature contains many case reports that describe ADRs related to dietary supplements. However, the exact incidence of ADRs with dietary supplements is impossible to determine because there is no required monitoring or reporting systems in place and many ADRs go unrecognized.

An interesting case involves the herb ephedra, also known as *ma huang*. This herb was marketed as a dietary supplement and promoted primarily for weight loss and enhancing athletic performance. It received a great deal of negative media attention after two professional athletes died during training sessions. It turned out that the athletes were using ephedra. Over a period of several years there were well over 100 reports to the FDA of life-threatening ADRs linked to ephedra, including heart attacks, strokes, seizures, and death.

Finally, in March 2004, the FDA banned sale of dietary supplements containing ephedra.[34] Still, the FDA could not prove that ephedra was the cause of these numerous ADRs. The FDA had to act based on the best available evidence. Because there are no reporting standards or requirements for manufacturers to collect data on their products' safety, it would be unlikely that the FDA would ever have enough data to scientifically prove causality.

the FDA's actions on ephedra will have long-lasting effects. It will ultimately set the precedent by which other cases against dietary supplements will be decided.

Currently, the only national mechanism for collecting data on ADRs related to dietary supplements is the FDA MedWatch program. This is the same program that collects data about adverse events with conventional drugs. The FDA's Center for Food Safety and Applied Nutrition (CFSAN) is developing a new comprehensive system for monitoring and tracking ADRs related to dietary supplements. It will be called the CFSAN Adverse Event Reporting System (CAERS). Once this program is in place, the FDA will be better able to determine which dietary supplement may represent a danger to the consumer.[35]

JCAHO AND ASHP GUIDELINES

The JCAHO requires that hospitals have an ADR reporting program.[19] The programs are generally a function of the pharmacy and therapeutics (P&T) committee and the department of pharmacy. The JCAHO encourages the reporting of serious ADRs to the FDA.

The American Society of Health-System Pharmacists (ASHP) also encourages pharmacists to take a leadership role in establishing a reporting system and in monitoring ADEs. ASHP has published very specific guidelines as part of its practice standards. The ADR standards can be found on the Internet at <<www.ashp.org/bestpractices/MedMis/MedMis_Gdl_ADR.pdf>>.[36]

IMPLEMENTING A PROGRAM

Prior to implementing an ADR program, the health care facility must educate its staff on the importance and significance of the program. The pharmacy department is in an excellent position to provide this education because of its involvement in the P&T committee, pharmacokinetic dosing, drug utilization evaluation (DUE), and drug distribution. The pharmacy department can be an excellent resource for developing an ADR program, as well as providing data about ADRs to the P&T committee.

The JCAHO and the ASHP standards can be used as a basis for starting an ADR monitoring program. In addition to the standards, the pharmacy and medical literature contain abundant examples of successful programs. Guidelines for starting a program include the following:

1. Develop definitions and classifications for ADRs that work for the institution. The definitions and classifications in this chapter provide a good starting point for discussion.
2. Assign responsibility for the ADR program within the pharmacy and throughout other key departments. A multidisciplinary approach is an essential factor. The program needs a leader and an advocate, which often comes from the pharmacy

department. But it also needs the involvement of nursing and medical departments in order to collect reports from all health professionals. Cooperation is important for a successful program. This can often be achieved through involvement of the P&T committee.

3. Develop forms for data collection and reporting or other mechanisms for reporting (some institutions use computer reporting, as well as hotline phone numbers).

4. Promote awareness of the program. Promote the awareness of ADRs and the importance of reporting such events.

5. Develop policies and procedures for handling ADRs being sent to the FDA. Indicate who is responsible for sending them. This is usually someone in the pharmacy department.

6. Establish mechanisms for screening and evaluating ADRs. These mechanisms should include retrospective reviews, concurrent monitoring, as well as prospective planning for high-risk groups. It is worthwhile to educate pharmacists to check for ADRs when they see orders for certain indicator drugs that are often used to treat an ADR (Table 17–2), orders to discontinue or hold drugs, and orders to decrease the dose or frequency of a drug.[37] Also, electronic screening methods to check for laboratory tests that are indicative of ADRs (e.g., drug levels, *Clostridium difficile* toxin assays, elevated serum potassium, and low white blood cell counts) can be helpful.[38]

7. Routinely review ADRs for trends. Monitor ADRs continuously and concurrently. Report all findings to P&T committee.

8. Develop preventive interventions. Develop strategies for decreasing the incidence of ADRs (depending on the opportunities presented by the ADRs reported). *Please note,* this vital step has often been ignored in the literature; however, for an ADR program to be part of the quality assurance process, it must be included, wherever possible.

TABLE 17–2. ADR INDICATOR DRUGS

Antidiarrheal agents
Atropine (except preoperatively)
Dextrose 50% (IV push)
Diphenhydramine (except at bedtime)
Epinephrine (IV push)
Flumazenil
Naloxone
Potassium supplement (diuretic or digoxin patients)
Protamine
Sodium polystyrene sulfonate (patients on potassium sparing diuretics or ACE inhibitors)
Topical steroids
Vitamin K

TECHNOLOGY

Information systems and high-end technology may play an important role in monitoring, identifying, and minimizing ADRs. Information systems are available that can identify and alert practitioners to potential ADRs and detect potential drug-drug interactions that may contribute to ADRs. One system was developed at Brigham and Women's Hospital to detect potential ADRs. The system was programmed to detect a combination of patient-specific factors and medications that may indicate a patient who has the potential to experience an ADR. For example, patients taking medications that require renal function-based dosing who have elevated serum creatinine may be flagged as patients at risk for development of an ADR. Various other screening rules were also programmed. This system was compared to voluntary stimulated reporting and retrospective chart review. The electronic system detected more ADRs than spontaneous reports, but fewer than chart review. Interestingly, the errors detected by the computer system were different than those detected by chart review, indicating that a combination of ADR and ADE detection systems may provide the best results. As expected, using the computer system saved work time, requiring one-fifth as many person-hours as the chart review method.[39]

In another study, a similar ADE detection system identified potential ADEs in 64 of every 1000 admissions. The prescribing physician did not recognize 44% of the ADEs detected by the system.[40] Computer systems that detect clinically significant drug-drug interactions may also be relevant for reducing ADRs. Although software is readily available for this purpose, one survey indicates that only slightly more than half of the hospitals are using drug interaction software integrated with their drug distribution system. Despite this finding, most pharmacists believe that drug interaction software does or would increase their ability to detect clinically significant drug-drug interactions that may contribute to ADRs.[41]

The health care industry is lagging behind other industries in the implementation of high-end technology information systems.[42] Health care organizations will likely be required to invest in that technology to significantly improve the quality of care and stay competitive in the health care market.[39,42]

Pharmacists can play a vital role in developing, maintaining, and promoting ADR monitoring programs. These programs can provide valuable information about ADRs within the institution, as well as provide information that can be forwarded to the FDA. ADR monitoring programs have been developed that impact positively on patient care and have been shown to improve communication channels, as well as provide additional education on adverse events. An ADR program should have a multidisciplinary approach and provide a mechanism to impact the quality of patient care. Although the examples concentrated on hospital practice, the concepts are applicable to any practice area and all pharmacists should be involved in ADR reporting to improve both knowledge about drugs and individual patient care.

Medication Errors

Patients depend on health systems and health professionals to help them stay healthy. As a result, frequently patients receive drug therapy with the notion that these medications will help them lead a more healthy life. In fact, the initiation of drug therapy is the most common medical treatment received by patients.[43] In virtually all cases, patients and their health care providers understand that when medications are given, there are some known and some unknown risks. Patients also experience significant unexpected drug-related morbidity and mortality. These events may occur in up to 6.5% of hospitalized patients.[9] As many as 19% of disabling medical injuries are caused by ADEs, 45% of which are related to medication errors.[2] Errors in the medication use process, including errors in medication prescribing, dispensing, administering, and monitoring, are responsible for 14% of drug-related deaths.[44] In the early 1980s, an average of one medication error per patient per day was reported.[45] A review of medication error-related deaths from 1983 to 1993 has shown an increase from 2876 deaths in 1983 to 7391 deaths in 1993, a 2.57-fold overall increase. Medication error-related deaths in outpatients had an 8.48-fold increase and in inpatients there was a 2.37-fold increase during the same period.[4]

"First do no harm" is a common adage very familiar to most health care practitioners. It is the responsibility of all health professionals and health systems to maintain this philosophy and contribute to the minimization of medication errors. Because the medication use process is complex and involves multiple individuals representing several health professions and some nonprofessionals, communication and teamwork among the various professions are a necessity. Because society perceives pharmacists to be responsible for the safe and effective use of drugs,[44] however, the pharmacy profession needs to take a prominent role in the maximization of safe medicine use as a core responsibility of pharmaceutical care.[46]

DEFINITIONS

In general terms, "an error is a failure to perform an intended action that was appropriate given the circumstances."[47] The pharmacy and medical community have taken this rather simple general definition and applied the language of the professions to define what precisely constitutes an error in a medical environment within the scheme of medication misadventures and ADEs. The National Coordinating Council for Medication Error Reporting and Prevention (NCC MERP), an organization composed of 19 national organizations and individual members, including the FDA, American Medical Association (AMA), American Pharmacists Association (APhA), United States Pharmacopoeia (USP), and several others (Table 17–3), has developed a detailed definition of what constitutes a medication error.

> Any preventable event that may cause or lead to inappropriate medication use or patient harm while the medication is in the control of the health care professional, patient, or consumer.

TABLE 17–3. NATIONAL COORDINATING COUNCIL FOR MEDICATION ERROR REPORTING AND PREVENTION MEMBER ORGANIZATIONS

American Association of Retired Persons
American Healthcare Association
American Hospital Association
American Medical Association
American Nurses Association
American Pharmaceutical Association
American Society of Health-System Pharmacists
American Society for Healthcare Risk Management
Department of Veterans Affairs
Generic Pharmaceutical Industry Association
Institute for Safe Medication Practices
Joint Commission on the Accreditation of Healthcare Organizations
National Association of Boards of Pharmacy
National Council of State Boards of Nursing
Pharmaceutical Research and Manufacturers of America and U.S. Pharmacopoeia
U.S. Food and Drug Administration
U.S. Pharmacopoeia

Such events may be related to professional practice, health care products, procedures, and systems, including prescribing; order communication; product labeling, packaging, and nomenclature; compounding; dispensing; distribution; administration; education; monitoring; and use.[1]

As previously mentioned, medication errors fall within the broad category of medication misadventures. In cases where the medication error results in injury to a patient, that error also falls into the medication misadventure subcategory of ADEs (see Figure 17–1).[1]

Based on the NCC MERP definition, an error may occur as a result of not adequately counseling or educating a patient on proper use of medication. When, for example, a patient inappropriately uses a metered-dose inhaler for asthma and fails to receive the full amount of the medication, a medication error has occurred. The error may be secondary to a lack of education or may have occurred despite adequate counseling and education. Independent of the cause, based on the above definition, a medication error did occur.

Based on this definition, medication errors also occur when a prescriber writes an incorrect dose on a prescription pad. Even if the prescriber is called by a dispensing pharmacist to clarify and change the order and the patient eventually receives an appropriately dosed medication, an error did occur in the process. An adverse outcome does not necessarily have to occur to classify an event as a medication error.[47]

The "five rights" is a commonly used, but less precise, method of evaluating medication errors. Each medication dose that is administered must comply with these five rights to be free of error: (1) right patient, (2) right drug, (3) right dose, (4) right time, and (5) right route.

The five rights are a tool to assist health care professionals at every step in the medication use process to minimize the occurrence of errors.[48] Each professional, when prescribing, dispensing, or administering, should clarify that the five rights are in order before furthering the process of medication use. The five rights also provide an easy and understandable way to identify when medication errors occur. Whenever the five rights are not met, a medication error has occurred. However, when using this very simplified method of looking at medication errors, many of the more common errors, such as dose omissions, may be missed.

The precise definitions for medication errors may vary among institutions. The general principles will be similar, but there may be differences in what qualifies as a reportable error. For example, at one institution it may be determined that an error has occurred when a dose is not received by a patient within 15 minutes of the scheduled time. At another institution, there may be more flexibility, with errors reported only if medication is not administered until more than 30 minutes beyond the scheduled time. Also, some institutions may not report errors that do not affect the patient. For example, institutions may not report an inappropriately written prescription if that error is caught by a pharmacist or nurse before the medication reaches the patient. Instead, a pharmacist or nurse may report it as a professional intervention. Although, according to the NCC MERP definition, it would technically count as an error.

CLASSIFICATION

Defining medication errors is important. It is necessary to develop definitions so that organizations and institutions can identify and track errors. After medication errors have been identified, it is also important to classify the errors. Classification helps to determine where errors are occurring and the severity of the errors, and assists with development of measures to improve the medication use process and minimize the occurrence of such errors.

Medication errors can be classified in a variety of ways. Some medication error reporting systems focus on the type of error. For example, organizations might be interested in whether the error was a dispensing, administering, or prescribing error. Other systems may be more interested in the outcome of the error. These systems focus on what effect, if any, the error had on a patient. For example, organizations may want to know if an extended hospital stay was necessary as a result of the error or if a patient died or suffered a disabling injury. Medication errors may also be subclassified. For example, errors may be further classified based on the profession committing the error or the particular drug involved in the error. Each of these systems will be described in more detail in the following sections.

ERROR TYPE

Probably the most common way to classify errors is to identify them by type. This classification focuses on whether an error was related to dispensing, administering, prescribing, or patient compliance. ASHP has provided definitions for various types of errors in 11 categories.[45,49]

1. *Prescribing error:* Errors in this category are fairly broad, but generally focus on inappropriate drug selection, dose, dosage form, or route of administration. Examples may include ordering duplicate therapies for a single indication, prescribing a dose that is too high or too low for a particular patient, writing a prescription illegibly, prescribing an inappropriate dosage interval, or ordering a drug to which the patient is allergic.[45]

    In one study, the most common type of prescribing error (56.1%) was related to an inappropriate dose (either too high or too low). The second most common prescribing error was related to prescribing an agent to which the patient was allergic (14.4%). Prescribing inappropriate dosage forms was the third most common error (11.2%).[43] Other relatively common prescribing errors have included failing to monitor for side effects and serum drug levels, prescribing an inappropriate medication for a particular indication, and inappropriate duration of therapy.[50]

2. *Omission error:* An omission error occurs when a patient does not receive a scheduled dose of medication. This is considered to be the second most common error in the medication use process, behind wrong time errors.[51]

3. *Wrong time error:* What constitutes a wrong time error may vary considerably among institutions. In general, this type of error occurs when a dose is not administered in accordance with a predetermined administration interval. Most institutions realize that it is often impossible to be totally accurate with the administration interval and typically 15 to 30 minutes outside that interval is acceptable. Institutions must establish a policy to indicate what exactly constitutes an error in this category.

4. *Unauthorized drug error:* This type of error occurs when patients receive a drug that was not authorized by an appropriate prescriber. This might include giving the wrong patient a medication.

5. *Improper dose error:* This type of error is different from that which occurs when a prescriber orders an inappropriate dose of a medication. This error occurs when the dose administered is different than what was prescribed, assuming that the prescribed dose was appropriate.

6. *Wrong dosage form error:* This error is also different from the type described in the prescribing error section. This error occurs when a patient receives a dosage form different from that prescribed, assuming the appropriate dosage form was originally ordered.

7. *Wrong drug preparation error:* When medications require some type of preparation, such as reconstitution, this type of error may occur. These kinds of errors may also occur in the compounding of various intravenous admixtures and other products.

8. *Wrong administration technique:* These errors occur when a drug is given to a patient inappropriately. An example is when an intravenously administered agent is given at an excessive rate or when an agent meant for intramuscular administration is given intravenously.

9. *Deteriorated drug error:* This error occurs when drugs are administered that have expired or have deteriorated prematurely due to improper storage conditions.

10. *Monitoring error:* These errors occur when patients are not monitored appropriately either after they have received a drug or before they received a drug. For example, if a patient is placed on warfarin therapy and adequate blood tests are not performed to assess the patient's response, resulting in a life-threatening hemorrhage, a monitoring error has occurred. Further, in a community pharmacy, if a pharmacist fails to review a patient's medication history prior to dispensing a medication, resulting in a significant drug-drug interaction, a monitoring error has occurred.

11. *Compliance error:* This type of error occurs when patients use medications inappropriately. Although it may seem that health care professionals have little responsibility here, proper patient education and follow-up may play a significant role in minimizing this type of error. This type of error may be a direct result of insufficient patient counseling from a dispensing pharmacist, a prescribing physician, or both.

These types of medication errors are not mutually exclusive. Multiple types of errors may occur during a single administration of a drug and a single adverse patient outcome may be the result of more than one type of error.[49]

OUTCOME OR SEVERITY

Although the classifications of errors frequently are based on type, most errors are also classified by the final result or outcome of an error. Even though errors may occur based on the types described above, there is not always an adverse outcome. It is important for institutions to monitor both the types of errors that occur and the outcomes associated with them. Most reporting systems request information regarding type and outcome of a medication error. Institutions may use information about outcomes to focus their error minimization efforts on the types of errors resulting in the most serious outcomes.

The NCC MERP has proposed a medication error index that serves to categorize errors based on the severity or outcome of the error. This index is divided into four main categories and nine subcategories as follows:[45,52]

1. No error

   Category A: Circumstances or events that have the capacity to cause error.

2. Error, no harm

   Category B: An error occurred, but the medication did not reach the patient.

Category C: An error occurred that reached the patient, but did not cause the patient harm.

Category D: An error occurred that resulted in the need for increased patient monitoring, but caused no patient harm.

3. Error, harm

Category E: An error occurred that resulted in the need for treatment or intervention and caused temporary patient harm.

Category F: An error occurred that resulted in initial or prolonged hospitalization and caused temporary patient harm.

Category G: An error occurred that resulted in permanent patient harm.

Category H: An error occurred that resulted in a near-death event (e.g., anaphylaxis and cardiac arrest).

4. Error, death

Category I: An error occurred resulting in patient death.

SUBCLASSIFICATIONS

Errors may need to be classified based on the professional involved with the error and the particular drug involved in the error. For example, if a health system notices that most of its errors are prescribing errors, that system may want to implement some training programs for physicians or develop new policies to help minimize those errors. If it is found that a particular dispensing error is increasing, an institution may ask for a review of the pharmacy procedures associated with that particular error.

It has also been found that certain drugs or classes of drugs are more commonly involved in errors than other drugs. For example, in hospitals, intravenous drugs are involved in 70% of medication errors. Medication errors resulting in pharmacist malpractice cases most often involve the drugs warfarin, corticosteroids, hypoglycemic agents, digoxin, amoxicillin, and phenytoin. Physician malpractice cases most commonly involve antibiotics, corticosteroids, and narcotics.[50] In one study evaluating prescribing errors, the agents most commonly involved included antibiotics (34.1%), cardiovascular agents (15.9%), gastrointestinal agents (7%), narcotics (5.7%), other analgesics (4.9%), and hormonal agents (4.1%).[43]

The classification of errors serves an important role. Health systems need detailed information on the extent, types, and consequences of medication errors to appropriately allocate efforts and resources to reduce their occurrence.

PSYCHOLOGY OF MEDICATION ERRORS: WHY DO ERRORS OCCUR?

Being human, health care professionals of all types have a propensity to commit errors in every area of their professional lives, including the medication use process. To understand why errors occur, it is necessary to examine the medication use system and the vital components in that system, health care professionals.

According to Senders, "An error is a psychological event with psychological causes..."[47] To better understand why health care professionals commit errors, we must look at the cognitive processes that occur at the time of the error. However, even the best understanding of the psychology of errors will not likely eliminate the problem entirely. Humans will most likely commit errors at an unacceptable rate despite our best efforts to understand and remedy their occurrence. With this in mind, it is necessary to develop systems of medication use that account for human error and have processes in place to identify and correct human error before medications reach patients.

At a very basic level, Dr. James Reason suggests that there are two broad types of errors committed: slips and mistakes. Slips generally occur when the professional's attention is diverted from the activity at hand, resulting in an inadvertent error, such as typing the wrong name on a label. A mistake occurs when an error is committed in problem solving due to inadequate knowledge or inappropriate information. For example, this is likely to occur when a seasoned practitioner makes therapeutic decisions based on personal experience rather than overwhelming research evidence.[45]

Davis[53,54] also suggests a broad categorization of causes of errors: (1) performance lapses, (2) lack of knowledge, and (3) lack or failure of safety systems. Davis's definitions parallel Reason's in that performance lapses could also be called slips and lack of knowledge falls into the mistakes category. Lack or failure of safety systems will be discussed in more detail in another section.

Personal and environmental factors are thought to interact to influence cognitive function that may lead to slips. There are several factors specific to the professional involved and their working environment that may contribute to their commiting an error. Grasha and O'Neill[55] have outlined some of the factors that may affect cognitive processes, resulting in lapses of performance.

1. *Excessive task demand:* Many dispensing pharmacists attribute their errors to this situation, complaining that their workload is so heavy and they are overloaded with tasks, making it difficult to work error free. In one survey, 68% of pharmacists rated "work overload" as a major contributing factor to the committal of dispensing errors.[56] Most pharmacists and experts in medication errors agree that work overload may be the most significant factor contributing to medication errors.[50,56]

2. *Personal characteristics:* Personal factors such as age, sensory deficits, or state of health may contribute to performance lapses. Personal levels of stress or fatigue may also have an impact. Someone who is bored at work may also be more error prone.

3. *Extra-organizational factors:* Factors, such as similar product names or packaging from pharmaceutical companies, may have an extensive impact on the committal of

errors with particular drugs. In one study, look-alike or sound-alike drugs were involved in 37% of medication errors.[57] As an example, this issue is currently being addressed for the sound-alike drugs celecoxib (Celebrex®), fosphenytoin (Cerebyx®), and citalopram (Celexa®). Complex insurance plans are also extraorganizational factors that may serve to complicate the medication use process and contribute to slips. The profession of pharmacy has been referred to as the most heavily regulated of all professions. Legal mandates for policing illegal prescriptions and other regulatory requirements are also good examples of extra-organizational factors.

4. *Work environment:* Poor working conditions may influence the rate of error committal. Poor illumination and high noise levels have been shown to affect the dispensing error rate in pharmacies.[55] Other factors in this category may include high ambient temperatures and frequent interruptions from the telephone or patients.

5. *Intra-organizational factors:* In the era of managed care, there is a significant emphasis on the bottom line. Policies and procedures demanding high output or mandating long working hours may significantly affect cognition and the ability to prevent error occurrence.

6. *Interpersonal factors:* Conflicts among coworkers or with patients may distract professionals from the tasks at hand and contribute to error commission. General interruptions from people may also fall into this category.

Some factors that may contribute to cognitive lapses and the commission of medication errors may fall into more than one of these categories. Furthermore, factors from multiple categories may occur simultaneously to contribute to error commission.

Health care professionals have indicated that other factors may also contribute to medication errors. Some of those factors are as follows.

1. *Lack of communication:* This factor may also fall under interpersonal factors listed above. Failure to communicate among fellow employees or among health care professionals has frequently been named as contributing to medication error. For example, an error may be more likely to occur if a pharmacist chooses not to clarify unclear physician orders. Poor physician handwriting and verbal orders are also significant factors.[51]

2. *Failure to comply with policy:* This is a common factor in dispensing and administering drugs. In one survey, 42 to 46% of pharmacists said that failing to check drugs before dispensing was a significant factor in dispensing errors.[56] Noncompliance with policy has also been associated with drug administration errors. Often nurses develop specific personal routines for administration of certain agents, which they perceive to be an improvement in the medication administration process, despite contrary policy.[51]

3. *Lack of knowledge:* This is a frequently cited factor in the committal of medication errors. Mistakes, rather than slips, are typically committed as a result of inadequate knowledge. Placing inexperienced recent graduates in positions where they cannot

interact with more experienced practitioners may increase medication errors. Non-specialists covering a service that is normally staffed by a specialist may also lead to errors.[54] Nurses untrained in pharmacology may be more unlikely to recognize potential inconsistencies in disease state and medication usage and doses, resulting in the possibility of increased medication errors reaching the patient.[51]

4. *Lack of patient counseling:* It has been said that the last safety check prior to dispensing medication should be counseling the patient. Talking to the patient allows the pharmacist to correlate the medication and dose with the patient's condition and helps the pharmacist to detect any errors that may have occurred in the medication use process. In one study, 89% of errors committed in a community pharmacy were detected during patient counseling.[50] However, errors may occur not only from lack of counseling, but also from providing incorrect information during patient counseling.[58] Providing incorrect information may also fall in the lack of knowledge category.

There are a variety of intrapersonal, interpersonal, and environmental factors that may contribute to errors in the medication use process. The examples provided above are a partial list of contributory factors at the level of the health care practitioner. These factors influence the occurrence of slips or performance lapses and mistakes committed by individuals. They do not address failure of a system or failure of a safety net as a whole process. The medication use process involves multiple health care professionals, nonprofessional staff, patients, and multiple physical environments. The safety net should work with all professionals and in all environments and may consist of multiple checks by individuals of other people's work, computer systems that screen for errors, barcode scanning systems, quality assurance measures, extra-organizational measures (e.g., to minimize ordering medications from companies with similar packaging), and multiple other systems. To adequately address the causes of errors, failures in the system must also be addressed. Although it is important to address the problem of individuals committing errors (e.g., increasing training and enforcing policy), adequately developed safety systems should be in place to significantly minimize the number of errors reaching patients. When errors do occur, it is necessary to address the event in the context of failure of the system or safety net.[59]

MEDICATION ERROR REPORTING

To err is human; to forgive is against company policy.

—John Senders, 1978[47]

Reporting medication errors, particularly severe or life-threatening errors, may have adverse consequences for both the individuals and the organization involved. Health care professionals have lost their jobs and been sued as a result of medication errors. As a result, health care professionals and health systems are reluctant to open themselves up to adverse outcomes associated with reporting medication errors.[50] As an example, in one hospital there were only 36 incident reports regarding medication errors over a yearlong reporting period. At the same institution, an observational study revealed that as many as 51,200 errors were likely to have actually occurred during that same reporting period.[45] In New York, a pharmacist had his license suspended after committing a single dispensing error that resulted in brain damage in a patient. In Nevada, a pharmacy was fined 2 weeks net profit for a dispensing error that resulted from understaffing.[50] A medical center in New Jersey was successfully sued for $12 million and fined by the state board of pharmacy after a medication error killed an infant.[60] In Colorado, three nurses were indicted on charges of criminal negligence after a medication administration error killed an infant.[61] In the current environment, the disincentives for error reporting seem to outweigh the incentives.[62]

The case in Colorado is particularly disheartening for experts in the field of medication misadventures. It demonstrates an example of a system failure that resulted in punishment of individual health care professionals. In this case, a 1-day-old baby was prescribed long-acting penicillin because its mother had acquired an infection. The medication was erroneously administered intravenously to the infant instead of intramuscularly, resulting in death of the infant. It was also found that a pharmacist had actually dispensed 10 times the appropriate dose. Cases similar to this one have been reported in the literature and had even occurred at that same institution, as reported a few weeks before this particular incident. Although this case is sad and disturbing, there was clearly a serious malfunctioning of the medication use process at this institution that allowed two serious errors to go unrecognized. District attorneys in Colorado pressed criminal charges against the nurses involved that could result in 3 to 5 years' imprisonment. The exact cause of this error is unknown, but it points to a lack of availability of clear and relevant drug information. It is also an example of blaming individuals for errors that may be the result of system breakdown.[61]

Despite the negative actions taken against individuals and organizations that commit medication errors, reporting errors is an absolute necessity for at least three reasons. First, to improve current medication use systems, the circumstances under which errors occur must be understood. Without adequate reporting, institutional and national self-evaluation would be impossible. Second, taking a proactive role in identifying errors and using that information to improve medication use systems may actually protect organizations from negligence claims. When errors are not reported, it may be interpreted as concealment.[50] In one study conducted at a Veterans Affairs Medical Center, it was shown that an institutional policy to immediately report medical errors to patients and their families and offer compensation resulted in liability payments among the lowest of 35 similar Veterans Affairs Medical Centers.[63] Finally, voluntary error reporting is necessary to avoid being placed on accreditation watch by the JCAHO. If the JCAHO discovers that a serious error occurred at an accredited organization that was not previously reported, the JCAHO will perform an immediate on-site survey and place the organization on accreditation watch. The JCAHO has recently made voluntary reporting appear less risky for organizations and individuals in an effort to increase medication error reporting. Under a relatively new policy, when an error occurs and is reported, the institution is now given an opportunity to investigate and implement corrective measures on its own. Previously, the JCAHO would immediately launch its own investigation and place the organization on accreditation watch. The JCAHO has also acknowledged that firing professionals involved with an error is not a proper response or consistent with quality improvement principles.[3] This new approach has been shown to increase reporting.[60] Time will tell if professionals and organizations continue to take this opportunity to conduct vigorous internal review to implement and improve systems to minimize medication errors.[62]

INSTITUTIONAL REPORTING

Individual institutions must develop a reporting system specific to their institution, designed to meet their specific needs. There are at least four methods for collecting reports of medication errors.[45,50] These methods may be used alone or in combination.

1. *Anonymous self-reports:* In this system, anyone detecting or committing an error can report it without associating their name with the error. It is essentially risk-free for the reporter and, therefore, it may increase the likelihood of having an error reported. Despite this theoretical advantage, there is still underreporting, particularly in cases that do not result in patient harm.[45]
2. *Incident reports:* This type of self-reporting system is the most commonly used. In this system, errors are written up as legal reports and are often used to satisfy the JCAHO requirements; however, errors are highly underreported.[45]
3. *Critical-incident technique:* Although not really a reporting system, this technique uses observations and interviews of professionals involved in medication errors to analyze and identify weaknesses in the system. This method uses errors reported by other systems in an attempt to provide solutions to existing medication use problems.[45]
4. *Disguised observation:* Instead of relying on individuals to report errors, this method places an observer among health care professionals to watch for the occurrence of errors. The purpose of the observation is unknown by the professionals. Errors are then recorded and reported. This method is more reliable than self-reporting, but is time-consuming and expensive.[45]

NATIONAL REPORTING

Reporting of medication errors is important for every practitioner without regard to their practice setting. However, institutional reporting is often emphasized because it is necessary in order to maintain the institution's accreditation status. In an effort to share institutional experiences in order to avoid the same errors being repeated at several institutions, national reporting systems for institutions have evolved. There is a great deal of controversy regarding legal concerns and reporting errors outside of respective institutions. It is thought by some in the legal community that reporting errors in any way may expose institutions to less legal protection.[3,50] Despite the objections of some in the legal community, national reporting must be done to share information among practitioners and institutions in an effort to increase the safety of patients. Several programs are available for this purpose.

1. *MedWatch:* This program was developed by the FDA Medical Products Reporting Program for the purpose of monitoring clinically significant ADEs and problems with medical products. MedWatch monitors quality, performance, and safety of medical products, devices, and medications. This program contributes to surveillance of medication errors that may be associated with product labeling and names.[45] The MedWatch program does not monitor reports of medication errors that are not specifically associated with a problematic product. For example, MedWatch will only collect reports about faulty products (e.g., improperly functioning devices that led to a medication error). Medication errors associated with strictly human error are not reported to MedWatch. For example, they don't collect reports of drug prescribing or administration errors. Significant reports may result in distribution of e-mail and "Dear Doctor" alerts to health care professionals. These announcements can also be viewed on the Internet at <<http://www.fda.gov/medwatch/safety.htm>>. Health care professionals and consumers can report ADEs and product problems by completing a MedWatch form (see Appendix 17–4) and mailing it to the FDA, by calling 1-800-FDA-1088, or reporting on-line at <<http://www.fda.gov/medwatch>>.

2. *USP-ISMP Medication Errors Reporting Program (MERP):* This program is a collaboration between the USP and the ISMP. Errors can be reported anonymously 24 hours a day by calling 1-800-23-ERROR. Report forms (Appendix 17–5) can also be mailed or submitted online at <<http://www.usp.org/>>. Reported errors are reviewed by USP and forwarded to the manufacturer and the FDA.[45,56]

3. *MedMARx:* This program was developed by the USP and is the only service that requires payment of a fee for use. However, this service provides much more than an anonymous method of reporting errors. It also allows subscribing organizations to report and monitor organization-specific errors online. Furthermore, organizations can compare their error rates with other subscribing organizations of similar type. The program also allows organizations to perform root cause analysis as required by the JCAHO when errors occur that result in patient harm.[64] More information regarding MedMARx can be found at <<http://www.usp.org>>.

At the institutional, organizational, or national level, medication error reporting systems generally require that a form be completed that describes the error, how it was treated, and its outcome. To standardize information associated with medication error reporting, the NCC MERP has developed a taxonomy for medication errors that may be applied in reporting and analyzing medication errors. This taxonomy ensures use of standard language and structure of information reported. Use of this taxonomy may help organizations develop reporting systems and analyze their specific medication errors. This 19-page document can be viewed and printed at <<http://www.nccmerp.org/pdf/taxo2001-07-31.pdf >>.

ERROR PREVENTION

The ultimate purpose for defining, classifying, analyzing, and reporting medication errors is to enable individuals and organizations to implement better systems that prevent medication errors. The ASHP has identified a multitude of risk factors associated with the occurrence of medication errors as outlined below.[49]

- Work shift—more errors occur during the day shift
- Inexperienced or inadequately trained staff
- Medical services with special needs (e.g., pediatrics and oncology)
- Higher number of medications per patient
- Environmental factors such as high levels of noise, poor lighting, and frequent interruptions
- High workload for staff
- Poor communication among health care providers
- Dosage form—more errors with injectable drugs
- Drug category—more errors with certain classes of drugs (e.g., antibiotics)
- Type of drug distribution systems—unit dose system is associated with fewer errors; high levels of floor stock are associated with increased errors
- Improper drug storage
- Calculations—increased errors with increased complexity and frequency of amount of calculations required
- Poor handwriting
- Verbal orders
- Lack of effective policies and procedures
- Poorly functioning oversight committees

Although this is not necessarily a comprehensive list, prevention strategies that successfully address these risk factors may be successful at minimizing the occurrence of medication errors. In the remainder of this section, some strategies for reducing medication errors will be described.

PRACTITIONER STRATEGIES

Individual health care practitioners play an integral role in the medication use process and must be familiar with factors that may contribute to medication errors. Although individuals are merely one part of a medication use system, each must take some responsibility for ensuring that their individual practices are consistent with the goal of reducing medication errors. Practitioners that recognize the potential for errors in various situations and implement personal practice habits to minimize errors can have a significant impact on error reduction. The following is a look at some things individual practitioners can do to minimize medication errors.

1. *Patient communication:* As previously discussed, interaction with the patient may significantly reduce medication errors. A pharmacist who counsels patients before handing out the medication is more likely to catch a dispensing error.[65] Similarly, nurses may minimize errors that reach a patient by asking the patient about allergies and describing the medication to the patient just prior to administration. Physicians may similarly contribute to better medication use by counseling a patient more thoroughly when writing the prescription.[49] When the pharmacist also counsels, there will be reinforcement of the information. Also, if the directions are different from the pharmacist compared to the physician, it may indicate that an error was committed somewhere in the medication use process.[65]

2. *Intraprofessional communication:* In addition to communicating with patients, health care professionals need to improve communication among themselves. Illegible writing, extensive verbal medication orders, and a "Lone Ranger" approach to practice have no place in a health system devoted to reducing medication errors. When a medication order is unclear, it is a necessity to clarify that order before the medication use process continues. Poor prescription writing is commonly cited as a cause for medication errors. Abbreviations should be avoided (this will be discussed in more detail later in the chapter). Lack of knowledge about the proper use of drugs is also frequently cited as a cause of prescribing errors.[9,66] Prescribers should ensure proper use of medications by consulting with pharmacists, other physicians, or the medical literature.[49]

3. *Education and training:* Lack of knowledge among all health care practitioners is commonly associated with medication errors. Health care professionals should stay abreast of current medical literature.[49] In the health care environment, the phrase "in my clinical experience..." is often used. Undoubtedly experience counts for a lot, but past experiences are no substitute for a thorough understanding of current medical literature.

Using evidence-based medicine can help in this regard. Please refer to Chap. 9 for further information.

4. *Reporting:* Health care professionals should recognize the necessity of medication error reporting. To enable other organizations and professionals to avoid the mistakes of others, reporting must be carried out consistently and routinely.

HEALTH SYSTEM STRATEGIES

The medication error literature emphasizes the importance of health system involvement in minimizing medication errors. It is not good enough for health systems to tell their employees to be more careful or to try to minimize errors. The medication use process involves multiple professional and nonprofessional staff that are prone to errors. Health systems must recognize that even the most highly trained and proficient practitioners will commit errors as a result of being human. In addition to individual responsibility, health systems must ensure that they provide the tools needed by all parties involved to help prevent medication errors. A medication error that reaches a patient is not the result of error committed by a single person, but a flaw in the medication use process. The following identifies some of the things health systems can do to help minimize medication errors.

1. *Environmental factors:* As discussed, there are numerous work place factors that may contribute to performance lapses and medication errors. Low lighting, high levels of noise, high temperatures, and stressful work environments are examples. Health systems should ensure that their facilities do not contribute to the commission of errors.[49]

2. *Policy:* Health systems should implement policies supportive of the effort to minimize medication errors. For example, policies that support the employment of adequate personnel for staffing and supervision should be implemented. High workloads and inadequate staffing directly correlate with medication errors.[51] Policies that demand multiple checks prior to dispensing or administering medication should also be implemented. Unit dose drug distribution systems are preferred.[44] Policies that limit floor stock and do not allow nonpharmacists to dispense medications should be implemented. Health systems must define medication errors and their classifications, and implement policies for monitoring and correcting such errors. Policies for medication error reporting should minimize risk to reporters of error and allow for the development of a system that supports improvement of the system rather than punishment of employees.[49]

   Policies to eliminate dangerous abbreviations can reduce errors. Abbreviations in medical charts and on prescriptions can lead to confusion and errors. In January 2004, the JCAHO instituted a new policy that requires hospitals and other facilities to create a list of unsafe abbreviations. These abbreviations are prohibited from being used in any record or medication order. For example, the abbreviation q.d. can be misread as qid. Instead "daily" should be written out. MS (for morphine sulfate) can be confused with $MgSO_4$ (for magnesium sulfate). U (for unit) can be misread as 0, 4, or cc.[67] For a complete list, refer to the following website: <<http://www.jcaho.org/accredited+organizations/patient+safety/04+npsg/04_faqs. htm#abbreviations>>.

3. *Failure mode and effect analysis:* This is a systematic approach to identifying potential errors and adverse outcomes before they occur. It has been adapted from the aerospace industry and can be applied to the medication use process. It is a system to prospectively review each step in the medication use process with the goal of improving safety and decreasing potential errors. With the use of failure mode and effect analysis, health systems should be able to design and implement medication use processes that have a significantly lower incidence of medication errors.[68]

4. *Drug and patient information:* Lack of information has been frequently cited as a cause of medication errors, particularly prescribing errors. Health systems should ensure that all health care providers have ready access to necessary patient-specific information and general drug information. Health systems may implement technology that allows viewing of a patient chart over a computer terminal or provides electronic medical references. Health systems may establish a drug information center where pharmacists are readily available to answer drug therapy questions. Considerable success has also been found in reducing medication errors when a knowledgeable pharmacist participates on medical rounds.[10]

5. *Training:* It is important for health care professionals to stay up-to-date regarding drug therapy. Health systems should contribute to this effort by supporting educational programs for their employees.[49]

6. *Reporting:* Health systems should implement nonpunitive systems for medication error reporting. Accurate error monitoring will help organizations implement successful medication use processes that minimize adverse outcomes associated with medication errors.

7. *Technology:* The health care industry seems to be behind other industries in the area of informatics.[42] To significantly improve quality of care and minimize medication errors, health systems need to make a substantial investment in information technology and in training health professionals to use new technology.[69] Health care practitioners need to have ready access to medical and drug information, patient data, and an automated medication order system. The lack of drug and patient information, as described, has been associated with a large number of prescribing errors. Automated dispensing equipment and software that screens for drug-drug interactions and proper dosing can reduce errors.[70,71] Implementation of electronic prescribing, also known as physician order entry, would minimize many problems with illegible writing and abbreviations and would save time for pharmacists and physicians.[72] Furthermore, electronic prescribing has been shown to significantly reduce the number of serious medication errors.[73] It's already being used in many institutions nationwide. Instead of handwriting orders that

are then transcribed by a nurse, prescribers use an electronic system to select a drug name, dose, and dosing regimen. It's an effective tool that is now endorsed by the Institute for Safe Medication Practices. While electronic prescribing helps resolve one type of error, it can create other types. These systems might actual increase the rate of drug selection errors. Because prescribers of medication are picking from a list, there is an increased change of selecting the wrong drug, strength, or formulation. Pharmacists need to be extra alert for potential errors in drug selection when electronic prescribing systems are in place.

Bar coding is another technology that can greatly recue medication errors, particularly dispensing and administration errors. In 2004, the FDA passed a rule requiring linear bar codes on most prescription and over-ther-counter drugs and blood products used in the hospital setting. In some cases, these systems can reduce medication error rates by up to 85%. The way the systems work is simple. Each medication that is dispensed gets a bar code. Each patient in the hospital also gets a bracelet to wear that has a bar code. When the medication is dispensed the bar code on the medication is scanned to ensure that it matches the order that was entered. When the medication gets to the patient both the medication and the patient bracelet are scanned. The computer system checks to determine if in fact the correct medication is being given to the correct person.[74] A slightly different technology that is used in this same way is radio frequency identification (RFID), which employs a chip that can be read by an electronic device. In the future, this chip may be embedded in the medication, medication packaging, and/or the patient.

NATIONAL PRIORITY

Medication error prevention may be more important now than ever before for health systems. The Healthcare Financing Administration (HCFA) has initiated new quality of care measures to ensure that health systems participating in the Medicare and Medicaid programs are minimizing medication errors. The new conditions of participation are now less focused on procedures and more focused on outcomes. Citing modern drug information systems and drug packaging as significant tools to reduce medication errors, the HCFA expects health systems to document a medication error rate of 2% or less.[75]

In 1998, the Institute of Medicine (IOM) formed the Quality of Healthcare in America Committee that was charged with developing a strategy to improve quality in health care. In their published report, *"To Err is Human: Building a Safer Health System,"* the Committee highlights what is currently known about the extent of medical errors, what contributes to medical errors, and recommendations to minimize errors and improve the quality of health care in the United States. The report can be found in full-text on the Internet at http://books.nap.edu/html/to_err_is_human/. The Committee's recommendations include the following:[4]

1. *Creation of a Center for Patient Safety.* This center would fall within the control of the Agency for Healthcare Research and Quality (AHRQ) and would be responsible for setting national goals for patient safety, tracking progress toward those goals, and reporting progress to the President of the United States and Congress. The Center would also contribute to better understanding of errors in health care and identify methods for preventing errors by funding research activities and information dissemination programs.

2. *Development of a national mandatory reporting system.* This system would initially focus on hospital mandatory reporting of deaths and serious harm secondary to medical error to state governments. State governments would then share information with other states as coordinated by the Center for Patient Safety. Eventually, other institutional settings, including ambulatory care settings, would also have the same requirements. Furthermore, standards would be developed for reporting, including uniform reporting nomenclature and taxonomy.

3. *Encouragement of voluntary reporting systems.* The Center for Patient Safety would encourage increased participation in voluntary reporting programs and fund pilot projects for reporting systems.

4. *Extend peer-review protection to information about medical errors used to improve organizational quality and safety.* The Committee suggests that the United States Congress ensure confidentiality in cases of medical error that do not result in serious harm to a patient by enacting specific legislation to protect that information. This will create an environment conducive to increased reporting of certain kinds of errors that will help organizations fix flaws in their systems.

5. *Performance standards for health care organizations should focus more on patient safety.* The Committee suggests that licensing and accreditation standards should eventually be implemented that require patient safety programs as a minimum standard. Purchasers of health care (i.e., insurance companies) should then provide incentives for demonstration of continuous improvement in patient safety.

6. *Performance standards for health care professionals should focus more on patient safety.* Health care professional licensing bodies (e.g., state boards of pharmacy) should begin to require periodic reexamination to ensure competence and understanding of safety practices. Licensing or credentialing bodies should develop ways to identify practitioners that are unsafe. Professional organizations should develop and offer training to health care professionals and disseminate informative publications regarding patient safety. Safety issues should also be incorporated into practice guidelines. Professionals and professional organizations should collaborate on issues of patient safety.

7. *The FDA should focus more attention on the safe use of drugs.* The Committee suggests that the FDA should develop standards for drug packaging and labeling to minimize medication errors associated with labeling and sound-alike drugs. The FDA,

pharmaceutical industry, and health care professionals should work together to identify and remedy safety issues associated with problematic labeling and naming.

8. *Health care organizations and professionals should make continually improved patient safety a serious pursuit with defined executive responsibility.* Patient safety programs should be developed with well-described and understood standards and a nonpunitive system for reporting and analyzing errors. Interdisciplinary team training programs should be completed.

9. *Health care organizations should implement medication safety practices proven to reduce errors.* All health care organizations should implement programs for improving safety of the medication use process based on published recommendations shown to reduce medication errors.

The recommendations of the Committee are broad and do not address many of the finer points that health care organizations must deal with to implement a safer environment for patients. However, the recommendations provide a map to improved patient safety for organizations to pursue. The Committee suggests reevaluation of the same issues again in 5 years to assess progress toward improved patient safety and decreased medical errors.

Conclusion

Medication misadventures are a serious problem in the U.S. health care system. Recognition of the problem is an important first step in developing strategies to minimize their occurrence. Reporting of medication misadventures is an absolute necessity to gauge our progress and direct our efforts.

An editorial appearing in the *American Journal of Health-System Pharmacy* encourages institutions to recognize the role that pharmacists play in minimizing errors.[76] Adequate staffing by qualified pharmacists who actively participate in all aspects of the medication use process, including prescribing, dispensing, and administering, has been shown to significantly decrease medication errors.[10] Institutions are urged to use pharmacists to their full potential, by more actively employing pharmacists in clinical settings where they can collaborate with other health care professionals, so that they may strengthen efforts to reduce medication errors.

Pharmacists have the responsibility of ensuring the safe and effective use of medications. Although other health care providers and health care systems must significantly contribute to this effort, pharmacists, as champions of the medication use process, must take a leading role. Several studies have already demonstrated the tremendous benefit pharmacists can provide to patients through reduction of medication misadventures. As a mandate of pharmaceutical care, pharmacists need to continue to contribute to improving patient care by actively pursuing improvements in the medication use process.

Study Questions

1. Describe the relationship of medication misadventures, adverse drug events, adverse drug reactions, and medication errors.

2. Define adverse drug reaction.

3. Describe the JCAHO requirements for adverse drug reaction reporting.

4. List 10 reasons why physicians may not report adverse drug reactions.

5. Describe a successful adverse drug reaction program.

6. Explain how technology might improve adverse drug reaction programs.

7. Explain the "five rights."

8. Who is responsible for minimizing medication errors?

9. Why should pharmacists take a leading role in minimizing adverse drug events?

10. Identify three national medication error reporting programs.

11. Explain why it is important to analyze the medication use process when errors occur rather than blaming individuals.

12. Describe strategies practitioners and health systems can use to minimize medication errors.

REFERENCES

1. American Society of Health-System Pharmacists. Suggested definitions and relationships among medication misadventures, medication errors, adverse drug events, and adverse drug reactions. Am J Health Syst Pharm. 1998;55:165–6.

2. Rich DS. A process for interpreting data on adverse drug events: determining optimal target levels. Clin Ther. 1998;20(Suppl C): c59–C71.

3. Rich DS. The Joint Commission's revised sentinel event policy on medication errors. Hosp Pharm. 1998;33:881–5.

4. Institute of Medicine. To err is human: building a safer health system. Washington, DC: National Academy Press; 1999.

5. White TJ, Arakelian A, Rho JP. Counting the costs of drug-related adverse events. Pharmacoeconomics. 1999;15:445–58.

6. Johnson JA, Bootman JL. Drug-related morbidity and mortality. A cost-of-illness model. Arch Intern Med. 1995;155:1949–56.

7. Classen DC, Pestotnik SL, Evans S, Loyd JF, Burke JP. Adverse drug events in hospitalized patients. JAMA. 1997;277:301–6.

8. Ernst FR, Grizzle AJ. Drug-related morbidity and mortality: updating the cost-of-illness model. J Am Pharm Assoc. 2001;41:192–9.

9. Lesar TS, Briceland L, Stein DS. Factors related to errors in medication prescribing. JAMA. 1997;277:312–7.

10. Leape LL, Cullen DJ, Clapp M, Burdick E, Demonaco HJ, Erickson JI, et al. Pharmacist participation on physician rounds and adverse drug events in the intensive care unit. JAMA. 1999;282:267–70.

11. Making health care safer: a critical analysis of patient safety practices. Evidence Report/Technology Assessment: No. 43. AHRQ Publication No. 01-E058, 2001. Rockville (MD): Agency for Healthcare Research and Quality. Available from: http://www.ahrq.gov/clinic/ptsafety

12. Beney J, Bero LA, Bond C. Expanding the roles of outpatient pharmacists: effects on health services utilisation, costs, and patient outcomes. Cochrane Database Syst Rev. 2000(3):CD000336.

13. Wong YL. Adverse effect of pharmaceutical excipients in drug therapy. Ann Acad Med. 1993;22:99–102.

14. Calis KA, Young LR. Clinical analysis of adverse drug reactions: a primer for clinicians. Hosp Pharm. 2004;39:697–712.

15. Forster AJ, Halil RB, Tierney MG. Pharmacist surveillance of adverse drug events. Am J Health Syst Pharm. 2004;61:1466–72.

16. Swanson KM, Landry JP, Anderson RP. Pharmacy-coordinated, multidisciplinary adverse drug reaction program. Top Hosp Pharm Manage. 1992;12:49–59.

17. Lazarou J, Pomeranz BM, Corey PN. Incidence of adverse drug reactions in hospitalized patients: a meta-analysis of prospective studies. JAMA. 1998;279:1200–5.

18. Fincham JE. An overview of adverse drug reactions. Am Pharm. 1991;NS31:435–41.

19. Rich DS. New JCAHO medication management standards for 2004. Am J Health Syst Pharm. 2004;61:1349–58.

20. Lamy PP. Adverse drug effects. Clin Ger Med. 1990;6:293–307.

21. Karch FE, Lasagna L. Toward the operational identification of adverse drug reactions. Clin Pharmacol Ther. 1977;21:247–54.

22. Naranjo CA, Busto U, Sellers EM, Sandor P, Ruiz I, Roberts EA, et al. A method of estimating the probability of adverse drug reactions. Clin Pharmacol Ther. 1981;30:239–45.

23. Kramer MS, Leventhal JM, Hutchinson TA, Feinstein AR. An algorithm for the operational assessment of adverse drug reactions: I. Background, description, and instructions for use. JAMA. 1979;242:623–32.

24. Hutchinson TA, Leventhal JM, Kramer MS, Karch FE, Lipman AG, Feinstein AR. An algorithm for the operational assessment of adverse drug reactions: II. Demonstration of reproducibility and validity. JAMA. 1979;242:633–8.

25. Jones JK. Adverse drug reactions in the community health setting: approaches to recognizing, counseling, and reporting. Fam Comm Health. 1982;5(2):58–67.

26. Michel DJ, Knodel LC. Comparison of three algorithms used to evaluate adverse drug reactions. Am J Hosp Pharm. 1986;43:1709–14.

27. Lane DA. The bayesian approach to causality assessment: an introduction. Drug Inf J. 1986;20:455–61.

28. What is a serious adverse event? [Cited 2000 Feb 28]: [1 screen]. Available from: http://www.fda.gov/medwatch/report/desk/advevnt.htm

29. Faich GA, Dreis M, Tomita D. National adverse drug reaction surveillance: 1986. Arch Intern Med. 1988;148:785–7.

30. Stang PE, Fox JL. Adverse drug events and the Freedom of Information Act: an apple in Eden. Ann Pharmacother. 1992;26:238–43.

31. Rogers AS, Israel E, Smith CR, Levine D, McBean AM, Valente C, et al. Physician knowledge, attitudes, and behaviour related to reporting adverse drug events. Arch Intern Med. 1988;148:1596–1600.

32. MedWatch: The FDA Medical Products Reporting Program. FDA Med Bull. 1993;23:insert.

33. Hoffman RP. Adverse drug reaction reporting—problems and solutions. J Mich Pharm. 1989;27:400–3, 407–8.

34. Food and Drug Administration. Dietary supplements containing ephedrine alkaloids final rule summary [accessed 2004 Mar 21]. Available from: http://www.fda.gov/oc/initiatives/ephedra/february2004/finalsummary.html

35. Center for Food Safety and Applied Nutrition. Announcing CAERS—The CFSAN Adverse Event Reporting System. 2002 Aug 29 [accessed 2004 Mar 28]. Available from: http://www.cfsan.fda.gov/~dms/caersltr.html.

36. ASHP guidelines on adverse drug reaction monitoring and reporting. Am J Hosp Pharm. 1989;46:336–7.

37. Saltiel E, Johnson E, Shane R. A team approach to adverse drug reaction surveillance: success at a tertiary care hospital. Hosp Form. 1995;30:226–32.

38. Classen DC, Pestotnik SL, Evans RS, Burke JP. Computerized surveillance of adverse drug events in hospital patients. JAMIA. 1991;266:2847–51.

39. Jha AK, Kuperman GJ, Teich JM, Leape L, Shea B, Rittenberg E, et al. Identifying adverse drug events: development of a computer-based monitor and comparison with chart review and stimulated voluntary report. JAMIA. 1998;5:305–14.

40. Raschke RA, Gollihare B, Wunderlich TA, GuidryJR, Leibowitz AI, Peirce JC, et al. A computer alert system to prevent injury from adverse drug events. JAMA. 1998;280:1317–20.

41. Dalton M, Chambers G, Halvachs F. Implementing an effective drug interaction reporting program. Hosp Pharm. 1999;34:31–42.

42. Felkey BG. Health system informatics. Am J Health Syst Pharm. 1997;54:274–80.

43. Lesar TS, Lomaestro BM, Pohl H. Medication-prescribing errors in a teaching hospital: a 9-year experience. Arch Intern Med. 1997;157:1569–76.

44. Kelly WN. Pharmacy contributions to adverse medication events. ASHP Online. 1999 [cited 1999 Sept 8]: [1 screen]. Available from:http://www.ashp.org/public/proad/mederror/pkel.html

45. Coleman IC. Medication errors: picking up the pieces. Drug Top. 1999;143:83–92.

46. Chenier GE, Vogel DP. Medication error prevention guidelines. Pharm Pract News. 1999:25–8.

47. Senders JW. Theory and analysis of typical errors in a medical setting. Hosp Pharm. 1993;28:505–8.

48. Institute for Safe Medication Practices. The "five rights." 1999 Aug 17 [1999 cited Sept]: [1 screen]. Available from: http://www.ismp.org/MSAarticles/FiveRights.html

49. American Society of Hospital Pharmacists. ASHP guidelines on preventing medication errors in hospitals. Am J Hosp Pharm. 1993;50:305–14.

50. Abood RR. Errors in pharmacy practice. US Pharm. 1996;21:122–32.

51. Pepper GA. Errors in drug administration by nurses. ASHP Online. 1999 [cited 1999 Sept 8]: [1 screen]. Available from: http://www.ashp.org/public/proad/mederror/pep.html

52. Dunn EB, Wolfe JJ. Medication error classification and avoidance. Hosp Pharm. 1997;32:860–5.

53. Davis NM. Performance lapses as a cause of medication errors. Hosp Pharm. 1996;31:1524–5.

54. Davis NM. Lack of knowledge as a cause of medication errors. Hosp Pharm. 1997;32:16–25.

55. Grasha AF, O'Neill M. Cognitive processes in medication errors. US Pharm. 1996;21:96–109.

56. Ukens C. Breaking the trust: exclusive survey of dispensing errors. Drug Top. 1992;136:58–69.

57. DeMichele D. Preventing medication errors. US Pharm. 1995;20:69–75.

58. Fitzgerald WL, Wilson DB. Medication errors: lessons in law. Drug Top. 1998;142:84–93.

59. Davis NM. Lack or failure of the safety net as a cause of medication errors. Hosp Pharm. 1997;32:143–4.

60. Glut of medication errors focuses pharmacists on event reporting. Drug Util Rev. 1998:201–6.

61. Cohen MR. ISMP medication error report analysis: the mistake of blaming people and not the process. Hosp Pharm. 1997;32:1106–11.

62. Leape LL, Woods DD, Hatlie MJ, Kizer KW, Schroeder SA, Lundberg GD. Promoting patient safety by preventing medical error. JAMA. 1998;280:1444–7.

63. Landis NT. Disclosure of errors may have financial benefit. Am J Health Syst Pharm. 2000;57:312.

64. Cousins DD. Developing a uniform reporting system for preventable adverse drug events. Clin Ther. 1998;20:C45–C58.

65. Proulx SM. Medication errors. US Pharm. 1997;22:73.

66. Jones EH, Speerhas R. How physicians can prevent medication errors: practical strategies. Clev Clin J Med. 1997;64:355–9.

67. Institute for Safe Medication Practices. ISMP list of error-prone abbreviations, symbols, and dose designations. ISMP Medication Safety Alert. 2003;8:3–4.

68. McNally KM, Page MA, Sunderland B. Failure-mode and effects analysis in improving a drug distribution system. Am J Health Syst Pharm. 1997;54:171–7.

69. Greiner AC, Knebel E, editors. Health professions education: a bridge to quality. Washington, DC: National Academy Press; 2004. Available from: http://www.nap.edu/openbook/0309087236/html/index.html

70. Neuenschwander M. Limiting or increasing opportunities for errors with dispensing automation. Hosp Pharm. 1996;31:1102–6.

71. McMullin ST, Reichley RM, Kahn MG, Dunagan WC, Bailey TC. Automated system for identifying potential dosage problems at a large university hospital. Am J Health Syst Pharm. 1997;54:545–9.

72. Davis NM, Cohen MR. Computer generated prescription orders. Am Pharm. 1995;NS35(9):10.

73. Bates DW, Leape LL, Cullen DJ, Laird N, Petersen LA, Teich JM, et al. Effect of computerized physician order entry and a team intervention on prevention of serious medication errors. JAMA. 1998;280:1311–6.

74. Food and Drug Administration. FDA Issues Bar Code Regulation. 2004 Feb 25 [accessed 2004 Mar 28]. Available from: http://www.fda.gov/oc/initiatives/barcode-sadr/fs-barcode.html

75. Wechsler J. Federal agencies seek to reduce drug errors, improve information on adverse events. Formulary. 1998;33:161–2.

76. Sellers JA. Too many errors, not enough pharmacists. Am J Health Syst Pharm. 2000;57:337.

18

Chapter Eighteen

Investigational Drugs

Bambi Grilley

Objectives

After completing this chapter, the reader will be able to

- List the major legislative acts that led to our current system of drug evaluation, approval, and regulation.
- List all of the requirements (as specified by the Office of Human Research Protections [OHRP]) for an institutional review board (IRB).
- Prepare appropriate pharmacy reviews of protocols for use by the IRB or other review committees when they evaluate new protocols.
- List the steps in the drug approval process.
- Describe the difference between a commercial investigational new drug (IND), treatment IND, an emergency IND, and an individual investigator IND.
- Define orphan drug status and list the advantages of classifying a drug as an orphan drug.
- Provide pharmacy support for clinical research including (but not limited to):
  - Ordering drug supplies for ongoing clinical trials.
  - Maintaining drug accountability records as required by the Food and Drug Administration (FDA).
  - Preparing drug and protocol data sheets for use by healthcare personnel in the hospital.
  - Preparing pharmacy budgets for sponsored clinical research.
  - Aiding study sponsors in designing and conducting clinical trials in their institution.
  - Assisting investigators in initiating and conducting clinical trials (including emergency use INDs).

It is estimated that $802 million is spent to get a new drug product to market in the United States.[1] For every 4000 products synthesized in the lab, only 5 will ever be tested in humans and only one of those will ever reach the market.[2] The FDA is the federal agency that decides which drugs, biologics, and medical devices are marketed in this country.[3] In fact, FDA-regulated products account for about 25 cents of every consumer dollar spent.[3] The centers of the FDA involved in regulating drugs, biologics, and medical devices used in humans are as follows:

- Center for Biologics Evaluation and Research (CBER)
- Center for Drug Evaluation and Research (CDER)
- Center for Devices and Radiological Health (CDRH)[4]

Since pharmacists are rarely involved in dispensing devices or radiologic products, this chapter will concentrate only on the regulations associated with CBER and CDER.

On average, the FDA approves two new molecular entities (NMEs) each month.[5] Since 1940, more than 1000 NMEs have been approved in the United States.[5] It is very important that the clinical trials on which the FDA will base their decisions be both scientifically accurate and complete. Pharmacists can play an important role in ensuring that the clinical trials conducted at their institutions meet the goals set forth by the study sponsor, the local investigator, and ultimately the FDA.

Currently, most investigational drug research is conducted by medical schools, hospitals, and organizations specifically designed to conduct clinical research trials. For this reason, the dispensing of investigational drugs rarely occurs in a community pharmacy setting. In some institutions, a pharmacist will be hired specifically to handle investigational drugs. More frequently, however, this role falls to a specified staff pharmacist or the drug information pharmacist. To successfully manage investigational drugs, the pharmacist must be a bookkeeper, inventory control manager, and, most importantly, an information disseminator. Before proceeding, it is necessary to define a number of terms that will be used in this chapter.

Definitions

- *Clinical investigation*: Any experiment in which a drug is administered or dispensed to one or more human subjects. An experiment is any use of a drug (except for the use of a marketed drug) in the course of medical practice. Although there are many other definitions, this is the FDA's definition and would seem the appropriate one to use given the nature of this topic. Please note that the FDA does not regulate the practice of medicine and prescribers are (as far as the agency is concerned) free to use any marketed drug for "off-label use."[6]

- *Clinical safety officer* (*CSO*): Also known as the regulatory management officer (RMO). This will be the sponsor's FDA contact person. Generally the CSO/RMO assigned to a drug's IND application will also be assigned to the New Drug Application (NDA).
- *Commercial IND*: An IND for which the sponsor is usually either a corporate entity or one of the institutes of the National Institutes of Health (NIH). In addition, CDER may designate other INDs as commercial if it is clear the sponsor intends the product to be commercialized at a later date.[7]
- *Control group*: The group of test animals or humans that receive a placebo (a dosage that does not contain active medicine) or active (a dosage that does contain active medicine) treatment. For most preclinical and clinical trials, the FDA will require that this group receive placebo (commonly referred to as the placebo control). However, some studies may have an active control, which generally consists of an available (standard of care) treatment modality. An active control may, with the concurrence of the FDA, be used in studies where it would be considered unethical to use a placebo. A historical control is one in which a group of previous patients is compared to a matched set of patients receiving the new therapy. A historical control might be used in cases where the disease is consistently fatal (i.e., acquired immunodeficiency syndrome [AIDS]).
- *Contract research organization* (*CRO*): An individual or organization that assumes one or more of the obligations of the sponsor through an independent contractual agreement.[6]
- *Drug master file* (*DMF*): A submission to the FDA that may be used to provide confidential detailed information about facilities, processes, or articles used in the manufacturing, processing, packaging, and storing of one or more human drugs.[8]
- *Drug product*: The final dosage form prepared from the drug substance.[9]
- *Drug substance*: An active ingredient that is intended to furnish pharmacologic activity or other direct effect in the diagnosis, cure, mitigation, treatment, or prevention of disease or to affect the structure or any function of the human body.[9]
- *Food and Drug Administration* (*FDA*): The agency of the U.S. government that is responsible for ensuring the safety and efficacy of all drugs on the market.[6,9]
- *Institutional Review Board* (*IRB*): A committee of reviewers that evaluates the ethical implications of a clinical study protocol.[10,11]
- *Investigational New Drug* (*IND*): A drug, antibiotic, or biologic that is used in a clinical investigation. The label of an investigational drug must bear the statement: "Caution: New Drug—Limited by Federal (or United States) law to investigational use."[6]
- *Investigational New Drug Application* (*INDA*): A submission to the FDA containing chemical information, preclinical data, and a detailed description of the planned clinical trials. Thirty days after submission of this document to the FDA by the sponsor,

clinical trials may be initiated in humans, unless the FDA places a clinical hold. When the FDA allows the studies to proceed, this document allows unapproved drugs to be shipped in interstate commerce.[6]

- *Investigator.* The individual responsible for initiating the clinical trial at the study site. This individual must treat the patients, assure that the protocol is followed, evaluate responses and adverse reactions, assure proper conduct of the study, and solve problems as they arise.[6]

- *New Drug Application (NDA):* The application to the FDA requesting approval to market a new drug for human use. The NDA contains data supporting the safety and efficacy of the drug for its intended use.[9]

- *New Molecular Entity (NME):* A compound that can be patented, that has not been previously approved.

- *Sponsor.* An organization (or individual) who takes responsibility for and initiates a clinical investigation. The sponsor may be an individual or pharmaceutical company, government agency, academic institution, private organization, or other organization.[6]

- *Sponsor-investigator.* An individual who both initiates and conducts a clinical investigation (i.e., submits the IND and directly supervises administration of the drug as well as other investigator responsibilities).[6]

- *Subject:* An individual who participates in a clinical investigation (either as the recipient of the investigational drug or as a member of the control group).[6]

History of Drug Development Regulation in the United States

For more than a century after the Declaration of Independence, drug products were not regulated in this country. Available drugs were often ineffective, but some were addictive, toxic, or even lethal. During this same period, doctors were not licensed and nearly anyone could practice medicine. The public was, for the most part, responsible for using common sense when evaluating which products they would use.

The evolution of drug regulations in this country is a study in human tragedy. Crises have instigated the development of many of the laws regulating drug development, preparation, and distribution.

The first federal law developed to deal with drug quality and safety was the Import Drug Act of 1848. This law was passed after it was discovered that American troops involved in the Mexican War had been supplied with substandard imported drugs. The act provided for the inspection, detention, and destruction or reexport of imported drug shipments that failed to meet prescribed standards.

The Pure Food and Drugs Act was passed in 1906. This law required that drugs not be mislabeled or adulterated and stated that they must meet recognized standards for strength and purity. Mislabeling in this context only referred to the identity or composition of drugs (not false therapeutic claims). False therapeutic claims were prohibited with the passing of the Sherley Amendment in 1912.

In 1937, sulfanilamide was released. This drug showed promise as an anti-infective agent and was prepared as an oral liquid. The vehicle used for this preparation was diethylene glycol (a sweet-tasting solvent similar to ethylene glycol, which was used as an automobile antifreeze). A total of 107 people died after taking this preparation. Within 1 year of this tragedy, the Food, Drug and Cosmetic Act of 1938 was enacted. This law required that the safety of drugs, when used in accordance with the labeled instructions, be proven through testing before they could be marketed. It was in this law that the submission of an NDA to the FDA was first described. The NDA was required to list the drug's intended uses and provide scientific evidence that the drug was safe. If after 60 days the FDA had not responded to the manufacturer regarding the NDA, the manufacturer was free to proceed with marketing of the product.

In 1951 the Durham-Humphrey Amendment was passed. This law divided pharmaceuticals into two distinct classes:

1. Over-the-counter (OTC) medications that could be safely self-administered.
2. Prescription (Rx) medications that had potentially dangerous side effects and, therefore, required expert medical supervision.

This law required the following statement be added to the labels for all prescription medications: "Caution: Federal Law prohibits dispensing without a prescription."

In 1962, another drug tragedy occurred that resulted in additional regulations. In that year, an inordinate number of pregnant women in Western Europe gave birth to children with severe deformities. These deformities were related to the use of the drug thalidomide. Although U.S. consumers were not directly affected by this tragedy, because thalidomide had not been released in the U.S. market, it was a compelling reason for the legislature to develop stronger laws regarding the testing of new drug products. The Kefauver-Harris Drug Amendment was passed the same year. This law specified that the manufacturer had to demonstrate proof of efficacy, as well as safety, prior to marketing any new drug. Additionally, this law required that drug manufacturers operate in conformity with current good manufacturing practices (CGMP). Finally, it stated that the FDA had to formally approve an NDA before the drug could be marketed.[12]

There are numerous other laws and regulations that affect drug products in the United States, but those mentioned above provide the legal foundation for the current regulation of drug products in this country. Based on these laws, the FDA has assumed a large role in assessing the safety and efficacy of drug products prior to their distribution in the United States.

As stated, the goal of the FDA is to provide American consumers with safe and effective therapy. Extensive debate regarding the need to reform the FDA has been ongoing in the United States for years. Critics of the FDA have long claimed that the approval process for drugs in this country is too costly and time consuming.[13] Interestingly, although a comparison of biotech drug approval times between the European Medicines Evaluation Agency (EMEA) and the United States reveals that biotechnology product approvals in Europe take less time than in the United States for the same product, certain categories of products were actually approved more quickly in the United States. Additionally, the EMEA does not have a mechanism to provide priority reviews for products and, thus, approval of those products takes longer in Europe than in the United States.[14] Nevertheless, the FDA and the federal government have initiated reforms designed to address criticism.[15] Recent reform acts include the Prescription Drug User Fee Act of 1992 (PDUFA), which was reauthorized in 1997 and 2002, and the Food and Drug Administration Modernization Act of 1997 (FDAMA). PDUFA redefined the time frames for NDA reviews and established revenues to fund the increased demands created by the new time frames.[16] The FDAMA, which reauthorized PDUFA, was much broader in scope and impacted not only the drug approval process, but also other aspects of the practices of pharmacy and medicine.[17] Finally, the FDA has undertaken many information technology initiatives to facilitate the regulatory review process. Included in these initiatives is the development of systems allowing for electronic submission, management, and review of regulatory information. Other attempts by the FDA to increase availability of investigational drugs and to expedite the drug approval process will be discussed later in this chapter.

Increasingly, drug companies are involved in global drug development. Historically, the regulatory requirements for drug approval varied from country to country, resulting in a significant amount of time and money being spent to receive multiple approvals. For this reason, the International Conference on Harmonization (ICH) has brought together officials from Europe, the United States, and Japan to develop common guidelines for ensuring the quality, safety, and efficacy of drugs. The FDA has been very involved in the development of the ICH guidelines.[18] The ultimate goal of these guidelines is to provide pharmaceutical firms a method to ensure simultaneous submission and rapid regulatory approval in the world's major markets. This would minimize duplication of effort, improve efficiency, and increase the quality and consistency of medical treatments available to patients worldwide.[19]

For gene therapy products, review and approval by the National Institutes of Health Office of Biotechnology Activities (NIH/OBA) and the Institutional Biosafety Committee are required in addition to review and approval by the FDA and IRB (discussed below). Submission requirements for the NIH/OBA are similar to those mandated by the FDA (covered later in this chapter). The review process for gene therapy products is a separate topic that will not be further addressed in this chapter. Individuals interested in regulatory requirements of gene therapy products can refer to review articles such as *Gene Transfer: Regulatory Issues and Their Impact on the Clinical Investigator and the GMP facility* published in Cytotherapy in 2003.[20]

In addition to the regulatory review of investigational drugs by the FDA, research protocols are also reviewed for ethical appropriateness by IRBs. The formalized process for protecting human subjects began with the Nuremberg Code. This code was used to judge the human experimentation conducted by the Nazis around the middle of the twentieth century. The Nuremberg Code states that "the voluntary consent of the human subjects is absolutely essential." The code goes on to specify that the subject must have the capacity to consent, must be free from coercion, and must comprehend the risks and benefits involved in the research.[21] The Declaration of Helsinki reemphasized the above points and distinguished between therapeutic and nontherapeutic research. This document was first developed in 1964 and has been revised multiple times, most recently in 2000.[22]

The National Institutes for Health (NIH), as part of the Department of Health and Human Services (DHHS), used these two documents to develop its own policies for the Protection of Human Subjects in 1966. These policies were raised to regulatory status in 1974 and established the IRB as a mechanism through which human subjects would be protected. The Belmont Report, released in 1978, further delineates the basic ethical principles underlying medical research on human subjects.[23] Title 45 Part 46 of the Code of Federal Regulations (CFR), which was released in 1981, was designed to make uniform the protection of human subjects in all federal agencies.[10] Title 21 Part 50 (approved in 1980) of the CFR sets forth guidelines for appropriate informed consent and Title 21 Part 56 (approved in 1981) of the CFR sets forth guidelines for the IRB.[11,24] Copies of these regulations can be obtained on the Internet at <<http://www.gpoaccess.gov/cfr/index.html.>>

These two documents are used by the FDA and the DHHS to evaluate the ethical conduct of clinical trials in the United States. Further information regarding the role of the IRB will be presented later in this chapter.

The Drug Approval Process

The first step in the drug approval process is preclinical testing. This testing is either *in vitro* or in animals. Before filing an IND, the sponsor must have developed a pharmacologic profile of the drug, determined its acute and subacute (14 to 90 days) toxicity in at least two species of animals. Chronic toxicity studies in animals can coincide with the use of the drug in clinical trials in humans (although they must be initiated at least 13 weeks in advance). The preclinical chronic toxicity studies must be of at least the same duration as any planned clinical trial (i.e., a 6-month study in humans requires at least 6 months of preclinical data).[12]

After the preclinical testing is completed, the sponsor will file an IND with the FDA. The IND is the application by the study sponsor to the FDA to begin clinical trials in humans.

Most often, the sponsor is a pharmaceutical company, but occasionally an individual investigator will file an IND and serve as a sponsor-investigator. The investigator IND is submitted when a physician plans to use an approved drug for a new indication (i.e., one that is outside the package labeling) or on occasion, for an unapproved product or for an NME. The IND requirements for the sponsor-investigator are the same as those for any other sponsor. For that reason, no differentiation will be made in the following discussion of the drug approval process.

The IND can be filed after the study sponsor has identified the pharmacologic profile of the drug and has results from both acute and short-term toxicity studies in animals. An IND is not required if the drug to be studied is marketed in the United States and all of the following requirements are met.

1. The study is not to be reported to the FDA in support of a new indication.
2. The study does not involve a different dose, route, or patient population that increases the risk to patients.
3. IRB approval and informed consent are secured.
4. The study will not be used to promote the drug's effectiveness for a new indication.

In situations where it is unclear whether an IND is required or not, a call to the FDA may be beneficial. If an IND is required, the application needs to contain the following information.

1. *Cover sheet*: Form 1571 (see Appendix 18–1). This form identifies the sponsor, documents that the sponsor agrees to follow appropriate regulations, and identifies any involved CRO. This is a legal document.
2. *Table of contents*
3. *Introductory statement*: States the name, structure, pharmacologic class, dosage form, and all active ingredients in the investigational drug; the objectives and planned duration of the investigation should be stated here.
4. *General investigational plan*: Describes the rationale, indications, and general approach for evaluating the drug, the types of trials to be conducted, the projected number of patients who will be treated, and any potential safety concerns; the purpose of this section is to give the FDA reviewers a general overview of the plan to study the drug.
5. *Investigator's brochure*: An information packet containing all available information on the drug including its formula, pharmacologic and toxicologic effects, pharmacokinetics, and any information regarding the safety and risks associated with the drug; it is important that this brochure be kept current and comprehensive; therefore, it should be amended as necessary. The investigator's brochure may be used by the investigator or other healthcare professionals as a reference during the conduct of the research study.

6. *Clinical protocol* (*note*: in general, phase I protocols are allowed to be less detailed than phase II and phase III protocols).
   - *Objectives and purpose*: A description of the purpose of the trial (a typical phase I objective would be to determine the maximum tolerated dose of the investigational drug, whereas a typical phase III objective would be to compare the safety and efficacy of the investigational drug to placebo or standard therapy).
   - *Investigator data*: Provides qualifications and demographic data of the investigators involved in the clinical trial (may be presented on form 1572 [see Appendix 18–2]).
   - *Patient selection*: Describes the characteristics of patients who are eligible for enrollment in the trial and states factors that would exclude the patient.
   - *Study design*: Describes how the study will be completed; if the study is to be randomized, this will be described here with a description of the alternate therapy.
   - *Dose determination*: Describes the dose (with possible adjustments) and route of administration of the investigational drug; if retreatment or maintenance therapy of patients is allowed, it will be detailed in this section.
   - *Observations*: Describes how the objectives stated earlier in the protocol are to be assessed.
   - *Clinical procedures*: Describes all laboratory tests or clinical procedures that will be used to monitor the effects of the drug in the patient; the collection of these data is intended to minimize the risk to the patients.
   - *IRB approval for protocol*: Documentation of this approval is not required as part of the IND application process; however, form 1571 does state that an IRB will review and approve each study in the proposed clinical investigation before allowing initiation of those studies.
7. *Chemistry, manufacturing, and control data*
   - *Drug substance*: Describes the drug substance including its name, biologic, physical, and chemical characteristics; the address of the manufacturer; the method of synthesis or preparation; and the analytical methods used to assure purity, identity, and the substance's stability.
   - *Drug product*: Describes the drug product including all of its components; the address of the manufacturer; the analytical methods used to ensure identity, quality, purity, and strength of the product; and the product's stability.
   - *Composition, manufacture, and control of any placebo used in the trial*: The FDA does not require that the placebo be identical to the investigational drug; however, it wants to ensure that the lack of similarity does not jeopardize the trial.
   - *Labeling*: Copies of all labels (drug substance, product, and packages).
   - *Environmental assessment*: Presents a claim for categorical exclusion from the requirement for an environmental assessment (a statement that the amount of

waste expected to reach the environment may reasonably be expected to be nontoxic).

8. *Pharmacology and toxicology data*
   - *Pharmacology and drug disposition*: Describes the pharmacology, mechanism of action, absorption, distribution, metabolism, and excretion of the drug in animals and *in vitro*.
   - *Toxicology*: Describes the toxicology in animals and *in vitro*.
   - A statement that all nonclinical laboratories involved in the research adhere to Good Laboratory Practice (GLP) regulations.

9. *Previous human experience*: Summary of human experiences, which includes data from the United States and, where applicable, foreign markets. Known safety and efficacy data should be presented (especially if the drug was withdrawn from foreign markets for reasons of safety or efficacy).

10. *Additional information*: Other information that would help the reviewer evaluate the proposed clinical trial should be included here. For example, if a drug has the potential for abuse, data on the drug's dependence and abuse potential should be discussed in this section.[25]

The Letter of Authorization (LOA) to cross-reference a Drug Master File, IND application, or NDA (referred to in item 9 on page 1 of form 1571) is required when the investigational product (or some component of the investigational product) being used in the research is being supplied by a manufacturer other than the study sponsor. The original holder of the IND/NDA/DMF prepares the LOA. An LOA is frequently required when two companies are working together toward development of a product.[8]

The IND should be amended as necessary. There are four types of documents that may be used to amend the IND. They are as follows:

1. *Protocol amendments*: Submitted when a sponsor wants to change a previously submitted protocol or add a new study protocol to an existing IND.[26]

2. *Information amendments*: Submitted when information becomes available that would not be presented using a protocol amendment, IND safety report, or annual report (for example, new chemistry data).[27]

3. *IND safety reports*: Reports clinical and animal adverse reactions; reporting requirements depend on the nature, severity, and frequency of the experience. The following definitions are used to help evaluate adverse reactions.
   a. *Serious adverse drug experience:* Any adverse drug experience occurring at any dose that results in any of the following outcomes: death, a life-threatening adverse drug experience, inpatient hospitalization or prolongation of existing hospitalization, a persistent or significant disability/incapacity, or a congenital anomaly/birth

defect. Important medical events that may not result in death, be life threatening, or require hospitalization may be considered a serious adverse drug experience when, based on appropriate medical judgment, they may jeopardize the patient or subject and may require medical or surgical intervention to prevent one of the outcomes listed in this definition.

b. *Unexpected adverse drug experience:* Any adverse drug experience that is not listed in the current labeling for the drug product. This includes events that may be symptomatically and pathophysiologically related to an event listed in the labeling, but differs from the event because of greater severity or specificity.

For serious and unexpected, fatal, or life-threatening adverse reactions associated with the use of the drug, the sponsor is required to notify the FDA by telephone or fax within 7 calendar days after the sponsor receives the information. The sponsor must also submit a written report within 15 calendar days. For clinical and nonclinical adverse events that are both serious and unexpected, the sponsor must notify the FDA in writing within 15 calendar days. The written reports should describe the current adverse event and identify all previously filed safety reports concerning similar adverse events. The written report may be submitted as a narrative or as form 3500A.[28]

4. *Annual reports:* Submitted within 60 days of the annual effective date of an IND; it should describe the progress of the investigation including information on the individual studies, summary information of the IND (summary of adverse experiences, IND safety reports, preclinical studies completed in the last year), relevant developments in foreign markets, and changes in the investigators brochure.[29]

Each submission to a specific IND is required to be numbered sequentially (starting with 000). A total of three sets (the original and two copies) of all submissions to an IND file (whether a new IND or revisions to an existing IND) are sent to the FDA.[25]

Once submitted to the FDA, the IND will be forwarded to the appropriate review division based on the therapeutic category of the product.[12] The FDA has 30 days after receipt of an IND to respond to the sponsor. The sponsor may begin clinical trials if there is no response from the FDA within 30 days.[30] The FDA delays initiation of a new study or discontinues an ongoing study by issuing a clinical hold. Clinical holds are most often used when the FDA identifies an issue (through initial review or through later submissions) that the agency feels poses a significant risk to the subjects. After this issue has been satisfactorily resolved, the clinical hold can be removed and the investigations can be initiated or resumed.[31]

There are four phases of clinical trials. Clinical studies generally begin cautiously. As experience with the agent grows, the dose and duration of exposure to the agent may also increase. The number of patients treated at each phase of study and the duration of the studies can vary significantly depending on statistical considerations, the prevalence of patients affected by the disease, and the importance of the new drug. However, some general guidelines regarding the four phases of clinical testing are presented below.

A phase I trial is the first use of the agent in humans. As such, these studies are usually initiated with cautious (low) doses and in small numbers of subjects. Doses may be increased as safety is established. A phase I study will usually treat 20 to 80 patients and last an average of 6 months to 1 year. The purpose of a phase I trial is to determine the safety and toxicity of the agent. Frequently these trials include a pharmacokinetic portion. These trials assist in identifying the preferred route of administration and a safe dosage range. When possible, these trials are initiated in normal, healthy volunteers. This allows for evaluation of the effect of the drug on a subject who does not have any preexisting conditions. In situations in which this is not practical, such as oncology drugs, in which the drug itself can be highly toxic, these drugs are usually reserved for patients who have exhausted all conventional options.

A phase II trial is one in which the drug is used in a small number of subjects who suffer from the disease or condition that the drug is proposed to treat. The purpose of a phase II trial is to evaluate the efficacy of the agent. Data from the phase I trial, *in vitro* testing, and animal testing may be used to identify which group of patients is most likely to benefit from therapy with this agent. Phase II trials usually treat between 100 and 200 patients and will average about 2 years in duration.

Phase III trials build on the experience gained during the phase II trials. The purpose of a phase III study is to further define the efficacy and safety of the agent. Frequently, in phase III studies, the new agent is compared to current therapy. These trials are usually multicenter studies, generally treat from 600 to 1000 patients, and usually last about 3 years. Some of the phase III trials will be "pivotal" studies and will serve as the basis for the NDA for a drug's marketing approval.

After phase III trials have been completed, the sponsor will submit an NDA to the FDA requesting approval of the drug for marketing. The FDA requires the completion of two well-designed, controlled clinical trials prior to submission to the FDA. However, the sponsor will include information gathered from all of the clinical trials to show that the drug is safe and effective and to describe the pharmacology and pharmacokinetics of the drug. The NDA will include all preclinical data, clinical data, manufacturing methods, product quality assurance, relevant foreign clinical testing (or marketing experience), and all published reports of experience with the drug (whether sponsored by the company or not). A proposed package insert will be supplied as well.[32]

The NDA will be distributed to the appropriate FDA drug review divisions. This is one of the same divisions described earlier in this chapter in the section discussing the IND evaluation process. As noted, these divisions are based on the therapeutic group of the drug. The same reviewer may be assigned to review the IND and the NDA.[12]

The speed at which the NDA will be processed is to some extent determined by the classification the drug receives during its initial review. Each drug is rated with a number—letter designation that evaluates two separate aspects of the drug. The number portion of the rating is associated with the uniqueness of the drug product (ranging from 1 for an NME to 7 for a drug that has already been marketed, but without an approved NDA). The letter portion of the rating is associated with the therapeutic potential of the drug product. The P (priority review) designation is given to drugs that represent a therapeutic advance with respect to available therapy, whereas an S (standard review) is given to drugs that have little or no therapeutic gain over previously available drugs.[33]

During the review process, the FDA may utilize one of its 15 prescription drug advisory committees to help review the NDA. These committees are composed of experts. They provide the agency with independent, nonbinding advice, and recommendations regarding the NDA.[12,33] Within 180 days of receipt of an NDA, the FDA will review the application and send the applicant an action letter (stating the NDA is either "approved," "approvable," or "not approvable"). When an approval letter is sent, the drug is considered approved as of the date of the letter (this rarely occurs with an original NDA). When an approvable letter is sent, it means that the application "substantially meets the requirements for marketing approval and the agency believes that it can approve the application if specific additional information or material is submitted or specific conditions are agreed to by the applicant."[34,35] The sponsor has 10 days to respond to the approvable letter (although an extension is usually granted if requested within the 10-day period).[36] A not approvable letter is sent when the FDA believes the NDA is insufficient for approval. The letter will describe the deficiencies in the application. Once again the sponsor has 10 days to respond to the letter. The sponsor can amend the NDA, withdraw the NDA, or request a hearing with the FDA to clarify whether grounds exist for denying approval of the application.[37]

After the drug has been approved, phase IV trials may be initiated. These trials are also referred to as postmarketing studies. They are conducted for the approved indication, but may evaluate different doses, the effects of extended therapy, or the drug's safety in patient populations that were not represented in premarketing clinical trials. These phase IV trials may be requested by the FDA or they may be initiated by the sponsor in an attempt to gather more data on the safety and efficacy of the drug or to identify a competitive advantage of the drug over other available therapies.[38]

The median NDA review process (from submission to approval) takes 7.7 months for priority NDAs, while the median approval time for standard NDAs was 15.4 months.[39] Although there has been a significant decrease in review times since the 1980s, for diseases (such as AIDS and cancer) where these investigational drugs may be the only therapy available, this time delay can still be a significant factor.[40] Therefore, in addition to the priority classification assigned at the time of NDA review, the FDA has also developed procedures to expedite the drug development and review process and has established methods for providing promising experimental drugs to desperately ill patients.

The treatment IND is one way the FDA has allowed for increased accessibility of experimental drugs for desperately ill patients. For a drug to qualify for use under a treatment IND, it must meet the following criteria:

1. The drug must be intended to treat a serious or immediately life-threatening disease.
2. There must be no satisfactory alternative therapy for the patient.
3. The drug must be under investigation in controlled clinical trials.
4. The sponsor must be actively pursuing FDA approval of the drug.

There are two different categories of treatment IND: immediately life-threatening conditions and serious conditions. The FDA defines immediately life-threatening conditions as those where death is likely to occur within a matter of months. In this situation, the FDA would allow treatment with the drug earlier than phase III, but not earlier than phase II. Serious conditions are defined as those in which the disease causes major irreversible morbidity (such as Alzheimer's disease). For use in treating serious conditions, the drug must meet tougher requirements for safety and efficacy. As a result, treatment INDs for serious illnesses are more likely to be granted during phase III trials or after all clinical trials have been completed. Provisions of the treatment IND regulations permit charging for the investigational drug under certain conditions. The amount the sponsor may charge for the investigational drug cannot exceed the amount necessary to recover costs associated with drug production, development, and distribution. Both drug sponsors and individual investigators are eligible to request FDA approval of a treatment IND. The drug sponsor may do so via submission of a treatment protocol, which states how and why the drug will be used. If the drug sponsor will not establish a treatment protocol and an investigator feels access to the drug is necessary, the investigator may submit a treatment IND for the drug, assuming the drug is available. The treatment IND that the investigator submits should contain all of the components of a treatment protocol as well as information about the investigator and a description of the steps taken by the investigator to obtain the drug under a treatment protocol from the drug sponsor.[41-43]

The parallel track is a way the FDA has allowed for increased accessibility of experimental drugs specifically for AIDS patients. Using this mechanism, drugs may be made available after completion of phase I studies to patients who are ineligible for enrollment in the clinical trials and are unable to benefit from current therapies. Regular controlled studies for safety and efficacy are still essential and the sponsors are required to monitor the impact of the parallel track on enrollment in ongoing clinical trials. To date this mechanism has been rarely utilized.[44,45]

The most recent effort to improve access to potentially beneficial products is known as the Cancer Initiative of 1996.[46] The most recent clarification of the initiative was released in 2004.[47] This policy was designed to address the needs of oncology patients. This initiative allows for the following:

1. Accelerating drug approval by using surrogate endpoints to approve oncology drugs. A surrogate endpoint of a clinical trial is "a laboratory measurement or a physical sign used as a substitute for a clinically meaningful endpoint that measures directly how a patient feels, functions, or survives. Changes induced by a therapy on a surrogate endpoint are expected to reflect changes in a clinically meaningful endpoint."[48]
2. Treating patients in the United States with drugs approved in other countries via expanded access protocols.
3. Expanding the number of consumer members on the advisory committees.
4. Reducing the number of INDs required to conduct studies of marketed oncology drugs.

There has been much interest in this program and it has shown promising results.[12]

Emergency use INDs are another way that the FDA allows access to investigational drugs for desperately ill patients. The emergency use IND allows shipment of a drug by the sponsor prior to the submission of an IND. This type of IND can only be used to treat individual patients with life-threatening diseases where all other options have been exhausted. The FDA must authorize the emergency use IND; however, prospective IRB approval is not required.[49,50]

The FDA has also attempted to expedite the review process for new drugs. One such initiative is the accelerated drug approval program. This program can be utilized if the drug is intended for the treatment of a serious or life-threatening condition and it demonstrates the potential to address unmet medication needs for the condition. The application would then be evaluated by weighing the risk/benefit relationship of the severity of the disease and alternatives to the new product. These products could be approved based on surrogate endpoints or on clinical endpoints other than survival or irreversible morbidity if the product can provide a meaningful therapeutic benefit to patients. In some cases, this approval could be given as early as post-phase II studies. Two pivotal phase II studies would be required before the NDA could be submitted. In these situations, the FDA can apply restrictions to the marketing and distribution of such products and significant postmarketing studies (phase IV) will be required because they would provide information regarding larger and more diverse patient populations than may be seen in the earlier phases of study.[51]

Finally, the FDA has attempted to improve the drug development and approval process by initiating a program of meeting with study sponsors to discuss and review the preclinical and clinical studies that will be necessary for drug development and approval. The purpose of these meetings is to help the sponsor minimize wasteful expenditures of time and money while still meeting the scientific objectives necessary for drug approval. For products designed to treat desperately ill patients, these meetings can occur prior to submission of the initial IND and at the end of phase I studies. Additionally, the FDA will meet with the sponsor of any IND at the end of phase II studies and prior to submission of the NDA.[52-55]

The Institutional Review Board

The IRB is a committee of at least five members formed to review proposed clinical trials and the progress of such studies to ensure that the rights and welfare of human subjects are protected. The IRB must contain at least one member who has specialized in a scientific area (usually this will be a physician) and at least one board member who has a specialty in a non-scientific area, such as law, ethics, or religion. Additionally, the IRB must contain at least one individual who is not affiliated with the institution where the research is being conducted. Membership of the IRB varies between institutions. Common members of IRBs include physicians, pharmacists, nurses, lawyers, clergy, and laypeople. The IRB is also responsible for ensuring that the proposed clinical trial is not in conflict with the institution's research policies or philosophy. The IRB and the study sponsor will have little if any direct contact. The primary investigator (PI) generally acts as the liaison between these two parties. The IRB should evaluate the research proposal to ensure that the following requirements are met.

- The risks to subjects are minimal.
- The expected risk/anticipated benefit ratio must be reasonable.
- Equitable subject selection is used.
- Informed consent must be received from each participant (or his or her representative).
- Informed consent must be documented in writing.
- Data must be monitored to ensure subject safety.
- Patient confidentiality must be maintained.
- If appropriate, additional safeguards against coercion must be included in studies that include vulnerable subjects (children, prisoners, pregnant women, mentally disabled people, or economically or educationally disadvantaged persons).

A notable exception to the requirements for written informed consent, as described above, has been provided for research done in emergency circumstances involving human subjects who cannot give informed consent because of their emerging, life-threatening medical condition (for which available treatments are unproven or unsatisfactory), and where the intervention must be administered before informed consent from the subject's legally authorized representative is feasible. In these situations the exception from informed consent requirements may proceed only after the sponsor has received prior written permission from the FDA (via IDE or IND approval) and from the IRB. In this type of research, both community consultation and public disclosure must be provided for the protocol.[56,57]

The IRB must, at a minimum, perform annual reviews of all ongoing clinical trials and evaluate adverse experiences to ensure that the criteria listed above continue to be met.[58,59]

The IRB must maintain documentation of all IRB activities including copies of all research proposals reviewed, minutes of IRB meetings, records of continuing review activities, copies of all correspondence between the IRB and the investigators, a list of IRB members, written procedures of the IRB, and statements of significant new findings provided to subjects. This documentation should be retained for at least 3 years. Records that pertain to research should be retained for 3 years after the research is completed.[60–62]

Some institutions divide their review of proposed clinical research into two separate processes. One of these is the review of the protocol for scientific worth (scientific review), and the other is the review of the protocol for ethical considerations (IRB review). For many years the role of the IRB and the effectiveness of the informed consent process have been questioned.[63–65] Federal officials and regulatory agencies continue to contemplate reform of the process to better meet the goals of providing study subjects with information from which they can make an educated decision regarding whether or not they wish to participate in a clinical trial. Information regarding the role the pharmacist can assume in both IRB and scientific reviews of protocols will be presented later in the chapter.

The Orphan Drug Act

The Orphan Drug Act was passed in 1983. This act provides incentives for manufacturers to develop orphan drugs. An orphan drug is one used for the treatment of a rare disease (affecting fewer than 200,000 people in the United States) or one that will not generate enough revenue to justify the cost of research and development. The Orphan Drug Act is administered by the FDA's Office of Orphan Products Development. The orphan drug designation provides the following incentives.

- *Tax incentives*: The sponsor is eligible to receive a 50% tax credit for money spent on research and development of an orphan drug; unfortunately, this is only beneficial to profitable companies as this credit cannot take the form of a tax refund.
- *Protocol assistance*: If a sponsor can show that a drug will be used for a rare disease, the FDA will provide assistance developing the preclinical and clinical plan for the product.
- *Grants and contracts*: The FDA budget may allot up to $12 million annually for grants and contracts to be used in developing orphan drugs. Clinical trials are awarded grants from $100,000 to $200,000 per year in direct costs for up to 3 years.
- *Marketing exclusivity*: The first sponsor to obtain marketing approval for a designated orphan drug is allowed 7 years of marketing exclusivity for that indication, but identical versions of the same product marketed by another manufacturer may be approved for other indications.

The Orphan Drug Act does not provide advantages for the drug approval process. Sponsors seeking approval for drugs that will be designated as orphan drugs must still provide the same safety and efficacy data as all other drugs evaluated by the FDA. Exceptions to the rules governing the number of patients who should be treated in the clinical trials may be made based on the scarcity of patients with the condition. Additionally, because in many cases there are no alternative therapies for the disease, the drug may be given a high review priority during the NDA process.[33,66,67]

Role of the Pharmacist

The pharmacist can play a vital role in the clinical research process by

- Being the PI on a study.
- Reporting adverse events.
- Preparing the IND.
- Serving on the IRB and, where applicable, on the Scientific Review Committee.
- Providing financial evaluations of investigational protocols.
- Disseminating information regarding both the protocol and the investigational drug to other healthcare personnel.
- Maintaining drug accountability records.
- Ordering, maintaining and, when necessary, returning drug supplies for ongoing clinical trials.
- Randomizing and, when necessary, blinding drug supplies for a clinical trial.

The pharmacist can serve as the PI on clinical research studies. The type of study for which a pharmacist is PI varies based on the expertise and experience of the pharmacist. Common types of studies for which pharmacists serve as PIs include pharmacoeconomic and pharmacology/pharmacokinetic studies. For some of these trials, a physician must be a co-investigator.

The pharmacist can assist the investigator by reporting clinical trial adverse events to the FDA. A discussion of the types of adverse events and the applicable reporting requirements was presented in the IND section of this chapter. Further information about the concept of adverse drug reaction reporting, including identification and classification of adverse events can be found in the adverse drug reaction section of Chap. 17.

The pharmacist can assist in preparing the IND by following the guidelines presented earlier in this chapter.

Preferably, the pharmacist should be a voting member of the IRB and, as such, may have some control over clinical trials initiated at the institution. More important, however, is the role the pharmacist may have in the scientific review of the protocol, whether this occurs as part of the scientific review board review or as part of the IRB review. When reviewing a protocol for scientific purposes, the pharmacist should verify that the protocol or associated documents such as the investigator's brochure contain the following information.

1. The name and synonyms of the study drug.
2. The chemical structure of the study drug.
3. The mechanism of action of the study drug.
4. The dosage range of the study drug (with appropriate rationale).
5. Animal toxicologic and pharmacologic information (when available, any known human toxicologic and pharmacologic information should also be presented).
6. How the drug will be supplied (dosage form and size).
7. The preparation guidelines for the drug (including stability and compatibility information when appropriate).
8. The storage requirements of the drug (both before and, when appropriate, after preparation).
9. The route of administration (and, if applicable, the rate of administration).

In addition, the pharmacist should confirm that any toxicities specified in the protocol are detailed for the patient in the informed consent of the protocol.

The pharmacist should also review the protocol for other potential problems (such as incompatibilities and inappropriate infusion devices). Frequently, nursing does not have an opportunity to review protocols prior to initiation and it falls to the pharmacist to ensure that the drug can be given as specified in the protocol. For complex protocols, it may be best to request secondary reviews by other specialists, such as the nurses who will be giving the doses or the pharmacists who will be preparing the doses. The pharmacist can review the protocol for clinical and scientific issues appropriate to his or her knowledge level and experience. Those pharmacists with research experience or a strong clinical background may, and probably should, comment on the study design or scientific merit of a particular protocol.

With the central role of financial considerations in today's research environment, pharmacists can also provide valuable insight into the costs associated with clinical research. Traditionally, the study sponsors would provide the investigational drug free of charge to the hospital (and to the patient), and the patient (or the third-party payer) would be responsible for paying for all other charges associated with therapy. Increasingly, third-party payers are reluctant to pay for investigational therapy. This leaves the patient, and subsequently the hospital, in a financially risky situation. A significant portion of costs associated with clinical research is pharmacy related (either supportive care medications or infusion devices, solutions, and so forth, that are used to administer the investigational drug). If, during the review process, the pharmacist can provide the investigator and the scientific review board with information regarding the potential cost of the research (at least as it relates to pharmacy charges), both the investigator and the review board can make a more educated decision regarding appropriation of resources for research purposes. When preparing an economic review of a protocol the pharmacist should pay specific attention to the following items.

1. Can the therapy be converted from inpatient to outpatient?
2. Can the method of infusion or the infusion device be changed to one that is more cost effective?
3. Does the treatment plan call for administration of compatible medications that could be mixed in the same container?
4. Is the supportive care adequate and not excessive (this is especially important with high-cost drugs, such as antiemetics and growth factors)?
5. Does the protocol have a high risk of reimbursement denial? This can be evaluated by reviewing the package insert, *American Hospital Formulary Service Drug Information, US Pharmacopeia—Drug Information (USP-DI),* and for oncology products, *Association of Community Cancer Centers Compendia-Based Drug Bulletin.* Other factors in reimbursement risk include the cost of the drug and the supportive care or tests associated with the drug. If the protocol does have a high risk of reimbursement denial, can free drug supplies offset part or all of this risk?

See Appendix 18–3 for an economic review template that can be used to evaluate this information.

The pharmacist can assist in disseminating information regarding both the protocol and the investigational drug by preparing data sheets that may be used by pharmacy and nursing personnel (and in some situations by physicians who may be unfamiliar with the research). This information can be distributed using various methods including paper, the hospital mainframe, and the intranet. The drug data sheet should include the following elements.

- Drug name (synonyms)
- Therapeutic classification
- Pharmaceutical data
- Stability and storage data
- Dose preparation guidelines (where applicable)
- Usual dosage range
- Route of administration
- Known side effects and toxicities
- Mechanism of action
- Status (phase of study)
- Study chairperson
- Date effective (and dates of revision)
- References

The protocol data sheet should include the following elements:

- Protocol number (as assigned by the institution)
- Protocol title
- Drug name(s) (synonym[s])
- Protocol description
  1. Objectives
  2. Study design
     a. Registration requirements
     b. Primary location of patients
     c. Type of study
  3. Treatment course (including retreatment criteria)
- Availability
  1. Supplier
  2. Status
  3. How supplied
- Storage, stability, and compatibility
  1. Intact drug
  2. Prepared drug (for injectables this should include both reconstitution and dilution guidelines)
- Dosage range
- Dose preparation guidelines
- Administration guidelines
- Special notes
- PI
- Research nurse

The PI and study sponsor should approve both the drug data sheet and the protocol data sheet before dissemination. This will help eliminate any potential errors and may reduce the liability the pharmacist assumes in preparing and distributing these documents. The pharmacist should assume primary responsibility for ordering and maintaining adequate drug supplies for conducting the clinical trial. All investigational drugs should be stored in the pharmacy. Usually, ordering can be done via telephone; however, sometimes study sponsors require written drug orders. If the drug under investigation is a controlled substance, a written order will definitely be required. Shipment and receipt of the drug can vary from 1 day to several weeks (or sometimes months for very specialized drug products). The pharmacist must be sufficiently knowledgeable regarding the rate of patient enrollment in the protocol and subsequent drug usage to ensure that the institution does not run out of drug. The pharmacist should also assume responsibility for returning unused drug supplies at the completion of the study. The sponsor may authorize on-site destruction of unused supplies provided this will not increase the risk to humans (or provide a risk to the environment). Many study sponsors will attempt to have the pharmacist save and return all used drug supplies as well. This is not a FDA requirement and for safety and space reasons should be discouraged.

Another role the pharmacist should assume is maintaining drug accountability records. These records can be maintained manually or on a computer. The records must document all drug shipments, returns, and dispensing to patients. At a minimum, these records should document:

- The date of the transaction.
- The patient initials and an identifying number.
- The dose.
- The number of vials of drug used or received.
- The lot number of the drug (if multiple lot numbers were used, each one should be documented).
- The initials of the individual who performed the transaction.

The National Cancer Institute (NCI) has prepared a sample drug accountability form that may be used as a guide (see Appendix 18–4).[68]

Computer systems that will maintain drug accountability records are available commercially. Personal computer–based, web-based, and mainframe-based systems exist. Some of these systems will also provide drug labels, drug and protocol information, summaries of investigational drug dispensing (useful in the preparation of productivity reports), and even monthly billing summaries to be used for posting charges to the study budget. A web-based system that is currently on the market is IDEA being marketed by DDOTS, Inc.[69] (<<http://www.ddots.com/>>) Another commercially available system is the IDS system being marketed by the Manhatten Group.[70] Obviously, the development of a personalized system that meets the specific needs of the institution or pharmacy is ideal. However, this can be costly, laborious, and time consuming. If a personalized system is developed, it is important to remember that the system must be able to maintain the integrity of the records and that a clear audit trail needs to be maintained. Ultimately, the decision to computerize drug accountability records and the selection of which system to use, is one that the pharmacist should make only after evaluating the needs of the institution/pharmacy and the available budget.[71-74]

Drug accountability records and drug supplies may be inspected at any time by the sponsor. The frequency of these inspections may vary according to the wishes of the sponsor. They may be monthly, quarterly, or annually. The FDA also has the right to inspect these records. The investigational drug pharmacist should play a key role in providing drug accountability information to either the FDA or the sponsor during an audit. If proper records are not being maintained, the sponsor or the FDA may discontinue the investigator's participation in the clinical investigation.

After the clinical trial is complete, records must be maintained at the study site for the following time periods:

- Two years after approval of the NDA or
- Two years after the FDA received notification that the investigation was discontinued.[75]

The pharmacist should also assume primary responsibility for randomizing and, where appropriate, blinding clinical trials. These two activities assist the sponsor in reducing or eliminating the bias of the clinical trial. A randomized study is one in which patients are randomly assigned (similar to flipping a coin) to different therapies. Usually the assignment is done using a computer-generated randomization list; however, a manual list may be used as well. The randomization groups may include a number of different therapy options (e.g., a study may have four different treatment arms with an equal number of patients assigned to each arm). The number of patients assigned to the different groups may vary as well (e.g., a study may have two different treatment regimens where patients will be assigned in a 2:1 ratio to the first treatment option). The investigator should not be aware which arm the patient has been assigned to before randomization. Therefore, the involvement of a third party (such as the pharmacist) is important. A blinded study is one in which, after the patient has been randomized, the drug is masked so that at least one of the involved parties (e.g., physician, nurse, patient, or pharmacist) is not aware of what the patient is to receive. In a single-blind study, the only individual who is not aware of what the patient is receiving is the patient himself. In a double-blind study, neither the nurse, doctor, or patient is aware of what the patient is receiving. The role of a pharmacist in a double-blind study is crucial, and sloppy work in this area destroys a clinical investigation. A triple-blind study is one in which the drug arrives at the pharmacy already blinded. In this scenario, the patient, nurse, doctor, and pharmacist are not aware of what drug the patient is to receive. Although this may seem simpler than a double-blind study, it is equally difficult because each patient has his or her own supply of medication and it is important that the supplies be dispensed appropriately. In a triple-blind study, the sponsor supplies the investigator with a mechanism for removing the blind from the patient (in case of emergency). It is critical that the pharmacist keep the master list. The protocol should state who has access to the master list and under what conditions this access should occur. If the FDA discovers that the investigator had access to this list, the study will be considered invalid.

Pharmacists should be willing and able to request reimbursement for the services they provide. Funds for these services are usually negotiated directly with the study sponsor before initiation of the protocol. The majority of pharmacies charge a base fee for each protocol initiated at its institution (these fees generally range from $50 to $3000 per protocol).

This base fee may be fixed or it may vary based on the size of the patient population, the complexity of the protocol, or the number of doses to be prepared. Some institutions also charge an annual renewal fee for ongoing clinical trials (ranging from $40 to $750). Most pharmacies will charge a separate fee for randomizing and blinding a clinical trial. This fee can be a one-time (per study) fee or it can be a per-patient fee (one-time fees range from $25 to $300 while per-patient fees range from $1 to $50). Some hospitals also charge dispensing fees per dose or per amount of time required to prepare a dose ($5 for oral doses up to $50 dollars for IV chemotherapy). Pharmacies can also charge a monthly fee for drug storage and inventory (ranging from $10 to $50 per month). This fee varies based on the amount of space and type of storage (freezer, room temperature, or refrigerator) required. The pharmacist can also charge a professional fee for services that exceed the standard services provided for in the base fee (range of $20 to $70 per hour). Examples of services that should be charged for separately include monitoring of patients, completing case report forms, and completing sponsor specific drug accountability records. These services are usually charged for using an hourly rate.[76–81]

Conclusion

Assisting in implementing and conducting clinical trials can be a satisfying role for the pharmacist. A large part of the role of the pharmacist will be providing protocol and drug information to the investigators and associated study personnel. An even more satisfying role is that of providing information to the study participants. The laws governing these trials can be complex, but they are understandable once the pharmacist has taken the time to study them. The pharmacist can and should play an integral role in the conduct of clinical trials at their institution.

Helpful Websites
- NIH/Office of Biotechnology Activities (OBA) <<http://www4.od.nih.gov/oba/Rdna. htm>>
- FDA <<http://www.fda.gov/>>
- FDA forms <<http://www.fda.gov/opacom/morechoices/fdaforms/fdaforms.html>>
- Archives of the Federal Register <<http://www.accessdata.fda.gov/scripts/oc/ohrms/ index.cfm>>
- Code of Federal Regulations <<http://www.gpoaccess.gov/cfr/index.html>>
- FDA Dockets Management Page <<http://www.fda.gov/ohrms/dockets/default. htm>>
- ICH<<www.ich.org>>

- NIH/OHRP <<http://www.hhs.gov/ohrp/>>
- CenterWatch <<http://www.centerwatch.com/>>

Study Questions

1. What are the steps in the drug approval process?

2. What type of information is contained in the investigator's brochure?

3. What type of information is gathered in a phase I, phase II, phase III, and phase IV trial? Why is this relevant to the drug approval process?

4. What is the purpose of the IRB?

5. What incentives does the Orphan Drug Act provide to the manufacturers? Does this accelerate the drug approval process?

6. What role does the pharmacist play in the clinical research process?

REFERENCES

1. Tufts Center for the Study of Drug Development. Tufts Center for the Study of Drug Development pegs cost of a new prescription medicine at $802 Million [article on the Internet]. 2000 Mar [cited 2004 Mar]. Available from: http://csdd.tufts.edu/.

2. Tufts Center for the Study of Drug Development. How new drugs move through the development and approval process [article on the Internet]. 2001 Nov 1 [cited 2004 Mar]. Available from: http://csdd.tufts.edu/.

3. Food and Drug Administration. Protecting consumers, promoting public health [presentation on the Internet]. Washington, DC; 2004 Aug [cited 2004 Sept 15]. Available from: http://www.fda.gov/oc/opacom/fda101/fda101text.html

4. Food and Drug Administration [homepage on the Internet]. Washington, DC: FDA Organization [cited 2004 Sept 15]. Available from: http://www.fda.gov/opacom/7org.html

5. CDER; Food and Drug Administration. Approval Times for Priority and Standard NME's Calendar Years 1993–2003. Washington, DC [updated 2003 Dec 31; posted 2004 Jan 21; cited 2004 Sept 15]. Available from: http://www.fda.gov/cder/rdmt/NMEapps93-03.htm

6. United States Federal Government Code of Federal Regulations. 21CFR312.3. Washington, DC [updated 2004 Apr 1; cited 2004 Sept 15]. Available from: http://www.gpoaccess.gov/cfr/index.html

7. CDER; Food and Drug Administration [procedure on the Internet]. IND process and review procedures [updated 1998 May 1; cited 2004 Sept 15]. Available from: http://www.fda.gov/.

8. CDER; Food and Drug Administration [presentation on the Internet]. Guideline for drug master files [updated 2004 May 26; cited 2004 Sept 15]. Available from: http://www.fda.gov

9. United States Federal Government Code of Federal Regulations. 21CFR314.3. Washington, DC [updated 2004 Apr 1; cited 2004 Sept 15]. Available from: http://www.gpoaccess.gov/cfr/index.html

10. United States Federal Government Code of Federal Regulations. 45CFR46. Washington, DC [updated 2004 Apr 1; cited 2004 Sept 15]. Available from: http://www.gpoaccess.gov/cfr/index.html

11. United States Federal Government Code of Federal Regulations. 21CFR56. Washington, DC [updated 2004 Apr 1; cited 2004 Sept 15]. Available from: http://www.gpoaccess.gov/cfr/index.html

12. Mathieu M. New drug development: a regulatory overview. 4th ed. Cambridge (MA): PAREXEL International Corporation; 1997.

13. Bruderle TP. Reforming the Food and Drug Administration: legislative solution or self-improvement. Am J Health Syst Pharm. 1996;53:2083–90.

14. Tufts Center for the Study of Drug Development. Impact report: European approval of New Biotech Drugs Outpaces US Approval. 2004 [cited 2004 Mar]. Available from: http://csdd.tufts.edu/.

15. Kessler DA, Hass AE, Feidin KL, Lumpkin M, Temple R. Approval of new drugs in the United States. JAMA. 1996;276:1826–31.

16. Food and Drug Administration. Prescription Drug User Fee Act of 1992 (amended 2002) [2004 Feb 10; cited 2004 Mar]. Available from: http://www.fda.gov

17. Food and Drug Administration. Food and Drug Administration Modernization Act of 1997. 1997 [cited 2004 Mar]. Available from: http://www.fda.gov

18. Reynolds T. European drug agency promises quicker approvals. JNCI. 1995;87:1050–1.

19. International Conference on Harmonization [website on the Internet]. History and future of ICH [revised 2000; cited 2004 Mar]. Available from: http://www.ich.org

20. Grilley B, Gee A. Gene transfer: regulatory issues and their impact on the clinical investigator and the GMP facility. Cytotherapy. 2003;5(3):197–207.

21. The Nuremberg Code. Trials of war criminals before the Nuremberg Military Tribunals under Control Council Law No. 10. Vol 2. Washington, DC: US Government Printing Office; 1989 Sept: 181–2.

22. The World Medical Association. Declaration of Helsinki [clarified 2000; cited 2004 Mar]. Available from: http://www.wma.net/e/policy/b3.htm

23. Food and Drug Administration. The Belmont report: ethical principles and guidelines for the protection of human subjects of research [updated 1998; cited 2004 Mar]. Available from: http://www.fda.gov/oc/ohrt/IRBS/belmont.html

24. United States Federal Government Code of Federal Regulations. 21CFR50. Washington, DC [updated 2004 Apr 1; cited 2004 Sept 15]. Available from: http://www.gpoaccess.gov/cfr/index.html

25. United States Federal Government Code of Federal Regulations. 21CFR312.23. Washington, DC [updated 2004 Apr 1; cited 2004 Sept 15]. Available from: http://www.gpoaccess.gov/cfr/index.html

26. United States Federal Government Code of Federal Regulations. 21CFR312.30. Washington, DC [updated 2004 Apr 1; cited 2004 Sept 15]. Available from: http://www.gpoaccess.gov/cfr/index.html

27. United States Federal Government Code of Federal Regulations. 21CFR312.31. Washington, DC [updated 2004 Apr 1; cited 2004 Sept 15]. Available from: http://www.gpoaccess.gov/cfr/index.html

28. United States Federal Government Code of Federal Regulations. 21CFR312.32. Washington, DC [updated 2004 Apr 1; cited 2004 Sept 15]. Available from: http://www.gpoaccess.gov/cfr/index.html

29. United States Federal Government Code of Federal Regulations. 21CFR312.33. Washington, DC [updated 2004 Apr 1; cited 2004 Sept 15]. Available from: http://www.gpoaccess.gov/cfr/index.html

30. United States Federal Government Code of Federal Regulations. 21CFR312.40. Washington, DC [updated 2004 Apr 1; cited 2004 Sept 15]. Available from: http://www.gpoaccess.gov/cfr/index.html

31. United States Federal Government Code of Federal Regulations. 21CFR312.42. Washington, DC [updated 2004 Apr 1; cited 2004 Sept 15]. Available from: http://www.gpoaccess.gov/cfr/index.html

32. United States Federal Government Code of Federal Regulations. 21CFR314.50. Washington, DC [updated 2004 Apr 1; cited 2004 Sept 15]. Available from: http://www.gpoaccess.gov/cfr/index.html

33. CDER; Food and Drug Administration [procedure on the Internet]. Drug Classification and Priority Review Policy. 1998 [cited 2004 Mar]. Available from: http://www.fda.gov

34. United States Federal Government Code of Federal Regulations. 21CFR314.100. Washington, DC [updated 2004 Apr 1; cited 2004 Sept 15]. Available from: http://www.gpoaccess.gov/cfr/index.html

35. United States Federal Government Code of Federal Regulations. 21CFR314.105. Washington, DC [updated 2004 Apr 1; cited 2004 Sept 15]. Available from: http://www.gpoaccess.gov/cfr/index.html

36. United States Federal Government Code of Federal Regulations. 21CFR314.110. Washington, DC [updated 2004 Apr 1; cited 2004 Sept 15]. Available from: http://www.gpoaccess.gov/cfr/index.html

37. United States Federal Government Code of Federal Regulations. 21CFR314.120. Washington, DC [updated 2004 Apr 1; cited 2004 Sept 15]. Available from: http://www.gpoaccess.gov/cfr/index.html

38. Bready BB. Conducting clinical trials in oncology. Cancer Bull. 1990;42:411–5.

39. Food and Drug Administration. FDA sees rebound in approval of innovative drugs in 2003 new innovation initiative anticipated to speed approvals in years ahead. FDA News. 2004 Jan 15.

40. Carpenter D, Chernew M, Smith D, Fedrick AM. Approval times for new drugs: does the source of funding matter? Health Aff. 2003;23(1):618–24.

41. United States Federal Government Code of Federal Regulations. 21CFR312.34. Washington, DC [updated 2004 Apr 1; cited 2004 Sept 15]. Available from: http://www.gpoaccess.gov/cfr/index.html

42. United States Federal Government Code of Federal Regulations. 21CFR312.35. Washington, DC [updated 2004 Apr 1; cited 2004 Sept 15]. Available from: http://www.gpoaccess.gov/cfr/index.html

43. United States Federal Government Code of Federal Regulations. 21CFR312.7. Washington, DC [updated 2004 Apr 1; cited 2004 Sept 15]. Available from: http://www.gpoaccess.gov/cfr/index.html

44. How FDA expedites evaluation of drugs for AIDS and other life-threatening illnesses. Wellcome Programs in Pharmacy. 1993 Jan.

45. Food and Drug Administration. Expanded access and expedited approval of new therapies related to HIV/AIDS [updated 1998 Mar 5; cited 2004 Mar]. Available from: http://www.fda.gov

46. CBER; Food and Drug Administration. Reinventing the regulation of cancer drugs: accelerating approval and expanding access [updated 1996 Mar; cited 2004 Mar]. Available from: http://www.fda.gov

47. CDER/CBER; Food and Drug Administration. Guidance for industry: IND exemptions for studies of lawfully marketed drug or biological products for the treatment of cancer [updated 2004 Jan; cited 2004 Mar]. Available from: http://www.fda.gov

48. Temple RJ. A regulatory authority's opinion about surrogate endpoints. In: Nimmo WS, Tucker GT, editors. Clinical measurement in drug evaluation. New York: Wiley; 1995.

49. United States Federal Government Code of Federal Regulations. 21CFR312.36. Washington, DC [updated 2004 Apr 1; cited 2004 Sept 15]. Available from: http://www.gpoaccess.gov/cfr/index.html

50. United States Federal Government Code of Federal Regulations. 21CFR56.104. Washington, DC [updated 2004 Apr 1; cited 2004 Sept 15]. Available from: http://www.gpoaccess.gov/cfr/index.html

51. United States Federal Government Code of Federal Regulations. 21CFR314.510-520 (subpart H). Washington, DC [updated 2004 Apr 1; cited 2004 Sept 15]. Available from: http://www.gpoaccess. gov/ cfr/index.html

52. United States Federal Government Code of Federal Regulations. 21CFR312.82. Washington, DC [updated 2004 Apr 1; cited 2004 Sept 15]. Available from: http://www.gpoaccess.gov/cfr/index.html

53. United States Federal Government Code of Federal Regulations. 21CFR312.41. Washington, DC [updated 2004 Apr 1; cited 2004 Sept 15]. Available from: http://www.gpoaccess.gov/cfr/index.html

54. United States Federal Government Code of Federal Regulations. 21CFR312.47. Washington, DC [updated 2004 Apr 1; cited 2004 Sept 15]. Available from: http://www.gpoaccess.gov/cfr/index.html

56. U.S. Government. Department of Health and Human Services. Waiver of informed consent requirements in certain emergency research. Fed Regist. 2000;61:51531–3.

57. Food and Drug Administration. Guidance for institutional review boards, clinical investigators, and sponsors: exception from informed consent requirements for emergency research. 2000 Mar 30.

58. United States Federal Government Code of Federal Regulations. 45CFR46.108. Washington, DC [updated 2004 Apr 1; cited 2004 Sept 15]. Available from: http://www.gpoaccess.gov/cfr/index.html

59. United States Federal Government Code of Federal Regulations. 21CFR56.109. Washington, DC [updated 2004 Apr 1; cited 2004 Sept 15]. Available from: http://www.gpoaccess.gov/cfr/index.html

60. Protecting human research subjects: institutional review board guidebook [updated 2001 Jun 21; cited 2004 Mar]. Available from: http://ohrp.osophs.dhhs.gov/irb/irb_guidebook.htm

61. United States Federal Government Code of Federal Regulations. 21CFR56.115. Washington, DC [updated 2004 Apr 1; cited 2004 Sept 15]. Available from: http://www.gpoaccess.gov/cfr/index.html

62. United States Federal Government Code of Federal Regulations. 21CFR46.115. Washington, DC [updated 2004 Apr 1; cited 2004 Sept 15]. Available from: http://www.gpoaccess.gov/cfr/index.html

63. Davis R. U.S.: Human medical tests lack oversight. USA Today. 1998 June 8; ect.A:1, 19–20.

64. Hochhauser M. Is "therapeutic misconception" being used to recruit subjects? ARENA Newsletter. Spring 2003;XVI:5–7.

65. Hochhauser M. "Therapeutic misconception" and "recruiting doublespeak" in the informed consent process. IRB: Ethics Hum Res. 2002 Jan–Feb; 24(1):240–1.

66. United States Federal Government Code of Federal Regulations. 21CFR316. Washington, DC [updated 2004 Apr 1; cited 2004 Sept 15]. Available from: http://www.gpoaccess.gov/cfr/index.html

67. CDER; Food and Drug Administration. OOPD frequently asked questions [updated 2004 Sept 10; cited 2004 Sept 15]. Available from: http://www.fda.gov/orphan/faq/.

68. National Cancer Institute. Investigator's handbook: a manual for participants in clinical trials of investigational agents (version 4). Sponsored by the Division of Cancer Treatment, National Cancer Institute. Bethesda (MD) [cited 2004 Mar]. Available from: http://ctep.cancer.gov/handbook/hndbk_12.html

69. DDOTS, Inc. [homepage on the Internet] [cited 2004 Mar]. Available from: http://www.ddots.com/idea_product_overview.cfm

70. Manhattan Group: Software and Solutions [homepage on the Internet] [cited 2004 Mar]. Available from: http://www.manhattangroup.com/ids.asp

71. Burnham NL, Elcombe SA, Skorlinski CR, Kosanke L, Kovach JS. Computer program for handling investigational oncology drugs. Am J Hosp Pharm. 1989;46:1821–4.

72. Grilley BJ, Trissel LA, Bluml BM. Design and implementation of an electronic investigational drug accountability system. Am J Hosp Pharm. 1991;48:2816.

73. Lakamp JE, Lunik MC, Wilson AL, Armbruster CJ. Using a hospital mainframe computer for pharmacy investigational drug study management. Top Hosp Pharm Manage. 1993;13:37–46.

74. Iteen SE, Cepaglia J. Investigational drug information through a hospital-wide computer system. Am J Hosp Pharm. 1992;49:2746–8.

75. United States Federal Government Code of Federal Regulations. 21CFR312.57. Washington, DC [updated 2004 Apr 1; cited 2004 Sept 15]. Available from: http://www.gpoaccess.gov/cfr/index.html

76. Rockwell K. Pharmacy-based investigational drug services: a national survey. Top Hosp Pharm Manage. 1993;13:1–15.

77. NYU School of Medicine: Office of Clinical Trials. Investigational drug services for NYU Hospitals Center and Bellevue Hospital [homepage on the Internet] [cited 2004]. Available from: http://www.med. nyu.edu/clinicaltrials/PatIDS.html

78. Research and Education Institute at Harbor-UCLA Medical Center [procedure on the Internet]. Investigational Drug Services [cited 2004 Mar]. Available from: http://www.rei.edu/Invest.htm

79. UTMB Department of Pharmacy. Investigational Drug Service (IDS) [procedure on the Internet] [cited 2004 Mar]. Available from: http://www.utmb.edu/rxhome/Inpatient_Pharmacy/IDS.htm

80. Rhode Island Hospital/The Miriam Hospital website. Pharmacy resources, services and fees for clinical investigational drug trial sponsored by pharmaceutical industry guidelines [procedure on the Internet] [cited 2004 Mar]. Available from: http://www.lifespan.org/research/forms/pharmsvc/ pharmsvcindustrytrials.pdf =

81. Duke Comprehensive Cancer Center website. Pharmaceutical Research Services [procedure on the Internet] [cited 2004 Mar]. Available from: http://cancer.duke.edu/Pharm/services.asp

Appendices

Appendices

2–1

Drug Information Response Quality Assurance Evaluation Form

Drug Information Service
Department of Pharmacy Services, MCVH
Quality Assurance Review

Month under review _____   Date of request _____
Primary responder _____   DIS staff supervisor _____

	Satisfactory	Unsatisfactory	N/A	Comment
Requestor's demographic data was complete	—	—	—	—
Background information inquiry was thorough	—	—	—	—
...was appropriate	—	—	—	—
Search question was clearly noted	—	—	—	—
...was succinct	—	—	—	—
Search strategy & reference selection were relevant	—	—	—	—
...were comprehensive	—	—	—	—
Literature & information retrieved were evaluated	—	—	—	—
...were interpreted	—	—	—	—
...were documented	—	—	—	—
Conclusions were appropriate per data collected	—	—	—	—
...data assimilation	—	—	—	—
Oral or verbal response was accurate	—	—	—	—
...complete	—	—	—	—
...succinct	—	—	—	—
...provided in a timely manner	—	—	—	—
Follow-up communication were clearly documented	—	—	—	—
...showed appropriate reaction	—	—	—	—

	Excellent		Acceptable	Unacceptable	
Summary (circle choice):	5	4	3	2	1

Recommendations:_____

Reviewer's initials:_____

Appendix 2–2

Drug Information Request/Response Form

REQUEST/RESPONSE FORM   DATE___/___/___
Drug Information Service—Department of Pharmacy Services   TIME ___:___
Medical College of Virginia Hospitals   (use military time)

DEMOGRAPHIC DATA:
Requestor_____'_____   Dept/Affiliation_____
Phone/Pager_____   Location/City_____
MCV-VCU____   Profession: Physician___   Nurse____   PA/NP___Student_____
NON-MCV____   Pharmacist____   Dentist_____   Other_____

Initial Question:_____
BACKGROUND INFORMATION (age, gender, weight, disease states, medications, lab values,
allergies, etc.)

ULTIMATE QUESTION:_____
                              Receiver_____   Respond by_____
Classification: (check only one category)
__Availability (strength,   __Compatibility/Stability/   __Therapy Eval./
   manufacturer, formul.)   Administration (rate/method)   Drug of Choice
__Identification   __Drug Interactions (drug,   __Dosage/Regimen Recomendations
__General Product   lab, disease, food)   __Adverse Effects
   Information   __Pharmaceutics (compounding, __Poisoning/Toxicology
__Laws/Policy &   formulations)   __Teratogenicity/Genetic Effects
   Procedure/P & T   __Pharmacokinetics (ADME/   __Lactation/Infant Risks
__Cost   levels/HD, PD, HPI)   __Other: _____
__Foreign/Investigational
__Referral: __Clin Pktcs __Poison Cntrl __Nutrn Supp __Library
__Other: _____
SEARCH STRATEGY: (Indicate resource and utility [+ or –]; record specific data on back)

FINDINGS/EVALUATION (see back):
RESPONSE:

Responder/Supervisor_____/_____   Written Response:__Y__N Date____/_____
Time:_____:_____   Time Spent: < 5_____ 5–30_____ 30–60_____ >60_____

┌──┐
│ __Quality Assurance __Statistics __Projects ___Pharmacy Trend Written Reference Search___ │
│ Verbal Reference Search____   Drug Information Service Consult____ │
└──┘

FOLLOW-UP INFORMATION: (also note attempts to contact, messages left)

2-3

Standard Questions for Obtaining Background Information from Requestors

Regardless of the type or classification of the question, the following information should be obtained:

1. The requestor's name.
2. The requestor's location and/or page number.
3. The requestor's affiliation (institution or practice), if a health care professional.
4. The requestor's frame of reference (i.e., title, profession/occupation, and rank).
5. The resources the requestor has already consulted.
6. If the request is patient specific or academic.
7. The patient's diagnosis and other medications.
8. The urgency of the request (negotiate time of response).

SPECIFIC*

The following questions should be asked when appropriate for calls of the following classes:

Availability of Dosage Forms

1. What is the dosage form desired?
2. What administration routes are feasible with this patient?
3. Is this patient alert and oriented.
4. Does the patient have a water or sodium restriction?
5. What other special factors regarding drug administration should be considered?

Identification of Product

1. What is the generic or trade name of the product?
2. Who is the manufacturer? What country of origin?
3. What is the suspected use of this product?

---

*Specific questions for only selected types of requests presented; other specific questions would be appropriate for other types of requests.

4. Under what circumstances was this product found? Who found the product?
5. What is the dosage form, color markings, size, and so on?
6. What was your source of information? Was it reliable?

General Product Information

1. Why is there a particular concern for this product?
2. Is written patient information required?
3. What type of information do you need?
4. Is this for an inpatient, outpatient, or private patient?

Foreign Drug Identification

1. What is the drug's generic name, trade name, manufacturer, and/or country of origin?
2. What is the dosage form, markings, color, strength, or size?
3. What is the suspected use of the drug? How often is the patient taking it? What is the patient's response to the drug? Is the patient male or female?
4. If the medication was found, what were the circumstances/conditions at the time of discovery?
5. Is the patient just visiting, or planning on staying?

Investigational Drug Information

1. Why do you need this information? Is the patient in need of the drug or currently enrolled in a protocol?
2. If a drug is to be identified, what is the dosage form, markings, color, strength, or size of the product?
3. Why was the patient receiving the drug? What was the response when the patient was on the drug? What are the patient's pathological conditions?
4. If a drug is desired what approved or accepted therapies have been tried? Was therapy maximized before discontinued?

Method and Rate of Administration

1. What dosage form or preparation is being used (if multiple salt forms are available)?
2. What is the dose ordered? Is the drug a one-time dose or standing orders?
3. What is the clinical status of the patients? Could the patients tolerate a fluid push of XX mL? Is the patient fluid or sodium restricted? Does the patient have congestive heart failure (CHF) or edema?
4. What possible delivery routes are available?
5. What other drugs are the patient receiving currently? Are any by the same route?

Incompatibility and Stability

1. What are the routes for the patient's medications?
2. What are the doses (in mg), concentrations, and volumes for all pertinent medications?

3. What are the infusion times/rates expected or desired?
4. What is the base solution or diluent used?
5. Was the product stored in a refrigerator or at room temperature? For how long?
6. Was the product exposed to sunlight? For how long?
7. Was the product frozen? For how long?
8. When was the product compounded/prepared?

Drug Interactions

1. What event(s) suggest that an interaction occurred? Please describe.
2. For the drugs in question, what are the doses, volumes, concentrations, rate of administration, administration schedules, and length of therapies?
3. What is the temporal relationship between the drugs in question?
4. Has the patient received this combination or a similar combination in the past?
5. Other than the drugs in question, what other drugs is the patient receiving currently? When were these started?

Drug-Laboratory Test Interference

1. What event(s) suggest an interaction occurred? Please describe.
2. For the drug in question, what is the dose, volume, concentration, rate of administration, administration schedule, and length of therapy?
3. What is the temporal relationship between drug administration and laboratory test sampling?
4. What other drugs are the patient receiving?
5. Has clinical chemistry (or the appropriate laboratory) been contacted? Are they aware of any known interference similar to this event?
6. Was this one isolated test or a trend in results?

Pharmacokinetics

1. What is the generic name, dose, and route of the drug?
2. What is the patient's age, gender, height, and weight?
3. What are the diseases being treated and the severity of the illness?
4. What are the patient's hepatic and renal functions?
5. What other medications are the patient receiving?
6. What physiologic conditions exist (e.g., pneumonia, severe burns, or obesity)?
7. What are the patient's dietary and ethanol habits?

Serum or Urine Therapeutic Levels

1. Is the patient currently receiving the drug? Have samples already been drawn? At what time?
2. What is the disease or underlying pathology being treated? If infectious in nature, what is the suspected/cultured organism?

3. If not stated in the question, what was the source of the sample (blood, urine, saliva; venous or arterial blood)?
4. What was the timing of the samples relative to drug administration? Over what period of time was the drug administered and by what route?
5. What were the previous concentrations for this patient? Was the patient receiving the same dose then?
6. How long has the patient received the drug? Is the patient at steady state?

Therapy Evaluation/Drug of Choice

1. What medications, including doses and routes of administration, are the patient receiving?
2. What are the patient's pathology(ies) and disease(s) severity?
3. What are the patient's specifics: age, weight, height, gender, organ function/dysfunction?
4. Has the patient received the drug previously? Was response similar?
5. Has the patient been compliant?
6. What alternative therapies has the patient received? Was therapy maximized for each of these before discontinuation? What other therapies are being considered?
7. What monitoring parameters have been followed (serum concentrations/levels, clinical status, other clinical lab results, objective measurements, and subjective assessment).
8. What is the patient's name and location?

Dosage Recommendations (Normal and Compromised)

1. What disease is being treated? What is the extent/severity of the illness?
2. What are the drugs being prescribed? What drugs have the patient received to date?
3. Does the patient have any insufficiency of the renal, hepatic, or cardiac system?
4. For drugs with renal elimination, what are the serum creatinine/creatinine clearance, blood urea nitrogen (BUN), and/or during output? Is the patient receiving peritoneal dialysis or hemodialysis?
5. For drugs with hepatic elimination, what are the liver function tests (LFTs), bilirubin (direct and indirect), and/or albumin?
6. For drugs with serum level monitoring utility, characterized the most recent levels per timing relative to dose and results.
7. Are these lab values recent? Is the patient's condition stable?
8. Does this patient have a known factor that could affect drug metabolism (ethnic background, such as Japanese or Chinese, or acetylator status)?

Adverse Effects

1. What is the name, dosage, and route for all drugs currently and recently prescribed?
2. What are the patient specifics (age, gender, height, weight, organ dysfunction, and indication for drug use)?
3. What is the temporal relationship with the drug?

4. Has the patient experienced this adverse relationship (or a similar event) with this drug (or similar agent) previously?
5. Was the suspected drug ever administered before? Why was it discontinued then?
6. What were the events/findings that characterize this adverse drug reaction (ADR) (include onset and duration)?
7. Has any intervention been initiated at this time?
8. Does the patient have any food intolerance?
9. Is there a family history for this ADR and/or drug allergy?

Toxicology Information

1. What is your name, relationship to the patient, and telephone number?
2. What are the patient specifics (age, gender, height, weight, organ dysfunction, and indication for drug use)?
3. Is this a suspected ingestion or exposure?
4. What is the product suspected to have been ingested? What is the strength of the product and the possible quantity ingested (e.g., how much was in the bottle)?
5. How long ago did the ingestion occur?
6. How much is on the child or surrounding floor?
7. How much was removed from the child's hands and mouth? Was the ingestion in the same room where the product was stored?
8. What has been done for the patient already? Has the poison control center or emergency room (ER) been called?
9. Do you have syrup of ipecac available? Do you know how to give it properly?
10. What is the patient's condition (sensorium, heart rate, respiratory rate, temperature, skin color/turgor, pupils, sweating/salvation, and so on)?
11. Does the patient have any known illnesses or organ dysfunction?

Teratogenicity

1. What was the drug the patient received and what was the dose? What was the duration of therapy?
2. Is the patient pregnant or planning to become pregnant?
3. When during pregnancy was the exposure (trimester or weeks)?
4. What are the patient specifics (age, height, weight, gender)?
5. What is the source of the case information?
6. Was the patient compliant?
7. For what indication was the drug being prescribed?

Drugs in Breast Milk

1. What was the drug the patient received and what was the dose? What was the duration of therapy?

2. How long has the infant been breast-feeding?
3. Has the infant ever received nonmaternal nutrition? Is bottle-feeding a plausible alternative?
4. What is the frequency of the breast-feeds? What is the milk volume?
5. How old is the infant?
6. Does the mother have hepatic or renal insufficiency?
7. What was the indication for prescribing the drug? Was this initial or alternate therapy?
8. Has the mother breast-fed previously while on the drug?

2-4

Appendix 2-4

Drug Information Request—An Example Completed Form

REQUEST/RESPONSE FORM
Drug Information Service-Department of Pharmacy Services
Medical College of Virginia Hospitals

DATE___/___/___
TIME ___:___
(use military time)

DEMOGRAPHIC DATA:
Requestor _Dr. Kolinski_____   Dept/Affiliation _Dermatology_____
Phone/Pager _555-1234_____   Location/City _MCV_____
MCV-VCU__   Profession _XX_ Physician   _Nurse   _PA/NP   _Student
NON-MCV__   __Pharmacist   _Dentist   _Other_____

Initial Question: _How do I get thalidomide?_____
BACKGROUND INFORMATION (age, gender, weight, disease states, medications, lab values, allergies, etc.)

male, 67yo patient with Behcet's disease × 5 years
        disease is progressing, destroying most of palate
        has heard thalidomide may be useful (recommendation from Louisiana)
        pt has received steroids, dapsone, colchicine, chlorambucil
        other patient background obtained and WNL
        MD, a dermatologist, has also heard of possibly using cyclosporine

ULTIMATE QUESTION: _What are (third-line) therapeutic recommendations for this patient?_ __
                          Receiver_____   Respond by_____
Classification: (check only one category)

_Availability (strength, manufacturer, formulary)	_Drug Interactions (drug, lab, disease, food)	_Adverse Effects
_Identification	_Pharmaceutics (compounding, formulations)	_Poisoning/Toxicology
_General Product Information	_Pharmacokinetics (ADME/ levels/HD, PD, HPI)	_Teratogenicity/ Genetic Effects
_Laws/Policy & Procedure/P & T	X Therapy Evaluation/ Drug of Choice	_Lactation/Infant Risks
_Cost	_Dosage/Regimen Recommendations	_Other: _____
_Foreign/Investigational		
_Compatibility/Stability/ Administration (rate/method)		

__Referral:__Clinical Pharmacokinetics__Poison Control__Nutrition Support__Library__Other:___
SEARCH STRATEGY: (Indicate resource and utility [+ or -]; record specific data on back)

This would start with general (tertiary) references, and proceed through secondary references to the primary literature.

FINDINGS/EVALUATION (see back): (back not shown)
RESPONSE:
Recommend CYA before thalidomide, considering response rates and commercial availability...
Responder/Supervisor_____/_____ Written Response:___Y___N Date___/___/___
Time:___:___ Time Spent:___<5___5–30___30–60___>60

__Quality Assurance __Statistics __Projects ___Pharmacy Trend Written Reference Search___
Verbal Reference Search____ Drug Information Service Consult____

FOLLOW-UP INFORMATION: (also note attempts to contact, messages left)

4-1

Appendix 4-1

Veterinary Informatics

Drug, Dosing, and Pharmacology Resources

In addition to the resources listed in Chapter 4, the following print and Internet resources are useful for obtaining information on veterinary pharmacology and toxicology subjects.

NATIONAL ANIMAL POISON CONTROL CENTER[1]

This website <<www.napcc.aspca.org>> focuses on animal toxicology and safety, and is the premier resource for pharmacists in a community setting who may receive poisoning questions about animals. The American Society for the Prevention of Cruelty to Animals (ASPCA) Animal Poison Control Center is a nonprofit organization dedicated to helping animals exposed to potentially hazardous substances by providing 24-hour veterinary diagnostic and treatment recommendations. A toll-free number is available for immediate assistance when faced with a toxicology problem (888-426-4435), and a fee of $50.00 is required. The Center has extensive experience in assisting veterinarians in poison management by providing immediate and specific treatment recommendations. The site also provides useful information on poison prevention. References to toxicology publications and general consultation are listed in this website.

VETERINARY PHARMACOLOGY AND THERAPEUTICS[2]

This textbook provides comprehensive information on the basic and applied principles of veterinary pharmacology and therapeutics. Information on mechanisms of action, pharmacodynamics, and pharmacokinetics is detailed.

SMALL ANIMAL CLINICAL PHARMACOLOGY AND THERAPEUTICS[3]

A useful pharmacology reference textbook focusing on pharmaceuticals for the prevention and treatment of small animal diseases. The book is divided into three sections detailing principles of drug therapy with special attention to clinical relevancy, the use of drugs from a categorical basis, and pharmaceutical use from a body systems approach.

EXOTIC ANIMAL FORMULARY[4]

This pocket guide provides quick, convenient access to essential pharmacology information for exotic animals. Indications and dosages for fish, reptiles, birds, rodents, amphibians, primates, and other exotic species are provided. The text contains tables, appendices, and a formulary containing commonly needed information for each exotic group.

THE EXOTIC ANIMAL DRUG COMPENDIUM: AN INTERNATIONAL FORMULARY[5]

This text provides a formulary reference for numerous exotic animal species (wildlife, laboratory animals, zoo animals, and exotic pets). The formulary contains 28 drug sections, with each section constructed as tables according to species, drug, dosage, and additional comments. Each listed dosage is accompanied by a notation as to how the dose was developed: pharmacokinetics research, clinical trials, anecdotal, or manufacturer. The book is written for veterinarians who care for exotic animal species and veterinary pharmacists who dispense the drugs.

JOURNAL OF THE AMERICAN VETERINARY MEDICAL ASSOCIATION

This periodical from the American Veterinary Medical Association is published twice a month and abstracts can be found on a MEDLINE® search. The journal is peer-reviewed and contains articles with a research or clinical focus. Regulatory issues and current topics in veterinary medicine are included in most issues.

COMPENDIUM ON CONTINUING EDUCATION FOR THE PRACTICING VETERINARIAN

This journal, a monthly publication of the Veterinary Learning Systems, contains peer-reviewed articles on veterinary pharmaceuticals and veterinary therapeutics. The table of contents is available online at <<www.vetlearn.com>>. The site provides a searchable archive of back issues and you can find specific articles by author and/or keywords.

USP, VETERINARY MEDICINE[6]

The site <<www.usp.org>> provides drug information, quality reviews, and veterinary news. The USP veterinary drug information monographs on antibiotic use in animals are available online at no cost. The site also provides information on drug standards for veterinary products and vaccine associated feline sarcomas.

Veterinary Disease State Resources

The following print and Internet resources are useful for obtaining information regarding veterinary disease states. There are also animal health websites that contain educational information written for owners.

THE MERCK VETERINARY MANUAL (MVM)[7]

The manual has served veterinarians and other animal health professionals as a concise and reliable animal health reference for over 45 years. The full-text electronic version is available for free online at <<www.merckvetmanual.com>>. A guide to abbreviations used in veterinary medicine is also included.

VET MED CENTER[8]

Vet Med Center's mission is to address and satisfy the information needs of the animal health care community.[9] This site <<www.vetmedcenter.com>> serves as a point of access for veterinary professionals and pet owners to comprehensive animal health information, reference materials, clinical databases, and news.[9] The site is searchable by specialty (cardiology, dermatology, ophthalmology), current news, or wellness topics. The drug formulary can also be searched. Most of the information focuses on canines and felines.

PET PLACE[10]

The site <<www.vetmedcenter.com>> has pet centers focusing on different species (dog, cat, bird, horses, fish, reptiles, and small mammals). The database includes articles on veterinary disease states and preventative medicine. The drug library search tool allows the user to find drug information on a specific pharmaceutical. There are also text and graphics describing medication administration techniques for dogs and cats.

PET EDUCATION[11]

This website <<www.peteducation.com>> contains a variety of information on many species, such as the dog, cat, birds, fish, reptiles, and small pets. The site features a category on drug information, with subcategories on antibiotics, eye medications, ear and skin medications, pain relievers, and wormers. It also offers information about the common veterinary prescription and OTC medications, supplements, and nutraceuticals used in dogs and cats.

PETS WITH DIABETES[12]

This website <<www.petdiabetes.org>> contains information on diabetes in small animals, particularly dogs and cats. The site offers general diabetes education and drug information. It also offers insight and information on home testing and complications. There are also resources to support owners of diabetic animals.

Legal and Regulatory

FOOD ANIMAL RESIDUE AVOIDANCE DATABANK (FARAD)[13]

FARAD is a repository of comprehensive residue avoidance information. FARAD uses a computer-based decision support system designed to provide livestock producers and veterinarians with practical information on how to avoid drug, pesticide, and environmental contaminant residue situations. Current label information, including withdrawal times on all drugs approved for use in food animals in the United States, is available. Contact FARAD at 1-888-USFARAD (1-888-873-2723). The FARAD informational website is <<www.farad.org>>.

Current Practice Resources

AMERICAN VETERINARIAN MEDICAL ASSOCIATION (AVMA)[9]

The site provides numerous links organized by discipline for locating information. There are links to public resources, as well as allied organizations and groups. There are also links to veterinary education and current issues. Under the resources tab, you can find the AVMA's position statement on compounded drugs.

DVM MAGAZINE

A very informative magazine found at <<www.dvmnewsmagazine.com>> that reports on current issues within the veterinary profession, disease state updates, breaking news, practice management, and new products and devices for small animal, food animal, and equine practitioners.

The following table lists some tertiary resources that may be useful for specific categories of veterinary drug information requests.

USEFUL VETERINARY RESOURCES BY CATEGORY OF REQUEST

Type of Request	Useful Tertiary Sources
Toxicology and pharmacology	National Animal Poison Control Center,[1] Veterinary Drug Handbook,[14] Veterinary Pharmacology and Therapeutics,[2] Small Animal Clinical Pharmacology[3]
Veterinary disease states	Textbook of Veterinary Internal Medicine,[15] Merck Veterinary Manual,[7] The 5-Minute Veterinary Consultant, Pet Place website,[10] Pet Education website
Drug doses and indications	Veterinary Drug Handbook, Compendium of Veterinary Products, The 5-Minute Veterinary Consultant, Merck Veterinary Manual, Small Animal Clinical Pharmacology, Exotic Animal Formulary,[5] Vet Med Center website[8]
Legal and regulatory	Food and Drug Administration Center for Veterinary Medicine website
Current topics in veterinary medicine	DVM News Magazine, American Veterinary Medical Association website,[9] Food and Drug Administration Center for Veterinary Medicine website

NOTE: Parts of the material in this Appendix and Chapter 4 appeared in an article entitled *Veterinary Information for Pharmacists*, January 2004, *US Pharmacist*. Used here with permission from the publisher of *US Pharmacist*.

REFERENCES

1. National Animal Poison Control Center [homepage on the Internet]. New York: Association for the Prevention of Cruelty to Animals; c2004 [updated 2004 Mar 4; cited 2004 Mar 4]. Available from: http://www.napcc.aspca.org
2. Adams HR, editor. Veterinary pharmacology and therapeutics. 8th ed. Ames, IA: Iowa State Press; 2001.
3. Booth DM, editor. Small animal clinical pharmacology and therapeutics. Philadelphia, PA: W.B. Saunders; 2001.
4. Carpenter JW, Mashima TY, Rupier DJ, editors. Exotic animal formulary. 2nd ed. Philadelphia, PA: W.B. Saunders; 2001.
5. Marx KL, Roston MA, editors. The exotic animal drug compendium: an international formulary. Trenton, NJ: Veterinary Learning Systems; 1996.
6. USP Veterinary Medicine [homepage on the Internet]. Rockville, MD: United States Pharmacopeia; c1997-2004 [updated 2003 Nov 30; cited 2004 Mar 4]. Available from: http://www.usp.org/veterinary
7. Merck Veterinary Manual [homepage on the Internet]. Whitehouse Station, NJ: Merck & Co; c2003 [updated 2003 Dec 31; cited 2004 Mar 4]. Available from: http://www.merckvetmanual.com
8. VetMedCenter [homepage on the Internet]. San Francisco, CA: VetMedCenter; c2000 [updated 2000 Dec 30; cited 2004 Mar 4]. Available from: http://www.vetmedcenter.com
9. American Veterinary Medical Association [homepage on the Internet]. Schamburg, IL: American Veterinary Medical Association; c1996–2004 [updated 2004 Mar 4; cited 2004 Mar 4]. Available from: http://www.avma.org

10. PetPlace.com [homepage on the Internet]. Weston, FL: Intelligent Content Corp.; c1999–2003 [updated 2003 Dec 30; cited 2004 Mar 4]. Available from: http://www.petplace.com

11. PetEducation.com [homepage on the Internet]. Drs. Foster & Smith Inc.; c1997–2004 [updated 2004 Mar 4; cited 2004 Mar 4]. Available from: http://www.petplace.com

12. Pets with Diabetes [homepage on the Internet]. Petdiabetes.org; c2000–2004 [updated 2004 Feb 28; cited 2004 Mar 4]. Available from: http://www.petdiabetes.org

13. The Food Animal Residue Avoidance Databank [homepage on the Internet]. U.S. Department of Agriculture; c1998 [updated 1998 Dec 30; cited 2004 Mar 4]. Available from: http://farad.org

14. Plumb DC. Plumb's veterinary drug handbook: desk. 5th ed. Ames, IA: Blackwell Publishing Professional; 2005.

15. Ettinger SJ, Feldman EC. Textbook of veterinary internal medicine. 6th ed. New York: Elsevier; 2005.

4-2

Appendix 4–2

Performing a PubMed® Search

PubMed® Search

PubMed® is a database that is maintained by the National Library of Medicine and is available to the public at no charge. This database is available online at <<http://www.ncbi.nlm.nih.gov/PubMed>>. The information indexed by PubMed® includes MEDLINE®, OLDMEDLINE (articles from the 1950s to the mid-1960s), as well as citations for additional life science journals.

This database is especially helpful when looking for off-label uses of medications. For example, if a prescriber contacts you asking for information about the efficacy of fluoxetine in treatment of anorexia nervosa, it may be appropriate to seek information from the primary literature. A PubMed® search might be a good place to start this search. When performing a search using PubMed® one can begin with just a key word, for example fluoxetine. As Figure 1 shows, just using the term fluoxetine yields in 5904 results. The results can be narrowed by entering a second key word, such as anorexia nervosa, and combining the two terms with the Boolean operator AND.

While the addition of a second search term (see Figure 2) did narrow the results, there are still 59 results that match these two terms. At this time, it may be wise to explore the limit option (see Figure 3) provided by the database. Limits allow the user to restrict the number of results returned for a search. Some databases allow searches to be limited by a variety of factors, including language of publication, year of publication, type of article (e.g., human study, review, and case report) or by type of journal where publication is found. Since the requestor is seeking efficacy data, it is appropriate to limit these search results to just clinical trials.

By limiting the results to only clinical trials, 16 citations of possible interest have been identified (Figure 4). It is now necessary to look at the abstracts for these citations (Figure 5) and determine if these are helpful to provide a response to the query. By clicking on the blue hyperlink, an abstract is displayed. This abstract summarizes the information in the article, as well as providing complete citation information for that specific article. If the publisher's website offers full text of an article, a link is provided at the top of the page to the journal website. Some journals charge a fee for access to the full-text article while others do not.

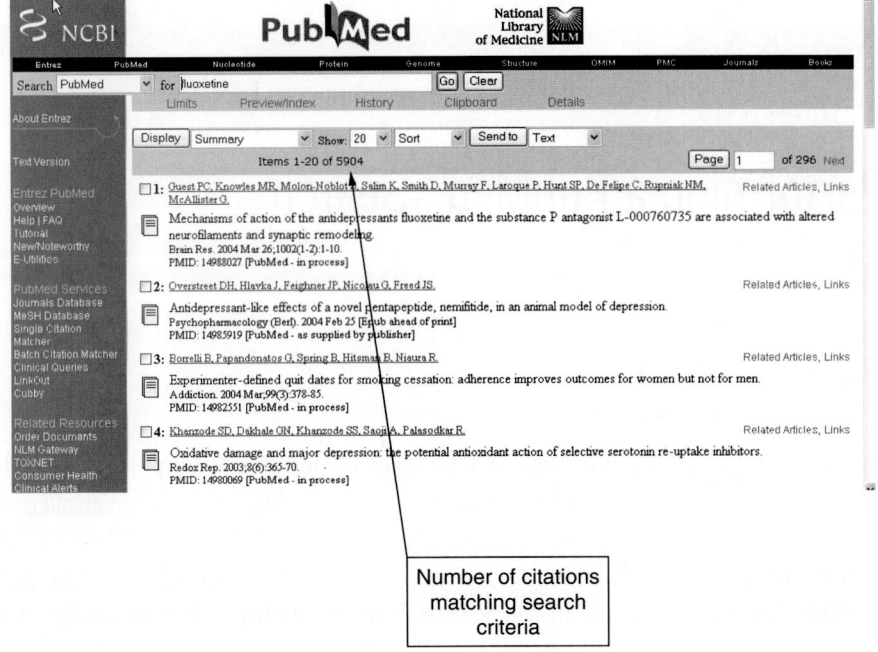

Figure 1. Key word search.

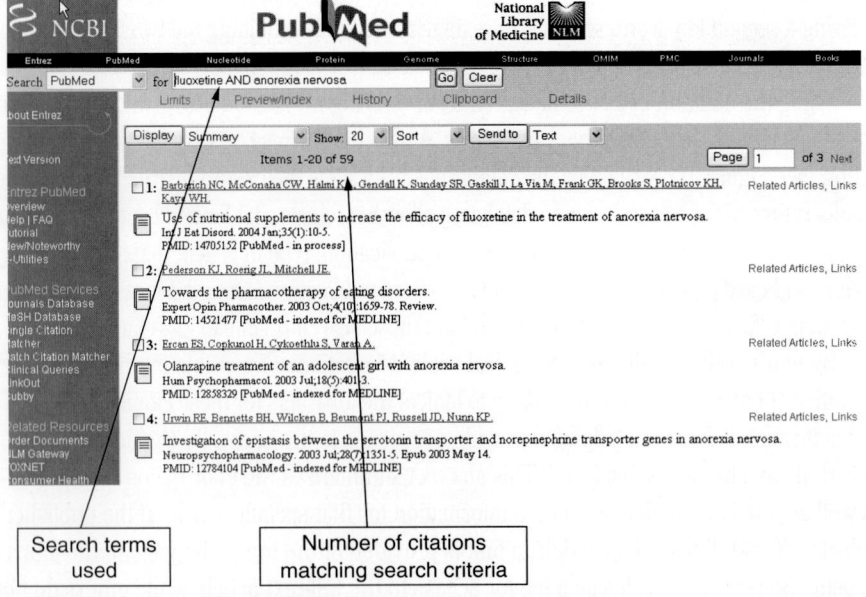

Figure 2. Multiple key word search.

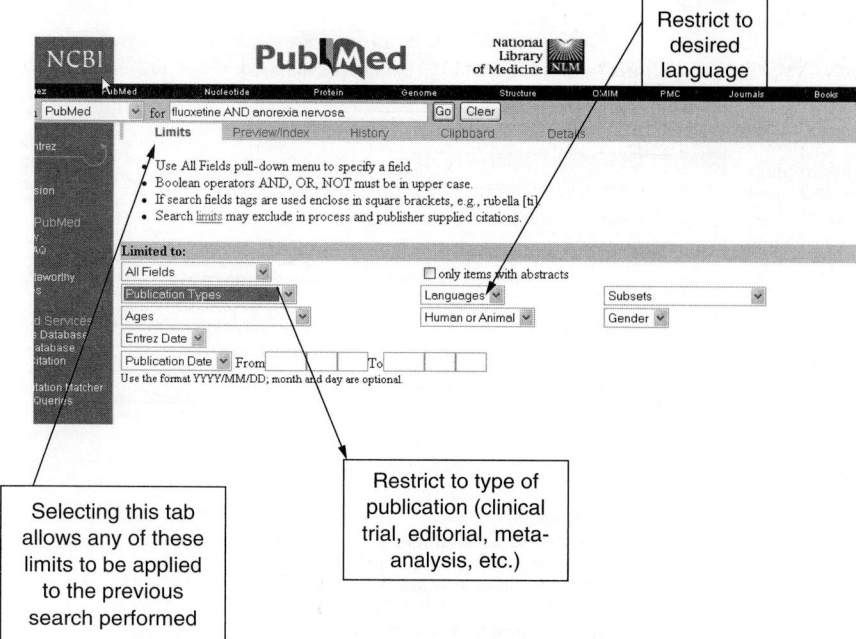

Figure 3. Limit screen.

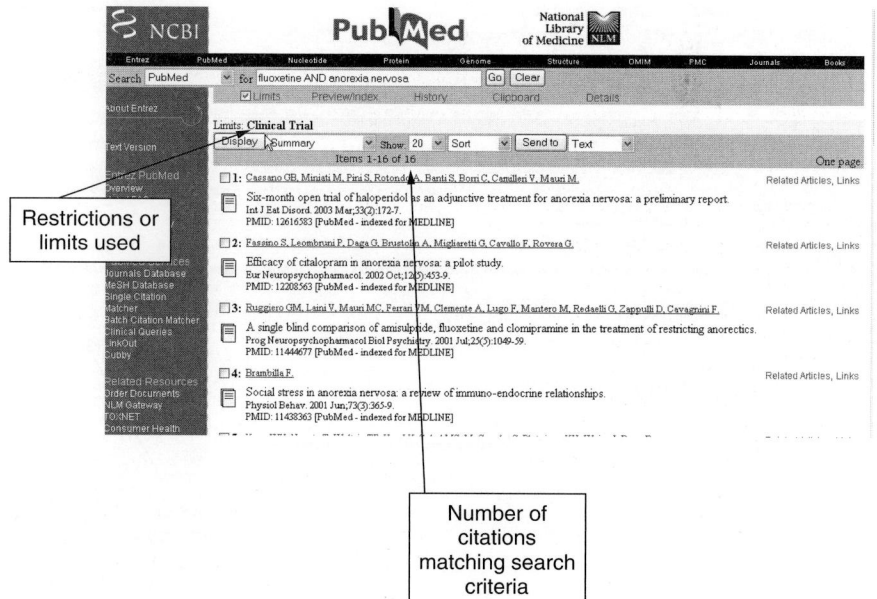

Figure 4. Results of search with restrictions.

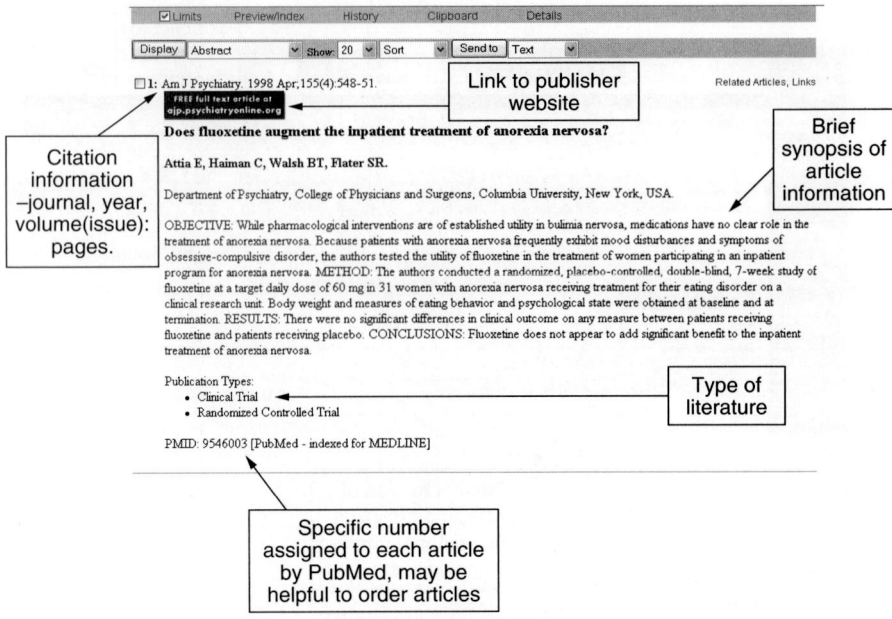

Figure 5. PubMed abstract.

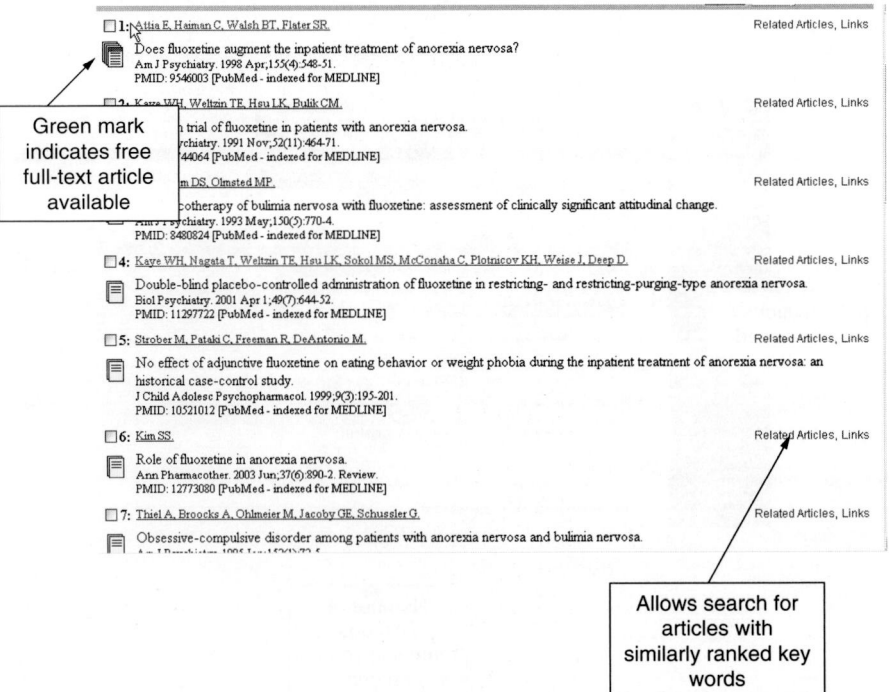

Figure 6. Related articles search.

Those journals not charging for an article are clearly marked as "free full text." You can then select that icon and go directly to a full-text PDF or html of the desired article.

One additional helpful feature offered by PubMed® is the "Related Articles" search (Figure 6). The database will first identify the key words or Medical Subject Headings (MeSH) associated with the article selected and then identify secondary words and terms. The database will then compare these terms (both primary and secondary terms) with other articles indexed in PubMed® to determine which other articles include similarly ranked terms and therefore might be of interest.

The best way to effectively search this database is by experience. However, PubMed® offers a tutorial to gain additional experience in how to most effectively conduct literature searches. This interactive tutorial session is available at <<http://www.nlm.nih.gov/bsd/pubmed_tutorial/m1001.html>>.

Selected Primary Literatures Sources

Journal Title	Publisher	ISSN	Areas Covered
American Journal of Health-System Pharmacy: AJHP	American Society of Health-System Pharmacists	1079-2082	Clinical and managerial areas of pharmacy practice in health systems
American Journal of Pharmaceutical Education	American Association of Colleges of Pharmacy	0002-9459	Scholarship and advancement of pharmacy education
Annals of Internal Medicine	American College of Physicians	0003-4819	Internal medicine, including management of disease states
Annals of Pharmacotherapy	Harvey Whitney Books Company	1060-0280	Safe, effective, and economical use of drugs
Antimicrobial Agents and Chemotherapy	American Society for Microbiology	0066-4804	Information regarding the use of antimicrobial agents
Archives of Internal Medicine	American Medical Association	0003-9926	Focus on the diagnosis and treatment of disease states
Clinical Pharmacokinetics	Adis International Limited	0312-5963	Focus on pharmacokinetic and pharmacodynamic properties of drugs
Clinical Pharmacology and Therapeutics	Mosby Year Book Incorporated	0009-9236	The effect of drugs on the human body
Drug Information Journal	Drug Information Association	0092-8615	Technology related to disseminating drug information
Drug Topics	Thomson Health care	0012-6616	Focus on issues impacting community pharmacy and on new drug therapies
Drugs	Adis International Limited	0012-6667	Pharmacotherapeutic aspects of both new and established drugs
Formulary	Advanstar Communications Incorporated	1082-801X	Contemporary issues in drug policy management and pharmacotherapy
Hospital Pharmacy	Facts & Comparisons Incorporated	0018-5787	Issues related to pharmacy in institutional settings

Journal Title	Publisher	ISSN	Areas Covered
JAMA (the Journal of the American Medical Association)	American Medical Association	0098-7484	New research and review information that impacts health care
Journal of Cardiovascular Pharmacology	Lippincott Williams & Wilkins	0160-2446	New information about the treatment of cardiovascular disease
The Journal of Clinical Pharmacology	Lippincott Williams & Wilkins	0091-2700	Clinical information about the safety, tolerability, efficacy, therapeutic use, and toxicology of drugs
Journal of Pharmaceutical Sciences	Wiley	0022-3549	Application of physical and analytical chemistry to pharmaceutical sciences
Journal of Pharmacology and Experimental Therapeutics	American Society for Experimental Pharmacology and Therapeutics	0022-3565	Covers interaction between chemicals and biological systems, as well as metabolism, distribution, and toxicology
Journal of Pharmacy and Pharmacology	Pharmaceutical Press	0022-3573	Addresses a variety of practice areas, including drug delivery systems, biomaterials and polymers, and implications of human genome on drug therapies
Journal of The American Pharmacists Association	American Pharmacists Association	1544-3191	News, information, and research in the area of pharmacotherapeutic management
Medical Letter on Drugs and Therapeutics	Medical Letter, Inc.	0025-732X	Provides information on new drug therapies and drugs of choice for disease management
New England Journal of Medicine	Massachusetts Medical Society	0028-646X	Results of recent research considered important to the practice of medicine
Pharmaceutical Research	Plenum Press	0724-8741	Emphasis on drug delivery, drug formulation, pharmacokinetics, pharmacodynamics, and drug disposition
PharmacoEconomics	Adis International Limited	1170-7690	Information regarding the economical use of drug therapies
Pharmacological Reviews	American Society of Pharmacology and Experimental Therapeutics	0031-6997	Current topics of interest including cellular pharmacology, drug metabolism and disposition, renal pharmacology, and neuropharmacology

Journal Title	Publisher	ISSN	Areas Covered
Pharmacotherapy	IOS Press	0277-0008	Published by American College of Clinical Pharmacy and focused on original research in clinical practice
Pharmacy Times	Romaine Pierson Publishing Incorporated	0003-0627	Focus on new drug therapies and patient counseling as it relates to community pharmacy
Therapeutic Drug Monitoring	Lippincott Williams & Wilkins	0163-4356	Fosters exchange of knowledge between fields of pharmacology, pathology, toxicology, and analytical
U.S. Pharmacist	Jobson Publishing Corporation	0148-4818	Information regarding the practice of community pharmacy

SOURCE: Fuller N, Allison A, Beattie M, et al. AACP core list of journals for libraries that serve schools and colleges of pharmacy 2003. American Association of Colleges of Pharmacy [online]; July 2003 [cited 2004 Mar 1]: [6 screens]. Available from: <<http://www.aacp.org/site/page.asp?TRACKID=&VID=1&CID=380&DID=3619>>.

6–1

Appendix 6–1

Questions for Assessing Clinical Trials

OVERALL ASSESSMENT

- Was the article published in a reputable, peer-reviewed journal?
- Are the investigator's training/education/practice site adequate for the study objective?
- Did the funding source bias the study?

TITLE/ABSTRACT

- Was the title unbiased?
- Did the abstract contain information not found within the study?
- Did the abstract provide a clear overview of the purpose, methods, results, and conclusions of the study?

INTRODUCTION

- Did the authors provide sufficient background information to demonstrate the rationale for the study?
- Were the study objectives clearly identified?
- What was the major null hypothesis and alternate hypothesis?

METHODS

- Was an appropriate study design used to answer the question?
- Were reasonable inclusion/exclusion criteria presented to represent an appropriate patient population?
- Was a selection bias present?
- Was subject recruitment described? If so, how were subjects recruited? Was it appropriate?
- Was institutional review board (IRB) approval obtained?

- Was subject informed consent obtained?
- Were the intervention and control regimens appropriate?
- What type of blinding was used? Was this type appropriate?
- Was randomization included? If so, what type was used? Was this appropriate?
- Who generated the allocation sequence, enrolled participants, and assigned participants to groups? Was this appropriate?
- Which ancillary treatments were permitted? Would they have affected the outcome?
- Was a run-in period included? How does this affect the results?
- Did the investigators measure compliance? How was compliance measured? Was this adequate?
- Was the primary endpoint appropriate for the study objective?
- Were secondary endpoints measured? If so, were they adequate for what was being studied?
- Were planned subgroup analyses planned? If so, were they appropriate?
- Was the method used to measure the primary endpoint appropriate?
- What type of data best describes the primary endpoint? Is this what was gathered?
- Were data collected appropriately?
- What number of patients was needed for the primary endpoint to detect a difference between groups (power analysis)? Was the necessary sample size calculated? Were there enough patients enrolled to reach this endpoint?
- What were the alpha (α) and beta (β) values? Were these appropriate?
- Were the statistical tests used appropriate?

RESULTS

- Were the number of patients screened, enrolled, administered treatment, completing, and withdrawing from the study reported? Were reasons for subject discontinuations reported? Were withdrawals handled appropriately?
- Was the trial adequately powered?
- Were the subject demographics between groups similar at baseline? If not, were the differences likely to have an affect on the outcome data?
- Were data presented clearly?
- Were the results adjusted to take into account confounding variables?
- Was intention-to-treat analysis used?
- Were estimated effect size, p values, and confidence intervals reported?
- Were the results statistically significant? Clinically different?
- Based on the results, could a Type I or Type II error have occurred?
- Can the trial results be extrapolated to the population?
- Was the null hypothesis accepted or rejected?

- Are subgroup analysis presented? Are these appropriate?
- Was ancillary therapy included? Did this affect the study results?
- Were therapy adverse effects included?

CONCLUSIONS/DISCUSSION

- Did the information appear biased or did the trial results support the conclusions?
- Were trial limitations described?
- Did the investigators explain unexpected results?
- Are the results able to be extrapolated to the population?
- Were the study results clinically meaningful?

REFERENCES

- Were the references listed well represented (e.g., current and well representing the literature)?
- Is a comprehensive list of published articles related to the trial objective presented?

7-1

7-1

Appendix 7–1

Beyond the Basics: Questions to Consider for Critique of Primary Literature

TRUE EXPERIMENT

- Refer to Chap. 6

N-OF-1 TRIAL

- Was assignment of active and control treatment to study periods randomized?
- Was the study blinded?
- Were multiple observation periods used?
- Were study endpoints clearly defined?

STABILITY STUDY

- Were study methodologies and test conditions clearly defined?
- Were validated assays used?
- Were assays validated using time-zero measurements and an adequate number of test samples taken?

BIOEQUIVALENCY STUDY

- Did the protocol define the characteristics of the subjects?
- Were confounding factors (e.g., smoking and alcohol use) identified and controlled?
- Was a crossover design used?
- Was the study randomized and blinded?

PROGRAMMATIC RESEARCH

- Were one of two options used for subject comparison: (1) comparison of subjects to those not using the program or service, (2) comparison of subjects before or after initiation of the program or service?

- Was the program or service clearly defined?
- Did the authors specify from whose perspective (e.g., patient, provider, physician, and third-party payer) the study was undertaken?
- If costs were analyzed, were all costs associated with provision of the program or service included in the analysis, including personnel, inflationary changes, and cost-savings for what might have been, had the intervention not occurred?
- Were clinically important outcome parameters used to assess effectiveness of the program or service?

FOLLOW-UP (COHORT) STUDY

- Were exposed and unexposed subjects similar in terms of demographic characteristics and susceptibility to disease states?
- Were subjects randomized to exposure or nonexposure, if possible?
- Were inclusion and exclusion criteria described in detail?
- Was the research question clearly stated?
- Were the same efforts to measure outcomes made in each group?
- Were 95% confidence intervals calculated?
- Were follow-up rates the same for the exposed and unexposed groups?

CASE-CONTROL STUDY

- Was predisposition of disease similar in cases and controls except for exposure to the risk factor?
- Were cases and controls matched?
- Was exposure to the risk factor similar to that which would occur in the general population?
- Did cases and controls undergo similar diagnostic evaluations?
- Were investigators who assessed patients or collected data blinded to the status of the subject as a case or control?
- Did the investigators compare cases with several different control groups?
- Were 95% confidence intervals calculated?

CROSS-SECTIONAL STUDY

- Did investigators ensure accuracy in data collection?
- If a survey or questionnaire was used, was it validated?
- Were the inclusion and exclusion criteria clearly defined and stated?
- Was selection of cases clearly described?

CASE STUDY, CASE REPORT, OR CASE SERIES

- Did the authors recognize the preliminary nature of the results (i.e., recommendations for clinical application of the results should be guarded)?

SURVEY STUDY

- Was the survey instrument valid and reliable? Was a pretest or pilot test conducted on the survey instrument?
- Was the sample size large enough to detect a difference between groups?
- Was the survey objective and carefully planned?
- Were data quantifiable?
- Was the sample representative of the target population?
- Was response rate high enough to reflect results that would be expected of the target population?
- Did the investigators determine whether nonresponders differed from responders?

POSTMARKETING SURVEILLANCE STUDY

- Was a large enough sample studied to reflect current uses of and side effects associated with the new drug therapy?
- Were appropriate methods used to measure clearly defined endpoints?

NONSYSTEMATIC REVIEWS (NARRATIVE REVIEWS)

- Was an extensive search for available studies undertaken?
- Did the authors use a variety of resources to identify studies for inclusion in the review article?
- Was the review article focused on a clearly defined patient population?
- Did the studies included in the review article use valid research methods?
- Did the author examine reasons for differences in study results and conclusions?
- Were outcomes of the studies clinically important?
- Did the author consider benefits and risks of the drug therapy?

SYSTEMATIC REVIEWS (QUALITATIVE OR QUANTITATIVE)

- Did the authors clearly define the research question?
- Was the review article focused on a clearly defined patient population?
- Was an extensive search for available studies undertaken?
- Did the authors consider using results from both published and unpublished studies in the analysis?

- Did the authors clearly define criteria for study inclusion in the analysis?
- Did the authors list studies that were included in and excluded from the analysis?
- Did the authors provide details concerning methodologies of studies used in the analysis?
  - ○ Were included studies addressing the same clinical question(s)?
  - ○ Did all included studies use appropriate doses, regimens, and routes of administrations for both treatments and comparators?
  - ○ Were all included studies of appropriate duration?
- Were tests of homogeneity performed and results reported?
- Were those individuals who selected studies for inclusion in the analysis blinded to the names of the original authors, place of publication of the study, and final study results?
- If a meta-analysis, were appropriate statistical tests used and the probability of Type I and Type II errors considered?
- If a meta-analysis, were 95% confidence intervals calculated?
- If a meta-analysis, were sensitivity analyses conducted?
- Was an effect size calculated?
  - ○ Are treatment effects clinically important?
- Was the source of funding provided and could it be a source of bias in the results?

PRACTICE GUIDELINES

- Is there an explicit description of the procedures used to identify, select, and combine evidence?
- Are the recommendations valid?
- Are the guidelines regularly reviewed and updated to incorporate new evidence as it becomes available?
- Was the guideline peer-reviewed?
- Can the recommendations be generalized to a larger population?
- Was the source of funding for the development of the guideline provided and could it bias the conclusions?
- If another group of experts were to independently develop a guideline on the same clinical situation, would the recommendations be the same (are the recommendations reliable)?

PHARMACOECONOMIC ANALYSIS

- Readers are referred to Chap. 8 for evaluation of these types of trials.

QUALITY OF LIFE STUDIES

- Are health related-quality of life (HR-QOL) instruments validated?
- If a series of HR-QOL measurements are used, does this result in a valid HR-QOL battery?
- Are HR-QOL instruments sensitive to changes in the patients' status as the trial progresses?
- Are important aspects of patients' lives measured, as determined by the patients themselves?
- Is timing of HR-QOL measurements to answer the research questions appropriately related to anticipated timing of the clinical effects?
- Were sequences of HR-QOL assessments conducted in the same order for all patients?
- Was mode of data collection (self-report vs. trained interviewer) appropriate for type of questions being asked?
  ○ If mode of data collection was a trained interviewer, could the interview location lead to biased answers?
- Were response rates to questionnaires reported?
- Are there missing data?
  ○ If missing data exist, is there a specific pattern that suggests author manipulation to provide desired results (missing data could have countered author's hypothesis)?
- If a multicenter trial, did all sites evaluate HR-QOL?
- Is the HR-QOL instrument valid for examining the specific disease in question?
- Are both positive and negative findings reported?
- Are adverse drug events and HR-QOL measurements considered separately?
- Is impact of treatment effects included with HR-QOL measurements?
- Is there evidence that culturally defined factors may have impacted patient HR-QOL measurements and/or the assessment of these measurements?

DIETARY SUPPLEMENT MEDICAL LITERATURE

- Which plant part was utilized?
- Was a standardized botanical extract utilized?
- Was the study product standardization appropriate?
- Was a specific plant species or specific salt form utilized?
- Was the study dose appropriate?
- Was the trial length appropriate to perceive treatment effects or differences?
- Was the sample size sufficient to detect a difference between groups if one exists?

9–1

Appendix 9–1

New Zealand Guidelines Group (NZGG)

Steps in Guideline Development

Flowchart:

- **Problem identification**
- Formation of guideline development team
- Suitability screen
- Is development of guideline an appropriate solution? — **No** → Project outcomes unlikely to benefit from a guideline being developed → **Share evidence** → Consider the options
- **Yes** → Proceed with guideline development process
- Question formulation
- Current data acquisition and literature searching
- Identify evidence
- Assess evidence
- Determine benefits & harms
- Balance sheet*
- Develop recommendations and algorithm
- Disseminate
- Implement
- Evaluate
- Improve

*Balance sheets with cost may be omitted if there are too many assumptions to be made

Appendix 9–2

National Institute for Clinical Excellence (NICE)

A summary of key stages of NICE guideline developement (for developers)

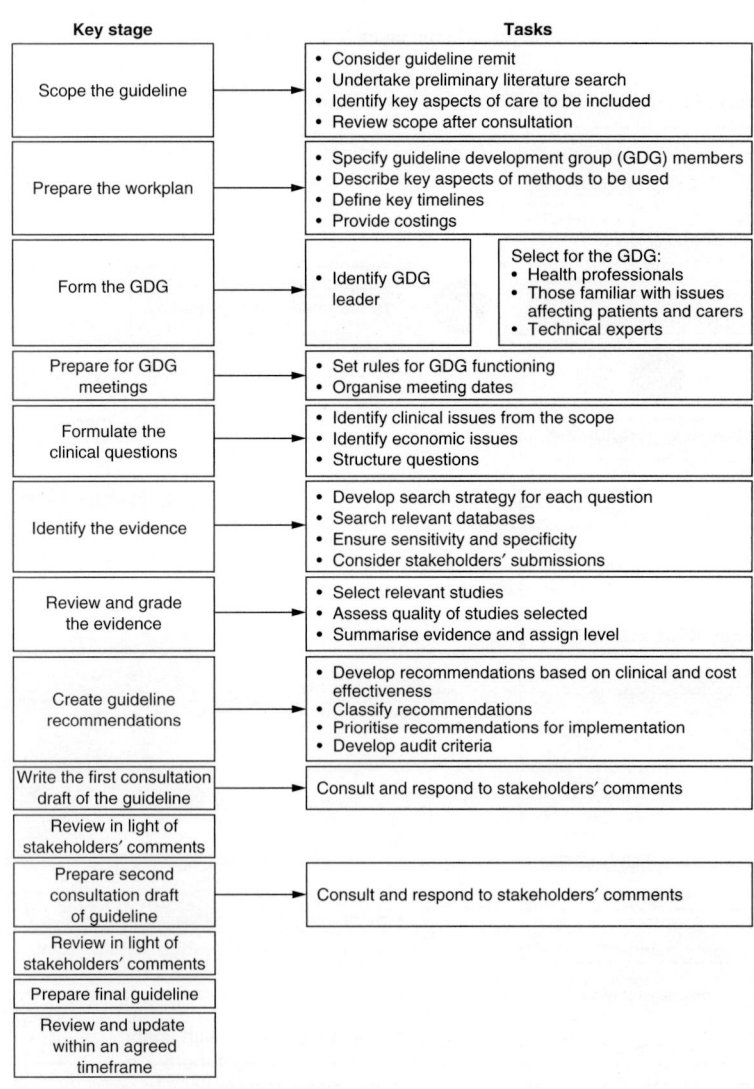

| Key stage | Tasks |

Scope the guideline
- Consider guideline remit
- Undertake preliminary literature search
- Identify key aspects of care to be included
- Review scope after consultation

Prepare the workplan
- Specify guideline development group (GDG) members
- Describe key aspects of methods to be used
- Define key timelines
- Provide costings

Form the GDG
- Identify GDG leader

Select for the GDG:
- Health professionals
- Those familiar with issues affecting patients and carers
- Technical experts

Prepare for GDG meetings
- Set rules for GDG functioning
- Organise meeting dates

Formulate the clinical questions
- Identify clinical issues from the scope
- Identify economic issues
- Structure questions

Identify the evidence
- Develop search strategy for each question
- Search relevant databases
- Ensure sensitivity and specificity
- Consider stakeholders' submissions

Review and grade the evidence
- Select relevant studies
- Assess quality of studies selected
- Summarise evidence and assign level

Create guideline recommendations
- Develop recommendations based on clinical and cost effectiveness
- Classify recommendations
- Prioritise recommendations for implementation
- Develop audit criteria

Write the first consultation draft of the guideline
Consult and respond to stakeholders' comments

Review in light of stakeholders' comments

Prepare second consultation draft of guideline
Consult and respond to stakeholders' comments

Review in light of stakeholders' comments

Prepare final guideline

Review and update within an agreed timeframe

Appendix 9–3

National Institute for Clinical Excellence (NICE) Topic Selection Criteria

NATIONAL INSTITUTE FOR CLINICAL EXCELLENCE

Topic suggestion and selection

Criteria for selecting topics for the advisory committee on topic selection

The Department of Health and the Welsh Assembly Government are responsible for selecting topics for the NICE technology appraisal and clinical guidelines work programmes. As part of the process of selecting topics to refer to NICE, the Advisory Committee on Topic Selection (ACTS) uses the criteria below to assess the suggestions put forward.

We recommend that healthcare professionals, patients and carers and the general public who suggest topics read these criteria before submitting their suggestion.

1. *Would guidance promote the best possible improvement in patient care given available resources? In particular, are one or more of the following criteria satisfied:*

   a. does the proposed guidance relate to one of the NHS clinical priority areas, or to other government health-related priorities such as reducing health inequalities

   b. does the proposed guidance address a condition which is associated with significant disability, morbidity or mortality in the population as a whole or in particular subgroups

   c. does the proposed guidance relate to one or more interventions that could significantly improve patients' or carers' quality of life and/or reduce avoidable morbidity or avoidable premature mortality, relative to current standard practice, or if used more extensively or more appropriately would do so

   d. does the proposed guidance relate to one or more interventions which if more extensively used would impact significantly on NHS or other societal resources (financial and other)

   e. does the proposed guidance relate to one or more interventions which could without detriment to patient care be used more selectively, thus freeing up resources for use elsewhere in the NHS?

2. *Will NICE be able to add value by issuing guidance, taking into account the following factors:*

NATIONAL INSTITUTE FOR CLINICAL EXCELLENCE
Topic suggestion and selection
Criteria for selecting topics for the advisory committee on topic selection   Page 1 of 2

a. is the evidence base sufficient to develop robust guidance across most or all of the interventions to be covered by the proposed guidance

b. is there evidence and/or reason to believe that there is or will be inappropriate practice and/or significant variation in clinical practice and/or variation in access to treatment (between geographical areas or social groups) in the absence of guidance?

3. *Would the most appropriate form of guidance consist of an appraisal, a clinical guideline, or a combination of the two, taking into account:*

a. the availability of an existing clinical guideline from NICE or from another authoritative source for the condition in question

b. the degree of urgency for guidance on any specific intervention for the condition in question

c. the possible complexity of the proposed guidance if formulated as an appraisal?

In general, the presumption is that guidance will take the form of a clinical guideline if no suitable guidance relating to the condition as a whole is available or in preparation. An appraisal should be considered if the perceived need relates to a particular intervention for a particular condition, and if either (a) there is an urgent need for guidance or (b) a clinical guideline for that condition is already available or in preparation.

4. *For new interventions, does the balance of advantage for patient care lie with appraisal at time of launch or at some specified future date, taking account of the following factors and the attached checklist:*

a. the possible impact on uptake or equity of access in the absence of guidance at time of launch

b. the likely robustness of the evidence base at time of launch;

c. the prospect of relevant additional data becoming available in the period immediately after launch

d. for surgical and related interventions, whether safety and efficacy have already been assessed (or will be assessed in the near future) by the Interventional Procedures Advisory Committee?

NATIONAL INSTITUTE FOR CLINICAL EXCELLENCE
Topic suggestion and selection
Criteria for selecting topics for the advisory committee on topic selection   Page 2 of 2

Appendix 9–4

Study Selection Process—Centre for Reviews and Dissemination (CRD)*

Flow Diagram of Study Selection Process

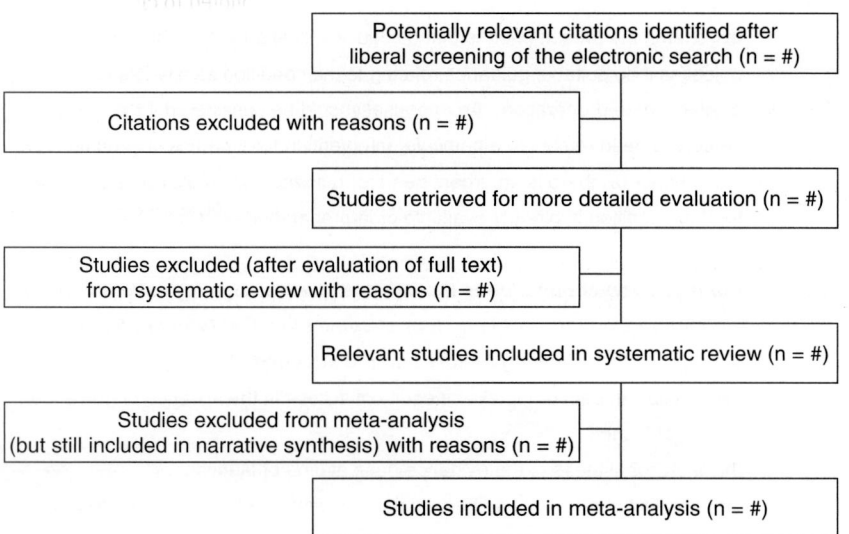

*Khan KS, ter Riet G, Glanville J, Showden AJ, Kleijnen J, eds. Undertaking systematic reviews of research on effectiveness CRD's guidance for those carrying out or commissioning reviews, 4th ed. CRD Report Number 4. University of York, York, UK: Centre for Reviews and Dissemination; 2001.

9–5

Study Selection Points—Centre for Reviews and Dissemination (CRD)

KEY POINTS ABOUT STUDY SELECTION

- Studies should be selected in an unbiased way, based on selection criteria that flow directly from the review questions, and that have been piloted to check that they can be reliably applied.
- Study selection is a staged process involving sifting through the citations located by the search, retrieving full reports of potentially relevant citations and, from their assessment, identifying those studies that fulfill the inclusion criteria.
- Parallel independent assessments should be conducted to minimize the risk of errors of judgment. If disagreements occur between reviewers, they should be resolved according to a predefined strategy using consensus and arbitration as appropriate.
- The study selection process should be documented, detailing reasons for inclusion and exclusion.

Study selection criteria (example)

Review question

In patients undergoing hip replacement, to what extent is the risk of post-operative infection reduced by antimicrobial prophylaxis?

Selection criteria	Inclusion criteria	Exclusion criteria
Population	▪ Patients undergoing hip replacement (primary or revision procedure)	Other operations
Interventions	▪ Antimicrobial prophylaxis compared to placebo or no prophylaxis	Lack of comparison
	▪ Comparison of different antimicrobials	
Outcome	▪ Surgical wound infection confirmed by appropriate microbiologic techniques	Infection not confirmed
Study design	▪ Randomised controlled trials	Non-randomised studies

Source: Khan KS, ter Riet G, Glanville J, Sowden AJ, Kleijnen J, eds. Undertaking systematic reviews of research on effectiveness CRD's guidance for those carrying out or commissioning reviews, 4th ed. CRD Report Number 4. University of York, York, UK: Centre for Reviews and Dissemination; 2001.

9-6

Appendix 9–6

Data Synthesis—Centre for Reviews and Dissemination (CRD)*

Key concepts in data synthesis for systematic reviews

DESCRIPTIVE DATA SYNTHESIS

A nonquantitative synthesis of the collated evidence to assess the extent of the evidence and to plan the quantitative synthesis. It allows a qualitative assessment of variation in study characteristics, quality, and results (heterogeneity). In some situations where there are numerous studies with consistent and large effects, it may be possible to discern effects solely from this synthesis.

QUANTITATIVE DATA SYNTHESIS

A synthesis using a group of statistical techniques to combine the results of the included studies (meta-analysis), to assess heterogeneity, and to quantitatively evaluate other aspects like publication bias. Meta-analysis is used to calculate a pooled estimate of effect and its confidence interval.

HETEROGENEITY

The variability or differences between studies in terms of key characteristics (clinical heterogeneity), quality (methodological heterogeneity), and effects (heterogeneity of results). Statistical tests of heterogeneity may be used to assess whether the observed variability in study results (effect sizes) is greater than that expected to occur by chance.

*Khan KS, ter Riet G, Glanville J, Sowden AJ, Kleijnen J, eds. Undertaking systematic reviews of research on effectiveness CRD's guidance for those carrying out or commissioning Reviews, 4th ed. CRD Report Number 4. University of York, York, UK: Centre for Reviews and Dissemination; 2001.

HOMOGENEITY

The degree to which the studies included in a review are similar. Studies are considered statistically homogeneous if their results vary no more than might be expected by the chance.

SENSITIVITY ANALYSIS

An analysis used to determine how the results of a systematic review change due to variations arising from uncertain decisions or assumptions about the data and the methods that were used.

PUBLICATION BIAS

A bias in the research literature where the likelihood of publication of a study is influenced by the significance of its results. For example, studies in which an intervention is not found to be effective may be less likely to be published. Systematic reviews that fail to identify such studies may overestimate the true effect of an intervention. In some subject areas (e.g., in alternative medicine), studies showing effectiveness may also suffer from publication bias.

9–7

Appendix 9–7

National Institute for Clinical Excellence (NICE)—Evidence Table Format for Intervention Studies

Bibliographic Reference	Study Type	Evidence Level	Number of Patients	Patient Characteristics	Intervention	Comparison	Length of Follow-up	Outcome Measures	Effect Size	Source of Funding	Additional Comments
Author, title, journal, volume, year, pages	Observational, cohort, case studies, and so forth	Report the classification with the SIGN or NICE systems	Total number of patients included in the study, including number of patients in each arm; with inclusion/ exclusion criteria, number of patients who started and completed	Relevant characteristics to the area of interest: age, gender, ethnic origin, comorbidity, disease status, community/ hospital-based	Intervention (treatment, procedure) studied. If important for the study, specify length of treatment. *Note: for diagnostic studies the intervention is the diagnostic test studied*	Placebo, alternative treatment. *Note: for diagnostic studies comparison of the test is with another test*	The length of time patients take part in the study, from first staging treatment until either a prespecified end-point (for example, death, specified length of disease-free remission) or the end of the data-gathering phase is reached. If the study is halted earlier than originally planned for any reason, this should also be noted here	All outcome measures, including associated harms. For studies with a diagnostic component there will be two interventions to consider-the diagnostic test used and the associated treatment. *Note: separate line for each outcome*	Absolute risk reduction and relative risk (reduction), number needed to treat, number needed to harm, odds ratios, as required. p values and confidence intervals whenever possible	Government funding (for example, National Health Service), voluntary charity (for example, Wellcome Trust), pharmaceutical company	Additional characteristics/ interpretations of the studies that the reviewer wishes to record. Important flaws in the study not identifiable from other data in the table. A range of additional questions or issues that will need to be considered, but do not figure in the results table

NOTE: An evidence table is a table summarizing the results of a collection of studies which, taken together, represent the evidence supporting a particular recommendation or series of recommendations in a guideline. Evidence table for intervention studies, National Institute for Clinical Excellence, February 2004.

9–8

Appendix 9–8

New Zealand Guidelines Group (NZGG)— Considered Judgment

CONSIDERED JUDGMENT FORM

Key Question	Evidence Table Ref.
1. Volume of evidence *Comment here on any issues concerning the quantity of evidence available on this topic and its methodological quality.*	
2. Consistency *Comment here on the degree of consistency demonstrated by the available evidence. Where there are conflicting results, indicate how the group formed a judgment as to the overall direction of the evidence.*	
3. Applicability *Comment here on the extent to which the evidence is directly applicable in the New Zealand setting. Comment here on how reasonable it is to generalize from the results of the studies used as evidence to the target population for this guideline.*	
4. Clinical impact *Comment here on the potential clinical impact that the intervention in question might have, e.g., size of patient population; magnitude of effect; relative benefit over other management options; resource implications; and balance of risk and benefit.*	
5. Other factors *Indicate here any other factors that you took into account when assessing the evidence base.*	

6. Evidence statement *Please summarize the development group's synthesis of the evidence relating to this key question, taking all the above factors into account, and indicate the evidence level which applies.*	**Evidence level**
7. Recommendation *What recommendation(s) does the guideline development group draw from this evidence? Please indicate the grade of recommendation(s) and any dissenting opinion within the group.*	**Grade of recommendation**

SOURCE: New Zealand Guidelines Group. *Handbook for the Preparation of Explicit Evidence-based Clinical Practice Guidelines*; 2001. Available at: www.nzgg.org.nz/development/documents/nzgg_guideline_handbook.pdf.

Appendix 9–9

Guidelines Advisory Committee (GAC) Levels of Evidence Grades of Recommendation

Levels of Evidence and Grades of Recommendation:
A Guidelines Advisory Committee (GAC) Comparison of Guideline Developer's Evidence Taxonomies

GAC Level of Evidence to Recommend	ACC/AHA	AHCPR	AHRQ	CTFPHC	CCOPGI	CPSO	ICSI	SIGN	USPTF
Excellent/Good Evidence to Recommend	Class I Class III	Grade A	Class I	Level I	Grade EV*	Level I Level II	Class A Class M*	1++/A 1+/A	Grade A
Fair Evidence to Recommend	Class II a	Grade B	Class II	Level II-1 Level II-2	Grade PE*	Level III	Class B Class C Class D*	1– 2++/B 2+/C	Grade B Grade D
Insufficient (Poor) Evidence to Recommend	Class II b	Grade C	Class III*	Level II-3	Grade O	Level IV	Class D**	2–3/D	Grade C Grade I
Consensus Opinion		Grade D	Class III**	Level III	Grade C Grade E Grade X	Level V	Class R Class X	4/D	

Notes:

M*: variable depending on study design. For example, meta analysis or systematic reviews based on randomized trials yield stronger evidence than other study designs.

Class D*: ICSI groups cross-sectional studies, case series and case reports as Class D evidence. The GAC considers cross-sectional studies to be fair evidence to recommend.

Class D**: ICSI groups cross-sectional studies, case series and case reports as Class D evidence. The GAC considers case series and case reports to be insufficient (Poor) evidence to recommend.

EV*: CCOPGI considers a comprehensive systematic review of the best available evidence to be evidence-based. The GAC considers systematic reviews excellent/good evidence, unless the systematic review is based on case series or case reports only. In the event that a systematic review was based on case series and case reports only, the GAC would consider the level of evidence to be insufficient (Poor).

PE*: CCOPGI considers a partially evidence-based recommendation to be based on a comprehensive review, but the method of selecting and evaluating evidence is less systematic or unspecified. The GAC considers partially evidence-based recommendations to be fair evidence, unless the partial review is based on case series or case reports only. In the event that a partial review was based on case series and case reports only, the GAC would consider the level of evidence to be insufficient (Poor).

Class III*: AHRQ groups case reports, uncontrolled case series and expert or consensus opinion as Class III evidence. The GAC considers case reports and uncontrolled case series as insufficient (Poor) evidence to recommend.

Class III**: AHRQ groups case reports, uncontrolled case series and expert or consensus opinion as Class III evidence. The GAC considers consensus opinion as its own category under "consensus".

(Continued)

713

Acronyms:

ACC/AHA: American College of Cardiology and the American Heart Association, Recommendations and Level of Evidence

AHCPR: Agency for Healthcare Policy and Research: Evidence Grading System

AHRQ: Agency for Healthcare Research and Quality: Strength of Evidence Rating

CCOPGI: Cancer Care Ontario Practice Guidelines initiative: Evidence-Based Categorization Scheme

CPSO: College of Physicians and Surgeons of Ontario

CTFPHC: Canadian Task Force on the Periodic Health Examination: Quality of Guidelines

ICSI: Institute for Clinical Systems Improvement: Evidence Grading System

SIGN: Scottish Intercollegiate Guidelines Network: Levels of Evidence

USPTF: U.S. Preventive Services Task Force: Classifications

From the Ontario Guidelines Advisory Committee. http://gacguidelines.ca/pdfs/LevelsOfEvidenceChart.pdf

9–10

National Institute for Clinical Excellence (NICE) Guideline Structure

GUIDELINE STRUCTURE

The full guideline contains all the recommendations, plus details of the methods used and the underpinning evidence. The structure and format of the full guideline are at the discretion of the National Collaborating Centre (NCC), but core elements should be as follows:

- Summary of recommendations and algorithm
- Introduction
  - Responsibility and support for guideline development
  - Funding
  - Guideline Developement Group membership
  - Patient and carer involvement
  - Epidemiologic data
  - Experience of those receiving care, or service use
  - Outcomes
  - Clinical issues
  - Aim and scope of the guideline
- Methods
  - Literature search strategy
  - Sifting and reviewing the literature
  - Synthesizing the evidence
  - Economic analysis
  - Assigning levels to the evidence
  - Areas without evidence and consensus methodology
  - Forming recommendations
  - Consultation
  - Related guidance: details of related NICE technology appraisals or clinical guidelines that are published or in preparation

- Guideline recommendations
  - Evidence statements
  - Recommendations
  - Audit criteria
  - Scheduled review of the guideline
  - Recommendations for research
- References
- Appendices, which may include:
  - Evidence tables (preferably on a CD-ROM)—details of search strategies

For examples of published guidelines refer to the NICE website: <<http://www.nice.org.uk/>>

9–11

Appendix 9–11

Scottish Intercollegiate Guidelines Network (SIGN) Consultation and Peer-Review

Scottish Intercollegiate Guidelines Network March 2004

```
        ┌──────────────────────────────────────┐
        │   Systematic literature review       │
   ┌────│   and draft recommendations          │
   │    └──────────────────────────────────────┘
   │                    │
┌──────────────────┐    ▼
│ Draft guideline  │  ┌──────────────────────────────────┐
│ available        │  │ Draft guideline presented        │
│ on SIGN web site │  │ and discussed at national open   │
│ for limited      │  │ meeting                          │
│ period           │  └──────────────────────────────────┘
└──────────────────┘                │
   │                                ▼
   │         ┌──────────────────────────────────┐
   └────────▶│ Feedback incorporated and draft  │
             │ guideline submitted to SIGN      │
             └──────────────────────────────────┘
                            │
                            ▼
             ┌──────────────────────────────────┐
             │ In-house editing and             │
             │ methodological checks            │
             └──────────────────────────────────┘
```

Systematic literature review and draft recommendations

Draft guideline available on SIGN web site for limited period

Draft guideline presented and discussed at national open meeting

Feedback incorporated and draft guideline submitted to SIGN

In-house editing and methodological checks

Peer review reports obtained

Draft circulated for information to various health service organizations

Comments compiled and discussed with development group chairman, in consultation with group

SIGN editorial group review guideline and peer review comments

Guideline development group members sign off final draft

Dissemination and implementation

Appendix 9–12

Grades of Recommendation Assessment Development and Evaluation(GRADE) System Advantages

COMPARISON OF GRADE AND OTHER SYSTEMS

Factor	Other Systems	GRADE	Advantages of GRADE System*
Definitions	Implicit definitions of quality (level) of evidence and strength of recommendation	Explicit definitions	Makes clear what grades indicate and what should be considered in making these judgments
Judgments	Implicit judgments regarding which outcomes are important, quality of evidence for each important outcome, overall quality of evidence, balance between benefits and harms, and value of incremental benefits	Sequential, explicit judgments	Clarifies each of these judgments and reduces risks of introducing errors or bias that can arise when they are made implicitly
Key components of quality of evidence	Not considered for each important outcome. Judgments about quality of evidence are often based on study design alone	Systematic and explicit consideration of study design, study quality, consistency, and directness of evidence in judgments about quality of evidence	Ensures these factors are considered appropriately
Other factors that can affect quality of evidence	Not explicitly taken into account	Explicit consideration of imprecise or sparse data, reporting bias, strength of association, evidence of a dose-response gradient, and plausible confounding	Ensures consideration of other factors

COMPARISON OF GRADE AND OTHER SYSTEMS

Factor	Other Systems	GRADE	Advantages of GRADE System*
Overall quality of evidence	Implicitly based on the quality of evidence for benefits	Based on the lowest quality of evidence for any of the outcomes that are critical to making a decision	Reduces likelihood of mislabeling overall quality of evidence when evidence for a critical outcome is lacking
Relative importance of outcomes	Considered implicitly	Explicit judgments about which outcomes are critical, which ones are important but not critical, and which ones are unimportant and can be ignored	Ensures appropriate consideration of each outcome when grading overall quality of evidence and strength of recommendations
Balance between health benefits and harms	Not explicitly considered	Explicit consideration of trade-offs between important benefits and harms, the quality of evidence for these, translation of evidence into specific circumstances, and certainty of baseline risks	Clarifies and improves transparency of judgments on harms and benefits
Whether incremental health benefits are worth the costs	Not explicitly considered	Explicit consideration after first considering whether there are net health benefits	Ensures that judgments about value of net health benefits are transparent
Summaries of evidence and findings	Inconsistent presentation	Consistent GRADE evidence profiles, including quality assessment and summary of findings	Ensures that all panel members base their judgments on same information and that this information is available to others
Extent of use	Seldom used by more than one organization and little, if any empirical evaluation	International collaboration across wide range of organizations in development and evaluation	Builds on previous experience to achieve a system that is more sensible, reliable, and widely applicable

*Most other approaches do not include any of these advantages, although some may incorporate some of these advantages.
Source: Reproduced from: Atkins D, Best D, Briss PA, Eccles M, Falck-Ytter Y, Flottorp S, et al., for the GRADE Working Group. Grading quality of evidence and strength of recommendations. BMJ. 2004;328:1490.

9-13

Appendix 9-13

Appraisal of Guidelines Research & Evaluation (AGREE) Instrument

AGREE INSTRUMENT ITEMS FOR EVALUATION*

Domain 1	Scope and Purpose
Item 1	The overall objective(s) of the guideline is (are) specifically described
Item 2	The clinical question(s) covered by the guideline is (are) specifically described
Item 3	The patients to whom the guideline is meant to apply are specifically described

Domain 2	Stakeholder Involvement
Item 4	The guideline development group includes individuals from all relevant professional groups
Item 5	The patients' views and preferences have been sought
Item 6	The target users of the guideline are clearly defined
Item 7	The guideline has been piloted among target users

Domain 3	Rigor of Development
Item 8	Systematic methods were used to search for evidence
Item 9	The criteria for selecting the evidence are clearly described
Item 10	The methods used for formulating the recommendations are clearly described
Item 11	The health benefits, side effects, and risks have been considered in formulating the recommendations
Item 12	There is an explicit link between the recommendations and the supporting evidence
Item 13	The guideline has been externally reviewed by experts prior to its publication
Item 14	A procedure for updating the guideline is provided

Domain 4	Clarity and Presentation
Item 15	The recommendations are specific and unambiguous
Item 16	The different options for management of the condition are clearly presented
Item 17	The key recommendations are easily identifiable
Item 18	The guideline is supported with tools for application

Domain 5	Application
Item 19	The potential organizational barriers in applying the recommendations have been discussed
Item 20	The possible cost implications of applying the recommendations have been considered
Item 21	The guideline presents key review criteria for monitoring and/or audit purposes

Domain 6	Editorial Independence
Item 22	The guideline is editorially independent from the funding body
Item 23	Conflicts of interest of guideline development members have been recorded

*This is a list of the 23 items used by the AGREE instrument. A more detailed description of each item and scoring instructions for use of this instrument is provided at the AGREE collaboration website: http://www.agreecollaboration.org. Each item is scored on a four point scale: 1 = strongly disagree, 2 = disagree, 3 = agree, and 4 = strongly agree. In addition, the AGREE instrument includes an "overall assessment" regarding a recommendation to use the guideline in practice. The overall assessment uses a three point scale: 1 = not recommended, 2 = recommended with provisos or modifications, 3 = strongly recommended.

9–14

Appendix 9–14

Conference on Guideline Standardization (COGS) Checklist

THE COGS CHECKLIST FOR REPORTING CLINICAL PRACTICE GUIDELINES

Topic	Description
1. Overview material	Provide a structured abstract that includes the guideline's release date, status (original, revised, updated), and print and electronic sources.
2. Focus	Describe the primary disease/condition and intervention/service/technology that the guideline addresses. Indicate any alternative preventive, diagnostic or therapeutic interventions that were considered during development.
3. Goal	Describe the goal that following the guideline is expected to achieve, including the rationale for development of a guideline on this topic.
4. Users/setting	Describe the intended users of the guideline (e.g., provider types and patients) and the settings in which the guideline is intended to be used.
5. Target population	Describe the patient population eligible for guideline recommendations and list any exclusion criteria.
6. Developer	Identify the organization(s) responsible for guideline development and the names/credentials/potential conflicts of interest of individuals involved in the guideline's development.
7. Funding source/ sponsor	Identify the funding source/sponsor and describe its role in developing and/or reporting the guideline. Disclose potential conflict of interest.
8. Evidence collection	Describe the methods used to search the scientific literature, including the range of dates and databases searched, and criteria applied to filter the retrieved evidence.
9. Recommendation grading criteria	Describe the criteria used to rate the quality of evidence that supports the recommendations and the system for describing the strength of the recommendations. Recommendation strength communicates the importance of adherence to a recommendation and is based on both the quality of the evidence and the magnitude of anticipated benefits or harms.
10. Method for synthesizing evidence	Describe how evidence was used to create recommendations, e.g., evidence tables, meta-analysis, and decision analysis.
11. Prerelease review	Describe how the guideline developer reviewed and/or tested the guidelines prior to release
12. Update plan	State whether or not there is a plan to update the guideline and, if applicable, an expiration date for this version of the guideline.
13. Definitions	Define unfamiliar terms and those critical to correct application of the guideline that might be subject to misinterpretation.
14. Recommendations and rationale	State the recommended action precisely and the specific circumstances under which to perform it. Justify each recommendation by describing the linkage between the recommendation and its supporting evidence. Indicate the quality of evidence and the recommendation strength, based on the criteria described in 9.

15. Potential benefits and harms	Describe anticipated benefits and potential risks associated with implementation of guideline recommendations.
16. Patient preferences	Describe the role of patient preferences when a recommendation involves a substantial element of personal choice or values.
17. Algorithm	Provide (when appropriate) a graphical description of the stages and decisions in clinical care described by the guideline.
18. Implementation considerations	Describe anticipated barriers to application of the recommendations. Provide reference to any auxiliary documents for providers or patients that are intended to facilitate implementation. Suggest review criteria for measuring changes in care when the guideline is implemented.

SOURCE: Shiffman RN, Shekelle P, Overhage M, Slutsky J, Grimshaw J, Deshpande AM. Standardized reporting of clinical practice guidelines: a proposal from the conference on guideline standardization. Ann Intern Med. 2003;139:493–498.

9-15

Appendix 9–15

Implementation Strategies

CLASSIFICATION OF PROFESSIONAL INTERVENTIONS FOR GUIDELINE IMPLEMENTATION*

- *Distribution of educational materials*: Distribution of published or printed recommendations for clinical care, including clinical practice guidelines, audiovisual materials, and electronic publications. The materials may have been delivered personally or through mass mailings.
- *Educational meetings*: Healthcare providers who have participated in conferences, lectures, workshops, or traineeships.
- *Local consensus processes*: Inclusion of participating providers in discussion to ensure that they agreed that the chosen clinical problem was important and the approach to managing the problem was appropriate.
- *Educational outreach visits*: Use of a trained person who met with providers in their practice settings to give information with the intent of changing the provider's practice. The information given may have included feedback on the performance of the provider(s).
- *Local opinion leaders*: Use of providers nominated by their colleagues as "educationally influential." The investigators must have explicitly stated that their colleagues identified the opinion leaders.
- *Patient-mediated interventions*: New clinical information (not previously available) collected directly from patients and given to the provider, e.g., depression scores from an instrument.
- *Audit and feedback*: Any summary of clinical performance of healthcare over a specified period. The summary may also have included recommendations for clinical

---

*Reproduced from: Grimshaw JM, Thomas RE, MacLennan G, Fraser C, Ramsay CR, Vale L, et al. Effectiveness and efficiency of guideline dissemination and implementation strategies. Health Technol Assess. 2004;8(6):iii–iv, 1–72.

action. The information may have been obtained from medical records, computerized databases, or observations from patients.

The following interventions are excluded:

- Provision of new clinical information not directly reflecting provider performance which was collected from patients, e.g., scores on a depression instrument and abnormal test results. These interventions should be described as patient mediated.
- Feedback of individual patients' health record information in an alternative format (e.g., computerized). These interventions should be described as organizational.

- *Reminders*: Patient- or encounter-specific information, provided verbally, on paper or on a computer screen, which is designed or intended to prompt a health professional to recall information. This would usually be encountered through their general education, in the medical records or through interactions with peers, and so remind them to perform or avoid some action to aid individual patient care. Computer-aided decision support and drugs dosage are included.
- *Marketing*: Use of personal interviewing, group discussion (focus groups), or a survey of targeted providers to identify barriers to change and subsequent design of an intervention that addresses identified barriers.
- *Mass media*: (1) Varied use of communication that reached great numbers of people including television, radio, newspapers, posters, leaflets and booklets, alone or in conjunction with other interventions; (2) targeted at the population level.

11–1

Appendix 11–1

Question Example

DRUG INFORMATICS CENTER

St. Anywhere Hospital

Name of inquirer	Dr. Meghan J. Malone	Date: XX/XX/XX
Address	2184 Fall St. Seneca Falls, NY 13148	Time received: XX:XX AM/PM
		Time required: 5 hours
		Nature of request: Therapeutics
Telephone number:	(315)555-1212	Type of inquirer: MD

Question

A young, adult male patient recently arrived from Japan and presented to the physician sparse medical records indicating he is suffering from tsutsugamushi disease. Because of the language difficulties, not much is known about the patient, other than he is taking drug X for the illness. Physical examination reveals a patient in some discomfort with elevated temperature, swollen lymph glands, and red rash. All other findings appear to be normal. (*Note:* the person answering this question obtained as much background as possible about the patient.) The physician has little information on the disease and would like to know whether drug X is the most appropriate treatment.

Answer

Tsutsugamushi disease is an acute infectious disease seen in harvesters of hemp in Japan.[1] It is caused by *Rickettsia tsutsugamushi*. Common symptoms of the disease include fever, painful swelling of the lymph glands, a small black scab in the genital region, neck, or axilla, and large dark-red papules. The disease is known by a number of other names, including aka-mushi disease, flood fever, inundation fever, island disease, Japanese river fever, and scrub typhus.[2–4] (*Note:* background information presented.) The standard treatment of the disease includes either drug X or drug Y, although there are several other less effective treatments.[5-7] In the remainder of this paper, a comparison of the two major drugs will be presented. (*Note:* clear objective for paper is presented.)

A thorough search of the available literature was conducted. Unfortunately, there were few textbooks available on this disease. A search of MEDLINE® (1966 to present) and EMBASE's *Drugs and Pharmacology* (1980 to present) produced a number of articles that were obtained and are reviewed below. (*Note:* this documents the type of search and acts as a lead-in to the remainder of the body of the paper.)

Smith and Jones[8] performed a double-blind, randomized comparison of the effects of drug X and drug Y in patients with tsutsugamushi fever. Patients were required to be between 18 and 70 years old, and could not have any concurrent infection or disorder that would affect the immune response to the disease (e.g., neutropenia, AIDS). Twenty patients received 10 mg of drug X three times a day for 15 days. Eighteen patients received 250 mg of drug Y twice a day for 10 days. The two groups were comparable, except that the patients receiving drug X were an average of 5 years younger ($p < 0.05$). Drug X was shown to produce a cure, both in terms of symptoms and cultures in 85% of patients, whereas drug Y only produced a cure in 55.5% of patients. The difference was statistically significant ($p < 0.01\%$). No significant adverse effects were seen in either group. Although it appears that drug X was the better agent, it should be noted that drug Y was given in its minimally effective dose, and may have performed better in a somewhat higher or longer regimen. (*Note:* evaluative comments made about article.)

(*Note:* other articles would be described at this point.)

Based on the literature found, it appears that drug Y is generally accepted as the better agent, except in those patients with severe renal insufficiency. Because this patient does not appear to be suffering from that problem, it is recommended that he receive a 3-week course of drug Y in a dose of 500 mg three times a day. Renal function should be monitored weekly. The patient should receive an additional week of therapy, if the symptoms have not been gone for the final week of therapy. (*Note:* this patient's situation was specifically addressed, rather than just presenting a general conclusion.)

Signature: _____

      Sandy Q. Pharmacist, PharmD

References

(Present references here.)

11-2

Abstracts

Abstracts are a synopsis (usually of 250 words or less) of the most important aspect of an article. They should be clear, concise, and complete enough for readers to have a reasonable understanding of the important portions of the article.[1] Since they are the most commonly read part of an article, they must be accurate and avoid the three most common errors: differences in information presented in the abstract and in the body of the article, information given in the abstract that was not presented in the article, and conclusions presented in the abstract that are not supported by information in the abstract.[2–4]

There are basically three types of abstracts that are seen in the literature. The first two (descriptive and informational) are somewhat traditional; however, they do not convey as much information as the third, structured abstracts. Structured abstracts were originally designed to convey more information and have only been in use since the 1980s. The type of abstract to be used depends on the type of information and the requirements of the particular place the work is being submitted or used.

In addition to writing an abstract, some journals ask that indexing terms be submitted. Whenever possible, Medical Subject Headings (MeSH) from the National Library of Medicine should be used for the indexing terms. Each of the abstracts will be discussed in more detail in the following sections.

DESCRIPTIVE ABSTRACTS

A descriptive abstract, as its name implies, simply describes the information found in an article. Few specific details are given and it would mostly be used in a review article. An example of this type of abstract is as follows:

> Lists of references that should be available, depending on location of the drug information service, are presented. These lists are specific to community, hospital, long-term care facility, and academic sites. Included are general references, indexing and abstracting services, and journals. Specialty references that would be useful in specific circumstances are also presented. In addition, the equipment necessary to access the computerized resources is shown for the individual references.

INFORMATIONAL ABSTRACTS

Informational abstracts concisely summarize the factual information presented in a study. This type of abstract is more applicable to clinical studies.

Key points to include in an informational abstract include:

- Study design (e.g., double-blind, crossover)
- Purpose
- Number of patients
- Dosages
- Results
- Conclusions

An example of this type of abstract is as follows:

> A double-blind, randomized comparison of the effects of drug X and drug Y was performed in patients with tsutsugamushi fever, in order to determine whether either drug was superior in efficacy or safety. Twenty patients received 10 mg of drug X three times a day for 15 days. Eighteen patients received 250 mg of drug Y twice a day for 10 days. The two groups were comparable, except that the patients receiving drug X were an average of 5 years younger ($p < 0.05\%$). Drug X was shown to produce a cure, both in terms of symptoms and cultures in 85% of patients, whereas drug Y only produced a cure in 55.5% of patients. The difference was statistically significant ($p < 0.01\%$). No significant adverse effects were seen in either group. Drug X was shown to be significantly better than drug Y in the treatment of tsutsugamushi fever.

STRUCTURED ABSTRACTS

Due to perceived deficiencies in abstracts,[5] including lack of sufficient information,[6] a new type of abstract was presented in 1987[7] and later updated in 1990.[8] This structured abstract was designed to present more information about clinical studies and possibly laboratory studies, as compared to the informational abstract presented earlier.[9,10] This type of abstract is not meant for case reports, studies of tissues or animals, opinion articles, and position papers.[8] Abstracts following this standard seem to be gaining in popularity and have been mandated by an influential group of journals (e.g., *New England Journal of Medicine*,[11] *Annals of Internal Medicine*,[8] *JAMA: Journal of the American Medical Association*,[9] *British Medical Journal*,[12] *Canadian Medical Association Journal*,[13] *Chest*[14]), sometimes in a somewhat modified form. This type of abstract has also been suggested in the pharmacy literature.[15] Although the overall acceptance and approval of this format of abstract appears to be good, there are some who disapprove.[16–18] Also, there is at least some data suggesting that structured abstracts do not always contain as much information as they should, if the published rules are followed[19] and that they do not necessarily contain any more useful information than traditional abstracts.[20]

It is worth noting that articles with structured abstracts are indexed with a greater number of terms in MEDLINE®, which may lead to ease of finding such articles on computer search.[21]

An abstract following this procedure would contain the following subheadings and information.

- *Objective*—The main objective and key secondary objectives.
- *Design*—The basic design of the study (e.g., randomized, double-blind, crossover, placebo-controlled) and duration of any follow-up.
- *Setting*—The location and level of clinical care available at that location (e.g., tertiary care hospital, ambulatory clinic).
- *Patients or other participants*—Description of the patients, including illnesses and key sociodemographic features and how they were selected for the study (including whether it was a random, volunteer, or other type of sample); it should also include number of patients that refused to enroll in the study, proportion of the patients completing the study, and the number of patients withdrawn due to adverse effects.
- *Intervention(s)*—A brief description of any treatment(s) or intervention(s).
- *Main outcome measure(s)*—The main study outcome measurements, as planned before data collection were begun; if most of the article covers other material (e.g., data or hypotheses not planned to be observed before the study was started), that should be made clear.
- *Results*—The method(s) by which patients were assessed and the main results of the study, including any blinding. Statistical significance (particularly confidence intervals, odds ratios, numerators, and denominators) and levels of significance should be mentioned. Absolute, rather than relative, differences are presented (e.g., "adverse effects were seen in 5% of patients in group A and 10% of patients in group B," rather than "group B had twice as many adverse effects"). Provide response rate in survey articles.
- *Conclusion(s)*—The key conclusion(s) directly supported by the evidence presented in the study and their clinical application(s). Should also include whether further study is necessary.

An example of this type of abstract is as follows:

Study objective: To compare the safety and efficacy of drug X and drug Y in the treatment of tsutsugamushi fever.

Design: Randomized, double-blind trial.

Setting: Tertiary care, military hospital located on Guam.

Patients: Sequential sample of 40 young (age 20–37), otherwise healthy male patients with tsutsugamushi fever. Patients randomly divided into two equal groups. Two patients were removed from the group receiving drug Y, due to transfer to U.S. mainland hospitals. The two groups were comparable, except that the patients receiving drug X were an average of 5 years younger ($p < 0.05\%$).

Interventions: Twenty patients received 10 mg of drug X three times a day for 15 days. Eighteen patients received 250 mg of drug Y twice a day for 10 days.

Main outcome measures: Physician and patients' global assessment of disease activity; 5-point scale from 0 (no symptoms) to 5 (severe disability). Presence or absence of organism on laboratory specimens.

Results: Drug X was shown to produce a cure, both in terms of symptoms and cultures in 85% of patients, whereas drug Y only produced a cure in 55.5% of patients. The difference was statistically significant ($p < 0.01\%$). No significant adverse effects were seen in either group.

Conclusions: Drug X was shown to produce significantly higher cure rates than drug Y in the treatment of tsutsugamushi fever, with no difference in adverse effects. Additional trials at different doses and lengths of therapy should be performed.

A method to prepare a structured abstract for a review article differs from the first example.[22] This method would only be applicable in specific situations, where a number of similar studies were evaluated together. It would not be useful in a situation where a number of dissimilar articles dealing with the same topic were discussed (e.g., a review of all therapies for a particular disease). Such an abstract would consist of the following items:

- *Purpose*—The main objective of the review article, including information about the population tested, how they were tested, and the outcome.
- *Data sources*—A brief summary of data sources and the time periods covered.
- *Study selection*—The number of studies covered in the article and how they were selected for inclusion.
- *Data extraction*—A description of the guidelines for abstracting data and how those guidelines were applied.
- *Data synthesis*—The main results of the review and the method to obtain the results are outlined.
- *Conclusions*—Important conclusions, including applications, and need for further study.

An example of this type of abstract would be as follows:

Purpose: To evaluate the effect of the antihistamine, drug X, on symptoms of allergy, as determined by physicians' and patients' global symptom assessment.

Data sources: Studies published from January 1980 to December 2004 were identified by computer searches of MEDLINE® and EMBASE—*Drugs and Pharmacology* and hand searching of bibliographies of the articles identified via the computer search.

Study selection: Fifty-three studies evaluating the effects of drug X in the treatment of allergy were located.

Data extraction: Descriptive data regarding the population, dosing, effects, and adverse effects were assessed, along with the study's quality.

Results of data analysis: Subjective and objective measures of effectiveness demonstrated that drug X decreased or eliminated allergic symptoms approximately 80% of the time in a variety of patient types (e.g., seasonal allergic rhinitis, perennial allergic rhinitis, anaphylaxis). The only adverse effects seen were dryness of mucous membranes and sedation, seen in approximately 5% and 2% of patients, respectively.

Conclusions: Drug X is an effective agent for the treatment of allergic reactions. It has a low incidence of typical antihistamine adverse effects. Further studies should be performed to verify the effectiveness of drug X in comparison to other drugs commonly used for anaphylaxis.

REFERENCES

1. Staub NC. On writing abstracts. Physiologist. 1991;34:276–7.
2. Pitkin RM, Branagan MA. Can the accuracy of abstracts be improved by providing specific instructions? A randomized controlled trial. JAMA. 1998;280:267–9.
3. Pitkin RM, Branagan MA, Burmeister LF. Accuracy of data in abstracts of published research articles. JAMA. 1999;281:1110–1.
4. Winker MA. The need for concrete improvement in abstract quality. JAMA. 1999;281:1129–30.
5. Huth EJ. Structured abstracts for papers reporting clinical trials. Ann Intern Med. 1987;106:626–7.
6. Narine L, Yee DS, Einarson TR, Ilersich AL. Quality of abstracts of original research articles in CMAJ in 1989. CMAJ. 1991;144:449–53.
7. Ad Hoc Working Group for Critical Appraisal of the Medical Literature. A proposal for more informative abstracts of clinical articles. Ann Intern Med. 1987;106:598–604.
8. Haynes RB, Mulrow CD, Huth EJ, Altman DG, Gardner MJ. More informative abstracts revisited. Ann Intern Med. 1990;113:69–76.
9. Rennie D, Glass RM. Structuring abstracts to make them more informative. JAMA. 1991;266:116–7.
10. Haynes RB. Dissent. More informative abstracts: current status and evaluation. J Clin Epidemiol. 1993;46:595–7.
11. Relman AS. New "Information for Authors"—and readers. N Engl J Med. 1990;323:56.
12. Lock S. Structure abstracts. Now required for all papers reporting clinical trials. BMJ. 1988;297: 156.
13. Squires BP. Structured abstracts of original research and review articles. CMAJ. 1990;143:619–22.
14. Soffer A. Abstracts of clinical investigations. A new and standardized format. Chest. 1987;92:389–90.
15. Kane-Gill S, Olsen KM. How to write an abstract suitable for publication. Hosp Pharm. 2004;39:289–92.
16. Spitzer WO. Second thoughts. The structured sonnet. J Clin Epidemiol. 1991;44:729.
17. Heller MB. Dissent. Structured abstracts: a modest dissent. J Clin Epidemiol. 1991;44:739–40.
18. Heller MB. Structured abstracts [letter]. Ann Intern Med. 1990;113:722.

19. Froom P, Froom J. Variance and dissent. Presentation. Deficiencies in structured medical abstracts. J Clin Epidemiol. 1993;46:591–4.

20. Scherer RW, Crawley B. Reporting of randomized clinical trial descriptors and use of structured abstracts. JAMA. 1998;280:269–72.

21. Harbourt AM, Knecht LS, Humphreys BL. Structured abstracts in MEDLINE®, 1989-1991. Bull Med Libr Assoc. 1995:83(2):190–5.

22. Mulrow CD, Thacker SB, Pugh JA. A proposal for more informative abstracts of review articles. Ann Intern Med. 1988;108:613–5.

11–3

Bibliography

Although there seems to be a different method to prepare a bibliography for every English class ever given, there is fortunately a standardized method to prepare a bibliography in medical writing. This method is used by the National Library of Medicine and has been incorporated into the "Uniform Requirements for Manuscripts Submitted to Biomedical Journals"[1,2] it has been used widely since the 1970s in both journals and other medical writing. This method will be presented here.

References in the bibliography are placed in the order they are first cited in the text of a document, and each reference is assigned a consecutive Arabic number. Those cited only in tables or figures are numbered according to the place the table or figure is identified in the text. References are not listed multiple times in the bibliography, if they are cited more than once in the text of the document. Instead, subsequent citations to the same reference use the original reference number. It should also be noted that *Ibid* is not used. The reference number in the text will be the Arabic number in parenthesis or, commonly, superscript. This number is often cited after the sentence that contains the fact being referenced. If there are several references used to prepare a specific sentence, they may be listed at the end of the sentence or throughout the sentence. Also, if the sentence is a lead-in to an abstract, the authors' names are commonly listed followed by the reference number. See the sentences below for examples.

- Drug X has been shown to cause green rash with purple spots.[2,3]
- Drug Y is useful in the treatment of hypertension,[4] congestive heart failure,[5] and arrhythmias.[6]
- Smith and Jones[7] studied the effects of...
- Brown et al.[9] treated... (please notice on this example, al. is followed by a period since it is an abbreviation, whereas et is a full Latin word, and there is no need for a comma after the first author's name)
- Brown and associates[9] treated... (this is used the same way as the previous example, but is preferred by some people over the use of et al.)

Before getting into the method for listing references and examples, it should be mentioned that there are a number of general rules to be followed. They are as follows.

- Citations are often not found in conclusions of documents. The conclusions are based on the information presented, and cited, earlier in the article.
- Avoid using abstracts as references, if at all possible. Sometimes the information was only published as an abstract, so it is necessary to cite the abstract in that situation.
- Do not use unpublished observations or personal communications as references. In the latter case, it is proper to insert references to written, but not oral, communications in parentheses in the text. Permission must be obtained from the author for the use of this material and this should only be used if the material is not available from a public source of information.
- If reference is made to an article that has been accepted by a journal, but not yet published, the phrase *In press* should be inserted where the year, volume, and page numbers would normally be listed. It is necessary to get permission to cite this type of article and verification of acceptance by the journal should be obtained.

Please note the following examples should provide adequate direction in how to cite most publications. However, if detailed directions and further examples are needed, the reader is referred to the following documents that are available free on the Internet:

Patrias K. National Library of Medicine recommended formats for bibliographic citation. [monograph on the Internet]. Bethesda (MD): National Library of Medicine; 1991 [cited 2004 Aug 18]. Available from: http://www.nlm.nih.gov/pubs/formats/recommended-formats.pdf

Patrias K. National Library of Medicine recommended formats for bibliographic citation. Supplement: Internet formats [monograph on the Internet]. Bethesda (MD): National Library of Medicine; 2001 [cited 2004 Aug 18]. Available from: http://www.nlm.nih.gov/pubs/formats/internet.pdf

JOURNAL ARTICLES

To cite a journal article, the following information should be given:

- Last name of author(s) and initials (each separated by commas, with a period at the end). If there are more than six authors, the first six should be listed, followed by the phrase *et al.*
- Title of article (do not use quotation marks, capitalize only the initial word of sentences and proper nouns in English) (followed by a period).
- Title source (abbreviated as found in the list of journals in *Index Medicus*—see http://www.nlm.nih.gov/tsd/serials/lji.html).
- Year (followed by a semicolon). Month and day of month can be listed after the year, but is optional in journals that have continuous pagination throughout the volume.

- Volume number (listing the issue number in parenthesis is optional, but necessary in journals that do not have continuous page numbers for the entire volume) (followed by a colon).
- Page numbers (If continuous, use first and last pages separated by a hyphen. If separate pages, list the pages separated by a comma. If a combination of continuous and separate pages, use both (e.g., 18–29, 33, 40) (followed by a period).

Example Citations

Standard Journal Article

Smythe M, Hoffman J, Kizy K, Dmuchowski C. Estimating creatinine clearance in elderly patients with low serum creatinine concentrations. Am J Hosp Pharm. 1994;51:198–204.

Beck DE, Aceves-Blumenthal C, Carson R, Culley J, Dawson K, Hotchkiss G, et al. Factors contributing to volunteer practitioner-faculty vitality. Am J Pharm Ed. 1993;57:305–12.

Robinson ET. The pharmacist as educator: implications for practice and education. Am J Pharm Ed. 2004;68(3):Article 72.

Optional Addition of a Database's Unique Identifier

Smythe M, Hoffman J, Kizy K, Dmuchowski C. Estimating creatinine clearance in elderly patients with low serum creatinine concentrations. Am J Hosp Pharm. 1994;51:198–204. [Cited in PubMed®; PMID 7899715.]

Organization as Author

Task Force on Specialty Recognition of Oncology Pharmacy Practice. Executive summary of petition requesting specialty recognition of oncology pharmacy practice. Am J Hosp Pharm. 1994;51:219–24.

Personal Authors and Organization as Author

Wiencke K, Louka AS, Spurkland A, Vatn M, The IBSEN Study Group, Schrumpf E, et al. Association of matrix metalloproteinase-1 and -3 promoter polymorphisms with clinical subsets of Norwegian primary sclerosing cholangitis patients. J Hepatol. 2004 Aug;41(2):209–14.

No Author Given

N.Y. court rules against Medicaid co-pay. Drug Topics. 1994;138(3):6.

Article not in English

Antoni N. Zur kritjk der irrtümlich sogenannten sehnen- und periostreflexe. Acta Psychiatrica Neurologica 1932;VII:9–19.

Volume with Supplement

Nayler WG. Pharmacological aspects of calcium antagonism. Short term and long term benefits. Drugs. 1993;46(Suppl 2):40–7.

Issue with Supplement

Graves NM. Pharmacokinetics and interactions of antiepileptic drugs. Am J Hosp Pharm. 1993;50(Suppl 5):S23–9.

Volume with Part

Katchen MS, Lyons TJ, Gillingham KK, Schlegel W. A case of left hypoglossal neurapraxia following G exposure in a centrifuge. Aviat Space Environ Med. 1990;61(Pt 2):837–9.

Issue with Part

Dudley MN. Maximizing patient outcomes of antiinfective therapy. Pharmacotherapy. 1993;13(2 Pt 2): 29S–33S.

Issue with No Volume

Slaga TJ, Gimenez-Conti IB. An animal model for oral cancer. Monogr J Nat Cancer Instit. 1992;(13):55–60.

No Issue or Volume

Payne R. Acute exacerbation of chronic cancer pain: basic assessment and treatments of breakthrough pain. Acute Pain Sympt Manage. 1998:4–5.

Pagination in Roman Numerals

Koretz RL. Clinical nutrition. Gastroenterol Clin North Am. 1998 June;27(2):xi–xiii.

Expressing Type of Article (as needed)

Goldwater SH, Chatelain F. Taking time to communicate [letter]. Am J Hosp Pharm. 1994;51:232, 234.
Talley CR. Reducing demand through preventive care [editorial]. Am J Hosp Pharm. 1994;51:55.

Article Containing a Retraction

Brown MD. Retraction. Am Heart J. 1986;111:623. Retraction of Slutsky RA, Olson LK. In: Am Heart J. 1984;108:543–7.

Article Retracted

Slutsky RA, Olson LK. Intravascular and extravascular pulmonary fluid volumes during chronic experimental left ventricular dysfunction. Am Heart J. 1984;108: 543–7. Retraction in: Am Heart J. 1986;111:623.

Article Republished with Corrections

Warkentin TE, Greinacher A. Heparin-induced thrombocytopenia and cardiac surgery. Ann Thorac Surg. 2003;76:2121–31. Corrected and republished from: Ann Thorac Surg. 2003;76:638–48.

Article Containing Comment

Relman AS. An error corrected, a conclusion withdrawn, and a lesson learned [comment]. N Engl J Med. 1990;323:1482–3. Comment on: N Engl J Med. 1989;320:376–9.

Article Commented On

Pintor C, Loche S, Cella SG, Müller EE, Bauman G. A child with phenotypic Laron dwarfism and normal somatomedin levels [see comments]. N Engl J Med. 1989;320:376–9. Comment in: N Engl J Med. 1990;323:1482–3.

Article with Published Erratum

Reitz MS Jr, Juo HG, Oleske J, Hoxie J, Popovic M, Read-Connole E, et al. On the historical origins of HIV-1 (MN) and (RF) [letter]. AIDS Res Hum Retroviruses 1992;8:1539–41. Erratum in: AIDS Res Hum Retroviruses 1992;8:1731.

BOOKS

To cite a book, the following information should be given (Please note, previously published styles incorrectly had a comma instead of a semicolon after the publisher[1]):

- Last name of author(s) and initials (each separated by a comma and followed by a period)
- Title of book (followed by period)
- Edition, other than first (followed by period)
- Place of publication (city) (followed by colon) (if the location is not clear with just a city name, the state or country may be placed in parenthesis after the city name and before the colon)
- Name of publisher (followed by semicolon)
- Year of publication (followed by period)

Example Citations

Personal Author(s)

Albright RG. A basic guide to online information systems for health care professionals. Arlington (VA): Information Resource Press; 1988.

Editor(s), Compiler(s) as Author

DiPiro JT, Talbert RL, Yee GC, Matzke GR, Wells BG, Posey LM, editors. Pharmacotherapy: a pathophysiologic approach. 5th ed. New York: McGraw-Hill; 2002.

No Specific Editor(s), Compiler, or Author Identified

Drug facts and comparisons. 1999 edition. St. Louis: Facts and Comparisons; 1998.

Organization as Author and Publisher

United States Pharmacopeial Convention, Inc. USAN and the USP dictionary of drug names. Rockville: United States Pharmacopeial Convention, Inc.; 1993.

Chapters in a Book or Full Text Computer Reference

Theesen KA, Stimmel GL. Disorders of infancy and childhood. In: DiPiro JT, Talbert RL, Hayes PE, Yee GC, Matzke GR, Posey LM, editors. Pharmacotherapy: a pathophysiologic approach. 2nd ed. Norwalk (CT): Appleton & Lange; 1993. p. 953–61.

Thompson GA, Kayahara C, DRUGDEX® Editorial Staff. Cluster headache-drug therapy. In: Rumack BH, Bird PE, Gelman CR, Clouthier M, Hutchison T, editors. DRUGDEX® Information System. Englewood: MICROMEDEX®, Inc.; 1998.

Duffy JP, Tong TG. Iron. In: Rumack BH, McCrory MR, Smith RD, editors. POISINDEX® Information System. Englewood: MICROMEDEX®, Inc.; 1999.

Conference Proceedings

Allebeck P, Jansson B, editors. Ethics in medicine. Individual integrity versus demands of society. Karolinska Institute Novel Conference Series. Proceedings of the Third International Congress on Ethics in Medicine; 1989; Stockholm. New York: Raven Press; 1990.

Conference Paper

Keyserlingk E. Ethical guidelines and codes—can they be universally applicable in a multi-cultural world? In: Allebeck P, Jansson B, editors. Ethics in medicine. Individual integrity versus demands of society. Karolinska Institute Novel Conference Series. Proceedings of the Third International Congress on Ethics in Medicine; 1989; Stockholm. New York: Raven Press; 1990. p. 137–49.

Scientific or Technical Report

Issued by funding/sponsoring agency

Shekelle P, Morton S, Maglione M (Southern California Evidence-Based Practice Center/RAND, Santa Monica, CA). Ephedra and Ephedrine for Weight Loss and Athletic Performance Enhancement: Clinical Efficacy and Side Effects. Volume 1. Evidence Report and Evidence Tables. Evidence Report/Technology Assessment Number 78. Rockville (MD): Agency for Healthcare Research and Quality; 2003 Mar. Report No. AHRQ-PUB-03-E022. Contract No. AHRQ-290-97-001.

Issued by performing agency

Shekelle P, Morton S, Maglione M. Ephedra and Ephedrine for Weight Loss and Athletic Performance Enhancement: Clinical Efficacy and Side Effects. Volume 1. Evidence Report and Evidence Tables. Evidence Report/Technology Assessment Number 78. Santa Monica: Southern California Evidence-Based Practice Center/RAND, 2003 Mar. Report No. AHRQ-PUB-03-E022. Contract No. AHRQ-290-97-001. Sponsored by the Agency for Healthcare Research and Quality.

Dissertation

Wellman CO. Pain perceptions and coping strategies of school-age children and their parents: a descriptive-correlational study [dissertation]. Omaha (NE): Creighton University; 1985.

Patent

Schwartz B, inventor. New England Medical Center Hospital, Inc., assignee. Method of and solution for treating glaucoma. U.S. patent 5,212,168. 1993 May 18.

OTHER MATERIAL

Examples

Newspaper Article

Fein EB. Rise in fetal tests prompts ethical debate. The New York Times 1994 Feb 5; Sect. A:1(col. 2).

Audiovisual Material

Universal precautions: AIDS and hepatitis B prevention for home health care [videocassette]. Garden Grove (CA): Medcom; 1992.

Computer File

A.D.A.M. animated dissection of anatomy for medicine [computer program]. Version 2.2. Windows version. Marietta (GA): A.D.A.M. Software, Inc.; 1993.

Dictionary

Stedman's medical dictionary. 27th ed. New York: Lippincott Williams & Wilkins; 2000. Asthenia. p. 158.

Unpublished Material

Malone PM. Topics in informatics. Adv Pharm. In press 2004.

Electronic Material

CD-ROM

Haux R, Kulikowski C. Yearbook 04 of medical informatics - towards clinical bioinformatics [CD-ROM]. Stuttgart (Germany): Schatteuer; 2004.

Journal Article on the Internet

Nemecz G. Evening primrose. US Pharmacist [serial on the Internet] 1998 Nov [cited 1998 Dec 10];23:[about 1 p.]. Available from: http://www.uspharmacist.com/NewLook/Docs/1998/Nov1998/EveningPrimrose.htm

Robinson ET. The pharmacist as educator: implications for practice and education. Am J Pharm Ed [serial on the Internet]. 2004 [cited 2004 August 13];68(3):[about 4 p.]. Available from: http://www.ajpe.org/aj6803/aj680372/aj680372.pdf

Monograph on the Internet

Hochadel MA. Phenytoin [monograph on the Internet]. Tampa (FL): Gold Standard Multimedia Inc.; 2004 [cited 2004 Aug 16]. Available from: http://cpip.gsm.com.cuhsl.creighton.edu/default1.asp

Homepage/Website

American Society of Health-System Pharmacists [homepage on the Internet]. Bethesda (MD): American Society of Health Systems Pharmacists; c1997–2004 [updated 2004 Aug 18; cited 2004 Aug 18]. Available from: http://www.ashp.org/.

Part of a Homepage/Website

American Society of Health-System Pharmacists [homepage on the Internet]. Bethesda (MD): American Society of Health Systems Pharmacists; c1997–2004 [updated 2004 Aug 18; cited 2004 Aug 18]. Compounding Resource Center; [about 1 screen]. Available from: http://www.ashp.org/.

Database on the Internet

PubMed® [database on the Internet]. Bethesda (MD): National Library of Medicine. 2004 [cited 2004 Aug 18]. Available from: http://www.ncbi.nlm.nih.gov/entrez/query.fcgi

Part of a Database on the Internet

MeSH Browser [database on the Internet]. Bethesda (MD): National Library of Medicine. 2004 - [cited 2004 Aug 18]. phenytoin; unique ID: D015201; [about 670 p] Available from: http://www.nlm.nih.gov/mesh/MBrowser.html Files update weekly.

Package Insert

Package inserts are commonly cited in professional writing; however, the "Uniform Requirements" do not address the format to use. The following is a common format that is similar to those presented in this appendix.

Prilosec® (omeprazole) delayed-release capsules [product information]. Wayne (PA): Astra Merck, June 1998.

REFERENCES

1. International Committee of Medical Journal Editors. Uniform requirements for manuscripts submitted to biomedical journals [monograph on the Internet]. Philadelphia: International Committee of Medical Journal Editors: 2003 [cited 2004 Aug 11]. Available from: URL: http://www.icmje.org
2. International Committee of Medical Journal Editors. Uniform requirements for manuscripts submitted to biomedical journals: sample references [monograph on the Internet]. Philadelphia: International Committee of Medical Journal Editors; 2003 [cited 2004 Aug 11]. Available from: URL: http://www.nlm.nih.gov/bsd/uniform_requirements.html

13-1

Sample Case Scenarios

FURTHER DEMONSTRATION OF CASE ANALYSIS

Case Study #1

Dr. Rich, a drug information pharmacist working for a managed care organization, is asked to review and strongly encouraged to deny coverage for an expensive drug therapy (infliximab) that was used to treat rheumatoid arthritis.

ANALYSIS

Step #1

Identification of relevant background information.

A. Factual details of the case: Dr. Rich discovers the following information through literature research and expert consultation, as well as through discussion with colleagues and supervisors:
1. Infliximab is not FDA indicated for treating rheumatoid arthritis.
2. A single dose will cost the payer several hundred dollars.
3. There is limited study and experience literature that documents therapeutic benefits of the therapy in treating rheumatoid arthritis.
4. Relatively few and nonserious adverse events were associated with use of the agent in the limited literature available for all studied indications.
5. There is some theoretical basis and laboratory evidence to raise concern over the potential for loss of efficacy and/or hypersensitivity reactions with repeated doses of infliximab.
6. The case manager has identified that the claimant patient has been tried on virtually all standard therapies with poor control over the past year; there are some other experimental therapies that have not been tried.

7. The prescribing rheumatologist is a faculty member and researcher at the state medical university.

8. The medical record showed that the claimant patient had been informed and agreed to the infliximab being prescribed for this unapproved indication.

B. Identification of who is affected by the ethical dilemma: Dr. Rich is aware that the following parties may be affected by this issue.

1. Herself

2. The claimant patient and his or her significant others

3. The payer organization

4. Other groups and individuals covered by the managed care organization whose rates may be affected by increased costs related to the drug therapy

5. The prescriber

6. Other potential patients who may be prescribed this drug or who may benefit from the knowledge gained by specialists first prescribing the agent

C. Consideration for the cultural perspectives of those affected by the dilemma: Dr. Rich is cognizant of the following cultural perspectives of the involved parties:

1. The financial and cost-benefit perspectives of the organization for which she works

2. Her own scientific perspective relative to the appropriate volume and weight of evidence relative to safety and benefits of new agents

3. The legal interpretation that allows physicians to prescribe approved products for unapproved uses

4. The research perspective of specialists who conduct exploratory evaluation of new agents for alternative indications

5. The typical cultural perspective of patient reliance on the recommendations of experts in the field that manages a particular disease

6. A fairly typical cultural perspective that research costs should not be born by the research subject (this perspective may or may not also be applied to the subject's insurer)

Depending on the authority of published and other accepted expert sources, the discovered facts of this case may resolve any supervisory conflict and/or ethical concerns. If Dr. Rich still feels that she is confronted by a moral dilemma, she may go on to the following steps in the process of ethical analysis.

Step #2

Identification and justification of the relevant moral rules and principles (action-guides) pertinent to the case at hand.

Action-guides that seem pertinent to this inquiry include:

1. *Veracity*—There seems to be a clear obligation on the pharmacist's part to tender a truthful recommendation, based on her professional evaluation of the available

resources. It may be hoped that the organization has guidelines in place that support and protect this employee responsibility.

2. *Fidelity*—This principle of moral duty also appears applicable; the question the pharmacist must answer is: To whom does she most owe her fidelity? To the claimant patient? To the organization for which she works? To the entire patient population served by the organization?

3. *Nonmaleficence and beneficence*—Both of those principles will probably be pertinent in the face of limited data on this drug indication. Potential dangers and benefits for both the patient and the other involved parties must be considered.

4. *Justice*—Dr. Rich may believe that this principle obligates her to consider what is fair to the claimant patient, but also to other insured groups and individuals. She will need to resolve any conflicts in these interests.

Step #3

How should these rules and principles be ranked or balanced against each other in order to resolve the ethical dilemma?

The pharmacist must consider the interests of all those affected parties she has identified previously. She will need to decide if she has greater obligation to certain of the affected parties. It is hoped that, as Dr. Rich prioritizes and balances these applicable action-guides, she gains more clarity about the appropriate course of action. One possible way to address these relevant rules and principles is shown in Figure 13–1.

SUMMARY

It is hoped that Dr. Rich will find that this process of analysis has helped her to reach better clarity about where her primary obligations lie, and to sort out the benefits and problems

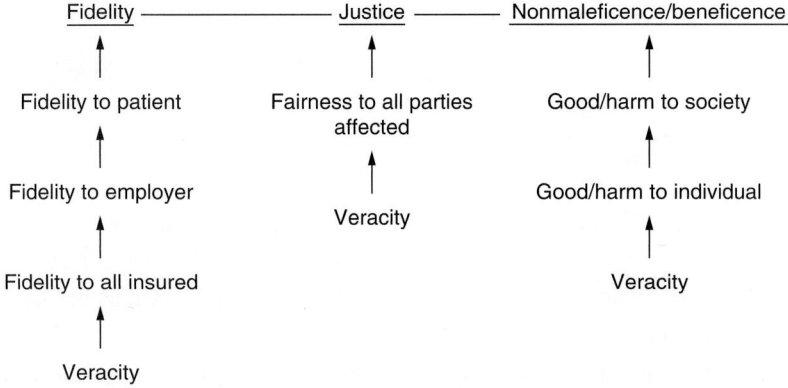

Figure 13–1

that should be considered in making the recommendation she decides is most appropriate. Her decision will be affected by a general orientation either toward a consequentialist theory of ethical obligation or toward deontological theory. Consequentialist theory judges on the basis of "good" versus "bad" outcome. Deontological theory places more importance on certain foundational principles, such as fidelity, with perhaps a greater emphasis on responsibility to the individual, or justice, which particularly emphasizes responsibilities to all involved parties and groups. In the example above, the alternative ways of balancing or prioritizing the pertinent rules and principles helps to clarify for the pharmacist that she must decide about her obligations to the individual client involved versus a larger group. The larger group could be her employer, organization, all plan participants, or even larger societal groups.

It is not likely that all will agree that this issue constitutes an ethical dilemma or on how to balance any pertinent rules and principles in this case. Ultimately, Dr. Rich will need to decide what constitutes the best resolution she can reach in this ethical dilemma.

Case Study #2

Mrs. Green, a new patient, calls the drug information center and asks Dr. Smith, the DI specialist, a question. She is concerned about whether she should take the metronidazole just prescribed for her by Dr. Mack, her family practitioner (who practices at the center where the DI center is located).

ANALYSIS

Step #1

Identification of relevant background information.

A. Factual details of the issue at hand. The pharmacist learns the following information through discussion with the patient:
   1. Mrs. Green is approximately 8 weeks pregnant; she wonders if this medication is safe for the baby.
   2. She says she is being treated for a recently acquired vaginal infection.
   3. She states that this is the first vaginal infection that she has had in several years.
   4. She mentions that she has only recently begun seeing Dr. Mack as her family just moved into town about 3 months ago.
   5. Mrs. Green indicates that Dr. Mack knows she is pregnant: he is managing her pregnancy.

6. She states that she asked him about the drug's safety, but he rather impatiently brushed off her questions by asking "don't you trust me?"

7. The pharmacist may decide that it is necessary to consult professional resources to evaluate whether the therapy appears to be appropriate. The pharmacist should not hesitate to ask the patient for some reasonable time period in which to investigate the pertinent information before providing an answer.

8. The pharmacist will need to consider whether any identified risks are likely to be known to the physician.

9. The pharmacist may decide that further facts must be obtained through direct discussion with the prescriber.

B. Identification of who is affected by the ethical issue. As the pharmacist reflects on this patient's inquiry, it is helpful to consider who might be impacted by his response:

1. Himself, relative to his own desire to do "right"; the relationship between him and his patient, the relationship between him and the physician.

2. The woman, relative to the consequences of any harm to her infant or of inadequate treatment of the infection, and relative to her future relationships with both the physician and the pharmacist.

3. The woman's infant, relative to the consequences of any teratogenic effects of the drug, or of inadequate treatment of the mother's infection.

4. The physician, relative to the consequences of prescribing a potentially inappropriate therapy during the woman's pregnancy, and relative to the effects of any drug information provided on the patient-physician relationship.

5. The woman's family, significant others, and society in general relative to the impacts of either delivery or abortion of a child with birth defects, or of inadequate treatment of the woman's infection.

C. Consideration for the cultural perspectives of those affected by the dilemma.

The pharmacist will consciously or unconsciously act within his own cultural and religious framework, and his understanding of his legal obligations. Awareness of his own perspective, as well as consideration of the cultural perspectives of others who may be affected, is important if he is to pursue a truly ethical course of action. To repeat Veatch's words differentiating ethical deliberations, "The deliberation takes into account the welfare of all involved or affected."[1] Each involved party's welfare is affected by his or her cultural perspective. Cultural, religious, and legal perspectives that the pharmacist must be aware of in this case might include:

1. Perspectives regarding parental responsibility to the unborn infant versus self

2. Perspectives and legal requirements relative to both the pharmacist's and physician's obligations to the patient and to her infant

3. Perspectives about the role and authority of the physician

Step #2

Identification and justification of the relevant moral rules and principles (action-guides) pertinent to the case at hand.

If the background facts of Mrs. Green's inquiry do not dismiss the pharmacist's ethical concerns, Dr. Smith will find it helpful to consider the various rules and principles discussed above in order to clarify the dimensions of his concern. It is most useful to first identify all potentially pertinent action-guides, and seek an understanding of how fundamentally each applies to the situation.

Ethical action-guides that seem pertinent to this inquiry include the following:

1. *Informed consent*—A moral rule supporting Mrs. Green's right to be informed and freely choose whether to take the metronidazole in relation to other available options.
2. *Respect for the patient-professional relationship*—This rule addresses Dr. Smith's obligation to support the professional relationship between Mrs. Green and Dr. Mack. It also requires Dr. Smith to respect his own professional relationship with the patient. Increasingly, pharmacists are interpreting this ethical rule to define their obligation to the patient as primary. Such an interpretation represents a departure for many pharmacists from a historical orientation of primary obligation to the physician.
3. *Veracity*—Addresses Dr. Smith's responsibility to tell the truth to Mrs. Green. This may be considered a basic principle of obligation within deontological theory, or a useful rule within consequentialist theory (to the extent that it promotes good).
4. *Nonmaleficence*—A basic principle of consequentialist theory that would found a decision to divulge information on minimizing the potential for harm.
5. *Beneficence*—This consequentialist principle would base the decision regarding what information to divulge on the potential to promote good. Beneficence and nonmaleficence can be considered together in judging the ethical response to Dr. Smith's dilemma.

   Dr. Smith must consider the potential benefits of the prescribed therapy for Mrs. Green, and address the potential harm resulting from exposure of her infant to the metronidazole. Consideration of other available alternatives for therapy is also pertinent. Frequently such consideration takes place, at least initially, in the face of inadequate and conflicting information. Dr. Smith will also need to decide what constitutes harm and good for Mrs. Green versus all others who may be affected.
6. *Fidelity/reciprocity*—A principle of obligation to an ethical covenant between Dr. Smith and Mrs. Green (within deontological theory), which may suggest a requirement for full disclosure of information. However, to the extent that this covenant asks that each party take on certain responsibilities and give up certain rights in order to achieve specific good outcomes full disclosure of potentially harmful information may not be required. For instance, if Dr. Smith were concerned that Mrs. Green may decide to

forgo any treatment and this could have strong potential of negative consequences for both Mrs. Green and her infant.

7. *Justice*—This principle is considered of intrinsic value within certain deontological theories, and addresses Mrs. Green's (and other affected parties') right to be given what is due—entitlement to information may be considered justice in this case. Certainly, Dr. Smith's time and expertise might be legitimately considered due to his patient.

8. *Autonomy*—This principle is directly applicable to Dr. Smith's dilemma, as was the related rule of informed consent, based on a belief in Mrs. Green's right to decide on issues that primarily affect her. The principle of autonomy has support within both deontological (as an intrinsic good) and consequentialist (if it is likely to promote good consequences) theories. However, competing interests (for example, Mrs. Green's and her child's), and the individual's capability to be truly autonomous (for example, the infant in this case), are factors that often complicate the application of this principle in medical ethics.

The reader may believe that other ethical rules or principles are pertinent to this case. If so, they should also be considered as the analysis proceeds.

Step #3

How should these rules and principles be ranked or balanced against each other in order to resolve the ethical dilemma?

This step may sometimes be accomplished rather easily through the use of moral intuition. At other times, careful consideration of ethical theory can suggest which are the more fundamental action-guides to be applied. In some cases, it may be necessary to balance similarly weighted principles against each other, identifying when the weight of one versus another might be considered greater.

The rules and principles that Dr. Smith considers pertinent in his dilemma over how to respond to Mrs. Green's inquiry could be ranked as shown in Figure 13–2.

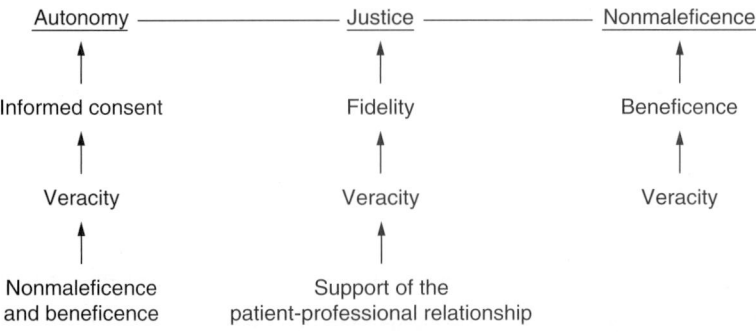

Figure 13–2

SUMMARY

In the case of Dr. Smith and Mrs. Green, autonomy, justice and nonmaleficience could be considered the primary principles that must be balanced against each other. Autonomy and justice are both valued principles within various deontological theories. Nonmaleficence and beneficence are the cornerstone principles of consequentialist theory. The principle of justice also seems to be inherent in the contract theory of medical ethics described by Veatch.[2] The other relevant rules and principles above support these primary principles and inform how they apply to specific ethical dilemmas. The Code of Ethics for Pharmacists (see Appendix 13–2) approved in 1994 provides further support for these fundamental principles and clearly indicates that Dr. Smith's primary obligation is to Mrs. Green rather than to Dr. Mack.[3,4] It may be surmised that all of the fundamental principles seem to support honestly discussing the benefits and risks of the therapy with the patient. However, if there were no good alternative therapies for Mrs. Green's infection, and Dr. Smith was concerned that probable noncompliance constituted a greater risk to her and/or her baby, the decision would become more difficult. Once Dr. Smith has considers the facts of the case, who will be affected by his action, the cultural perspectives and legal requirements for the affected parties, and the relevant action-guides he should have more clarity on what constitutes the ethical action. Finally, Dr. Smith's personal beliefs and values relative to these principles of patient autonomy, promotion of justice, and the importance of potential consequences will all affect his ultimate ethical decision. It must be emphasized that he will make some response, even if only by avoiding the patient's question.

Again, it is not likely that all will agree on this ranking or balancing of the pertinent rules and principles in this case, nor will there be universal agreement about what constitutes the right resolution to the ethical dilemma presented. It is necessary to remember that an ethical issue has been defined as one where most agree that there is a right answer, but cannot always agree on what that answer is.

Additional Case Studies

Additional sample case scenarios describing ethical dilemmas that might arise for pharmacists who are providing drug information.

CASE 1

A pharmacist is contacted by a patient inquiring about a medication his physician has recently prescribed for him called Obecalp (placebo spelled backwards).

(Excerpts discussing use of placeboes from texts by Veatch and Haddad are suggested reading prior to discussion of this case scenario.[5,6])

CASE 2

An unidentified caller asks for the name of a chemical that is understood to interfere with tests for marijuana in the blood or urine.

(A report on pharmacists providing information that might be used for questionable purposes is suggested reading prior to discussion of this case scenario.[7])

CASE 3

A local physician requests information on a potentially harmful homeopathic remedy and advice on how to deal with a family that is utilizing the product for their small children.

(A report on cultural perspectives and protection of vulnerable patients is suggested reading prior to discussion of this case scenario.[8])

CASE 4

While picking up a prescription, a patient requests detailed information about the medication, which she or he must begin immediately. Twelve other clients are waiting for service, and only 30 minutes remain before closing.

(Two reports addressing the impact of pharmacist provided direct guidance on patient satisfaction and FDA guidelines on the relative contributions of written information and oral counseling may be useful background reading for those discussing this case.[9,10])

CASE 5

A patient presents a new prescription to be filled. It is a prescription for tiagabine, a new anti-convulsant agent related to vigabatrin. Vigabatrin has never been approved for use in the United States due to reports of adverse effects on vision. Although this adverse event has never been reported with tiagabine, the agents affect gamma-amino butyric acid (GABA) in much the same way, and affects on GABA are thought to be the basis for the vision problem. The patient asks the pharmacist to address what adverse effects could occur with this agent. The pharmacist knows the patient to be an anxious individual with a history of noncompliance with his seizure medications, despite poorly controlled seizures.

(A report addressing this specific situation, as it relates to ethical dilemmas around counseling on potential adverse events is recommended reading prior to discussing this case.[11])

CASE 6

A pharmacist working for ABC Pharmaceuticals, a multinational drug manufacturer, is assigned to prepare a drug information piece for a new nonsteroidal anti-inflammatory drug to use as direct-to-consumer advertising. This piece will be utilized in several countries where the company sells products. The pharmacist is directed to include information on the potential gastrointestinal and renal toxicity of the agent in versions for countries where such information is legally required but, to omit this information for a version to be used in countries where there is no legal requirement to include this information.

(Two reports pertinent to this potential ethical dilemmas are recommended reading prior to discussing this case.[12,13])

CASE 7

A physician in the endocrinology department of the hospital asks the drug information specialist to assist with development of a report supporting the use of growth hormone in children with no growth hormone deficiency to treat short stature.

(A report by Haverkamp and Ranke is suggested reading prior to discussion of this case scenario.[14])

CASE 8

The drug information specialist is directed by the Director of Pharmacy (at the instigation of their hospital administration supervisor), to prepare a report for presentation to the pharmacy and therapeutics committee. The report is to recommend early dismissal and outpatient N-acetylcysteine treatment of patients with acetaminophen poisoning.

(A report by Dean et al. is suggested reading prior to discussion of this case scenario.[15])

CASE 9

A pharmacy clinician is asked to present an inservice for the pharmacy staff on a recently approved drug product that may have applicability for use in the facilities target population. The clinician is expected to present materials prepared by the manufacturer, which seem to be biased in favor of the product.

(Two reports on pharmaceutical promotion and the relationship between health professionals and the pharmaceutical industry are suggested reading prior to discussion of this case scenario.[16,17])

13-2

Appendix 13–2

Code of Ethics for Pharmacists

AMERICAN PHARMACEUTICAL ASSOCIATION, 1994

Pharmacists are health professionals who assist individuals in making the best use of medications. This Code, prepared and supported by pharmacists, is intended to state publicly the principles that form the fundamental basis of the roles and responsibilities of pharmacists. These principles, based on moral obligations and virtues, are established to guide pharmacists in relationships with patients, health professionals, and society.[18]

I. A pharmacist respects the covenantal relationship between the patient and pharmacist.

Considering the patient-pharmacist relationship as a covenant means that a pharmacist has moral obligations in response to the gift of trust received from society. In return for this gift, a pharmacist promises to help individuals achieve optimum benefit from their medications, to be committed to their welfare, and to maintain their trust.

II. A pharmacist promotes the good of every patient in a caring, compassionate, and confidential manner.

A pharmacist places concern for the well-being of the patient at the center of professional practice. In doing so, a pharmacist considers needs stated by the patient as well as those defined by heath science. A pharmacist is dedicated to protecting the dignity of the patient. With a caring attitude and a compassionate spirit, a pharmacist focuses on serving the patient in a private and confidential manner.

III. A pharmacist respects the autonomy and dignity of each patient.

A pharmacist promotes the right of self-determination and recognizes individual self-worth by encouraging patients to participate in decisions about their health. A pharmacist communicates with patients in terms that are understandable. In all cases, a pharmacist respects personal and cultural differences among patients.

IV. A pharmacist acts with honesty and integrity in professional relationships.

A pharmacist has a duty to tell the truth and to act with conviction of conscience. A pharmacist avoids discriminatory practices, behavior, or work conditions that

---

This code was approved by members of the American Pharmaceutical Association on October 27, 1994.[7]

impair professional judgment, and actions that compromise dedication to the best interests of patients.

V. A pharmacist maintains professional competence.

A pharmacist has a duty to maintain knowledge and abilities as new medications, devices, and technologies become available and as health information advances.

VI. A pharmacist respects the values and abilities of colleagues and other health professionals.

When appropriate, a pharmacist asks for the consultation of colleagues or other health professionals or refers the patient. A pharmacist acknowledges that colleagues and other health professionals may differ in the beliefs and values they apply to the care of the patient.

VII. A pharmacist serves individual, community, and societal needs.

The primary obligation of a pharmacist is to individual patients. However, the obligations of a pharmacist may at times extend beyond the individual to the community and society. In these situations, a pharmacist recognizes the responsibilities that accompany these obligations and acts accordingly.

VIII. A pharmacist seeks justice in the distribution of health resources.

When health resources are allocated, a pharmacist is fair and equitable, balancing the needs of patients and society.

REFERENCES

1. Veatch RM. Hospital pharmacy: what is ethical? (Primer). Am J Hosp Pharm. 1989;46:109–15.
2. Veatch RM. A theory of medical ethics. New York: Basic Books Publishers; 1981.
3. Vottero LD. Code of ethics for pharmacists. Am J Health Syst Pharm. 1995;52:2096, 2131.
4. Code of ethics adopted. Am Pharm. 1994;NS34(11):72.
5. Haddad AM, editor. Teaching and learning strategies in pharmacy ethics, 2nd ed. Binghamton (NY): Pharmaceutical Products Press; 1997.
6. Veatch RM, Haddad A. Case studies in pharmacy ethics. New York: Oxford University Press; 1999.
7. Uretsky SD, Kelly WN, Veatch RM. Pharmacist's responsibility for providing drug information to be used for questionable purposes. Am J Hosp Pharm. 1992;49:1725–30.
8. Carrese J, Brown K, Jameton A. Culture, healing, and professional obligations. Hastings Cent Rep. 1993;15–7.
9. Singhai PK, Gupchup GV, Raisch DW, Schommer JC, Holdworth MT. Impact of pharmacists' directive guidance behaviors on patient satisfaction. J Am Pharm Assoc. 2002;42(3):407–12.
10. Nightingale SL, McGinnis TJ. The role of the US Food and Drug Administration's patient information initiative in cost-effective drug therapy. Pharmacoeconomics. 1997;11(2):119–25.
11. Beran RG. Ethical dilemmas of potential adverse events. Med Law. 2001;20:385–91.
12. Herxheimer A, Lundborg CS, Westerholm B. Advertisements for medicines in leading medical journals in 18 countries: a 12-month survey of information content and standards. Int J Health Serv. 1993;23(1):161–72.

13. Lal A. Information contents of drug advertisements: an Indian experience. Ann Pharmacother. 1998;32:1234–8.
14. Haverkamp F, Ranke MB. The ethical dilemma of growth hormone treatment of short stature: a scientific theoretical approach. Horm Res. 1999;51:301–4.
15. Dean BS, Bricker JD, Krenzelok EP. Outpatient *N*-acetylcysteine treatment for acetaminophen poisoning: an ethical dilemma or a new financial mandate? Vet Hum Toxicol. 1995;38(3):222–4.
16. Monaghan MS, Galt KA. Student understanding of the relationship between the health professions and the pharmaceutical industry. Teach Learn Med. 2003;15(1):14–20.
17. Wilkes MS, Hoffman JR. An innovative approach to educating medical students about pharmaceutical promotion. Acad Med. 2001;76:1271–7.
18. Brown J. Ethical dilemmas: controversies in pain management. Adv Nurse Pract. 1997;69–72.

14–1

Pharmacy and Therapeutics Committee Procedure

Two policy and procedure operational statements are included here. The first is specifically written to centralize the formulary decision process for a multihospital health system: a formulary committee. The second, and closely related, operational statement is written as a model to function as the traditional pharmacy and therapeutics (P&T) committee for a hospital's medical staff. Both operational statements describe the functions of their related committees based on a certain degree of autonomy. Their membership is ultimately chosen by an administrative leader as a means to best isolate the committee from organizational as well as economic influences. The decision process for each operational statement is intended to create predictability and transparency. To implement this set of operational statements, each executive committee of a hospital in a multihospital system would pass the following resolution:

> The Medical Staff of Alpha Hospital agrees to delegate its Pharmacy and Therapeutic committee responsibilities to ALPHA OMEGA HEALTH based on the policy and procedures for a 'Hospital Formulary System' and a 'Hospital Pharmacy and Therapeutics Committee.

The two operational statements can also be combined to reflect the traditional functions of a single hospital, medical staff-based pharmacy and therapeutics committee. Also, there may be other arrangements where the two operational statements could provide the organizational environment for a closed health system, a pharmacy benefits manager, or one of the new organizational structures created by Federal Legislation in 2004 for the new financing of drug coverage in the United States.

POLICY TITLE: HOSPITAL FORMULARY SYSTEM

Purpose

To maintain a **HOSPITAL FORMULARY** and a Formulary Committee for all ALPHA OMEGA HEALTH Hospitals as a means to enhance the quality of health care for all patients served by ALPHA OMEGA HEALTH.

Policy

A. The Formulary Committee of ALPHA OMEGA HEALTH will periodically evaluate its performance as a means to improve its ability to support the Vision and Mission of ALPHA OMEGA HEALTH.

B. ALPHA OMEGA HEALTH will maintain one Formulary Committee and a Pharmacy and Therapeutics Committee (P&T COMMITTEE) at each ALPHA OMEGA HEALTH Hospital to implement this POLICY in accord with the applicable Medical Staff By-Laws and this POLICY.

C. The Formulary Committee of ALPHA OMEGA HEALTH will maintain a standard format for a **HOSPITAL FORMULARY** that is based on the provisions of this POLICY.

D. The Formulary Committee will develop and continually revise a list of therapeutic products, a **HOSPITAL FORMULARY,** that reflects the current clinical judgment of the Medical Staff of ALPHA OMEGA HEALTH Hospitals regarding the selection of the best therapeutic products for the health care of hospitalized patients. The Formulary Committee will evaluate the various alternative therapeutic products available and develop the **HOSPITAL FORMULARY** based on an evaluation of each therapeutic product's indications, effectiveness, risks, patient safety, and overall impact on health care costs.

E. The Formulary Committee will collaborate with the P&T Committee at each ALPHA OMEGA HEALTH Hospital to monitor compliance with the provisions of the **HOSPITAL FORMULARY**.

F. The Formulary Committee will support the quality improvement functions of ALPHA OMEGA HEALTH where necessary to improve the use of the **HOSPITAL FORMULARY**.

Procedure

A. Formulary Committee Development

1. The Formulary Committee will recommend, when appropriate, amendments to this POLICY AND PROCEDURE to the Chief Medical Officer of ALPHA OMEGA HEALTH. After revisions to any of these proposed amendments by the Chief Medical Officer, in collaboration with the Formulary Committee, the Chief Medical Officer will submit the amendments to the Executive Committee of the Medical Staff at each ALPHA OMEGA HEALTH Hospital for final approval.

2. The Officers of the Formulary Committee will prepare an Annual Membership Report to the Chief Medical Officer of ALPHA OMEGA HEALTH regarding participation of its members and any recommendations that may be important to maintain the expertise necessary for the affairs of the Formulary Committee.

3. The Officers of the Formulary Committee will prepare an Annual Report and submit it to the Professional Affairs Committee of ALPHA OMEGA HEALTH for approval. As a result of this review, the Professional Affairs Committee may make recommendations to the Formulary Committee for consideration regarding its affairs or to the Chief Medical Officer regarding amendments to this POLICY AND PROCEDURE.

B. Formulary Committee Organization

1. Regular Members

   a. Medical Staff Members

      i. There may be up to 16 Medical Staff members nominated annually by the Chief Medical Officer of ALPHA OMEGA HEALTH, each President or Chief of Staff from the Medical Staff of an ALPHA OMEGA HEALTH Hospital, or the Officers of the Formulary Committee. Any Medical Staff nominee must have demonstrated an active interest in evidence-based therapeutics, a willingness to be an active participant in the affairs of the Formulary Committee, and represent as a group, whenever possible, the specialties of: Family Practice, Internal Medicine, Pediatrics, Obstetrics and Gynecology, Hematology and Oncology, Cardiology, Infectious Disease, Pulmonology, and General Surgery.

      ii. From any nominees, 12-16 will be selected by the Chief Medical Officer of ALPHA OMEGA HEALTH on the basis of maintaining a reasonable balance among the following factors: hospital and outpatient-based physicians, primary care and disease focused physicians, physician liaison to the Medical Staff Executive Committee or P&T Committee of each ALPHA OMEGA HEALTH Hospital, and a balanced representation from the Medical Staffs of the ALPHA OMEGA HEALTH Hospitals.

   b. ADMINISTRATION MEMBER - The Chief Medical Officer of ALPHA OMEGA HEALTH, or designee who is a Medical Staff Member of an ALPHA OMEGA HEALTH Hospital, will be a Member of the Formulary Committee.

2. Special Members and Source of Selection

   a. The Chief Medical Officer of ALPHA OMEGA HEALTH will select Special Members as may be needed to provide administrative or technical support for the affairs of the Formulary Committee. The Special Members will include, at a minimum:

      i. Any pharmacist recommended by the pharmacist in charge at a Hospital Pharmacy of ALPHA OMEGA HEALTH and

      ii. At least one Registered Nurse from among the nursing staff of an ALPHA OMEGA HEALTH Hospital.

   b. The Chairperson of the Formulary Committee may select one or more Special Members from the personnel of ALPHA OMEGA HEALTH or the Medical

Staff of any ALPHA OMEGA HEALTH Hospital on a temporary basis as may be necessary for:

i. Technical support for the activities of the Formulary Committee or any Ad Hoc Subcommittee of the Formulary Committee or

ii. Information for the deliberations of the Formulary Committee regarding a proposal to add or delete an individual therapeutic product listed on the **HOSPITAL FORMULARY**.

3. Formulary Committee Officers

   a. The CHAIRPERSON will be selected by the Chief Medical Officer of ALPHA OMEGA HEALTH from among the Regular Members of the Formulary Committee. The Chairperson will:

   i. Manage the affairs of the Formulary Committee in a manner to (I) support the active, positive involvement of each Regular and Special Member; (II) acknowledge any conflict of interests; (III) initiate a replacement appointment of any Officer, Regular Member, or Special Member becoming inactive during a calendar year; (IV) appoint temporary Special Members; and (V) select the location for Meetings of the Formulary Committee;

   ii. Prepare the Annual Membership and Self-Evaluation reports; and

   iii. Appoint an Ad Hoc Subcommittee when necessary to study decisions in greater depth or to arrive at consensus recommendations for consideration by the Formulary Committee whose membership will be (1) 6 or less members from the Medical Staffs of the ALPHA OMEGA HEALTH Hospitals, (2) at least one member who is a Regular Member of the Formulary Committee, and (3) the Secretary, or designee, of the Formulary Committee.

   b. The VICE-CHAIRPERSON will be selected by the Chief Medical Officer of ALPHA OMEGA HEALTH from the Regular Members of the Formulary Committee. The Vice-Chairperson will assume the duties of the Chairperson during his or her absence.

   c. The SECRETARY will be selected by the Chief Medical Officer of ALPHA OMEGA HEALTH from among the Regular or Special Members of the Formulary Committee. The Secretary will assist the Chairperson in managing the affairs of the Formulary Committee by

   i. Preparing the minutes for each meeting of the Formulary Committee or any of its Ad Hoc Subcommittees.

   ii. Sending an agenda to the members prior to each meeting of the Formulary Subcommittee.

   iii. Maintaining a schedule for the annual regular review by the Formulary Committee of all therapeutic products listed on the **HOSPITAL FORMULARY**.

    iv. Coordinating the preparation of any Drug Monograph or any other report necessary for a meeting of the Formulary Committee by a Pharmacist In Charge, or designee, at an ALPHA OMEGA HEALTH Hospital.

4. Term of Appointment
   a. The Regular and Special Members will be appointed or reappointed each January for 1 year.
   b. Each Officer will be appointed or reappointed each January for 1 year.

5. Voting
   a. Each Regular Member will have one vote, and each Special Member will have not have a vote.
   b. Any two Regular Members present during a meeting of the Formulary Committee will constitute a quorum.
   c. The Regular Members present at a meeting of the Formulary Committee should recognize that a decision regarding a special issue may not be appropriate if certain Regular or Special Members having expertise related to the issue are not present. Based on attendance or any other pertinent reason, the Regular Members present at a meeting of the Formulary Committee should delay making any permanent decision when the appropriate expertise is not available during a meeting of the Formulary Committee.
   d. A simple majority of Regular Members voting will be required for any action of the Formulary Committee. Any abstention on the basis of a conflict of interests will be noted in the minutes for the meeting.

6. LIAISON: A Regular or Special Member may be appointed by the Chief Medical Officer of ALPHA OMEGA HEALTH to report on the affairs of the Formulary Committee during the deliberations of any other Committee of ALPHA OMEGA HEALTH.

7. MEETINGS: The meetings of the Formulary Committee will be
   a. Scheduled once a month for 1 hour or as may be planned by the Members of the Formulary Committee.
   b. Attended by Regular and Special Members only.
   c. Convened at a location arranged by the Chairperson.

8. COMMITTEE PROTOCOLS: The Formulary Committee may also arrange for the
   a. Procedures applicable to the resignation and replacement of any Regular Member, Special Member, or Officer during a calendar year.
   b. Management of any potential or actual conflict of interests affecting the participation of a Regular or Special Member during a meeting of the Formulary Committee.
   c. Use of alternative medications for the health care of a patient at any ALPHA OMEGA HEALTH Hospital.

d. Information necessary to request a change in the list of therapeutic products or other information described in the **HOSPITAL FORMULARY**.

e. Contents of a drug monograph that must be prepared before a therapeutic product not listed on the **HOSPITAL FORMULARY** is administered to a patient or before a therapeutic product is added to the **HOSPITAL FORMULARY**.

f. Management of any shortage of a therapeutic product listed in the **HOSPITAL FORMULARY** by the

   i. Timely notification of the Medical Staff at each ALPHA OMEGA HEALTH hospital, listing the specific dosage forms in limited or unavailable supply.

   ii. Development of alternative strategies for a patient's health care using therapeutic products currently available on the **HOSPITAL FORMULARY** when a therapeutic product becomes either not available or in limited supply.

   iii. Collaboration with the appropriate expertise within the Medical Staff of ALPHA OMEGA HEALTH Hospitals when a rationing protocol is necessary for a critical therapeutic product in limited supply.

   iv Review of any proposal for a rationing protocol by the Ethics Council of ALPHA OMEGA HEALTH when the Formulary Committee requests assistance before final approval to ensure that the appropriate ethical standards have been considered.

C. Hospital Formulary Format

1. Any therapeutic product used in the health care of a patient will be eligible for the **HOSPITAL FORMULARY.** This includes samples, prescription drugs as defined by the Federal Drug Administration, herbal or other alternative therapies administered topically or enterally, nutraceuticals, over-the-counter drugs, vaccines, diagnostic or contrast agents, radioactive agents, respiratory products, parenteral or enteral nutrients, blood products, intravenous solutions, and anesthetic gases. A therapeutic product may not be considered for the **HOSPITAL FORMULARY** if it would normally be considered a medical device, durable medical equipment, or implant.

2. The **HOSPITAL FORMULARY** will list the therapeutic products approved by the Formulary Committee in a format approved by the Formulary Committee. The format for the **HOSPITAL FORMULARY** will reflect the recommendations of nationally recognized organizations and include certain attributes, where appropriate, as described below.

a. Any restricted use provision will be defined by credentialing categories in use by the Medical Staffs of ALPHA OMEGA HEALTH Hospitals and be implemented when necessary to monitor or limit the use of a **HOSPITAL FORMULARY** therapeutic product known to be associated with

   i. An increased risk of a substantial adverse patient reaction

   ii. A highly specific therapeutic indication, or

   iii. An unusual impact on the over-all cost of health care.

    b. Specific patient education provisions will be added for any **HOSPITAL FOR-MULARY** therapeutic product known to require

       i. Special nutritional adjustments,

      ii. Prevention of substantial adverse effects or noncompliance, or

     iii. Unique requirements for informed consent.

    c. Continuing education provisions will be added when a Medical Staff Member or qualified hospital employee requires specialized knowledge prior to or during the administration of a given **HOSPITAL FORMULARY** therapeutic product. This is particularly applicable in the professional areas of oncology and cardiology.

    d. Special information may be added to assist the Medical Staff at each ALPHA OMEGA HEALTH HOSPITAL when necessary to improve the

       i. Level of compliance with prescribing only therapeutic products listed on the **HOSPITAL FORMULARY**

      ii. Acceptance of rational therapeutic concepts as a basis for planning health care intervention strategies

     iii. Acceptance of therapeutic interchange strategies involving therapeutic products not listed on the **HOSPITAL FORMULARY**.

  3. Each therapeutic product listed in the **HOSPITAL FORMULARY** will normally be stocked in each ALPHA OMEGA HEALTH Hospital's Pharmacy. The Formulary Committee may establish an alternative provision for inventory control of a **HOSPITAL FORMULARY** therapeutic product when the alternative provision will not interfere with the health care of an individual patient hospitalized at an ALPHA OMEGA HEALTH Hospital.

D. Hospital Formulary Maintenance

  1. A proposal for a change in a single therapeutic product listed on the **HOSPITAL FORMULARY** will require a specific set of steps before final approval by the Formulary Committee. These steps are defined below. The Formulary Committee may make a temporary exception to this provision when necessary to improve the quality of health care to patients at an ALPHA OMEGA HEALTH Hospital.

    a. Timely submission of a completed Formulary Request form to any pharmacist at an ALPHA OMEGA HEALTH Hospital by a Medical Staff member of an ALPHA OMEGA HEALTH Hospital or other professional employee of ALPHA OMEGA HEALTH.

    b. Review of the Formulary Request by a Pharmacist in charge, or designee, of an ALPHA OMEGA HEALTH Hospital's Pharmacy to be sure that it has been fully completed.

    c. Preparation of a Drug Monograph, as may be arranged by the Secretary of the Formulary Committee if a new therapeutic product has been proposed by the Formulary Request for the **HOSPITAL FORMULARY**.

    d. Preliminary review of the Formulary Request and any associated Drug Monograph by representative specialists affected by any proposed change in the **HOSPITAL FORMULARY**.

    e. Initial approval or disapproval of the Formulary Request at one meeting of the Formulary Committee, followed by review for comments at each ALPHA OMEGA HEALTH hospital's P&T Committee, before final approval or disapproval including any amendments to the Formulary Request at a subsequent meeting of the Formulary Committee.

2. The Formulary Committee will annually review all therapeutic products listed on the **HOSPITAL FORMULARY** according to a schedule of therapeutic classes as may be arranged throughout a calendar year by the Secretary of the Formulary Committee. The review of each class of therapeutic products will require a specific set of events before final approval. These steps are defined below.

    a. Review of a class of therapeutic products preliminarily by the Pharmacists in charge, or designees, of the ALPHA OMEGA HEALTH Hospital pharmacies prior to a meeting of the Formulary Committee regarding the possible need to

        i. Initiate a Formulary Request for a new addition to the **HOSPITAL FORMULARY,**

        ii. Deletion of a therapeutic product because of production defects, nonuse, lack of availability, recall, or replacement by another therapeutic product, or

        iii. A need to change information included in the **HOSPITAL FORMULARY** such as patient education, professional education, therapeutic interchange, or a restricted use provision;

    b. Preliminary review of the proposed revisions to the **HOSPITAL FORMULARY** by representative specialists affected by the proposed revisions; and

    c. Initial approval or disapproval of the therapeutic product class review at one meeting of the Formulary Committee, followed by review for comments at each ALPHA OMEGA HEALTH hospital's P&T Committee, before final approval or disapproval including amendments to the class review at a subsequent meeting of the Formulary Committee.

3. The Formulary Committee may authorize certain strategies by the ALPHA OMEGA HEALTH Hospital pharmacies that are necessary to offer the most appropriate therapeutic products for hospitalized patients. The Formulary Committee may authorize these special strategies when supported by its own decision and the support of each ALPHA OMEGA HEALTH hospital's P&T Committee. Certain specific strategies to be authorized by this POLICY AND PROCEDURE are listed below.

    a. A class review of **HOSPITAL FORMULARY** therapeutic products as described above may also be initiated when there is a Formulary Request for a therapeutic product that substantially affects the inclusion or supplementary information of other therapeutic products currently listed in the **HOSPITAL FORMULARY**.

b. The pharmacist in charge, or designee, at all ALPHA OMEGA HEALTH hospital pharmacies will arrange to prepare a preliminary or full Drug Monograph before any therapeutic product is dispensed that has not previously been ordered for a hospitalized patient at any ALPHA OMEGA HEALTH Hospital.

c. The Formulary Committee may provide for automatic therapeutic interchange between a therapeutic products that is not listed for another therapeutic product that is listed on the **HOSPITAL FORMULARY** when supported by appropriate scientific evidence and appropriately considered standards of practice.

d. The Formulary Committee may also select certain therapeutic products for the **HOSPITAL FORMULARY** that will be dispensed for certain indications or any indication even if prescribed with a "Do Not Substitute" designation. The Formulary Committee will use the same process for this designation as defined above for a new change in the **HOSPITAL FORMULARY**.

E. Hospital Formulary Compliance

1. The P&T Committee of each ALPHA OMEGA HEALTH hospital will be responsible for monitoring each Medical Staff physician's orders for a therapeutic product that is

    a. Not listed or does not have an automatic therapeutic interchange with a therapeutic product listed on the current **HOSPITAL FORMULARY**,

    b. For an indication not permitted by the **HOSPITAL FORMULARY**, or

    c. For an indication having a restricted use provision.

2. Any ALPHA OMEGA HEALTH hospital's P&T Committee may establish a Special Formulary as a means to temporarily support the efforts of it's Medical Staff in the health care of hospitalized patients having special requirements that are unique to that Hospital. The Special Formulary therapeutic products will be selected using the same process defined above for a change in the **HOSPITAL FORMULARY**. For a Special Formulary, the other Committees of the Hospital's Medical Staff will provide the advise and consent process. For any therapeutic product listed on an ALPHA OMEGA HEALTH Hospital's Special Formulary for 1 year or more, continued use of the Special Formulary status for the therapeutic product will require the approval of the Formulary Committee.

3. If a P&T Committee votes to not accept a decision of the Formulary Committee, the Chairperson, or designee, of the P&T Committee will be invited to a subsequent meeting of the Formulary Committee. At this formulary meeting, the Formulary Committee will attempt to develop a strategy for resolving the conflict

between the original decision of the Formulary Committee and the respective P&T Committee. In the event that a resolution is not achieved, the issue may be appealed by either Committee to the Professional Affairs Committee for a final decision within 3 months of the appeal.

F. Quality Improvement

1. The Formulary Committee will maintain access to the decisions of other hospital's formulary or P&T committees as a resource for the basis in managing difficult decisions regarding the **HOSPITAL FORMULARY.** The hospitals chosen should reflect regional as well as national locations.

2. The Formulary Committee will regularly assess the pending availability of new therapeutic products in the future that will likely require the preparation of a Formulary Request and drug monograph.

3. The Formulary Committee will regularly monitor the possible evolution of a shortage involving the availability of a therapeutic product listed on the **HOSPITAL FORMULARY**.

4. The Formulary Committee may recommend to each P&T Committee certain quality improvement projects, such as a Drug Use Evaluations for a certain product that would reflect the health care at all ALPHA OMEGA HEALTH Hospitals.

5. The Formulary Committee will monitor all Black Box Warnings or other Advisories issued by the Food and Drug Administration or pharmaceutical manufacturing company. The Formulary Committee will use the monitoring process as a basis to collaborate with each ALPHA OMEGA HEALTH hospital's P&T Committee as a means to promote patient safety.

6. The Formulary Committee will maintain a newsletter regarding its decisions and distribute it to each member of the Medical Staff of all ALPHA OMEGA HEALTH hospitals.

7. The Formulary Committee will collaborate with the P&T Committee at each ALPHA OMEGA HEALTH hospital to develop educational strategies for the ALPHA OMEGA HEALTH professional employees and each Hospital's Medical Staff that builds support for the principles and priorities used to maintain the **HOSPITAL FORMULARY**.

8. The Formulary Committee will offer consultation when requested or directed by the Board of Directors of ALPHA OMEGA HEALTH, its Committees, or any other ALPHA OMEGA HEALTH Committee regarding therapeutic products in the investigation, protocols, standard order sets, or quality assessment of health care.

9. The Formulary Committee will offer a means to coordinate the standardization of POLICY AND PROCEDURE's for the Pharmacy Departments of ALPHA OMEGA HEALTH hospitals.

POLICY TITLE: "HOSPITAL PHARMACY AND THERAPEUTICS COMMITTEE"

Purpose

To maintain a Pharmacy and Therapeutics Committee as a means to enhance the quality of health care for all patients served by the Alpha Medical Center

Policy

A. The Pharmacy and Therapeutics Committee of Alpha Medical Center will periodically evaluate its performance as a means to improve its ability to support the Vision and Mission of ALPHA OMEGA HEALTH.

B. The Alpha Medical Center will maintain a Pharmacy and Therapeutics Committee (P&T COMMITTEE) to implement this POLICY in accord with the applicable Medical Staff By-Laws and this POLICY.

C. The P&T Committee may maintain a SPECIAL FORMULARY at the Alpha Medical Center based on the provisions of the "Hospital Formulary System" POLICY AND PROCEDURE of ALPHA OMEGA HEALTH.

D. The P&T Committee will monitor compliance with the provisions of the **HOSPITAL FORMULARY**.

E. The P&T Committee will support the quality improvement functions of ALPHA OMEGA HEALTH where necessary to improve the use of the **HOSPITAL FORMULARY**.

F. The P&T Committee will review and approve any POLICY AND PROCEDURE of the Alpha Medical Center Pharmacy.

Procedure

A. Pharmacy and Therapeutics Committee Development

1. The P&T Committee will recommend, when appropriate, amendments to this POLICY AND PROCEDURE to the Administrator of Alpha Medical Center. After revisions to any of these proposed amendments by the Administrator, in collaboration with the P&T Committee, the Administrator will submit the amendments to the Executive Committee of the Alpha Medical Center Medical Staff for final approval.

2. The Officers of the P&T Committee will prepare an Annual Membership Report to the Administrator of the Alpha Medical Center regarding participation of its Members and any recommendations for changes in its membership that may be important to maintain the expertise necessary for the affairs of the P&T Committee.

3. The Officers of the P&T Committee will prepare an Annual Report and submit it to the Executive Committee of the Alpha Medical Center Medical Staff for approval. As a result of this review, the Executive Committee may make recommendations to the P&T Committee for consideration regarding its affairs or to the Administrator regarding amendments to this POLICY AND PROCEDURE.

B. Formulary Committee Organization

  1. Regular Members and Source of Selection

    a. Medical Staff Members

      i. There may be up to 8 Medical Staff members nominated annually by the Administrator, or designee, of Alpha Medical Center, the President of the Medical Staff of the Alpha Medical Center, or the Officers of the P&T Committee. Any Medical Staff nominee must have demonstrated an active interest in evidence-based therapeutics, a willingness to be an active participant in the affairs of the P&T Committee, and represent as a group, whenever possible, the specialties of: Family Practice, Internal Medicine, Pediatrics, Obstetrics and Gynecology, Hematology and Oncology, Cardiology, Infectious Disease, Pulmonology, and General Surgery.

      ii. From any nominees, 8 will be selected by the Administrator, or designee, of Alpha Medical Center on the basis of maintaining a reasonable balance among the following factors: hospital and outpatient-based physicians, primary care and disease focused physicians, physician continuity from year to year, and physician liaison to the Medical Staff Executive Committee of the Alpha Medical Center or the Formulary Committee of ALPHA OMEGA HEALTH.

    b. PHARMACY MEMBERS: The Administrator, or designee, of Alpha Medical Center will select two pharmacists that will include the pharmacist in charge of the Hospital's Pharmacy.

    c. NURSING SERVICE MEMBER: The Administrator, or designee, of Alpha Medical Center will select one Registered Nurse from the nursing service.

  2. Special Members and Source of Selection

    a. The Administrator, or designee, of Alpha Medical Center may select Special Members as needed to provide administrative or technical support for the affairs of the P&T Committee.

    b. The Chairperson of the Formulary Committee may select one or more Special Members from the personnel of the Alpha Medical Center or its Medical Staff on a temporary basis as may be necessary for:

      i. Technical support for the activities of the P&T Committee or any Ad Hoc Subcommittee or

      ii. Information for the deliberations of the P&T Committee regarding a proposal to add or delete an individual therapeutic product listed on the **HOSPITAL FORMULARY.**

  3. P&T Committee Officers and Source of Selection

    a. The CHAIRPERSON will be selected by the Administrator, or designee, of the Alpha Medical Center from the physician Regular Members of the P&T Committee. The Chairperson will:

   i. Manage the affairs of the P&T Committee in a manner to (1) support the active, positive involvement of each Regular and Special Member; (2) acknowledge any conflict of interests; (3) initiate a replacement appointment of any Officer, Regular Member, or Special Member becoming inactive during a calendar year; (4) appoint temporary Special Members; and (5) Select the location for Meetings of the P&T committee.

   ii. Prepare the Annual Membership and Self-Evaluation reports

   iii. Appoint an Ad Hoc Committee when necessary to study decisions in greater depth or to arrive at consensus recommendations for consideration by the P&T Committee whose membership will be (1) 6 or less members from the Medical Staff of the Alpha Medical Center, (2) at least one member who is a physician Regular Member of the P&T Committee, and (3) the Secretary, or designee, of the P&T Committee.

b. The VICE-CHAIRPERSON will be selected by the Administrator of the Alpha Medical Center from among the physician Regular Members of the P&T Committee. The Vice-Chairperson will assume the duties of the Chairperson during their absence.

c. The SECRETARY will be selected by the Administrator of the Alpha Medical Center from among the Regular or Special Members of the P&T Committee. The Secretary will assist the Chairperson in managing the affairs of the P&T Committee by

   i. Preparing the minutes for each meeting of the P&T Committee or any of its Ad Hoc Committees.

   ii. Sending an agenda to the Members prior to each meeting of the P&T Committee.

   iii. Maintaining liaison with the other committees of the Medical Staff.

   iv. Maintaining a schedule for the annual quality assurance activities of the P&T Committee.

   v. Assisting in the preparation of any Drug Monograph or any other report necessary for a meeting of the Formulary Committee of ALPHA OMEGA HEALTH.

4. Term of Appointment

   a. The Regular and Special Members will be appointed or reappointed each January for 1 year.

   b. Each officer will be appointed or reappointed each January for 1 year.

5. Voting

   a. Each Regular Member will have one vote, and each Special Member will not have a vote.

   b. Any two physician Regular Members present during a meeting of the Formulary Committee will constitute a quorum.

    c. The Regular Members present at a meeting of the P&T Committee should recognize that a decision regarding a special issue may not be appropriate if certain Regular or Special Members having expertise related to the issue are not present. Based on attendance or any other pertinent reason, the Regular Members present at a meeting of the P&T Committee should delay making any permanent decision when the appropriate expertise is not available during a meeting of the P&T Committee.

    d. A simple majority of Regular Members voting will be required for any action of the P&T Committee. Any abstention on the basis of a conflict of interests will be noted in the Minutes for the meeting.

6. Liaison - A Regular or Special Member may be appointed by the Administrator to report on the affairs of the P&T Committee during the deliberations of any other Committee of the Alpha Medical Center.

7. Meetings - The meetings of the P&T Committee will be:

    a. Scheduled once a month for 1 hour or as may be planned by the Members of the P&T Committee

    b. Attended by Regular and Special Members only

    c. Convened at a location arranged by the Chairperson.

8. Committee Protocols - The P&T Committee may also arrange for the:

    a. Use of definitions applicable to the resignation and replacement of any Regular Member, Special Member, or Officer during a calendar year as may be established by the Formulary Committee of ALPHA OMEGA HEALTH

    b. Management of any potential or actual conflict of interests affecting the participation of a Regular or Special Member during a meeting of the P&T Committee as may be determined by the Formulary Committee of ALPHA OMEGA HEALTH.

C. Hospital Formulary Development

1. The P&T Committee will review for comment at each meeting any therapeutic product recommended for addition or deletion to the **HOSPITAL FORMULARY** by the Formulary Committee of ALPHA OMEGA HEALTH.

2. The P&T Committee will review for comment at each meeting any class review of therapeutic products by the Formulary Committee of ALPHA OMEGA HEALTH and their recommendations for changes in the **HOSPITAL FORMULARY.**

D. Hospital Formulary Compliance

1. The P&T Committee will monitor each Medical Staff physician's orders for a therapeutic product that is

    a. Not listed or does not have an automatic therapeutic interchange with a therapeutic product listed on the current **HOSPITAL FORMULARY,**

    b. For an indication not permitted by the **HOSPITAL FORMULARY**

    c. For an indication having a restricted use provision.

2. The P&T Committee may establish a Special Formulary for therapeutic products not listed on the **HOSPITAL FORMULARY** as means to temporarily support the efforts of the Medical Staff for hospitalized patients having special requirements that are unique to Alpha Medical Center. The Special Formulary therapeutic products will be selected using the same process defined by the ALPHA OMEGA HEALTH Formulary Committee for the **HOSPITAL FORMULARY**. For a Special Formulary, the other Committees of the Alpha Medical Center's Medical Staff will provide the advise and consent process. For any therapeutic product listed on Special Formulary for 1 year or more, continued use of the Special Formulary status for the therapeutic product will require the approval of the Formulary Committee.

3. If the Alpha Medical Center P&T Committee votes to not accept a decision of the Formulary Committee, the Chairperson, or designee, of the P&T Committee will attend a subsequent meeting of the Formulary Committee. At this Formulary Meeting, the Formulary Committee will attempt to develop a strategy for resolving the conflict between the original decision of the Formulary Committee and the P&T Committee of the Alpha Medical Center. In the event that a resolution is not achieved, the issue may be appealed by either the Formulary Committee or the Alpha Medical Center P&T Committee to the Professional Affairs Committee for a final decision within 3 months of the appeal.

E. Quality Improvement
   1. The P&T Committee will regularly review the decisions of the ALPHA OMEGA HEALTH Formulary Committee as a means to evaluate any issues requiring the development of carefully considered implementation requirements at the Alpha Medical Center, such as the shortage of a therapeutic product.
   2. The P&T Committee will maintain an annually revised schedule for Drug Use Evaluations as may be established through consultation with other Medical Staff Committees.
   3. The P&T Committee or an Ad Hoc Subcommittee will review all Medication Error Reports.
   4. The P&T Committee will quarterly review all Adverse Medication Reaction Reports.
   5. The P&T Committee will participate in the development of standard order sets as may be requested by a member, a group of members, or a committee of the Medical Staff. Generally, the P&T Committee will not have primary responsibility of the a standard order set unless specifically requested by the Executive Committee of the Medical Staff.
   6. The P&T Committee will prepare an annual report to the Executive Committee regarding the overall level of prescribing compliance with the **HOSPITAL FORMULARY.**

7. The P&T Committee in collaboration with the Formulary Committee will monitor all Black Box Warnings or other Advisories issued by the Food and Drug Administration or pharmaceutical manufacturing company. The Formulary Committee will use the monitoring process as a basis to collaborate with each P&T Committee of ALPHA OMEGA HEALTH as a means to promote patient safety.

8. The P&T Committee will suggest information to the Formulary Committee for inclusion in the **HOSPITAL FORMULARY** newsletter.

9. The P&T Committee may make recommendations to the Medical Staff of Alpha Medical Center regarding the health care of hospitalized patients regarding the use of the **HOSPITAL FORMULARY** based on the outcome of certain studies undertaken by the P&T Committee. These studies will exclude any direct identification of patient names or medical records.

F. Pharmacy Department Policy and Procedure

1. The P&T Committee will periodically review and approve the POLICY AND PROCEDUREs of the Alpha Medical Center Pharmacy Department.

2. The review and approval will be, whenever possible, coordinated with the operational statements of the other Pharmacy Departments of ALPHA OMEGA HEALTH hospitals.

Appendix 14–2

Formulary Request Form

PHARMACY—FORMULARY COMMITTEE
Formulary Addition Request

NOTE: Both sides of this form must be completed in order for consideration by the Formulary Committee at its next regularly scheduled meeting. You may submit additional information based on the outline of this request if more space is required. If you are not a member of the committee, you must also complete a Conflict of Interest Statement and attach it to this request.

Generic Name _____ **Brand Name** _____

Indications - Describe the FDA-approved or potential off-label uses which have prompted this request.

Dosing - Describe the specific strength and administration form of this product necessary for this request.

Comparative Efficacy - Describe how this agent relates to other products in terms of effectiveness.

Contraindications and Warnings - Describe any substantial issues related to this product.

Adverse Effects - List any substantial issues related to this product.

Expected Outcomes - Describe how this product would substitute or add to the current formulary products.

Cost of Therapy - Describe how this product would change the overall cost of medical care.

Impact on Inpatient Care Processes - Describe any special requirements on a hospital for use of this product such as nursing/medical staff education, standards of care, discharge planning, certification, or standard order sets.

Impact on Outpatient Care Processes - Describe any special requirements on ambulatory care for use of this product such as compliance, follow-up, or monitoring.

Other Considerations - Describe any information not applicable to the above categories.

Requested By - Must be a Formulary Committee Member or Hospital Medical Staff Member.

Printed Name_____

Signature_____

Response - For record keeping by the Formulary Committee.

    Received by a Formulary Committee Member date_____

    Initial Formulary Committee consideration date_____

    Final Formulary Committee consideration date_____

Action Taken

Notification of Medical Staff Member submitting request date

_____

_____

Appendix 14–3

P&T Committee Meeting Attributes[1,2,3]

I. Timing
   A. Regular—The choice is often between monthly or bimonthly. Overall, a long-term commitment to one schedule that does not vary is ideal. A practical variation might include monthly meetings except August and December, in order to adjust for times when it is difficult to get quorum because of vacations and holidays. To support a regular meeting cycle, any cancellation on a sudden, unexpected basis must be avoided, virtually without exception. Finally, a 2- to 3-year experience with a given schedule would be necessary to permit members an opportunity to work a membership commitment into their own schedule.
   B. Monthly work cycle—Virtually all holidays occur in association with the first or last week of any month during the calendar year. Similarly, Mondays and Fridays frequently have distractions caused by the associated weekend demands. Thus, the second or third Tuesday-Wednesday-Thursday of the calendar month are often the best choice for a regular meeting.
   C. Daily work cycle—Given the character of the discussion above, the start of the morning or afternoon would be ideal for a meeting. The afternoon timing could be associated with a light lunch prior to starting the meeting.
II. Meeting Room Character
   A. Location—A location that minimizes the travel barriers encountered by all the members of the committee is best. In a multihospital organization, this choice may not be ideal if a perception of interhospital territoriality would create a perception of bias in the decisions of the committee. There have also been suggestions regarding the use of teleconferencing.[4] As this becomes a more widely accepted professional tool in the future, the barriers of travel time could be eliminated as a means to incorporate a higher degree of expertise within the members of the committee.
   B. Size—The room should have a rectangular table, or tables set up in a U-shaped layout if there are too many members for a single table, with chairs on all sides

and enough room for additional chairs next to the walls for guests who might be attending a meeting. The room should allow a comfortable fit for a table that is large enough for the usual attendance as well as appropriate audiovisual equipment. Overall, the room or table should not be so large that the usual attendees might feel isolated and, thus, less engaged in the agenda of any meeting. Similarly, a full turnout would crowd the room giving greater emphasis to the character of the deliberations.

C. Seating—This can be highly defined as is seen in cases with assigned seats having a name card displayed on the table for each member. The benefits of universal identity of the members would thus be enhanced, especially if they are generally unknown to each other because of the size of an institution or hospital group. More commonly, there may be no fixed seating arrangements, which better supports collaboration and open discussion. A decision by the chairperson to sit in different locations would further emphasize this approach to a seating tradition. It is also often good for pharmacy personnel to disperse themselves throughout the room to avoid a feeling of us vs. them in discussions.

REFERENCES

1. Doyle M, Straus D. How to make meetings work: the new interaction method. New York: Berkeley Publishing Group; 1993.
2. Nair KV, Coombs JH, Ascione FJ. Assessing the structure, activities, and functioning of P&T committees: a multisite case study. P&T. 2000;25(10):516–28.
3. Balu S, O'Connor P, Vogenberg FR. Contemporary issues affecting P&T committees. Part 2: beyond managed care. P&T. 2004;29:780–3.
4. Boedeker B. Virtual pharmacy & therapeutics meetings. The Harry S. Truman VA Hospital experience. Columbia (MO): Harry S. Truman Memorial Veteran's Hospital; 1999 Mar [cited 2004 Jan 27]. Available from: http://www.gasnet.org/esia/1999/march/virtual.html

14–4

Example P&T Committee Minutes

ORGANIZATION, INC.

Pharmacy and Therapeutics Committee Meeting

January 21, 2004

Scheduled at 07:00 AM

These minutes are privileged and not subject to disclosure or legal discovery proceedings under (Statute Number)

I. **Call to order.** The members or guests present or members absent are indicated below:

(legal names, usually with degrees)

The meeting was called to order by the chairperson at 7:00 AM. The physician members present represented a quorum. The minutes for the previous meeting were presented to the members. The section regarding a report of the chairperson from a discussion with the Executive Committee about illegible handwriting and unapproved abbreviations was specifically reviewed by the chairperson. The minutes did not describe the Executive Committee's request that the P&T committee quarterly forward five to eight examples of physician progress notes that reflect these two issues. The Executive Committee decided to have the president of the medical staff have individual contact with the medical staff members involved. A motion was made to approve the amended minutes and seconded. There being no further discussion, the motion was approved unanimously. After the vote, there was a brief discussion of the impending transition to a total electronic medical record with physician order entry and its ability to reduce transcribing errors. The physician members expressed concern regarding the ease of order entry. No further action was taken.

II. Pharmacy and Therapeutics Committee Organizational Affairs

A. Policy and Procedure Amendments: The chairperson submitted a draft revision of the entire policy and procedure for the P&T committee in response to new standards of the JCAHO and previously discussed requirements for the functions of the committee. The committee reviewed the proposed draft and agreed informally to reconsider it at the next meeting after the chairperson has had a chance to meet with the Chief Medical Officer regarding any other amendments that may be necessary.

B. Committee Procedures

    1. Conflict of Interest Disclosure: The chairperson gave the members the forms necessary to declare any potential or actual conflicts of interest according to the procedure established previously by the committee. The chairperson briefly reviewed this process and emphasized that conflicts of interest were only unacceptable when not acknowledged or no action is taken to resolve them during a meeting of the committee.

    2. Formulary Request format—no change

    3. Alternate Medication Use—no change

    4. Drug Monograph—no change

C. Committee membership—no action; end of year report due December 4.

D. Annual Report—Draft Report due January 5.

E. Ad hoc committees—none currently

F. Budget—reports due February, May, August, November

III. Formulary System

A. Formulary Maintenance

    1. Formulary additions/deletions

        a. IV lansoprazole (Protonix®)

        b. Fondaparinux (Arixtra®)

        c. Valdecoxib (Bextra®)

        d. Escitalopram (Lexapro®)

    2. Formulary Class Reviews

        28:04   General anesthetic agents

        72:00   Local anesthetic agents

        86:00   Smooth muscle relaxants

        24:00   Cardiovascular agents

    3. Nonformulary usage report

    4. Review of standing orders/guidelines/Caremaps TPN order sheet

IV. Drug Use and Quality Improvement

A. Medication error report—No report

B. Adverse medication reaction report — No report

C. Drug Usage Evaluation report—No report

D. Medication recall—No report

V. Hospital Pharmacy Policies—No report

VI. Current Medication Shortages—None

14–5

Appendix 14–5

Chairperson Skills

Experience

KNOWLEDGE OF FORMULARY ISSUES

This occurs ideally as a result of prior experience on the committee for several years pharmacy and therapeutics (P&T) committee meetings are often associated with an individual hospital, group of hospitals, a staff model health maintenance organization, or an insurance-related pharmacy benefit management (PBM) process. A chairperson's experience in each of these areas would be ideal.

PROFESSIONAL PRACTICE

It could be suggested that at least 10 years is required for a pharmacist, nurse, administrator, or physician to have a sense of the overall trends evolving within health care. Within a P&T committee, the chairperson would need this background to best respond to the biases that each member might bring to the deliberations. It is beneficial if the members have had mutual experience with the chairperson at a direct patient care level.

LEADERSHIP

The chairperson is likely to be the most essential person for the overall success of a P&T committee. This is most directly related to the organization truism that it is nearly impossible to hold a committee responsible for anything except when a committee is acting as the ultimate authority for an organization. Thus, the value of a P&T committee is related to its ability to serve the common interests of the entire organization affected by its actions. If the costs of the P&T committee members' time are considered, the committee's activities are the result of a very expensive effort. To best utilize this expertise, a chairperson must be skilled at mobilizing these resources in a manner that bests supports the overall efforts of the organization to which it is attached. A previously demonstrated ability to create this role for a committee is the most valuable attribute for use in choosing a committee's chairperson.

Meeting Strategies _____

PUNCTUALITY

Given the busy schedules of the members, it is necessary to start and end on time. To open a meeting, it is best to lay out the agenda including any new additions and briefly discuss any items that will require a special discussion. Within 2 to 3 minutes, the chairperson and each member should have an understanding of the scope of the meeting ahead.

FAIRNESS

Often, the health care process vacillates unpredictably between deductive and inductive reasoning processes. External observers are often baffled by this interplay. Related to this, it is suggested that a strict use of the Robert's Rules of Order for a meeting agenda may not facilitate the spontaneity for committee members that usually underlies their involvement in the character of health care. It is the responsibility of the chairperson to guide this process and seek out the opinions that the members have for a given issue. Also, if the knowledge necessary to make the best judgment for a given issue does not exist for a decision on the issue, it is important that the chairperson be able to facilitate a consensus that develops a means to rectify the deficiency.

INVOLVEMENT

Some members may not normally wish to participate spontaneously during a meeting. It is up to the chairperson to ask these members a specific question that would allow them a meaningful opportunity to participate in a given discussion. Occasionally, the chairperson might ask each member present about their opinion for a final decision being faced by the committee. This strategy should begin at one place around the table, moving to each member present clockwise around the meeting room.

Appendix 14–6

Conflict of Interest Declaration

Formulary Addition Request Conflict of Interest Statement

Generic Name_____ Trade Name_____

Substantial Involvement with a Competing Organization - ☐ Yes ☐ No
Please describe if:

1) A member of a health insurance company or another health system pharmacy and therapeutics committee.
2) Another health system medical staff officer.
3) A member of a group practice primarily affiliated with another health system.

Substantial Involvement with a Company which Manufactures the Product or Competes with the Product's Company - ☐ Yes ☐ No
Please describe if:

1) Receiving financial income or support in the last 12 months of more than $100 for research, attendance at a company-supported seminar, travel to an out-of-town meeting, or participation in a company-sponsored speaker's bureau.
2) Receiving pharmaceutical products from the company in the last 12 months for personal or family use, gifts for family or personal use, or samples for use other than as a courtesy for patients.
3) Maintaining in the last 12 months a substantial ownership of stock (>10% of outstanding shares) in the company having >30% of its revenue from sales to this organization, its affiliated organizations, or another local health system.

Substantial Inside Information - ☐ Yes ☐ No
Please describe if there are other outside relationships for which involvement in this request may be actually or potentially perceived as affecting the decision of the committee such as:

1) Having a substantial position of authority in another organization which might affect a member of the committee for employment or medical staff privileges.
2) Disclosing information about this request to another organization directly or indirectly which might give this organization, the other organization, or the requester an unfair advantage.
3) Receiving substantial assistance from the company or its representative which manufactures the requested product in the preparation of this Formulary Addition Request.

NOTE: This must be submitted along with the actual request form if the person submitting the request is not a member of the Formulary Committee. A copy of the Formulary Committee's Policy on Conflict of Interest Management is attached.

14–7

Appendix 14–7

Pharmaceutical Assistance Programs

Amy E. Archer

Core Characteristics of Pharmaceutical Assistance Programs

The inability to pay for prescription medications is a prevailing problem in the United States. The National Center for Health Statistics estimates that 43.6 million Americans did not have health insurance coverage in 2003.[1] Inability to afford insurance premiums is one of the most common reasons for the lack of coverage. Other factors include age, employers no longer offering health insurance benefits to employees, and unemployment. An aging population and an increase in the numbers of patients with major disease states have contributed to the growing number of prescriptions being filled in the United States. Seventy-five of the top 200 prescription drugs filled in 2002 do not yet have a generic on the market.[2] These products can be particularly expensive to buy without a prescription drug coverage benefit. The high price of obtaining brand name drugs places a financial burden on uninsured patients and, in many cases, patients are unable to afford to take their medications. The inability to pay for prescription medications leads to patient noncompliance and inappropriate drug use, both of which contribute to rising health care costs. The prevalence of this problem within the U.S. health care system highlights the need for programs through which uninsured patients may receive necessary medications. Various drug manufacturers have established medication assistance programs that aid impoverished and indigent patients in obtaining prescription medications. There are currently over 260 manufacturer-sponsored medication assistance programs that provide aid in obtaining more than 1300 brand name prescription drug products.[3] The objective of this appendix is to provide an overview of pharmaceutical assistance programs, as well as to provide examples of how to identify sponsor companies and enrollment procedures.

Free Internet-Based Information Sources

Several websites provide basic information to patients and health care professionals on the availability of medication assistance programs. The NeedyMeds website (<<www.needymeds. com>>)[3] is one of the most comprehensive sources of information about medication assistance programs, and is available to both patients and health care providers. The website includes the following information:

- Medication lists of drug products that may be available through assistance programs
- A list of medication assistance programs and their related manufacturers
- A list of manufacturers' information including address, telephone and fax numbers, and medication assistance programs offered (the website notes that there may not be an assistance program for every medication and manufacturer listed)
- Application forms in a downloadable and printable format for some assistance programs
- A list of pharmaceutical discount card programs and some of the requirements to enroll
- Links to Medicaid sites
- Links to information on state programs for aid
- Links to drug information sources
- Basic information regarding requirements for enrollment in medication assistance programs
- Federal Poverty Guidelines (updated annually)
- A NeedyMeds manual for health care providers and patient advocates supplying most of the information that can be found on the website (this manual ranges in price from $60 in a pdf format to $100 for a printed version in a binder)
- A packet of patient assistance program application forms for duplication (this packet is available for a $50 charge and is meant for health care providers and patient advocates as an accompaniment to the NeedyMeds manual)

NeedyMeds does not actively participate in any enrollment processes for patients. It is solely a site for information on how patients and patient advocates can pursue help with obtaining medications. The organization provides its information to patients for free; the only fees charged by NeedyMeds are for the manual and printed applications. These costs are charged only to social workers and health care professionals who do not have ready access to the Internet and therefore want to obtain materials to have on hand in print or electronic format.

The Rx Assist website (<<www.rxassist.org>>)[4] provides free information to patients and prescribers on available medication assistance programs, both private and public. This website includes a search engine to find information on available programs, an information packet for patients to download that describes where to look for assistance, as well as software for health care providers. The Rx Assist Plus software is a patient tracking database, as well as a tool to help fill out applications for assistance programs and manage the application process. It is available for a base price of $800. A discounted price of $200 is available to tax-exempt government agencies and nonprofit organizations, as well as practicing clinicians who serve underinsured patients.

Another source of free information on available patient assistance programs is the Pharmaceutical Research and Manufacturers of America (PhRMA) website (<<www.helpingpatients.org>>).[5] PhRMA provides a search engine built into the website to help patients, health care professionals, or caregivers to find potential assistance programs. There are also links to publications, current issues related to medications, an application wizard to help fill out and print applications, information on new medicines in development, and a directory of PhRMA-sponsored manufacturers who provide medication assistance programs.

Fee-Based Internet Information Sources

Two fee-based organizations that provide information services to patients are the Medicine Program (<<www.themedicineprogram.com>>)[6] and the Free Medicine Foundation (<<www.freemedicinefoundation.com>>).[7] These sites conduct research into available medication assistance programs based on information that patients supply by completing an application. Each application requires the applicant's name, address, telephone number, the name of each prescription medication being taken, and the name and address of each doctor who has written a prescription for the medications on the list. Patients complete the application and mail it to the address provided on the website. Patients are then mailed a customized packet and letter for the doctor asking for help in completing a specific patient assistance program application. The doctor is responsible for specifying prescriptions and drug dosages, as well as mailing the completed forms to the appropriate program sponsor. Program sponsors usually mail a 3-month supply of medication to the doctor, who is then responsible for distributing it to the patient. It is unclear from the websites whether the assistance programs are constructed to process refills beyond the initial supply of medicine. The processing fee for each site is $5 per prescription drug requested, which is refunded to the patient in the event that a patient's request for a medication is denied.

Information through Direct Manufacturer Contact

Another way to determine whether pharmaceutical companies will offer assistance in obtaining medications is to directly contact them. Publications such as *Drug Facts and Comparisons* and the *Physicians' Desk Reference* often contain contact information for pharmaceutical manufacturers. The Internet can also be a tool to look up contact information for drug manufacturers. Many manufacturers provide links on their websites to information about the patient assistance programs that they offer. Pfizer is one example of a drug manufacturer that provides free information to patients and patient advocates about programs that improve patient access to medications (<<www.pfizer.com>>).[8] The company website provides links to all Pfizer-sponsored assistance programs, as well as details about enrollment requirements and individual phone numbers that can be used to call for an application.

Pharmaceutical Assistance Program Enrollment Requirements

The majority of the medication assistance programs available to patients have very similar requirements for enrollment. Patients must meet the following criteria in order to be considered for most of the medication assistance programs that are sponsored by drug manufacturers:

- The applicant has no insurance coverage for outpatient prescription drugs.
- The applicant does not qualify for a government program which provides for prescription medications (such as Medicaid).
- The applicant's income is at such a low level that financial hardship occurs when the patient is required to purchase prescription medications at retail prices.

Most drug assistance programs require proof of income from the applicant and may or may not include a request for a copy of tax forms from the Internal Revenue Service (IRS). Individual programs have varying set limits that the applicant's income must fall within. Many are based on the Federal Poverty Guidelines, which change every year (see <<www.needymeds.com>> for a yearly update on Federal Poverty Guidelines).[3] The process for obtaining applications for available programs varies for each company and individual program. Some companies will mail applications directly to patients, while other companies will only send or fax applications directly to a health care provider. Many programs require the prescriber to complete certain sections of the application. Programs may or may not require an actual paper prescription for the medications requested. When hardcopy prescriptions are required, the quantity written on the prescription must match the total quantity of medication that is provided by the company as aid (i.e., if a company provides a 3-month supply of medicine, the prescription must also be written for a 3-month supply).

Patient Assistance Program Characteristics

Individual medication assistance programs vary in how they provide medications to their patient applicants. Several programs will only send medication directly to health care providers, who are then responsible for dispensing the drugs to their patients. A few programs either directly send medication to the applicants or send a voucher that can be used to obtain the medication from a retail pharmacy with no co-pay. Manufacturers will provide anywhere from a 30-day to a 4-month supply depending on the company and the medication. Refills are also handled by different methods depending on the program and drug manufacturer. Some assistance programs will refill medications simply on patient or health care provider request. Other programs require a completely new application in order to obtain a refill of medication. Most programs do not place a limit on the number of prescriptions or amount of a given medication that may be supplied, provided that the applicant continues to meet the program enrollment requirements. It is important to note that once enrollment approval is granted it does not extend indefinitely. Many programs require reapplication every several months or annually, even if there have been no changes in patient financial status.

Drug Discount Card Programs

A few companies offer opportunities to obtain medications at a discounted price through prescription card programs. Examples of popular drug discount cards are as follows:

- Lilly Answers Card (<<www.lillyanswers.com>>)[9]
- Members Rx Discount Card (<<www.membersadvantage.net>>)[10]
- The Orange Card (<<us.gsk.com/card>>)[11]
- Together Rx Card (<<www.together-rx.com>>)[12]

Requirements for enrollment vary depending on the program. The majority of discount programs require some kind of upper limit on income level, as well as requiring that the applicant not have any prescription drug coverage. The discounts provided through the card may either be a low flat fee of $12 to $15 per 30-day supply of medicine or a discount ranging from 20 to 40% depending on the medication and the company providing aid.

As of June 2004, many Medicare recipients gained access to Medicare-approved drug discount cards under the Medicare Prescription Drug Improvement and Modernization Act of 2003. The discount cards are available voluntarily to all recipients of Medicare Part A or Part B who do not receive prescription drugs through Medicaid. Savings on brand name drugs range from 16% to over 30% off of usual retail prices; savings for generic drugs range between 30% and 60% or more.[13] Discount cards are available through private companies and many limit coverage to particular geographic areas. Card fees range from zero to a maximum of $30 per year. Enrollment forms are obtained by contacting the company providing the discount card. Applicants are only eligible for one card at a time and must stay with their selected card through the remainder of the calendar year unless the sponsor company ends coverage or the enrollee moves to a new geographic area. The Medicare website (<<www.medicare.gov>>)[14] provides drug price comparisons between each available card per geographic region, as well as answers to frequently asked questions and an information booklet on the application process.

Pharmaceutical Assistance Program Limitations

One main limitation on the use of manufacturer-sponsored medication assistance programs is the time involved in applying for coverage and then obtaining the medications. Most program applications require a significant amount of input from both the patient and the health care provider. Patient input usually requires obtaining and preparing documentation that includes proof of income and proof that no other insurance benefit exists. Provider input may require a letter of medical necessity, as well as handwritten prescriptions and providing information about the applicant. There is an additional time factor regarding the processing of each application by the drug manufacturer. The time lag due to application processing may be a significant factor in obtaining needed medication due to the sheer numbers of both applications and individual drugs being used. The time involved in the application process limits the ability to obtain medicines needed for acute problems. The manufacturers may supply brand name medications to treat conditions such as infections but the medications may not be supplied in a timely manner to effectively treat an acute illness or injury. Medication assistance programs may therefore only be truly useful for obtaining maintenance medications, rather than medicines being used on a short-term or acute basis.

Another limitation on the use of medication assistance programs is the type of medications that are being covered. The majority of programs sponsored by pharmaceutical companies only cover their brand name drug products. Manufacturers may offer some type of aid for obtaining trade name drug products that have very recently lost their patent exclusivity. There do not appear to be many programs available to help patients obtain prescription medications that are readily available in generic forms, however. Generic prescription drugs are usually less expensive than their brand name counterparts, but there are still many patients who may not be able to afford to acquire them from a retail pharmacy. Roughly 125 of the top 200 prescription drugs filled in 2002 are available generically.[2] Therefore, the drug assistance programs may only be available for a small percentage of drugs being prescribed.

A further limitation on the use of medication assistance programs involves the education and skills of the people who are applying for this kind of aid. Applicants may not understand all of the requirements for enrollment and may need additional help to complete applications for aid. Ideally, applicants would have some kind of patient advocate helping them to complete necessary paperwork, but this may not be the case. Any deficiencies that applicants may have in understanding the instructions and terminology on the applications could place limitations on receiving aid from pharmaceutical companies.

One of the most important limitations on the use of medication assistance programs is health care provider refusal to participate in the process. Prescribers are increasingly busy in their practices and many either refuse to complete application forms due to time constraints or charge their patients extra for the service. Prescriber input is a necessity for a majority of pharmaceutical assistance programs. Patients who cannot convince their health care providers to participate in the application process may not be able to receive assistance in obtaining their medications.

Conclusion

Medication assistance programs can be a valuable, although temporary, resource for patients who have insufficient resources to obtain prescription drugs. Patient assistance programs can be identified either by directly contacting the manufacturer of a drug product or by utilizing Internet sites that provide comprehensive information about available programs. Enrollment into many types of pharmaceutical assistance programs often requires patient income information and provision of information by health care providers. Patients may independently complete the enrollment process for some programs, while other programs require a health care provider or patient advocate to initiate and complete program applications. Medication assistance programs vary in the types of aid they provide, ranging anywhere from discounted co-pays to free medications. They are often the most useful when a health care professional is directly involved in the process.

While many assistance programs exist, it is important to recognize their limitations. Factors such as income restrictions and health care provider involvement are possible barriers in the provision of aid to impoverished individuals and families. The time and effort involved in the application process can also provide an additional barrier to aid. The time factor involved may make the provision of maintenance or chronic medications easier to accomplish, while the provision of medicines for acute illness and injury is often not feasible. The entire process of acquiring aid from pharmaceutical companies appears to be the most useful when the patient has the assistance of an organized and dedicated staff of individuals who have understanding and experience with this type of endeavor. The type of aid supplied by pharmaceutical companies may be the most beneficial for clinics and hospital settings that are already familiar with helping indigent individuals and providing indigent programs. Voluntary organizations that seek to help impoverished and indigent patients with acute medical needs may not have the time, experience, or resources to effectively use manufacturer assistance programs to provide medications to those that they serve.

REFERENCES

1. National Center for Health Statistics/Centers for Disease Control and Prevention [homepage on the Internet]. Hyattsville (MD): U.S. Department of Health and Human Services; c2004 [updated 2004 June 30; cited 2004 Aug 29]. Available from: http://www.cdc.gov/nchs/pressroom/04news/insur2003.htm

2. Rx List [homepage on the Internet]. San Francisco (CA): Rx List LLC; c2004 [updated 2004; cited 2004 Aug 29]. Available from: http://www.rxlist.com/top200.htm

3. NeedyMeds [homepage on the Internet]. Philadelphia (PA): NeedyMeds, Inc. and Pediatrics for Parents, Inc.; c2004 [updated 2004; cited 2004 Aug 29]. Available from: http://www.needymeds.com

4. Rx Assist [homepage on the Internet]. Volunteers in Healthcare; c1999-04 [updated 2004; cited 2004 Aug 29]. Available from: http://www.rxassist.org

5. HelpingPatients [homepage on the Internet]. Pharmaceutical Manufacturers of America; c2004 [updated 2004; cited 2004 Aug 29]. Available from: http://www.helpingpatients.org

6. The Medicine Program [homepage on the Internet]. The Medicine Program; c2004 [updated 2004; cited 2004 Aug 29]. Available from: http://www.themedicineprogram.com

7. Free Medicine Foundation [home page on the Internet]. Doniphan: Free Medicine Foundation; c2003–04 [updated 2004; cited 2004 Aug 29]. Available from: http://www.freemedicinefoundation.com

8. Pfizer [homepage on the Internet]. New York: Pfizer Inc; c2002–04 [updated 2004; cited 2004 Aug 29]. Available from: http://www.pfizer.com

9. Lilly Answers [homepage on the Internet]. Indianapolis (IN): Eli Lilly and Company; c1994-04 [updated 2004; cited 2004 Aug 29]. Available from: http://www.lillyanswers.com/en/index.html

10. Members Advantage [homepage on the Internet]. Cincinnati (OH): Select Benefits Global Marketing Corp.; c2004 [updated 2004; cited 2004 Aug 29]. Available from: http://www.membersadvantage.net

11. Orange Card [homepage on the Internet]. GlaxoSmithKline (GSK) US; c2001-03 [updated 2003 Dec 3; cited 2004 Aug 29]. Available from: http://us.gsk.com/card

12. Together Rx [homepage on the Internet]. Together Rx, LLC; c2003 [updated 2003; cited 2004 Aug 29]. Available from: http://www.together-rx.com

13. Medicare Reform [homepage on the Internet]. Centers for Medicare and Medicaid Services/ Department of Health and Human Services; c2004 [updated 2004; cited 2004 Aug 29]. Available from: http://www.medicare.gov/MedicareReform/maddc_Facts_3steps.asp

14. Medicare [homepage on the Internet]. Centers for Medicare and Medicaid Services/Department of Health and Human Services; c2004 [updated 2004; cited 2004 Aug 29]. Available from: http://www. medicare.gov

15-1

Appendix 15–1

Format for Drug Monograph

INSTITUTION NAME HEADING

Generic Name: Can include other common, nonofficial names, e.g., TPA for alteplase.

Trade or Brand Name: If more than one, indicate company that each is from.

Manufacturer (or source of supply): Include website address.

Therapeutic Category: For example, thrombolytic agent for alteplase.

Classification: Note—other classifications, such as the VA class, can also be used.
- AHFS Number and Classification: If not in the book yet, see the list in the front of American Hospital Formulary Service—Drug Information book and figure out the most appropriate classification.
- FDA Classification see Tables 15–1 through 15–4: Include specific FDA website URL concerning approval.
- Status: Prescription, nonprescription, and/or controlled substance schedule (if applicable).

Similar Agents: A list of common treatments used for the same indication(s).

Summary: Includes a short summary of advantages and disadvantages of the drug, particularly in relation to other drugs or treatments used for each major indication, and any other significant information.

Recommendations: Indicate whether or not the drug should be added to the Drug Formulary of an institution, assuming they would have patients that would be treated for illnesses where this drug might be used. Also indicate specific formulary status for the drug (i.e., uncontrolled, monitored, restricted, and conditional—see ASHP guidelines) and whether the drug will replace any other product that might already be on the formulary. In addition, present any information on how the drug is to be placed in any clinical guidelines. For third-party payer monographs, information will need to be included regarding the payment tier.

Page one consists of the above information

Pharmacologic Data
- Mechanism of action (usually brief)
- Bacterial spectrum (if applicable)

Therapeutic Indications
- Food and Drug Administration (FDA)-approved indications (see package insert)—clearly indicate which indications are FDA approved.
- Potential unlabeled uses (list only if they are considered to be acceptable medical practice, although it is allowable to mention others that are early in investigation with a statement that the drug should not be used for them or that they require more study)—clearly indicate they are not FDA approved.
- How the drug, and similar drugs, fit into clinical guidelines.
- Clinical comparison (abstract at least two studies; see Appendix 11–1 for more abstract guidelines. Include human efficacy studies and, where available, studies comparing the product to standard therapy. *Note:* if there are other supportive studies for an indication, they can be covered briefly, if desired, along with the major study covered in detail. Be sure to note any deficiencies in the studies). Also, pharmacogenomic information may need to be included here and elsewhere.

Bioavailability/Pharmacokinetics: A table summarizing the following, in comparison to the comparator agent(s) can be very useful.
- Absorption
- Distribution
- Metabolism
- Excretion

Dosage Forms
- Forms and strengths: Compare to other agents (consider a table), since new products often have a limited number of dosage forms/routes as compared to established products. Purity and composition information should be included for herbal and alternative medications.
- Explain any special information needed for preparation and storage, in comparison to other products. Sometimes a product will be so difficult to prepare or have such a limited shelf-life after preparation that it is not worth stocking.

Dosage Range
- Adults
- Children
- Elderly
- Renal or hepatic failure

- Special administration requirements
- Any anticipated problems in supplies (i.e., shortages) or restrictions in distribution (e.g., physician needs to be certified to prescribe)

Known Adverse Effects/Toxicities
- Frequency and type (a table comparing the drug to others can be a clear and concise way of expressing this information)
- Prevention of toxicity
- Risk and benefit data

Special Precautions: Usually includes pregnancy and lactation

Contraindications

Drug Interactions: A simple one- or two-sentence statement for each—usually separate various interactions into separate short paragraphs and compare to other drugs.
- Drug-drug
- Drug-food
- Drug-laboratory

Patient Safety Information
- Includes medication error information

Patient Monitoring Guidelines
- Includes effectiveness, adverse effects, compliance, and other appropriate items

Patient Information
- Name and description of the medication
- Dosage form
- Route of administration
- Duration of therapy
- Special directions and precautions
- Side effects
- Techniques for self-monitoring
- Proper storage
- Refill information
- What to do if a dose is missed

Cost Comparison: Use Average Wholesale Price (AWP) and institutional prices, and make sure there is a comparison with any similar products at equivalent doses—a pharmacoeconomic analysis (see Chap. 8) is the best method of comparing drugs in this section; remember to include any required concomitant therapy. Providing a spreadsheet file with information to consider different circumstances may be helpful.

Date Presented to Pharmacy and Therapeutics Committee, and Name and Title of the Person Preparing the Document

References

- Follow guidelines as described in Appendix 11–3.

15-2

Example Drug Monograph

Note: This example is based on fictional products and is condensed. It shows examples of most sections in a real drug monograph, but often does not go into all of the details (e.g., a table of adverse effects is seen, but only a couple items are listed, whereas, a full drug monograph would list at least all common and/or serious reactions).

St. Anywhere Medical Center
Pharmacy & Therapeutics Committee
Drug Evaluation Monograph

Generic Name: artiblood
Brand Name: MegaBlood
Manufacturer: MegaPharmics
Classification: AHFS 16:00 Blood Derivatives
FDA Classification:1A
Status: Prescription Only

Summary

Artiblood is a new perfluorocarbon that has many similarities to the only other product in its class, fakered. Both products have the ability to temporarily replace the oxygen-carrying function of red blood cells in patients in whom use of whole blood or packed red blood cells is impossible due to medical or religious reasons. In general, artiblood was found to be more efficacious than fakered; however, it also has been shown to produce a greater number of adverse effects. The adverse effects are mostly gastrointestinal in nature; however, the increased INR can be a problem in some patients. Artiblood is not metabolized in the body, whereas fakered is approximately 50% metabolized to inactive components. These differences are generally not clinically significant, since the dose of either product is unlikely to need adjustment. Fakered is available in several different volume bags, allowing the dose to be matched more closely to the anticipated patient need. While the cost of fakered appears to be lower, a pharmacoeconomic analysis shows that artiblood would produce the greatest cost savings for the institution.

Recommendations

It is recommended that artiblood be added to the Drug Formulary for use restricted to those who cannot use natural blood replacement products because of religious reasons or because suitable blood types are not available.

Pharmacologic Data

Artiblood is a type of perfluorocarbon similar to fakered. These products have the unique ability to freely bind with or give up oxygen, depending on the partial pressures of the gas where the product is located (i.e., in the lungs there is an abundance of oxygen, so the product adsorbs oxygen; in the tissues there is a relative deficiency of oxygen, so the product gives up the gas).[1,2] The products do not have direct immunologic properties, nor do they have the ability to aid in blood clotting, although there may be some affect on blood clotting (either interference by coating platelets or precipitation of the clotting pathway mechanism).[3]

In addition to oxygen-carrying capabilities, the products have some plasma volume expansion properties. Artiblood has a similar effect to Dextran 40,[1] whereas fakered's properties are relatively insignificant.[4] Maximum plasma volume expansion occurs within several minutes of administration and lasts for approximately one day in normal patients. This results in increased central venous pressure, cardiac output, stroke volume, blood pressure, urinary output, capillary perfusion, and pulse pressure. Microcirculation is improved.

Therapeutic Indications

Indications

Artiblood is FDA approved for the short-term replacement of the oxygen-carrying capabilities of blood in patients who cannot use normal whole blood.[1] In addition, the product has been used successfully in cardiac catheter procedures, although this use is not FDA approved.[5] There is some early research into the use of the product as a plasma expansion product, but there is not enough information to support this use.[6]

Fakered is approved only for use in cardiac catheterization,[2] although it is commonly used as a blood replacement product in patients who cannot or will not use whole blood products.[7]

Evidence-Based Clinical Guidelines

A search of the literature was performed to identify evidence-based clinical guidelines. This included MEDLINE®, EMBASE Drugs and Pharmacology, the National Guideline Clearinghouse website, the American College of Cardiology website, and approximately a dozen Internet search engines; however, no applicable guidelines were identified.

Clinical Studies

Max and Sugar[6] conducted a comparison trial of artiblood (500 mL/day administered once over 1 hour—80 patients) and fakered (750 mL administered once over 90 minutes—82 patients) in patients (18–80 years of age) suffering from massive blood loss (>1 L), who could not use whole blood due to religious beliefs (e.g., Jehovah's Witnesses). In the artiblood group, all patients were undergoing open-heart surgery, as were 78 of the patients in fakered group. The remainder of the fakered group consisted of gunshot patients. Patients with renal insufficiency (creatinine clearance <50 mL/min) or diagnosed with liver dysfunction were eliminated from consideration. Both groups were similar, except that the artiblood group had more smokers, which may have had an affect on oxygen requirements. Withdrawals from the artiblood group were for the following reasons: death due to failure of heart-lung machine (1 patient), noncompliance with protocol (10 patients), worsening symptoms (3 patients), and side effects (1 patient: vomiting). The authors noted that protocol compliance problems were due to inappropriate staff education and were not related to the drug itself. In the fakered group, withdrawals were due to side effects (1 patient: diarrhea, 1 patient: nausea, 1 patient: abdominal cramps) and noncompliance with protocol (2 patients). The patients were assessed on the following items: oxygen and carbon dioxide content of the blood (samples drawn immediately before and after administration, and every 4 hours for 24 hours), coagulation profile of patient (drawn within 2 hours before and after administration), affect on normal blood chemistry profiles (SMA-20) (drawn within 2 hours before and after administration), and time to discontinuation of supplemental oxygen to the patient. Adverse effects were also noted. Results were analyzed using appropriate statistical methods. Artiblood was found to increase the oxygen- carrying capabilities of the blood in comparison to fakered ($p < .01$), although fakered did significantly improve oxygen-carrying capabilities over baseline ($p < .05$). While fakered had minimal affect on blood chemistry and coagulation profile, it was noted that INRs were increased in patients receiving artiblood ($p < .001$). Other adverse effects, mostly gastrointestinal in nature, were more common with fakered, although the symptoms typically disappeared within 2 hours of administration. Other measured characteristics seemed similar between the two groups. The authors concluded that artiblood was the superior agent, due to increased oxygen-carrying capabilities. The authors downplayed adverse effects, although the effects on INRs do appear worrisome. (Other studies would be covered here for all likely uses within an institution.)

Bioavailability/Pharmacokinetics[16–18]

Absorption

Absorption is not applicable, since these agents are administered by IV infusion.

Distribution

Artiblood is found in the blood stream, with little being distributed to the tissues. Approximately 5% of fakered is found in the liver, with the rest being in the bloodstream.

Metabolism

Artiblood is not metabolized in the body, whereas approximately 50% of fakered is broken down to inactive components and is excreted in the bile.

Elimination

Artiblood has a half-life of 5 to 15 hours. It is excreted unchanged in the urine. The longer half-life is seen in patients with renal insufficiency. Since the drug is usually given as a single dose, renal insufficiency does not pose a significant problem. Fakered has a half-life of 4 to 7 hours in normal patients. Significant renal or hepatic impairment may double the half-life.

Dosage Forms

Large Volume Parenteral

- Artiblood: 500 mL IV bags
- Fakered: 500, 750, and 1000 mL IV bags

No other forms or strengths available. Artiblood will have limited availability for the next 6 months due to the ability of the manufacturer to produce an adequate amount to satisfy demands. No problems in availability are expected after that point.

Dosage Range

The normal dose of artiblood for blood replacement is 500 mL, which may be repeated once after 4 hours. Doses may be cut in half for patients weighing less than 50 kg. No dosage adjustments are necessary in renal or hepatic impairment. The product has not been tested in patients younger than 12 years of age and is not recommended in that population. No dosage adjustment is necessary in the elderly.[1]

Fakered is given in doses of 500 mL to 1 L, with a maximum daily dose of 1.5 L. The dose is adjusted based on clinical response of the patient. The product can be used in patients as young as 6 years of age; however, the initial dose is 250 mL.[2]

Known Adverse Effects/Toxicities

The two agents are compared in the following table

Adverse Effect	Artiblood (% of Patients)	Fakered (% of Patients)
Gastrointestinal		
Nausea	20	7
...	...	...

Special Precautions

Neither drug has been studied long-term, therefore, the effects are not known in that situation.

Both products are considered Pregnancy Category C. Tests in pregnant animals have shown adverse effects and no adequate, well-controlled studies have been conducted in humans. There is no information available on the excretion of the drug in human milk. Overall, when considering use in pregnant or lactating women, the physician must consider the benefits versus the risks.

Safety and effectiveness of artiblood in children have not been established, although fakered may be used in children at least 6 years old.

Contraindications

Both agents are contraindicated in patients with hypersensitivities to the drug or any component of the dosage form.

Drug Interactions

Drug-Drug Interactions

Affects of heparin or low-molecular weight heparins may be significantly increased by either artificial blood replacement agent, although the affect by artiblood tends to be greater. There is no effect on either artiblood or fakered, although the heparin may improve circulation of the products to underperfused tissues. (Other interactions for both drugs would be listed and compared.)

Drug-Food Interactions

None are known or expected, since these agents are given intravenously and do not undergo enterohepatic recirculation.

Drug-Laboratory Test Interactions

INRs can be increased by both agents, although the effect is more noticeable with artiblood. (Other interactions for both drugs would be listed and compared.)

Patient Safety

This product has a good patient safety profile, with relatively minor adverse effects (e.g., nausea). Since the product has no coagulation or immunologic activity, health care providers must be aware that it is only used for temporary help in oxygen-carrying capabilities.

Patient Monitoring Guidelines

Monitor patient for objective evidence of effectiveness (e.g., oxygen content of blood and clinical effects). Obtain baseline INR and normal chemistry values, and monitor regularly. Monitor for adverse effects.

Patient Information

In a patient receiving the product due to trauma, it is likely that he or she will not be able to be given information. In that case, provide the information to the next of kin or guardian. Inform patients that the product is an intravenous product that does not contain any blood products. The patient or family should know that he or she may receive this product once or more during the first day after surgery. The patient or family should be informed that the drug has few noticeable adverse effects other than some gastrointestinal upset; however, the physician or pharmacist should be consulted if anything unusual occurs. The patient or family should know that some blood tests will be regularly performed to exclude the possibility of adverse effects. The nurse will keep the drug refrigerated until approximately 30 minutes before infusion. Warnings about missed doses are irrelevant.

Cost Comparison

General Pricing Information

	AWP	Daily Dose*	St. AMC	Daily Dose*
Artiblood 500 mL	$2500/bag	$2500	$2310/bag	$2310
Fakered 500 mL	$1000/bag	$1000	$800/bag	$800
Fakered 750 mL	$1500/bag	$1500	$1200/bag	$1200
Fakered 1000 mL	$2000/bag	$2000	$1600/bag	$1600

*Assume used one bag of each strength.

Pharmacoeconomic Analysis

- Problem definition: The objective of this analysis is to determine which artificial blood product should be included on our drug formulary.
- Perspective: This will be from the perspective of the institution.
- Specific treatment alternatives and outcomes: There are two drugs to be compared, artiblood and fakered. It will be assumed that natural blood products are not an alternative, since the ability to use natural products would preclude consideration of the artificial products. The outcomes to be measured are hospital costs.
- Pharmacoeconomic model: A cost-benefit analysis will be performed. A cost-utility analysis would be desirable, but insufficient information is available. *Note:* no published pharmacoeconomic analysis is available. The following table is based on information obtained from the literature concerning efficacy, adverse effects, monitoring, and so forth and uses St. AMC costs, since outside prices would be irrelevant.

	Cost per Patient	Benefit-to-Cost Ratio	Net Benefit
Cost of artiblood (including administration, monitoring, adverse reactions, and so forth)	$5120	$7430/$5120 = 1.45:1	$7430–$5120 = $2310
Benefits of artiblood (money saved by early patient discharge from ICU)	$7430		
Cost of fakered (including administration, monitoring, adverse reactions, and so forth)	$4000	$4500/$4000 = 1.125:1	$4500–$4000 = $500
Benefits of fakered (money saved by early patient discharge from ICU)	$4500		

NOTE: The above information is a summary of information, including averages, decision analysis, and sensitivity analysis that would be used in a pharmacoeconomic evaluation. While the details could be presented here, that may be distracting and confusing to some readers—a decision must be made as to whether all of the details will be presented. See Chap. 8 for details on how to prepare a pharmacoeconomic analysis of a drug being evaluated by the P&T Committee.

SOURCE: Presented by John Q. Doe, Pharm.D. to the Pharmacy and Therapeutics Committee on February 30, 20XX.

REFERENCES

References would be listed in the order in which they are cited in the text—see Appendix 11–3 for format and details.

16-1

Comparison of Quality Assurance and Total Quality Management in Health Care

Comparison	TQM Approach	QA Approach
Purpose	Improve quality of all services/products for all patients and customers	Improve quality of patient care
Scope	All systems and processes (clinical and nonclinical)	Clinical systems and processes
	Actions directed to improving processes	Actions directed toward improving people
Leadership	All clinical and nonclinical leadership	Physicians and clinical leadership
Aims	Continuous improvements if no problems are identified	Problem solving
	Focus on common causes of failed quality	Identify individuals whose performance or outcomes are outside expectations
Focus	Process improvement and people	Individuals (peer-review)
	Improve performance of everyone	Training or elimination of unacceptable few
	Prevention and process design	Inspection
	Customers are everyone involved in the system	Customers are patients, professionals, and review organizations
Customers and requirements	Measures based on customers and professionals	Measures established by health professionals
Methods	Brainstorming	Audits
	Nominal group technique	Nominal group technique
	Force field analysis	Hypothesis testing
	Coaching/mentoring	
	Flowcharts	
	Pareto charts	

	Cause and effect diagrams Run chart Control chart Histogram Scatter diagram Stratification Quality function deployment	
People involved	Everyone	Quality assurance committee/staff
	Actions are decided by a team with no time constraints	Actions decided by committees appointed for a specified time period
Outcomes	Improves performance for everyone involved in the process	Improves individual performance
	Reduces threats	Creates defensiveness
	Promotes team effort and eliminates territoriality	
Continuing activities	Continual process improvement through monitoring	Monitors when deviations and actions occur

Appendix 16–2

Tools Used in Quality Improvement

FLOWCHARTS

Flowcharts illustrate the steps of a process and how the steps are related to each other. They can be used to describe the process, increase a team's knowledge of the entire process, identify weaknesses or breakdown points in the current process, or design a new process. An example of a flowchart outlining how adverse reactions might be addressed within an organization appears on the next page.

PARETO CHART

Pareto charts are vertical bar graphs with the data presented so that the bars are arranged from left to right on the horizontal axis in order of decreasing frequency. This arrangement helps to identify which problems to address in what order. By addressing the data represented in the tallest bars (e.g., the most frequently occurring problems or contributing factors), efforts can be focused on areas where the most gain can be realized. Pareto charts are commonly used to identify issues to address, delineate potential causes of a problem, and

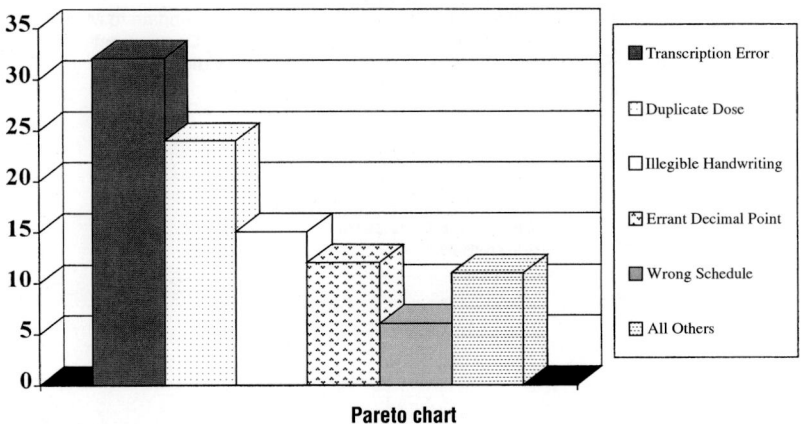

Pareto chart

Flowchart: Suspected Adverse Drug Reactions

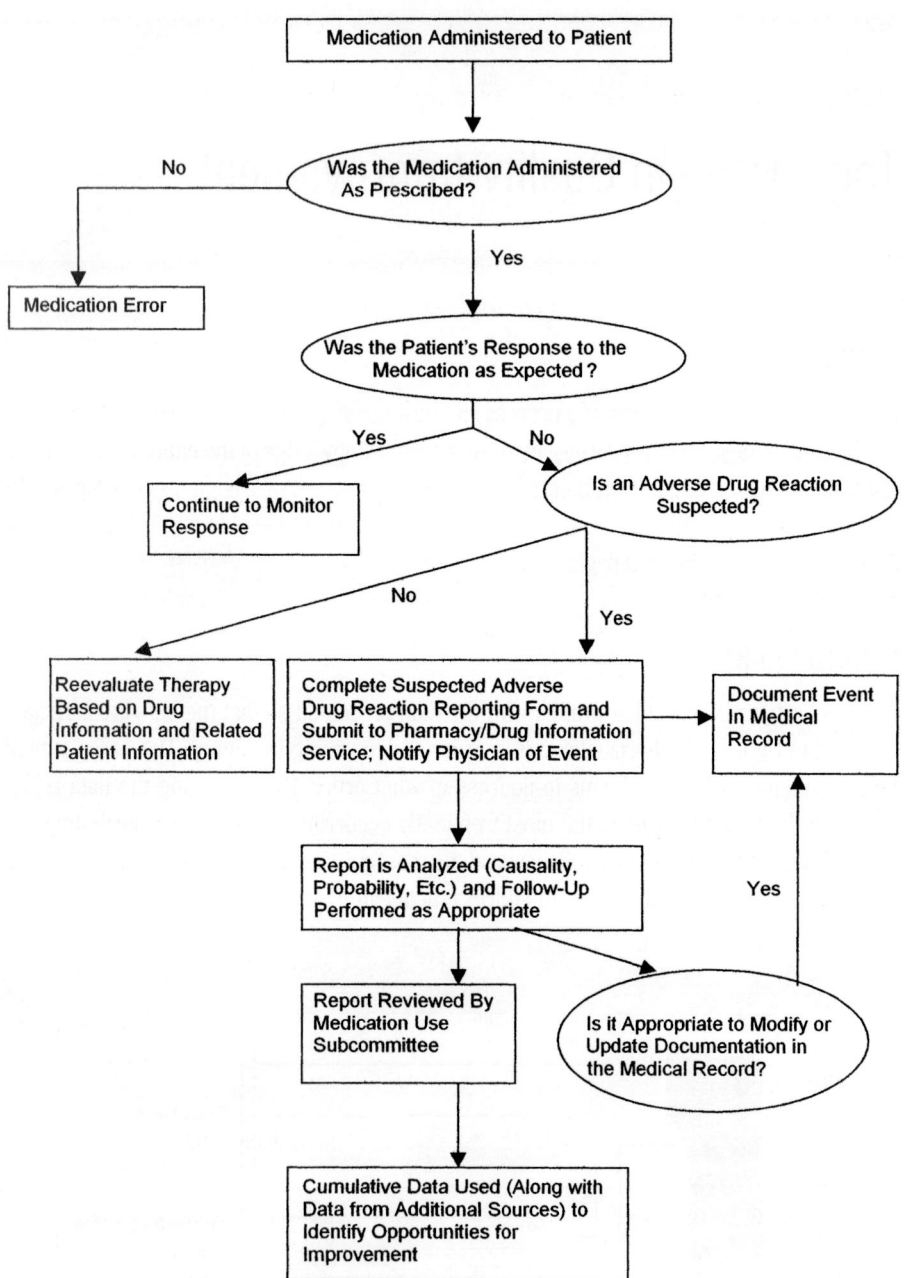

monitor improvements in processes. An example of a Pareto chart appears on page 798. This example illustrates frequently occurring factors contributing to improper dose medication errors. By focusing on transcription errors as a contributing factor on which to focus quality improvement efforts, the quality improvement team will generally gain more than by tackling the less frequent problems.

FISHBONE OR CAUSE AND EFFECT DIAGRAM

Fishbone or cause and effect diagrams represent the relationship between an outcome (represented at the head of the fish) and the possible causes of the outcome (represented as the bones of the fish). The bones of the fish should represent causes and not symptoms of the issue. Fishbone diagrams are commonly used to identify components of a process to address, delineate potential causes of a problem, or identify practitioner groups that participate in producing an outcome and should be represented in the group addressing quality issues in the process(es). An example of a fishbone chart appears below.

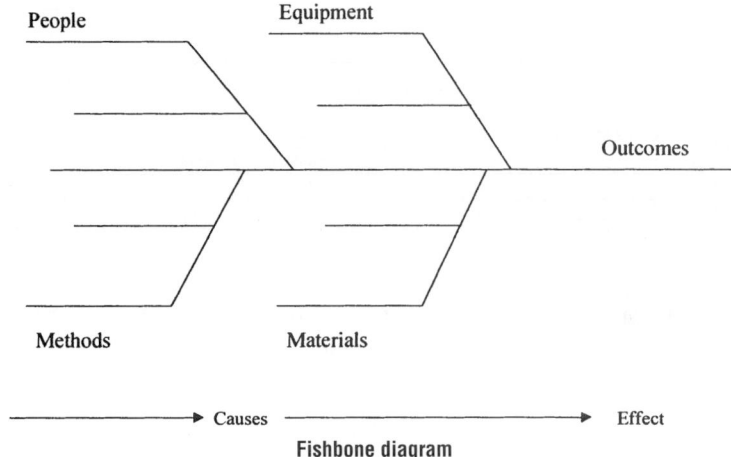

Fishbone diagram

CONTROL CHARTS

Control charts are run charts or line graphs with defined allowable limits of variation. Data are plotted on the graph as they become available, with new data points connected to older data by a continuous line. The x axis is usually a measure of time. The control limits help to identify which variations in data are important. Control limits are statistically determined based on average ranges and sample size. Fluctuation in data points above and below the average is expected and is referred to as "common variation" or "common cause" as long as they remain between the control limits. Data points above the upper control limit or below the lower control limit are referred to as "special variation" or "special cause." Special cause variation indicates that something different is going on outside the normal operation of the process. Also, a series of data points above or below average may indicate a trend in performance that may need to be addressed. As variability in a process is reduced by quality improvement efforts, control limits should be recalculated (and narrowed) based on ongoing data. An example of a control chart appears below. Calls from pharmacists to prescribers in response to questions or issues related to new medication orders are represented over a 6-month period. Data from the month of July indicate a significant increase in the number of calls made. A quality improvement team evaluating these data would then attempt to identify what contributed to this increase. A potential cause in many institutions might be the influx of new medical housestaff into the organization each July. One potential intervention to reduce this special cause is to improve the orientation of new practitioners to the medication use process within the organization.

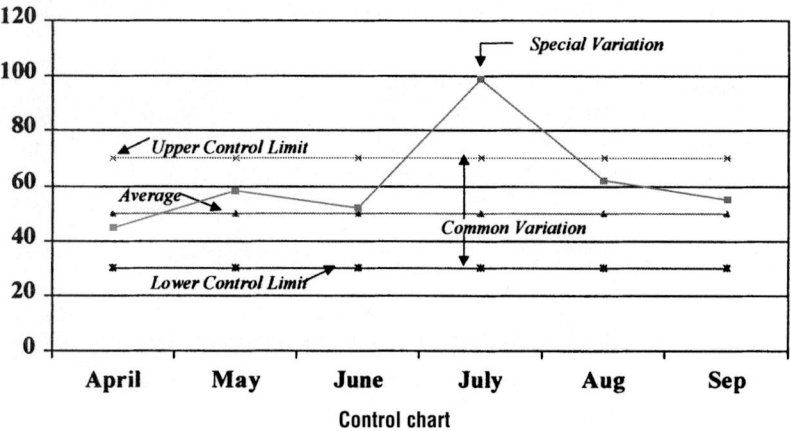

Control chart

16-3

Appendix 16-3

Examples of Approaches to Quality Improvement

SMART PROBLEM SOLVING PROCESS

Statement: Written statement outlining problem or opportunity for improvement
Selection of problem
Definition of problem in measurable terms

Measurement: Collection of baseline data based on most influential factors
Determine what needs to be known about the problem
Develop data collection method, compile data

Analysis: Analyze data and identify causes
Outline root causes of problems
Evaluate collected data to identify causes of specific outcomes

Remedy: Generate solutions and implement action
Identify action(s) needed to address root causes and implement

Test: Assess impact of corrective action(s)
Reassess (collect data) to determine if improvement has occurred

FOCUS-PDCA

Find a Process to Improve

Review of data, brainstorming a list of processes, and/or customer feedback can be used to identify processes in need of improvement.

Organize the Team

Team membership should include those who participate in the process and who are most familiar with its day-to-day function.

Clarify the Current Process

It is essential that team members understand how the process currently works. Flowcharts are useful tools to achieve this objective.

Understand the Current Process

Once the process is understood, causes of variation are identified. These could also be described as breakdowns of flaws in the process. Fishbone diagrams are useful tools to identify causes of variation.

This step also includes data collection on the process and more specifically, the variations identified. Check sheets, Pareto charts, histograms, and control charts are useful to display data.

Solution

Possible improvement solutions are then identified. Brainstorming and nominal group technique can be useful in this step.

Plan the Improvement

Plan who, what, when, where, and how solutions will be implemented. Also, determine what data will be needed to verify that the improvement has occurred.

Do the Improvement

Following appropriate coordination and training, implement the improvement solution.

Check the Results

Collect data to evaluate the effectiveness of the solution. These results should be compared to baseline data (obtained in the Understand the Current Process step). The same tools mentioned above can be useful in displaying this data.

Act on Results

If results were as expected, the new process should be standardized. If the results were not as expected, return to the Solution step to select an alternative solution and continue through the remaining steps. This cycle is repeated until the process improvement is achieved.

TEN-STEP PROCESS

1. Assign responsibility for monitoring and evaluation.
2. Delineate scope of care and service provided by the organization.
3. Identify important aspects of care and service provided by the organization.
4. Identify indicators, data sources, and collection methods to monitor important aspects of care.
5. Establish means to trigger evaluation (e.g., trends or patterns of use and thresholds).
6. Collect and organize data.
7. Initiate evaluation of care (as indicated by triggers set in step 5).
8. Take actions to improve care and service.
9. Assess the effectiveness of actions, maintain the improvement, then document improvements in care.
10. Communicate results to relevant individuals and groups.

16–4

Appendix 16–4

Example of a Quality Improvement Activity Plan

The following components should be included in the presentation of a proposal.

1. A description of the aspect of care to be assessed including historical background if appropriate (e.g., if this is a follow-up to a previous evaluation).
2. A description of the group responsible for developing the criteria, indicators, guidelines, and so on to be used in the evaluation.
3. The proposed criteria or indicators and performance expectations.
4. A summary of the data collection methods, case identification methods, timeframe for data collection, and minimal cases to be evaluated.
5. The proposed reporting channels and frequency of reports.

EXAMPLE OF CRITERIA AND REQUEST FOR APPROVAL

Medication Use Evaluation Criteria

Antiemetic Use in the Prophylaxis of Chemotherapy-Induced Nausea and Vomiting

Request for Approval by Medication Use Evaluation Committee

Purpose of evaluation: The purpose of this medication use evaluation (MUE) is to evaluate the use of antiemetic therapy in the prevention of chemotherapy-induced nausea and vomiting. This agent was selected for evaluation based on its essential role in the management of this patient population, potential inappropriate use, and increased cost relative to other antiemetic agents. This class of medications has not been evaluated within the organization for at least 5 years.

Criteria: A multidisciplinary group including physicians, clinical nurse specialists, staff nurses from the oncology unit, and pharmacists developed the attached criteria. They are submitted for approval by the MUE Committee.

Data Collection: Data will be collected on all patients with orders for this agent written throughout a period of approximately 30 days beginning in mid-January. A minimum of 50 cases will be reviewed. Pharmacists and clinical nurse specialists will collect data concurrently from the medical record. Patients will be identified by means of the pharmacy information system.

Results: Results will be presented to this Committee. Information will also be shared with the Cancer Care Committee and Hospital Quality Improvement Council. Prescriber-specific results will be confidentially provided to Medical Staff Support for use in the reappointment/recredentialing process.

MEDICATION USE EVALUATION CRITERIA

ANTIEMETIC USE IN THE PROPHYLAXIS OF CHEMOTHERAPY-INDUCED NAUSEA AND VOMITING

Name _____ **Rm** _____ **Age** _____ **Sex** _____ **Wt** ____ **Ht** _____

Allergies _____ **Service** _____

Chemo/Dose/Date/Time _____ **Attending MD:** _____

Medication Use Process Elements	S(%)	Exceptions

Prescribing

A. Indication—antiemetic (IV or PO)

1. No other drug and nondrug causes of preexisting nausea and vomiting identified — 95 — (A2a) Pt receiving other less emetic cancer chemotherapy regimen and not responsive to other antiemetics

2. Prevention of acute nausea and vomiting during the first 24 hours following the initiation of highly or moderately highly emetogenic cancer chemotherapy regimens: — 95 — to other antiemetics
Chemo/dose:
Other antiemetic/dose:
(A2b) Pt has had significant documented adverse reactions to alternative antiemetics and is receiving a regimen with a lesser emetogenic potential

   (a) Highly emetogenic (>90%): cisplatin, dacarbazine, mechlorethamine, streptozocin, cytarabine (>500 mg/m^2);

   (b) Moderately high (60 to 90%): carmustine, lomustine, cyclophosphamide, dactinomycin, plicamycin, procarbazine, methotrexate (>200 mg/m^2)

3. Prevention of anticipatory nausea and vomiting associated with any chemotherapy regimen

Dispensing/Administering

A. Dosage—IV antiemetic

  1. 0.4 mg/kg infused over 15 minutes begun 30 minutes prior to initiation of chemotherapy regimen; then two additional doses given 4 and 8 hours after first dose of therapy, or — 95 — Dosage reduced by 50% in patients with significant renal dysfunction (i.e., measured or estimated creatinine clearance < 25 mL/min)

  2. A single 85 mg dose infused over 15 minutes begun 30 minutes prior to initiation of chemotherapy regimen

B. Dosage—oral antiemetic
20 mg administered 30 minutes before chemotherapy is initiated, second dose 8 hours after first dose. Continue therapy twice a day for 1 to 2 days after completion of therapy — 95

Monitoring

Adverse Effects — Preventive and/or responsive management:

  1. Headache — < 15 — Identify other drug and nondrug causes

  2. Diarrhea — < 15 — Provide supportive and symptomatic therapy

  3. Constipation — < 10

  4. Sedation — < 10

Outcome Measures

  1. Prevention of nausea and emesis — 95 — (2) Medical contraindications:

  2. Cancer chemotherapy course not interrupted by nausea and vomiting — 95 — (a) to continuation of chemotherapy.
(b) patient expired.
(c) lost to follow-up.

Example Report—Prescriber-Specific Results

Prescriber-specific reports from medication use evaluation activities should be provided for use in the reappointment/recredentialing process. It is important that these reports contain sufficient information to facilitate peer-review. A summary of all cases involving the prescriber should be included in the report including a brief description of cases in which criteria were not met. A mechanism to access the medical record (e.g., a medical record number) should be provided to allow chart review if needed. An example appears below.

PRESCRIBER-SPECIFIC INFORMATION FOR USE IN REAPPOINTMENT/RECREDENTIALING

Source: Medication Use Evaluation (MUE) Committee

Evaluation Topic: Antiemetic Medication Use Evaluation

Dates of Evaluation: January

Data Enclosed:

    a. Summary of overall results reviewed by MUE Committee and actions taken by the Committee (see attached)

    b. Criteria used in evaluation (see attached, approved by MUE Committee prior to data collection)

    c. Prescriber-specific results (below)

1. Table outlining patient case number, medical record number, diagnosis, attending physician (by first letters of last name followed by ID #), and criteria not met (when applicable) for all patients managed by this attending physician during the evaluation period.
2. Any other prescriber-specific correspondence from the Committee.

Results for Attending Physician #12345

Attending #	Case #	Medrec #	Diagnosis	Criteria Not Met
12345	43	54321	OVARIAN CA	
12345	44	43215	BREAST CA	Dosing
12345	55	32154	SMALL CELL CA/ LIVER METS	Dosing
12345	58	15432	MET BREAST CA	Outcome
12345	59	53215	MET BREAST CA	
12345	71	42153	AML	Outcome
12345	121	15342	OVARIAN CA	

Summary of cases where dosing criteria not met
- Case #44 did not meet dosing criteria. Patient received 85 mg IV antiemetic on chemotherapy day 1 (cisplatin and VP16) then 85 mg in 24 hours on day 2 (VP 16 only).
- Case #55 did not meet dosing criteria. Patient received 85 mg IV antiemetic on chemotherapy day 1 (cisplatin and VP16) then 85 mg in 24 hours on day 2 (VP 16 only).

MUE Committee action taken (specific to this prescriber): letter written to prescriber.

Summary of cases where outcome criteria not met
- Case #58 did not meet outcome criteria (i.e., prevention of nausea and vomiting). Patient experienced nausea/vomiting × 1 less than 24 hours following antiemetic dose (85 mg IV × 1).
- Case #71 did not meet outcome criteria (i.e., prevention of nausea and vomiting). Patient received 85 mg IV antiemetic qd × 6 days. On 6th day had one episode nausea.

MUE Committee action taken (specific to this prescriber): none.

16-6

Appendix 16-6

Example of MUE Results

MEDICATION USE EVALUATION

Summary of Overall Results

Antiemetic: January

Background: This topic was selected based on high use, potential misuse, and high cost of these agents. Criteria for this evaluation were approved at the MUE Committee's December meeting. Please refer to attached criteria for additional information.

Total Patients Evaluated (All Indications for Use) = 52

Element	Standard	Results	Compliance
Prescribing			
Indication for use	95%	Overall results	
		Treatment/prevention of nausea/ vomiting associated with chemotherapy	100% (52/52)
		Highly emetogenic chemotherapy	46/46
		Anticipatory N/V associated with chemotherapy	6/6
Dispensing/ Administering			
Dosing	95%	Overall results	71% (37/52)
		Highly emetogenic chemotherapy	31/46
		Anticipatory N/V associated with chemotherapy	6/6
Monitoring			
Adverse Drug Reaction(s)	≤10 to 25% (varies with ADR)	Overall results	4% (2/52)
		Headache: 1 patient	
		Constipation: 1 patient	

Element	Standard	Results	Compliance
Outcome			
Prevention of nausea and emesis	95%	Overall Results	92% (46/50)*
		Highly emetogenic chemotherapy	41/44
		Anticipatory N/V associated	5/6
		with chemotherapy	
Chemotherapy course not interrupted	95%	Overall Results (All Indications)	100% (52/52)

*Includes only patients in whom outcome was documented. Outcome was not assessed in two patients who were discharged immediately following administration of chemotherapy.

Summary of Results

Prescribing: Criteria for indication of use were met in all cases.

Dispensing/Administering: Criteria for dosing was met in 37 of 52 cases with all cases involving anticipatory nausea and vomiting meeting criteria.

In 15 cases, patients receiving the antiemetic prior to highly emetogenic chemotherapy received doses not included in the approved criteria. Five of these patients received doses based on an investigational protocol. This dose is now under consideration by the FDA for approval and preliminary results (available only in abstract form) were recently presented at the American Society of Clinical Oncology meeting. Results with the new dosing regimen have been comparable to those with the currently approved doses.

In seven cases not meeting dosing criteria, patients received a single dose prior to chemotherapy consistent with the criteria. However, an additional dose was administered 24 hours after the first dose. These orders were written by two prescribers.

Two cases did not meet dosing criteria because the dose was not adjusted based on renal dysfunction. In both cases, the estimated creatinine clearance was between 20 and 25 mL/min and nephrotoxic drugs were not being administered concurrently. In both cases, the estimated creatinine clearance increased to 30 mL/min or more by day 2 of the admission (probably due to rehydration of the patient). Neither patient experienced adverse effects.

One dose was not administered within the appropriate timeframe. In this case, the antiemetic dose was administered just 5-minutes prior to the initiation of chemotherapy administration. The nurse administering the antiemetic documented administration on the way to the patient's room. When she arrived, the patient was not in the room. The dose was administered after he was located, approximately 25 minutes later. The nurse did not correct the actual administration time until after the chemotherapy was administered by a second nurse.

Recommendations:
1. Add new dosing regimen to dosing criteria.
2. Send letters to prescribers giving extra dose.

3. Renal dosing was not significantly outside guidelines. Mention findings in report to be published in quality improvement newsletter, but do not take prescriber-specific action.
4. The dose administered late was reported via an incident report; no further action by this group is required at this time.

Monitoring: The rate of adverse drug reactions was less than that reported in the literature. This might be reflective of underreporting and under-documenting of adverse drug events.

Recommendations:
1. The Adverse Drug Event Task Force is currently implementing a new process to improve reporting and documentation. No specific action by this group is required at this time.

Outcome: Ninety-two percent of patients did not experience nausea or vomiting. Outcome was assessable in 50 patients; two patients were discharged immediately following the administration of chemotherapy.

The patient who received his antiemetic dose just 5-minutes prior to chemotherapy experienced moderate nausea and no vomiting. Otherwise, the occurrence of nausea and vomiting was not related to problems with administration or dosing.

Recommendations:
1. 92% success rate is acceptable based on literature, no action is necessary.

General Recommendations:
1. After approval, implement recommendations presented above.
2. Publish results in the Quality Improvement Newsletter following review by the Cancer Care Committee and the Quality Improvement Committee.
3. Perform a follow-up evaluation focusing on dosing issues.
4. Initiate planned assessment of this agent's use in postoperative nausea and vomiting as soon as possible.

Note: An example of a prescriber-specific report for reappointment/recredentialing appears in Appendix 16–5.

Appendix 16–7

Quality Evaluation: Response to Drug Information Request

Request #	Date of Request				
Response by (circle one):	DI Staff Resident Student				
Caller (circle one):	MD RPh Nurse Other:				
Assessment of Search and Response to Request					
		Yes	**No**	**NA**	**Standard %**[*]
1. Is requestor's demographic information complete?					100
2. Background information is: A. thorough B. appropriate to request					100
3. Is the question clearly stated?					100
4. Search strategy/references: A. appropriate references were used B. search was sufficiently comprehensive C. is search strategy clearly documented					100
5. Response was: A. appropriate for the situation B. sufficient to answer the question C. provided in a timely manner D. integrated with available patient data E. supported by appropriate materials supplied to requestor					100
6. If complete response could not be provided within timeframe requested, was requestor advised as to the status of the request and the anticipated delivery of the final response?					100

[*] If performance falls below 90% in any category during any month, the service director will coordinate an assessment of the process and report findings and actions taken to the Pharmacy Quality Improvement Council.

Comments:

Reviewed by: _____

Appendix 17–1

Kramer Questionnaire*

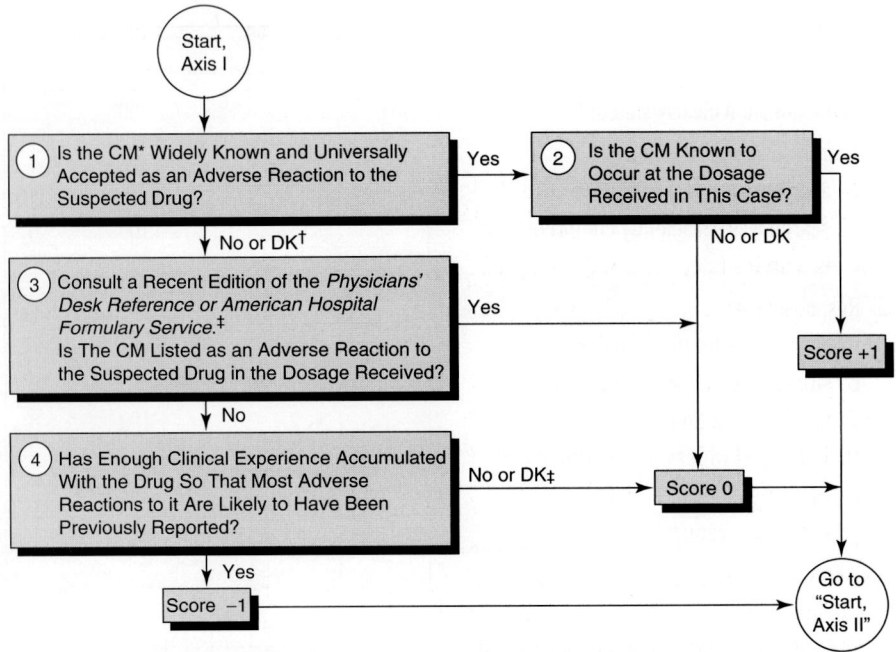

*Abbreviation CM indicates clinical manifestation, the abnormal sign, symptom, or laboratory test, or cluster of abnormal signs, symptoms, and tests, that is being considered as a possible adverse drug reaction.

†Abbreviation DK indicates do not know. This answer should be given when no data are available for the question being answered or when the quality of the data does not allow a firm "Yes" or "No" response.

‡When these are not available, an equivalent reference source may be used.

Figure 1. Axis I. Previous general experience with drug.

*Kramer MS, Leventhal JM, Hutchinson TA, Feinstein AR. An algorithm for the operational assessment of adverse drug reaction: I. background, descriptions, and instructions for use. JAMA 1979; 242(7):623–32.

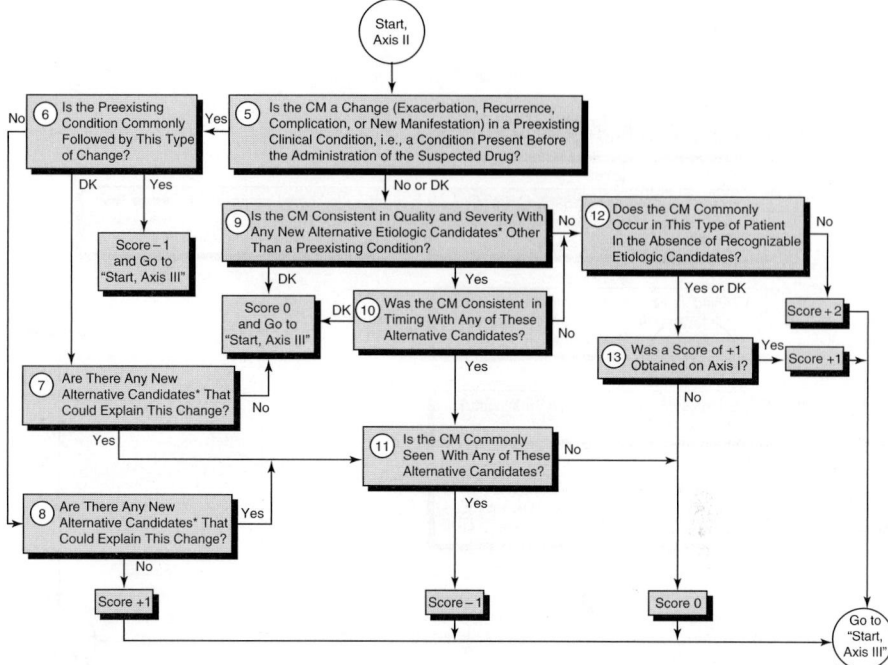

Figure 2. Axis II. Alternative etiologic candidates. For explanation of abbreviations, see Axis I.

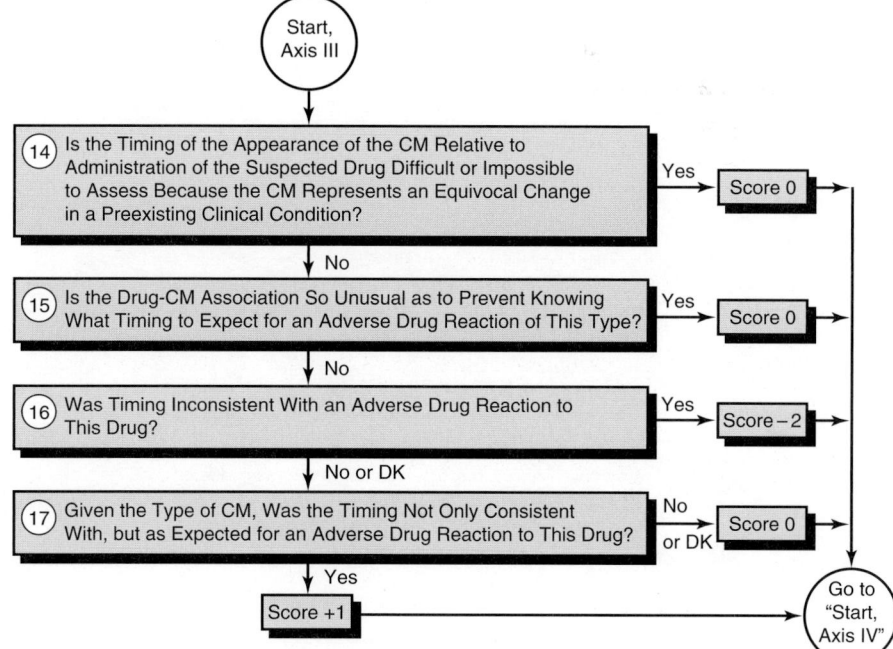

Figure 3. Axis III. Timing of events. For explanantion of abbreviations, see Axis I.

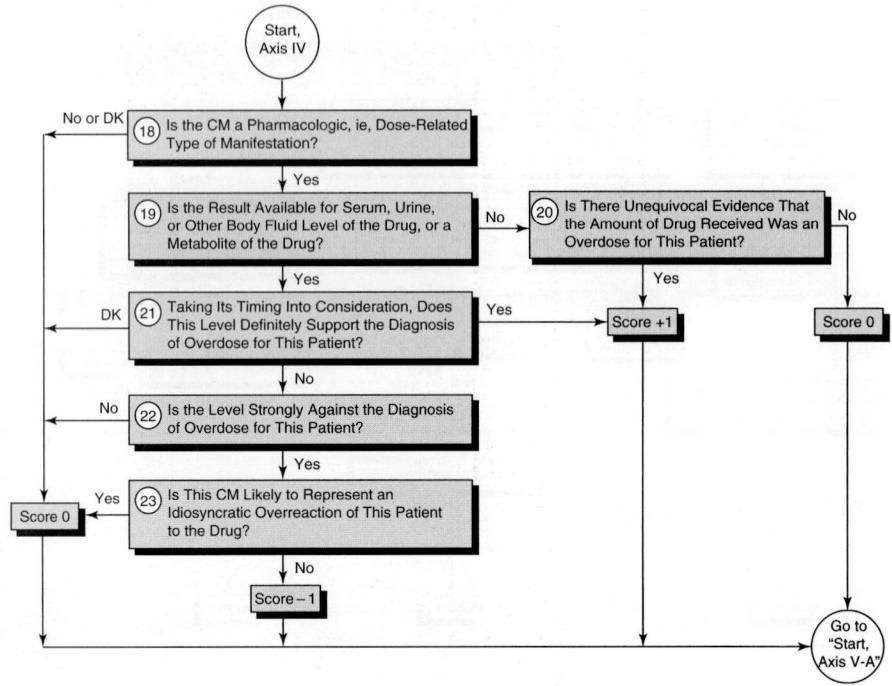

Figure 4. Axis IV. Drug levels and evidence of overdose. For explanantion of abbreviations, see Axis I.

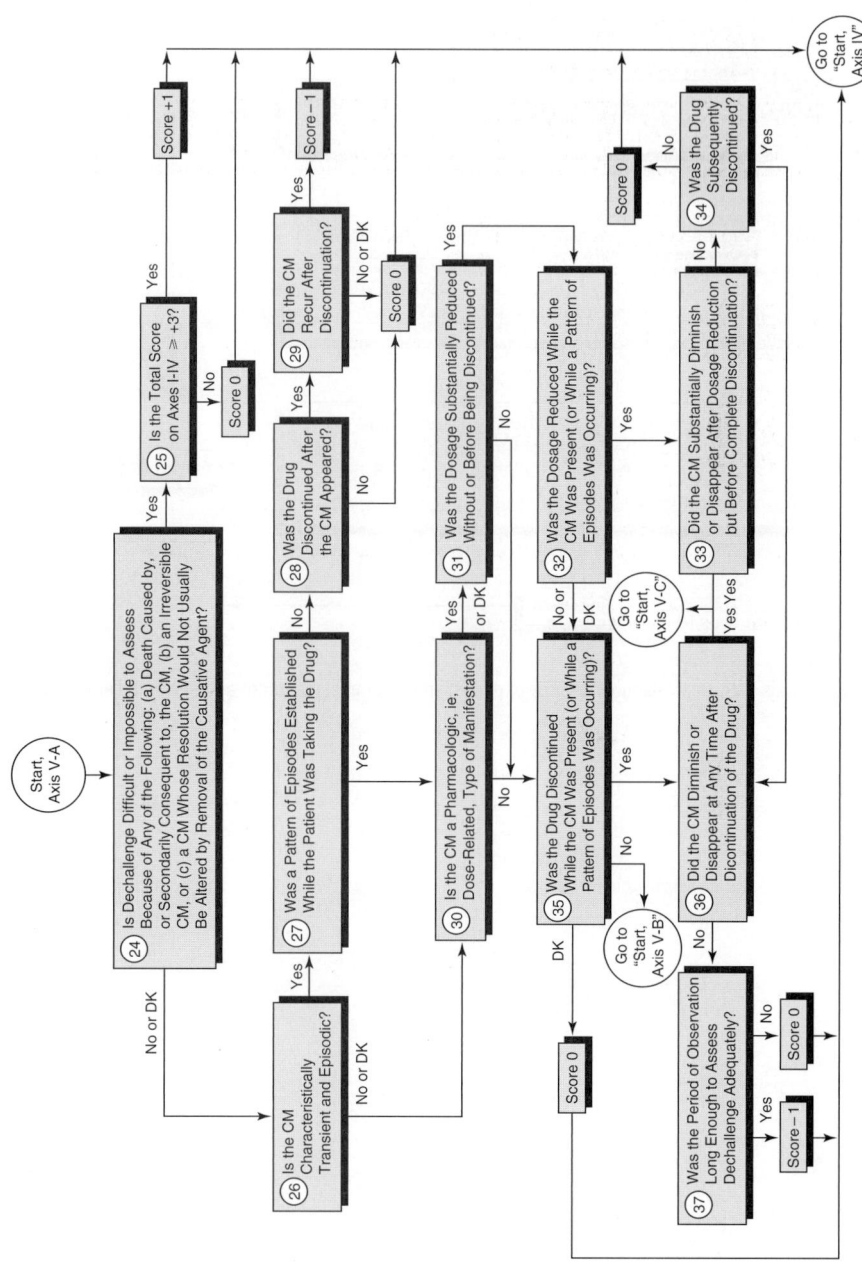

Figure 5A. Axis V-A. Dechallenge: Difficult assessments. For explanation of abbreviations, see Axis I.

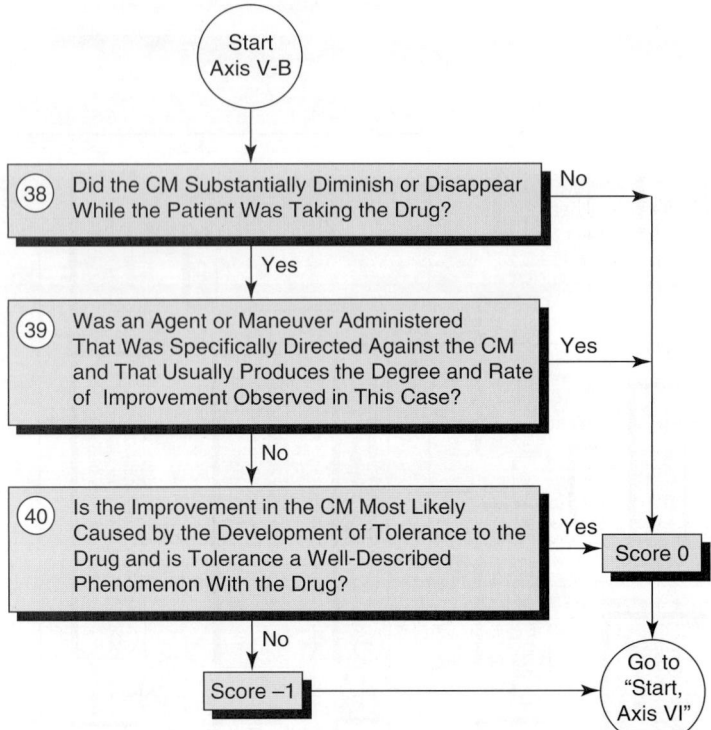

Figure 5B. Axis V-B. Dechallenge: Absence of dechallenge. For explanation of abbreviation, see Axis I.

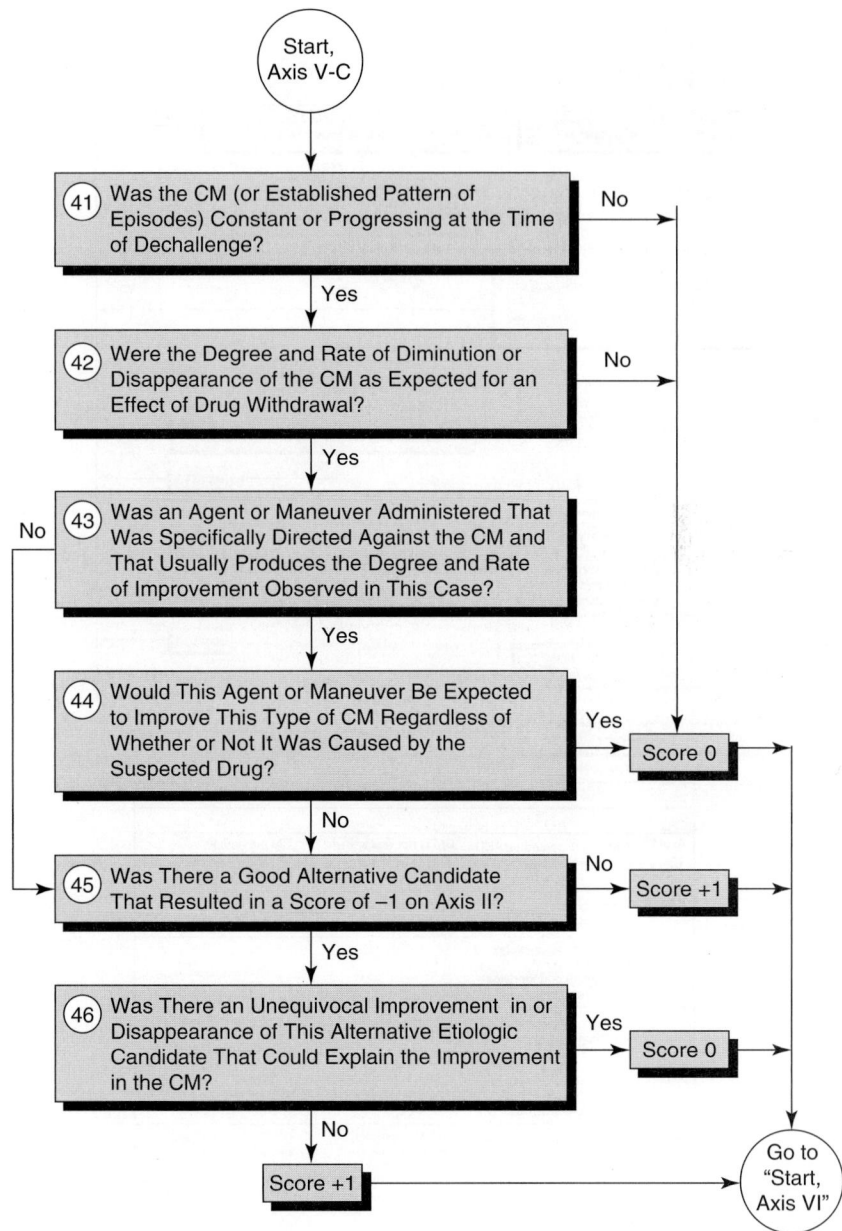

Figure 5C. Axis V-C. Dechallenge: Improvement after dechallenge. For explanation of abbreviation, see Axis I.

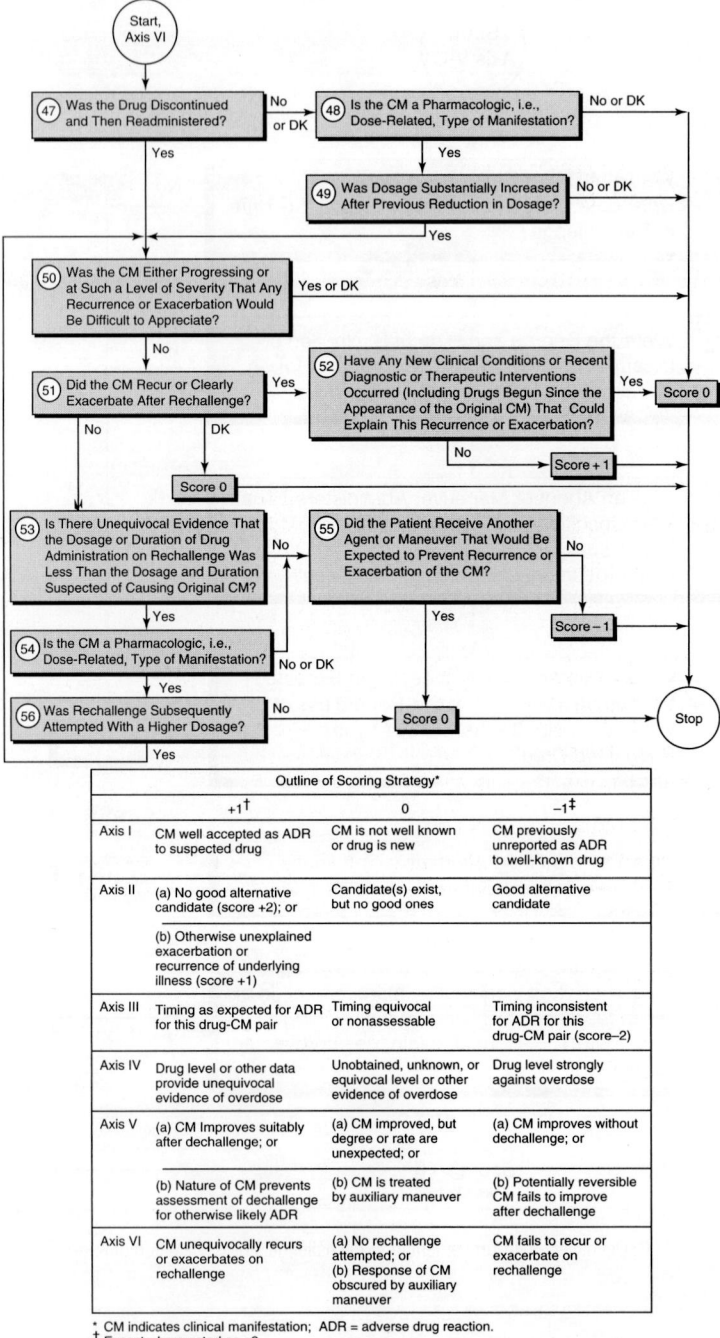

Figure 6. Axis VI. Rechallenge. For explanation of abbreviation, see Axis I.

17–2

Appendix 17–2

Naranjo Algorithm*

To assess the adverse drug reaction, please answer the following questionnaire and give the pertinent score.

	Yes	No	Don't know	Score
1. Are there previous conclusive reports on this reaction?	+1	0	0	
2. Did the adverse event appear after the suspected drug was administered?	+2	–1	0	
3. Did the adverse reaction improve when the drug was discontinued or a specific antagonist was administered?	+1	0	0	
4. Did the adverse reaction reappear when the drug was readministered?	+2	–1	0	
5. Are there alternative causes (other than the drug) that could on their own have caused the reaction?	–1	+2	0	
6. Did the reaction reappear when a placebo was given?	–1	+1	0	
7. Was the drug detected in the blood (or other fluids) in concentrations known to be toxic?	+1	0	0	
8. Was the reaction more severe when the dose was increased, or less severe when the dose was decreased?	+1	0	0	
9. Did the patient have a similar reaction to the same or similar drugs in any previous exposure?	+1	0	0	
10. Was the adverse event confirmed by any objective evidence?	+1	0	0	

Total Score_____

Score Interpretation
___Definite: ≥9
___Probable: 5 to 8
___Possible: 1 to 4
___Doubtful: ≤0

*Naranjo CA, Busto U, Sellers EM, Sandor P, Ruiz I, Roberts EA, et al. A method of estimating the probability of adverse drug reactions. Clin Pharmacol Ther. 1981;30(2):239–45.

Appendix 17–3

Jones Algorithm*

START HERE:**

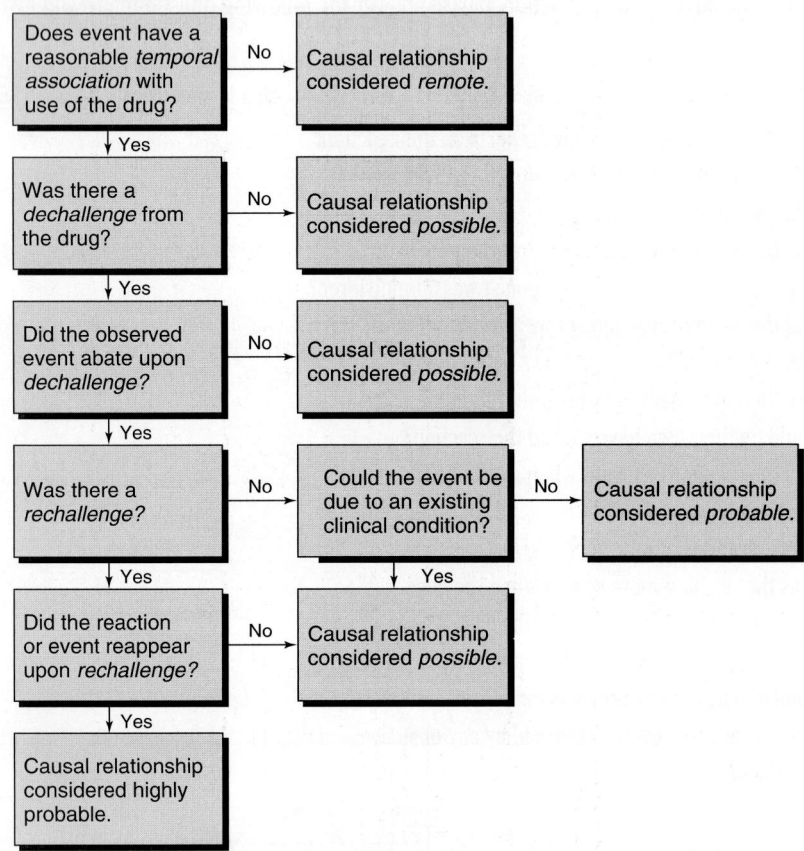

**Each drug is carried through independently; if > 1 drug was dechallenged or rechallenged simultaneously causality for all is ≤ possible.

QUESTIONS:

1. Did the reaction follow a reasonable temporal sequence?
2. Did the patient improve after stopping the drug?
3. Did the reaction reappear on repeated exposure (rechallenge)?
4. Could the reaction be reasonably explained by the known characteristics of the patient's clinical *state?*

*Jones JK. Adverse drug reactions in the community health setting: approaches to recognizing, counseling, and reporting. Clin Comm Health. 1982;5(2):58–67.

Appendix 17–4

MedWatch Form

U.S. Department of Health and Human Services

Form Approved: OMB No. 0910-0291, Expires: 10/31/08
See OMB statement on reverse.

MEDWATCH

The FDA Safety Information and
Adverse Event Reporting Program

For VOLUNTARY reporting of
adverse events, product problems and
product use errors

Page _____ of _____

FDA USE ONLY

Triage unit
sequence #

PLEASE TYPE OR USE BLACK INK

A. PATIENT INFORMATION

1. Patient Identifier	2. Age at Time of Event, or Date of Birth:	3. Sex	4. Weight
In confidence		☐ Female ☐ Male	_____ lb or _____ kg

B. ADVERSE EVENT, PRODUCT PROBLEM OR ERROR

Check all that apply:

1. ☐ Adverse Event   ☐ Product Problem (e.g., defects/malfunctions)
   ☐ Product Use Error   ☐ Problem with Different Manufacturer of Same Medicine

2. Outcomes Attributed to Adverse Event
(Check all that apply)

☐ Death: _____ (mm/dd/yyyy)
☐ Life-threatening
☐ Hospitalization - initial or prolonged
☐ Required Intervention to Prevent Permanent Impairment/Damage (Devices)

☐ Disability or Permanent Damage
☐ Congenital Anomaly/Birth Defect
☐ Other Serious (Important Medical Events)

3. Date of Event (mm/dd/yyyy)   4. Date of this Report (mm/dd/yyyy)

5. Describe Event, Problem or Product Use Error

6. Relevant Tests/Laboratory Data, Including Dates

7. Other Relevant History, Including Preexisting Medical Conditions (e.g., allergies, race, pregnancy, smoking and alcohol use, liver/kidney problems, etc.)

C. PRODUCT AVAILABILITY

Product Available for Evaluation? (Do not send product to FDA)

☐ Yes   ☐ No   ☐ Returned to Manufacturer on: _____ (mm/dd/yyyy)

D. SUSPECT PRODUCT(S)

1. Name, Strength, Manufacturer (from product label)

#1
#2

2. Dose or Amount	Frequency	Route
#1		
#2		

3. Dates of Use (If unknown, give duration) from/to (or best estimate)

#1
#2

4. Diagnosis or Reason for Use (Indication)

#1
#2

6. Lot #	7. Expiration Date
#1	#1
#2	#2

5. Event Abated After Use Stopped or Dose Reduced?

#1 ☐ Yes ☐ No ☐ Doesn't Apply
#2 ☐ Yes ☐ No ☐ Doesn't Apply

8. Event Reappeared After Reintroduction?

#1 ☐ Yes ☐ No ☐ Doesn't Apply
#2 ☐ Yes ☐ No ☐ Doesn't Apply

9. NDC # or Unique ID

E. SUSPECT MEDICAL DEVICE

1. Brand Name

2. Common Device Name

3. Manufacturer Name, City and State

4. Model #	Lot #	5. Operator of Device
Catalog #	Expiration Date (mm/dd/yyyy)	☐ Health Professional ☐ Lay User/Patient
Serial #	Other #	☐ Other:

6. If Implanted, Give Date (mm/dd/yyyy)   7. If Explanted, Give Date (mm/dd/yyyy)

8. Is this a Single-use Device that was Reprocessed and Reused on a Patient?
☐ Yes   ☐ No

9. If Yes to Item No. 8, Enter Name and Address of Reprocessor

F. OTHER (CONCOMITANT) MEDICAL PRODUCTS

Product names and therapy dates (exclude treatment of event)

G. REPORTER (See confidentiality section on back)

1. Name and Address

Phone #   E-mail

2. Health Professional?	3. Occupation	4. Also Reported to:
☐ Yes ☐ No		☐ Manufacturer ☐ User Facility ☐ Distributor/Importer

5. If you do NOT want your identity disclosed to the manufacturer, place an "X" in this box: ☐

FORM FDA 3500 (10/05)   Submission of a report does not constitute an admission that medical personnel or the product caused or contributed to the event.

ADVICE ABOUT VOLUNTARY REPORTING
Detailed instructions available at: http://www.fda.gov/medwatch/report/consumer/instruct.htm

Report adverse events, product problems or product use errors with:

- Medications *(drugs or biologics)*
- Medical devices *(including in-vitro diagnostics)*
- Combination products *(medication & medical devices)*
- Human cells, tissues, and cellular and tissue-based products
- Special nutritional products *(dietary supplements, medical foods, infant formulas)*
- Cosmetics

Report product problems - quality, performance or safety concerns such as:

- Suspected counterfeit product
- Suspected contamination
- Questionable stability
- Defective components
- Poor packaging or labeling
- Therapeutic failures (product didn't work)

Report SERIOUS adverse events. An event is serious when the patient outcome is:

- Death
- Life-threatening
- Hospitalization - initial or prolonged
- Disability or permanent damage
- Congenital anomaly/birth defect
- Required intervention to prevent permanent impairment or damage
- Other serious (important medical events)

Report even if:

- You're not certain the product caused the event
- You don't have all the details

How to report:

- Just fill in the sections that apply to your report
- Use section D for all products except medical devices
- Attach additional pages if needed
- Use a separate form for each patient
- Report either to FDA or the manufacturer *(or both)*

Other methods of reporting:

- 1-800-FDA-0178 – To FAX report
- 1-800-FDA-1088 – To report by phone
- www.fda.gov/medwatch/report.htm – To report online

If your report involves a serious adverse event with a device and it occurred in a facility outside a doctor's office, that facility may be legally required to report to FDA and/or the manufacturer. Please notify the person in that facility who would handle such reporting.

If your report involves a serious adverse event with a vaccine call 1-800-822-7967 to report.

Confidentiality: The patient's identity is held in strict confidence by FDA and protected to the fullest extent of the law. FDA will not disclose the reporter's identity in response to a request from the public, pursuant to the Freedom of Information Act. The reporter's identity, including the identity of a self-reporter, may be shared with the manufacturer unless requested otherwise.

The public reporting burden for this collection of information has been estimated to average 36 minutes per response, including the time for reviewing instructions, searching existing data sources, gathering and maintaining the data needed, and completing and reviewing the collection of information. Send comments regarding this burden estimate or any other aspect of this collection of information, including suggestions for reducing this burden to:

Department of Health and Human Services *Food and Drug Administration - MedWatch* *10903 New Hampshire Avenue* *Building 22, Mail Stop 4447* *Silver Spring, MD 20993-0002*	*Please DO NOT* *RETURN this form* *to this address.*	*OMB statement:* *"An agency may not conduct or sponsor, and a person is not required to respond to, a collection of information unless it displays a currently valid OMB control number."*

U.S. DEPARTMENT OF HEALTH AND HUMAN SERVICES
Food and Drug Administration

FORM FDA 3500 (10/05) (Back)   Please Use Address Provided Below – Fold in Thirds, Tape and Mail

----

DEPARTMENT OF
HEALTH & HUMAN SERVICES

Public Health Service
Food and Drug Administration
Rockville, MD 20857

Official Business
Penalty for Private Use $300

BUSINESS REPLY MAIL
FIRST CLASS MAIL   PERMIT NO. 946   ROCKVILLE MD

MEDWATCH
The FDA Safety Information and Adverse Event Reporting Program
Food and Drug Administration
5600 Fishers Lane
Rockville, MD 20852-9787

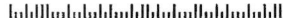

Appendix 17–5

USP-ISMP Medication Error Reporting Program (MERP) Form

USP MEDICATION ERRORS REPORTING PROGRAM
Presented in cooperation with the Institute for Safe Medication Practices
USP is an FDA MEDWATCH partner

Reporters should not provide any individually identifiable health information, including names of practitioners, names of patients, names of healthcare facilities, or dates of birth (age is acceptable).

Date and time of event:

Please describe the error. Include description/sequence of events, type of staff involved, and work environment (e.g., code situation, change of shift, short staffing, no 24-hr. pharmacy, floor stock). If more space is needed, please attach a separate page.

Did the error reach the patient?　☐ Yes ☐ No

Was the incorrect medication, dose, or dosage form administered to or taken by the patient?　☐ Yes ☐ No

Circle the appropriate Error Outcome Category (select one—see back for details): A　B　C　D　E　F　G　H　I

Describe the direct result of the error on the patient (e.g., death, type of harm, additional patient monitoring).

Indicate the possible error cause(s) and contributing factor(s) (e.g., abbreviation, similar names, distractions, etc.).

Indicate the location of the error (e.g., hospital, outpatient or community pharmacy, clinic, nursing home, patient's home, etc.).

What type of staff or healthcare practitioner made the initial error?

Indicate if other practitioner(s) were also involved in the error (type of staff perpetuating error).

What type of staff or healthcare practitioner discovered the error or recognized the potential for error?

How was the error (or potential for error) discovered/intercepted?

If available, provide patient age, gender, diagnosis. Do not provide any patient identifiers.

Please complete the following for the product(s) involved. (if more space is needed for additional products, please attach a separate page.)

	Product #1	Product #2
Brand/Product Name (If Applicable)		
Generic Name		
Manufacturer		
Labeler		
Dosage Form		
Strength/Concentration		
Type and Size of Container		

Reports are most useful when relevant materials such as product label, copy of prescription/order, etc., can be reviewed.
Can these materials be provided?　☐ Yes ☐ No　　Please specify:

Suggest any recommendations to prevent recurrence of this error, or describe policies or procedures you instituted or plan to institute to prevent future similar errors.

	( )	( )
Name and Title/Profession	Telephone Number	Fax Number
Facility/Address and Zip		E-mail
Address/Zip (where correspondence should be sent)		

Your name, contact information, and a copy of this report are routinely shared with the Institute for Safe Medication Practices (ISMP). Copies of reports will be sent to third parties such as the manufacturer/labeler, and to the Food and Drug Administration (FDA). You have the option of including your name on these copies.

In addition to releasing my name and contact information to ISMP, USP may release my identity to these third parties as follows (check boxes that apply):

☐ The manufacturer and/or labeler as listed above　☐ FDA　☐ Other persons requesting a copy of this report　☐ Anonymous to all third parties

Signature	Date

Return to: USP CAPS 12601 Twinbrook Parkway Rockville, MD 20852-1790	Submit via the Web at www.usp.org/mer Call Toll Free: 800-23-ERROR (800-233-7767) or FAX: 301-816-8532	Date Received by USP	File Access Number

PSF116G

WEPDF
©USPC 2003

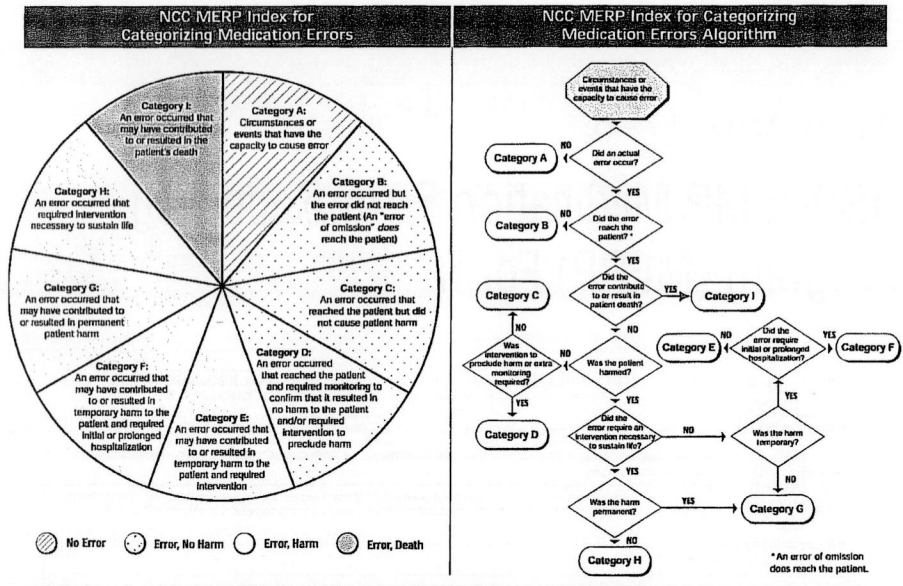

NCC MERP Index for Categorizing Medication Errors / NCC MERP Index for Categorizing Medication Errors Algorithm

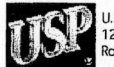 No Error   Error, No Harm   Error, Harm   Error, Death

© 2003 National Coordinating Council for Medication Error Reporting and Prevention

Full-size copies are available: INDEX—www.nccmerp.org/010612_color_index.pdf; ALGORITHM—www.nccmerp.org/010612_color_algo.pdf

National Coordinating Council for Medication Error Reporting and Prevention Definitions

Harm
Impairment of the physical, emotional, or psychological function or structure of the body and/or pain resulting therefrom.

Monitoring
To observe or record relevant physiological or psychological signs.

Intervention
May include change in therapy or active medical/surgical treatment.

Intervention Necessary to Sustain Life
Includes cardiovascular and respiratory support (e.g., CPR, defibrillation, intubation, etc.).

 U.S. Pharmacopeia
12601 Twinbrook Parkway
Rockville, MD 20852-1790

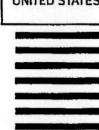

NO POSTAGE
NECESSARY
IF MAILED
IN THE
UNITED STATES

BUSINESS REPLY MAIL
FIRST-CLASS MAIL PERMIT NO 39 ROCKVILLE MD

POSTAGE WILL BE PAID BY ADDRESSEE:
DIANE D COUSINS RPh
THE USP CENTER FOR THE ADVANCEMENT OF PATIENT SAFETY
12601 TWINBROOK PARKWAY
ROCKVILLE MD 20897-5211

18-1

Appendix 18-1

Investigational New Drug Application

Form Approved: OMB No. 0910-0014.
Expiration Date: January 31, 2006
See OMB Statement on Reverse.

DEPARTMENT OF HEALTH AND HUMAN SERVICES
FOOD AND DRUG ADMINISTRATION

INVESTIGATIONAL NEW DRUG APPLICATION (IND)
(TITLE 21, CODE OF FEDERAL REGULATIONS (CFR) PART 312)

NOTE: No drug may be shipped or clinical investigation begun until an IND for that investigation is in effect (21 CFR 312.40).

1. NAME OF SPONSOR

2. DATE OF SUBMISSION

3. ADDRESS *(Number, Street, City, State and Zip Code)*

4. TELEPHONE NUMBER *(Include Area Code)*

5. NAME(S) OF DRUG *(Include all available names: Trade, Generic, Chemical, Code)*

6. IND NUMBER *(If previously assigned)*

7. INDICATION(S) *(Covered by this submission)*

8. PHASE(S) OF CLINICAL INVESTIGATION TO BE CONDUCTED:
☐ PHASE 1   ☐ PHASE 2   ☐ PHASE 3   ☐ OTHER
(Specify)

9. LIST NUMBERS OF ALL INVESTIGATIONAL NEW DRUG APPLICATIONS (21 CFR Part 312), NEW DRUG OR ANTIBIOTIC APPLICATIONS *(21 CFR Part 314)*, DRUG MASTER FILES *(21 CFR Part 314.420)*, AND PRODUCT LICENSE APPLICATIONS *(21 CFR Part 601)* REFERRED TO IN THIS APPLICATION.

10. ***IND submission should be consecutively numbered. The initial IND should be numbered "Serial number: 0000." The next submission (e.g., amendment, report, or correspondence) should be numbered "Serial Number: 0001." Subsequent submissions should be numbered consecutively in the order in which they are submitted.***

SERIAL NUMBER

11. THIS SUBMISSION CONTAINS THE FOLLOWING: *(Check all that apply)*
☐ INITIAL INVESTIGATIONAL NEW DRUG APPLICATION (IND)   ☐ RESPONSE TO CLINICAL HOLD

PROTOCOL AMENDMENT(S):
☐ NEW PROTOCOL
☐ CHANGE IN PROTOCOL
☐ NEW INVESTIGATOR

INFORMATION AMENDMENT(S):
☐ CHEMISTRY/MICROBIOLOGY
☐ PHARMACOLOGY/TOXICOLOGY
☐ CLINICAL

IND SAFETY REPORT(S):
☐ INITIAL WRITTEN REPORT
☐ FOLLOW-UP TO A WRITTEN REPORT

☐ RESPONSE TO FDA REQUEST FOR INFORMATION   ☐ ANNUAL REPORT   ☐ GENERAL CORRESPONDENCE

☐ REQUEST FOR REINSTATEMENT OF IND THAT IS WITHDRAWN, INACTIVATED, TERMINATED OR DISCONTINUED   ☐ OTHER
(Specify)

CHECK ONLY IF APPLICABLE

JUSTIFICATION STATEMENT MUST BE SUBMITTED WITH APPLICATION FOR ANY CHECKED BELOW. REFER TO THE CITED CFR SECTION FOR FURTHER INFORMATION.
☐ TREATMENT IND 21 CFR 312.35(b)   ☐ TREATMENT PROTOCOL 21 CFR 312.35(a)   ☐ CHARGE REQUEST/NOTIFICATION 21 CFR 312.7(d)

FOR FDA USE ONLY

CDR/DBIND/DGD RECEIPT STAMP	DDR RECEIPT STAMP	DIVISION ASSIGNMENT:
		IND NUMBER ASSIGNED:

FORM FDA 1571 (3/05)   PREVIOUS EDITION IS OBSOLETE.   PAGE 1 OF 2

PSC Media Arts (301) 443-1090   EF

12.
CONTENTS OF APPLICATION
This application contains the following items: *(Check all that apply)*

- [ ] 1. Form FDA 1571 *[21 CFR 312.23(a)(1)]*
- [ ] 2. Table of Contents *[21 CFR 312.23(a)(2)]*
- [ ] 3. Introductory statement *[21 CFR 312.23(a)(3)]*
- [ ] 4. General investigational plan *[21 CFR 312.23(a)(3)]*
- [ ] 5. Investigator's brochure *[21 CFR 312.23(a)(5)]*
- [ ] 6. Protocol(s) *[21 CFR 312.23(a)(6)]*
  - [ ] a. Study protocol(s) *[21 CFR 312.23(a)(6)]*
  - [ ] b. Investigator data *[21 CFR 312.23(a)(6)(iii)(b)]* or completed Form(s) FDA 1572
  - [ ] c. Facilities data *[21 CFR 312.23(a)(6)(iii)(b)]* or completed Form(s) FDA 1572
  - [ ] d. Institutional Review Board data *[21 CFR 312.23(a)(6)(iii)(b)]* or completed Form(s) FDA 1572
- [ ] 7. Chemistry, manufacturing, and control data *[21 CFR 312.23(a)(7)]*
  - [ ] Environmental assessment or claim for exclusion *[21 CFR 312.23(a)(7)(iv)(e)]*
- [ ] 8. Pharmacology and toxicology data *[21 CFR 312.23(a)(8)]*
- [ ] 9. Previous human experience *[21 CFR 312.23(a)(9)]*
- [ ] 10. Additional information *[21 CFR 312.23(a)(10)]*

13. IS ANY PART OF THE CLINICAL STUDY TO BE CONDUCTED BY A CONTRACT RESEARCH ORGANIZATION? [ ] YES [ ] NO

IF YES, WILL ANY SPONSOR OBLIGATIONS BE TRANSFERRED TO THE CONTRACT RESEARCH ORGANIZATION? [ ] YES [ ] NO

IF YES, ATTACH A STATEMENT CONTAINING THE NAME AND ADDRESS OF THE CONTRACT RESEARCH ORGANIZATION, IDENTIFICATION OF THE CLINICAL STUDY, AND A LISTING OF THE OBLIGATIONS TRANSFERRED.

14. NAME AND TITLE OF THE PERSON RESPONSIBLE FOR MONITORING THE CONDUCT AND PROGRESS OF THE CLINICAL INVESTIGATIONS

15. NAME(S) AND TITLE(S) OF THE PERSON(S) RESPONSIBLE FOR REVIEW AND EVALUATION OF INFORMATION RELEVANT TO THE SAFETY OF THE DRUG

I agree not to begin clinical investigations until 30 days after FDA's receipt of the IND unless I receive earlier notification by FDA that the studies may begin. I also agree not to begin or continue clinical investigations covered by the IND if those studies are placed on clinical hold. I agree that an Institutional Review Board (IRB) that complies with the requirements set fourth in 21 CFR Part 56 will be responsible for initial and continuing review and approval of each of the studies in the proposed clinical investigation. I agree to conduct the investigation in accordance with all other applicable regulatory requirements.

16. NAME OF SPONSOR OR SPONSOR'S AUTHORIZED REPRESENTATIVE

17. SIGNATURE OF SPONSOR OR SPONSOR'S AUTHORIZED REPRESENTATIVE

18. ADDRESS *(Number, Street, City, State and Zip Code)*

19. TELEPHONE NUMBER *(Include Area Code)*

20. DATE

(WARNING: A willfully false statement is a criminal offense. U.S.C. Title 18, Sec. 1001.)

Public reporting burden for this collection of information is estimated to average 100 hours per response, including the time for reviewing instructions, searching existing data sources, gathering and maintaining the data needed, and completing reviewing the collection of information. Send comments regarding this burden estimate or any other aspect of this collection of information, including suggestions for reducing this burden to:

Department of Health and Human Services
Food and Drug Administration
Center for Drug Evaluation and Research
Central Document Room
5901-B Ammendale Road
Beltsville, MD 20705-1266

Department of Health and Human Services
Food and Drug Administration
Center for Biologics Evaluation and Research (HFM-99)
1401 Rockville Pike
Rockville, MD 20852-1448
Please DO NOT RETURN this application to this address.

"An agency may not conduct or sponsor, and a person is not required to respond to, a collection of information unless it displays a currently valid OMB control number."

Appendix 18–2

Statement of Investigator

DEPARTMENT OF HEALTH AND HUMAN SERVICES FOOD AND DRUG ADMINISTRATION **STATEMENT OF INVESTIGATOR** *(TITLE 21, CODE OF FEDERAL REGULATIONS (CFR) PART 312)* (See instructions on reverse side.)	Form Approved: OMB No. 0910-0014. Expiration Date: January 31, 2006. *See OMB Statement on Reverse.* NOTE: No investigator may participate in an investigation until he/she provides the sponsor with a completed, signed Statement of Investigator, Form FDA 1572 (21 CFR 312.53(c)).

1. NAME AND ADDRESS OF INVESTIGATOR

2. EDUCATION, TRAINING, AND EXPERIENCE THAT QUALIFIES THE INVESTIGATOR AS AN EXPERT IN THE CLINICAL INVESTIGATION OF THE DRUG FOR THE USE UNDER INVESTIGATION. ONE OF THE FOLLOWING IS ATTACHED.

   ☐ CURRICULUM VITAE   ☐ OTHER STATEMENT OF QUALIFICATIONS

3. NAME AND ADDRESS OF ANY MEDICAL SCHOOL, HOSPITAL OR OTHER RESEARCH FACILITY WHERE THE CLINICAL INVESTIGATION(S) WILL BE CONDUCTED.

4. NAME AND ADDRESS OF ANY CLINICAL LABORATORY FACILITIES TO BE USED IN THE STUDY.

5. NAME AND ADDRESS OF THE INSTITUTIONAL REVIEW BOARD (IRB) THAT IS RESPONSIBLE FOR REVIEW AND APPROVAL OF THE STUDY(IES).

6. NAMES OF THE SUBINVESTIGATORS *(e.g., research fellows, residents, associates)* WHO WILL BE ASSISTING THE INVESTIGATOR IN THE CONDUCT OF THE INVESTIGATION(S).

7. NAME AND CODE NUMBER, IF ANY, OF THE PROTOCOL(S) IN THE IND FOR THE STUDY(IES) TO BE CONDUCTED BY THE INVESTIGATOR.

FORM FDA 1572 (3/05)   PREVIOUS EDITION IS OBSOLETE.   PAGE 1 OF 2

PSC Media Arts (301) 443-1090   EF

8. ATTACH THE FOLLOWING CLINICAL PROTOCOL INFORMATION:

☐ FOR PHASE 1 INVESTIGATIONS, A GENERAL OUTLINE OF THE PLANNED INVESTIGATION INCLUDING THE ESTIMATED DURATION OF THE STUDY AND THE MAXIMUM NUMBER OF SUBJECTS THAT WILL BE INVOLVED.

☐ FOR PHASE 2 OR 3 INVESTIGATIONS, AN OUTLINE OF THE STUDY PROTOCOL INCLUDING AN APPROXIMATION OF THE NUMBER OF SUBJECTS TO BE TREATED WITH THE DRUG AND THE NUMBER TO BE EMPLOYED AS CONTROLS, IF ANY; THE CLINICAL USES TO BE INVESTIGATED; CHARACTERISTICS OF SUBJECTS BY AGE, SEX, AND CONDITION; THE KIND OF CLINICAL OBSERVATIONS AND LABORATORY TESTS TO BE CONDUCTED; THE ESTIMATED DURATION OF THE STUDY; AND COPIES OR A DESCRIPTION OF CASE REPORT FORMS TO BE USED.

9. COMMITMENTS:

I agree to conduct the study(ies) in accordance with the relevant, current protocol(s) and will only make changes in a protocol after notifying the sponsor, except when necessary to protect the safety, rights, or welfare of subjects.

I agree to personally conduct or supervise the described investigation(s).

I agree to inform any patients, or any persons used as controls, that the drugs are being used for investigational purposes and I will ensure that the requirements relating to obtaining informed consent in 21 CFR Part 50 and institutional review board (IRB) review and approval in 21 CFR Part 56 are met.

I agree to report to the sponsor adverse experiences that occur in the course of the investigation(s) in accordance with 21 CFR 312.64.

I have read and understand the information in the investigator's brochure, including the potential risks and side effects of the drug.

I agree to ensure that all associates, colleagues, and employees assisting in the conduct of the study(ies) are informed about their obligations in meeting the above commitments.

I agree to maintain adequate and accurate records in accordance with 21 CFR 312.62 and to make those records available for inspection in accordance with 21 CFR 312.68.

I will ensure that an IRB that complies with the requirements of 21 CFR Part 56 will be responsible for the initial and continuing review and approval of the clinical investigation. I also agree to promptly report to the IRB all changes in the research activity and all unanticipated problems involving risks to human subjects or others. Additionally, I will not make any changes in the research without IRB approval, except where necessary to eliminate apparent immediate hazards to human subjects.

I agree to comply with all other requirements regarding the obligations of clinical investigators and all other pertinent requirements in 21 CFR Part 312.

INSTRUCTIONS FOR COMPLETING FORM FDA 1572
STATEMENT OF INVESTIGATOR:

1. Complete all sections. Attach a separate page if additional space is needed.

2. Attach curriculum vitae or other statement of qualifications as described in Section 2.

3. Attach protocol outline as described in Section 8.

4. Sign and date below.

5. FORWARD THE COMPLETED FORM AND ATTACHMENTS TO THE SPONSOR. The sponsor will incorporate this information along with other technical data into an Investigational New Drug Application (IND).

10. SIGNATURE OF INVESTIGATOR	11. DATE

(WARNING: A willfully false statement is a criminal offense. U.S.C. Title 18, Sec. 1001.)

Public reporting burden for this collection of information is estimated to average 100 hours per response, including the time for reviewing instructions, searching existing data sources, gathering and maintaining the data needed, and completing reviewing the collection of information. Send comments regarding this burden estimate or any other aspect of this collection of information, including suggestions for reducing this burden to:

Department of Health and Human Services	Department of Health and Human Services	
Food and Drug Administration	Food and Drug Administration	"An agency may not conduct or sponsor, and a
Center for Drug Evaluation and Research	Center for Biologics Evaluation and Research (HFM-99)	person is not required to respond to, a collection
Central Document Room	1401 Rockville Pike	of information unless it displays a currently valid
5901-B Ammendale Road	Rockville, MD 20852-1448	OMB control number."
Beltsville, MD 20705-1266		

Please DO NOT RETURN this application to this address.

FORM FDA 1572 (3/05)   PAGE 2 OF 2

18-3

Appendix 18–3

Protocol Medication Economic Analysis

Date:
Protocol title:
Study chairperson:

Hospital Cost Analysis

Drug	Hospital Cost per Cycle*	Number of Cycles	Total Cost per Patient	Number of Patients	Total Protocol Cost	Annual Cost
Primary Therapy						
Supportive Care						

*When applicable, doses calculated on 1.7 m^2 or 70 kg at initial dose level and costs include infusion fluids, administration sets, and tubing.

Patient Charge Analysis

Drug	Patient Charge per Cycle*	Number of Cycles	Total Charge per Patient	Number of Patients	Total Patient Billing
Primary Therapy					
Supportive Care					

*When applicable, charges include infusion fluids, administration sets, and tubing.

Reimbursement Risk

Drug	FDA Labeled	Compendium

Comments

Summary
_____
_____

18-4

Appendix 18-4

Investigational Drug Accountability Record

Form approved
OMB No. 0925-0240
Expires: 6/30/91

National Institutes of Health
National Cancer Institute

Investigational Drug Accountability Record

PAGE NO. _____

CONTROL RECORD ☐

SATELLITE RECORD ☐

Name of Institution | Protocol No. (NCI)

Drug Name, Dose Form and Strength

Protocol Title | Dispensing Area

Investigation

Line No.	Date	Patient's Initials	Patient's I.D. Number	Dose	Quantity Dispensed or Received	Balance Forward / Balance	Manufacturer and Lot No.	Recorder's Initials
1.								
2.								
3.								
4.								
5.								
6.								
7.								
8.								
9.								
10.								
11.								
12.								
13.								
14.								
15.								
16.								
17.								
18.								
19.								
20.								
21.								
22.								
23.								
24.								

NIH-2564
9-85

Glossary

Abstracting service   A database that provides abstracts and citations for journal articles.

Absolute risk reduction   The difference in the percentage of subjects developing the adverse event in the control group versus subjects in the intervention group. Also refers to the number of subjects spared the adverse event by taking the intervention compared to the control.

Abstracts   A synopsis (usually of 250 words or less) of the most important aspect(s) of an article.

Academic detailing   Process by which a healt hcare educator visits a physician to provide a 15 to 20 minute educational intervention on a specific topic. Information provided is based on the physician's prescribing patterns and evidence-based medicine.

Action-guides   A term coined by Beauchamp and Childress to refer to a hierarchical approach to analysis of an ethical issue when forming particular judgments about the issue.

Adjunctive therapy   Inclusion of a treatment that can affect the study outcome, but is equally distributed between both the intervention and control groups (e.g., controlled diet in a study measures lipid reduction therapy).

Adverse drug event (ADE)   Any injury caused by a medicine. This includes adverse drug reactions and medication errors.

Adverse drug reaction (ADR)   The Food and Drug Administration's (FDA) definition of ADRs is: "any adverse event associated with the use of a drug in humans, whether or not considered drug related, including the following: adverse event occurring in the course of the use of a drug product in professional practice; an adverse event occurring from drug overdose, whether accidental or intentional; an adverse event occurring from drug abuse; an adverse event occurring from drug withdrawal; and any significant failure of expected pharmacologic action." Adverse drug reactions also include drug interactions. Several other definitions are available; many of those are discussed in Chap. 17.

Agenda for change   An initiative adopted by the JCAHO in 1986 intended to improve standards by focusing on key functions of quality of care, to monitor the performance of health care organizations using indicators, to improve the relevance and quality of the survey process, and to enhance the accuracy and value of JCAHO accreditation.

Aggregator   A piece of software that is used to automatically collect information from RSS and weblog sites, which allows the user to look at material from many of those sites at one time and in one place.

Alpha (level of significance)   The probability of a false positive result in a study.

Analytic research   Quantitative research conducted in a controlled environment to determine cause and effect relationships.

Ancillary therapy   Inclusion of a treatment, which can directly affect the study outcome, that is not equally distributed between the intervention and control groups (e.g., antacid use in a study measuring reduction of heartburn symptoms between two acid-suppressive agents).

A priori   In reference to clinical trials, to do something prior to initiation of the study.

Article proposal   A letter asking the publisher whether he or she would be interested in possibly publishing something on a particular topic written by the person(s) who are inquiring.

Aspect of care   A term used in quality assurance programs to indicate the title that describes the area being evaluated.

Attributable risk   A statistical technique used in follow-up studies to determine the risk associated with exposure to a certain factor and the resultant developement of a disease state. Attributable risk estimates the number of disease cases per number of exposures to the factor.

Beta   The probability of a false negative result in a study.

Bioequivalence studies   Research that evaluates whether products are similar in rate and extent of absorption.

Bibliography   A list of references, usually seen at the end of a professionally written document.

Black Letter Rules   Principles of law that are known generally to all and are free from doubt and ambiguity. Also known as hornbook law, since they are in a format that would probably be enunciated in a hornbook.

Blinding   The procedures used in a clinical study to ensure that the investigator, subject, or both are unaware of which treatment is being administered. In a single-blind study, either the investigator or the subject does not know the treatment being received and in a double-blind study both the investigator and the subject are unaware of the treatment being received. Triple-blinding refers to the subjects, investigators, and the investigators analyzing the study results (either interim or final) being unaware of the treatment being received.

Blog   See weblog.

Body area network (BAN)   A multiple device, interconnected computer system carried on a person. Sometimes referred to as a wearable computer.

Boolean operators (logical operators)   Words used to combine search terms (i.e., AND, OR, and NOT) when using computerized databases.

Case law   The aggregate of reported cases; the law pertaining to a particular subject as formed by adjudged cases.

Case-control study   A retrospective study where a group of subjects (i.e., cases) with a particular characteristic (e.g., disease) is compared to a group (i.e., controls) without the characteristic to determine the influence of certain factors on development of the characteristic. Also, called a trohoc study.

CD-ROM   See compact disc-read only memory.

Clinical investigation   Any experiment in which a drug is administered or dispensed to one or more human subjects. Relating to investigational drugs, an experiment is any use of a drug (except for the use of a marketed drug) in the course of medical practice. While there are many other definitions, this is the Food and Drug Administration's definition and would seem the most appropriate one to use given the nature of this topic. Please note that the Food and Drug Administration does not regulate the practice of medicine and prescribers are (as far as the agency is concerned) free to use any marketed drug for "off-label use."

Clinical practice guidelines   The United States Department of Health and Human Services, Public Health Service, Agency for Health Care Policy and Research (AHCPR) defines clinical practice guidelines as "systematically developed statements to assist practitioner and patient decisions about appropriate health care for specific clinical circumstances."

Clinical Safety Officer (CSO)   Also known as the Regulatory Management Officer (RMO). This will be the sponsor's Food and Drug Administration contact person. Generally, the CSO/RMO assigned to a drug's Investigational New Drug Application will also be assigned to the New Drug Application.

Clinical significance   The clinical importance of data generated in a study, irrespective of statistical results. Usually refers to the application of study results in clinical practice. Also, can be called clinical meaningfulness.

Closed formulary   A drug formulary that restricts the drugs available within an institution or available under a third-party plan.

Coauthor   Any individual who writes a portion of an article, chapter, book, and so forth. This includes individuals other than the primary author, whose name is normally listed first on a publication.

Cohort study   See follow-up study.

Community rule   See locality rule.

Compact disc-read only memory (CD-ROM)   A storage and retrieval system for large quantities of computerized data. Modern computers usually cannot only read the data on these disks, but usually can write new data to disks designed to accept that new data.

Comparative negligence   The allocation of responsibility for damages incurred between the plaintiff and defendant, based on relative negligence of the two; the reduction of the damages to be recovered by the negligent plaintiff in proportion to his fault.

Compliance   A measure of how well instructions are followed. In a study, compliance refers to how well a patient follows instructions for medication administration and how well the investigator follows the study protocol.

Computer network   An interconnection of computers and computer-related devices (e.g., printers and modems) that allows the devices to interchange data, electronic mail, programs, and other files. In addition, a network allows sharing of peripheral devices, such as printers, modems, fax boards, and so forth. Normally, this interconnection is via a dedicated wiring system (other than telephone/modem communication), however, wireless connections are becoming common.

Concurrent indicator   An indicator used in any quality assurance program that determines whether quality is acceptable while an action is being taken or care is being given.

Confidence intervals   A measurement of the variability of study data. A 95% confidence interval is a numerical range that contains the true value for the population 95% of the time.

Consequentialist theories   Those moral theories that describe actions or decisions as morally right or wrong based on their consequences.

Continuous quality improvement (CQI)   The term given to the methodologies used in the process of Total Quality Management (TQM). Efforts to improve quality are part of each participant's responsibilities on an ongoing basis.

Contract Research Organization (CRO)   An individual or organization, which is the sponsor of a investigational new drug (IND) or new drug application (NDA), which assumes one or more of the obligations of the sponsor through an independent contractual agreement.

Control group   The group of test animals or humans that receive a placebo or active control. For most preclinical and clinical trials, the Food and Drug Administration will require that this group receive placebo (commonly referred to as the placebo control). However, some studies may have an active control that generally consists of an available (standard of care) treatment modality. An active control may, with the concurrence of the Food and Drug Administration, be used in studies where it would be considered unethical to use a placebo. A historical control is one in which a group of previously treated patients is compared to a matched set of patients receiving the new therapy. A historical control might be used in cases where the disease is consistently fatal (e.g., AIDS).

Controlled clinical trial   Prospective study that directly compares an intervention to a control to measure a difference in effect (outcome); best study design to measure a cause and effect relationship between the intervention and outcome.

Controls   A treatment (placebo, active, historical) used for comparison in a study to measure a difference in effect against an investigational agent. The investigator usually wishes to determine superiority of a new treatment over the control in terms of efficacy and safety.

Copayment   Payment made by an individual who has health insurance at the time the service is received to offset the cost of care. Copayments may vary depending on the service rendered.

Cost-benefit study   A study where monetary value is given for both costs and benefits associated with a drug or service. The results are expressed as a ratio (benefit to cost) and the ratio is used to determine the economic value of the drug or service.

Cost-effectiveness study   A study where the cost of a drug or service is compared to its therapeutic impact. Cost-effectiveness studies determine the relative efficiency of various drugs or services in achieving desired therapeutic outcomes.

Cost-minimization study   A study that compares costs of drugs or services that have been determined to have equivalent therapeutic outcomes.

Cost-utility study   A study that relates therapeutic outcomes to both costs of drugs or services and patient preferences and measures cost per unit of utility. Utility is the amount of satisfaction obtained from a drug or service.

Coverage error   See sampling error.

Coverage rules   Criteria for specific drugs determined by the health plan in conjunction with the pharmacy and therapeutics committee that is used to determine if a prescription is covered. Criteria are based on evidence-based medicine.

Criteria   A statement of the activity to be measured and evaluated. Also see indicator.

Crossover study   A study where each subject receives all study treatments, and endpoints during the various treatments are compared.

Cross-sectional study   A study where measurements are taken at a single point in time.

CQI   See continuous quality improvement.

Dechallenge   In relation to adverse drug reactions, this occurs when the drug is taken away or the dose is reduced and the patient is monitored to determine if the ADR abates or decreases in intensity.

Deep pocket   Practical consideration that involves the naming of additional codefendants in personal injury lawsuits to provide assurance to the plaintiff that there will be sufficient assets to pay the judgment.

Delta   The amount of difference in the outcome variable that the investigators wish to detect between intervention and control groups in a study.

Deontological theories   Proposes that intrinsic qualities of an act or decision assert its moral rightness or wrongness rather than consequences.

Descriptive research   Quantitative research that describes naturally occurring events.

Descriptive statistics   Statistics that describe data such as medians, modes, and standard deviations.

DIC   See drug information center.

Digital video disk (DVD)   Also known as Digital Versatile Disk. A disk that physically resembles a CD-ROM, but allows the storage of much larger amounts of data. It requires a special reading/writing device in a computer, although this device may also be combined with that used for CD-ROMs. DVDs have been used to a large extent to store and replay movies; however, they are now being used on computers to store large amounts of computer data, particularly large multimedia files.

DIS   See drug information service.

Drug formularies   See formulary.

Drug formulary system   See formulary system.

Drug informatics   A technologically advanced version of drug information. This often denotes the electronic management of drug information.

Drug information   The provision of unbiased, well-referenced, and critically evaluated information on any aspect of pharmacy practice.

Drug information center (DIC)   A physical location where pharmacists have the resources (e.g., books, journals, and computer systems) to provide drug information. This area is generally staffed by a pharmacist specializing in drug information, but may be used by a variety of the pharmacy staff or other individuals.

Drug information service (DIS)   A professional service providing drug information. This service is normally located in a drug information center.

Drug interaction   The Food and Drug Administration defines this as "a pharmacologic response that cannot be explained by the action of a simple drug, but is due to two or more drugs acting simultaneously."

Drug master file (DMF)   Reference on file with the Food and Drug Administration that contains information regarding the drug. There are five different types of DMF. The one that is most commonly used when filing an IND is the CMC-DMF (Chemistry, Manufacturing, and Controls-Drug Master File), which contains information regarding the chemistry, manufacturing, and controls of the drug.

Drug product   The final dosage form, prepared from the drug substance.

Drug regimen review (DRR)   The monthly evaluation of nursing home charts by pharmacists.

Drug substance   Bulk compound from which the drug product is prepared.

Drug use/usage evaluation (DUE)   See medication use evaluation.

Drug utilization review (DUR)   A program related to outpatient pharmacy services designed to educate physicians and pharmacists in identifying and reducing the frequency and patterns of fraud, abuse, gross overuse, or inappropriate or medically unnecessary care. DUR is typically retrospective in nature and utilizes claims data as its primary source of information.

Duty   A moral or legal obligation.

Editorial   Commentary usually prepared by an expert identifying the strengths and limitations plus application of the results of a clinical trial that is published in the same journal issue as the study.

Electronic mail (e-mail)   Brief messages sent from one computer to another, similar in use to interoffice memos. This serves as a quick, informal method of written communication. Also, e-mail may be used to send other items, such as word processing files, graphics, video, and so forth to others.

E-mail   See electronic mail.

Endpoint   A parameter measured in a clinical study. The primary endpoint is the major variable analyzed and reflects the main objective of the study. Secondary endpoints are additional variables of interest monitored during clinical studies.

Ethical theories   Integrated bodies of principles and rules that may include mediating rules that govern cases of conflicts.

Ethics (defined by AACP)   Philosophical inquiry into the moral dimensions of human conduct.

Ethics (defined by Beauchamp and Childress)   A generic term for several ways of examining the moral life.

Exclusion criteria   Characteristics of subject's that, if present, prohibit entrance into the study.

Exploratory research   Research of a qualitative nature in which the investigators examines an unknown area to generate hypotheses.

Extemporaneous compounding   The practice of compounding prescriptions from a list of several ingredients, usually performed by a pharmacist.

False negatives   Individuals with the disease that were incorrectly identified as being disease-free by the test.

False positives   Individuals without the disease that were incorrectly identified as having the disease by the test.

File transfer protocol (FTP)   A method to transfer files from one computer to another.

Follow-up study   A study where subjects exposed to a factor and those not exposed to the factor are followed forward in time and compared to determine the factor's influence on disease state development. Also called a cohort study.

Food and Drug Administration (FDA)   The agency of the U.S. government that is responsible for ensuring the safety and efficacy of all drugs on the market. This agency approves drugs for marketing.

Formulary   A continually revised list of medications that are readily available for use within an institution or from a third-party payer (e.g., insurance company and government) that reflects the current clinical judgment of the medical staff or the payer.

Formulary system   A method used to develop a drug formulary. It is sometimes even thought of as a philosophy.

Galley proofs   A copy of a written work as it is to be published. The purpose of this document is to allow the author(s) to make a final check to insure everything is correct before actual publication.

Health Insurance Portability and Accountability Act of 1996 (HIPAA)   This act includes privacy restrictions for electronic health records.

Health Maintenance Organization (HMO)   Form of health insurance whereby the member prepays a premium for the HMO's health services, which generally includes inpatient and outpatient care.

Health plan employer data and information set (HEDIS)   A set of performance measures used to compare managed health care plans.

Health-related quality of life (HR-QOL)   A general term for the impact of many dimensions of health status (such as physical, social and cognitive functioning, mental health, symptom tolerance, overall well-being, and so forth) on quality of life.

HIPAA   See Health Insurance Portability and Accountability Act of 1996.

Historical data   Data used in research that was collected prior to the decision to conduct the study (e.g., medical records, insurance information, and Medicaid databases).

HMO   See Health Maintenance Organization.

Homogenicity tests   Tests used when conducting a meta-analysis to determine the similarity of studies whose results were combined for the analysis.

https   A secure form of http, used to transmit confidential information, such as credit card numbers.

Hypertext transfer protocol (http)   A method by which information is encoded and transmitted on the World Wide Web.

Hypothesis   The researchers' assumptions regarding probable study results. The research hypothesis or alternative hypothesis (H_A) is the expectations of the researchers in terms of study results. The null hypothesis (H_0) is the no difference hypothesis, which assumes equality amongst study treatments. The null hypothesis is the basis for all statistical tests and must be rejected in order to accept the research hypothesis.

Incidence rate   Measures the probability that a healthy person will develop a disease within a specified period of time. It is the number of new cases of disease in the population over a specific time period.

Inclusion criteria   Characteristics of subjects that must be present in order for subjects to be entered into the study.

Indexing service   A searchable database of biomedical journal citations.

Indicator   A statement of a measurable item in the area being evaluated which signals whether the area being evaluated is or is not of sufficient quality.

Indicator drug   A drug that, when prescribed, may offer evidence that an adverse effect to a drug may have occurred. Pharmacists can then investigate further to determine whether there really was an adverse effect. Examples are found in Chap. 17.

Inferential statistics   Statistics (i.e., parametric and nonparametric tests) that determine the statistical importance of differences between groups and allow conclusions to be drawn from the data.

Informed consent   The document signed by a subject, or the subject's representative, entering into a trial that informs him or her of his or her rights as a research subject, plus potential benefits and risks of the trial. This document indicates that the person is willing to participate in the study.

Inherent drug risks   Are unique to the drug and usually identified in the package insert, but do not include probable or common side effects.

Institutional Review Board (IRB)   A group of individuals from various disciplines (e.g., laypeople, physicians, pharmacists, nurses, and clergy) who evaluate protocols for clinical studies to assess risks to the research participants and benefits to society. Approval of a local IRB (i.e., an IRB located in the community in which the study is to be conducted) is necessary prior to initiation of a clinical study involving patients.

Intention-to-treat analysis   Analysis of all subject results randomized in a clinical trial regardless of whether they completed or dropped out of the study.

Interim analysis   Evaluation of data at specified time points before scheduled termination or completion of a study.

Internet   A worldwide computer network.

Interval data   Data in which each measurement has an equal distance between points, but an arbitrary zero (e.g., temperature in Fahrenheit).

Interventional study   A study where the investigator introduces a factor and examines the factor's influence on certain variables or outcomes.

Investigational new drug (IND)   A drug, antibiotic, or biologic that is used in a clinical investigation. The label of an investigational drug must bear the statement: "Caution: New Drug—Limited by Federal (or United States) law to investigational use."

Investigational new drug application (INDA)   A submission to the FDA containing chemical information, preclinical data, and a detailed description of the planned clinical trials. Thirty days after submission of this document to the FDA by the sponsor, clinical trials may be initiated in humans (unless a clinical hold is placed by the FDA). When the FDA allows the studies to proceed, this document allows unapproved drugs to be shipped in interstate commerce.

Investigator   The individual responsible for initiating the clinical trial at the study site. This individual must treat the patients, assure that the protocol is followed, evaluate responses and adverse reactions, solve problems as they arise, and assure proper conduct of the study.

JCAHO   The Joint Commission on Accreditation of Healthcare Organizations.

Joint and several liability   Refers to the sharing of liabilities among a group of people collectively and also individually. If the defendants are jointly and severally liable, the injured party may sue some or all of the defendants together, or each one separately, and may collect equal or unequal amounts from each.

Kurtosis   Refers to how flat or peaked the curve appears. A curve with a flat or board top is referred to as platykurtic while a peaked distribution is described as leptokurtic.

Law   Involves written rules set by the whole society, or its representatives, that address the responsibilities of that society's members.

Letter to the editor   Comments from readers of a study or other article published in a journal. These are published in a later issue of the same journal and usually have a reply from the original study/article author(s). Occasionally, short reports of a case or small study may be reported this way.

Listserver   A service offered by some e-mail systems that allows a member of the listserver to send an e-mail message to one particular Internet address where it will be sent to all members of the listserver. This acts as a dynamic distribution list for e-mail messages.

Local area network (LAN)   A group of computers connected in a way that they may share data, programs, and or equipment over a small geographic area (e.g., building, department).

Locality rule   Legal doctrine created in the latter part of the nineteenth century that stated that the local defendant practitioner would have his or her standard of performance evaluated in light of the performance of other peers in the same or similar communities. Also known as community rule.

Logical operator   A term such as AND, OR, NOT, NEAR, or WITH that can be used in searching a computer database. See Chap. 5 for more detailed information.

Mail service drug program   Program that provides free home delivery for up to a 90-day supply of maintenance prescription drugs.

Mainframe computer   A large centralized computer that is used via computer terminals or other devices. This term is becoming blurred as smaller computer systems gain greater capabilities.

Managed Care Organization (MCO)   Health care provider who contracts with participating providers to provide a variety of services to enrolled members.

MCO   See Managed Care Organization.

Mean (arithmetic mean)   The most common measure of central tendency for data measured on an interval or ratio scale and is best described as the average numerical value for the data set. Calculated as the sum of the observations divided by the number of observations.

Measurement error   Error that occurs when the interviewer influences the collection of data or when the survey item itself is unclear from the respondent's point of view. Also called response bias.

Measures of association Calculation and interpretation of nominal study results using relative risk (RR), relative risk reduction (RRR), absolute risk reduction (ARR), and numbers needed to treat (NNT).

Median The middle value in a set of ranked data. In other words, the value such that half of the data points fall above it and half fall below it. In terms of percentiles, it is the value at the fiftieth percentile.

Medical executive committee A committee that acts as the administrative body of a medical staff in an institution. It is responsible for overseeing all aspects of care within the institution. This committee may be known by other names at specific institutions.

Medical subject headings (MeSH terms) A thesaurus of official indexing terms used when searching some of the databases of the National Library of Medicine (e.g., MEDLINE® and TOXLINE®).

Medication error Any preventable event that has the potential to lead to inappropriate medication use or patient harm.

Medication misadventure Any iatrogenic hazard or incident associated with medications. It includes adverse drug events (ADEs), adverse drug reactions (ADRs), and medication errors.

Medication use evaluation (MUE) The component of a health care organization's quality improvement program that should examine all aspects of medication use including prescribing, dispensing, administration, and monitoring of medication use. Prior to 1986, this function was commonly referred to as drug use (or usage) evaluation (DUR).

MedLARS See medical literature analysis and retrieval system.

Medical literature analysis and retrieval system (MedLARS) The computerized information retrieval system at the National Library of Medicine.

MedWatch The FDA Medical Products Reporting Program that monitors clinically significant adverse drug events and problems with medical products. Information is found at <<http://www.fda.gov/medwatch>>.

Meta-analysis A type of review where conclusions are based on the summarization of results obtained from combining and statistically evaluating data from previously conducted studies. Also called a quantitative systematic review.

Middle technical style A writing style used by professionals addressing professionals in other fields. It tends to be formal and avoids use of the first person (e.g., I and us). Technical jargon is avoided in this writing style.

Mode The most frequently occurring value or category in the set of data. A data set can have more than one mode.

Modified systematic approach A seven-step approach to answering drug information requests that includes (1) secure demographics of requestor, (2) obtain background information, (3) determine and categorize ultimate question, (4) develop strategy and conduct search, (5) perform evaluation, analysis and synthesis, (6) formulate and provide response, and (7) conduct follow-up and documentation.

Morbidity Detrimental consequences (other than death) related to a treatment, exposure, or disease state.

MUE See medication use evaluation.

Narrative review See nonsystematic review.

N-of-1 study A controlled study conducted in a single subject where periods of exposure to a treatment are compared to periods of exposure to a placebo to determine the effects of the treatment on various variables and outcomes in the subject.

NCQA See National Committee for Quality Assurance.

National Committee for Quality Assurance (NCQA) An organization dedicated to assessing and reporting on the quality of managed care plans; it surveys and accredits managed care organizations much like the JCAHO accredits hospitals.

Negative formulary A drug formulary that starts out with every marketed drug product and specifically eliminates products that are considered inferior, unnecessary, unsafe, too expensive, and so forth.

Negligence Failure to exercise that degree of care that a person of ordinary prudence or a reasonable person would exercise under the same circumstances. Elements of a negligence case include (1) duty breached, (2) damages, (3) direct causation, and (4) defenses absent.

New drug application (NDA) The application to the FDA requesting approval to market a new drug for human use. The NDA contains data supporting the safety and efficacy of the drug for its intended use.

NNT See number needed to treat.

Nominal data Data that is categorical (e.g., yes/no or male/female).

Noninherent drug risks Are created by the particular drug in combination with some extrinsic factor that the pharmacist should reasonably know about.

Nonparametric statistics Statistical tests used to analyze data that is not normally distributed, such as nominal and ordinal data.

Nonresponse bias See nonresponse error.

Nonresponse error Error that occurs when a significant number of subjects in the sample do not respond to the survey and when responders differ from nonresponders in a way that influences, or could influence, the results. Also, called nonresponse bias.

Nonsystematic review A review article that summarizes previously conducted research, but does not provide a description of the systematic methods used to identify the research included in the article. Also, called a narrative review.

Null hypothesis   See hypothesis.

Number needed to treat (NNT)   The number of patients who need to be treated for every one patient who benefits from a treatment. NNT is calculated as the reciprocal of absolute risk reduction.

OBRA '90   See Omnibus Reconciliation Act of 1990.

Observational study   A study where the investigator analyzes naturally occurring events.

Odds ratios   A statistical technique used in case-control studies to determine the risk of exposure to a factor on development of a certain characteristic or disease state. Odds ratios estimate relative risk.

Omnibus Reconciliation Act of 1990 (OBRA '90)   A statute (Public Law 101-508) focused on drug benefits provided under Medicaid. The statute requires pharmacists to conduct drug utilization review (DUR) including prescription screening, patient counseling, and documentation of interventions.

Online   The process of connecting to a remote computer via modem or network.

Open formulary   A formulary that allows any marketed drug to be ordered in an institution or under a third-party plan. Can be considered an oxymoron.

Ordinal data   Data measured on an arbitrary scale that reflects a ranking (e.g., 1+ and 2+ edema).

ORYX   A JCAHO initiative to mandate the use of performance measurement tools to monitor outcomes and to integrate this data into the accreditation process.

Outcome indicators   Quality assurance indicators that review whether the final desired result was obtained from whatever action was being reviewed.

Overview   A general term for a summary of the literature. Includes nonsystematic (narrative), systematic (qualitative), and qualitative (meta-analyses) reviews.

p value   A number (probability) that is generated during use of inferential statistics. The p value indicates whether a statistical difference exists between groups. If the p value is less than or equal to alpha or the level of significance, the difference is statistically significant. If the p value is greater than alpha, the difference is not statistically significant. Also, refers to the probability of rejecting a true null hypothesis.

Parallel study   A study where two or more groups receive different treatments and the outcomes are compared.

Parameter   A measurement that describes part of the population.

Parametric statistics   Statistical tests used to analyze data with a normal (e.g., bell-shaped) distribution. Commonly used to analyze ratio and interval data.

Parenteral admixtures   Solutions containing drug products for intravenous (IV) administration.

Patient pocket formulary   Pocket-sized drug formulary listing top therapeutic drug classes, preferred products within those classes, cost index for the products, and other pertinent information.

PBM   See pharmacy benefit management companies.

Peer-review A quality assurance program that centers on the evaluation of specific individuals by other similar professionals. Also, the process where a group of experts review a manuscript for accuracy and appropriateness for publication in a biomedical journal.

Per protocol analysis Assessment of the study results in only those subjects completing the entire study duration.

Pharmacy benefit design Contract that specifies the level of coverage and types of pharmaceutical services available to the health plan member.

Pharmacy benefit management (PBM) companies Organizations that manage pharmaceutical benefits for managed care organizations, medical providers, or employers.

Pharmacy network Select pharmacies and pharmacy chains where members of a health plan have to go to get their prescriptions filled, usually at a lower cost.

Pharmaceutical care The responsible provision of drug therapy for the purpose of achieving definite outcomes that improve a patient's quality of life.

Pharmacoeconomics The study of the economic impact of drug therapies or services.

Pharmacy and therapeutics (P&T) committee A group in an institution or company that oversees any and/or all aspects of drug therapy for that institution or company. In hospitals, it is usually a sub-committee of the Medical Staff. May be known by a variety of similar names, such as pharmacy and formulary committee, drug and therapeutics committee (DTC), or formulary committee.

Placebo A pharmaceutical preparation that does not contain a pharmacologically active ingredient, but is otherwise identical to the active drug preparation in terms of appearance, taste, and smell.

Poison information A specialized area related to and overlapping drug information. By definition, it is the provision of information on the toxic effects of an extensive range of chemicals, as well as, plant and animal exposures.

Poison information center A place that specializes in research, management, and dissemination of toxicity information. A physician usually directs it, although a pharmacist directs many activities on a day-to-day basis. Often, pharmacists and nurses provide staffing of these centers.

Policy A broad general statement that takes into consideration and describes the goals and purposes of a policy and procedure document.

Popular technical style A writing style used by professionals addressing laypeople. This is less formal than writing addressed to professionals.

Population Every individual in the entire universe with the characteristics or disease states under investigation. Because entire populations are generally very large, a sample representative of the population is usually selected for an investigation.

Positive formulary A drug formulary that starts out with no drug products and specifically adds products, after appropriate evaluation, that are needed by the institution or company.

Postmarketing surveillance study A study designed to examine drug use and frequency of side effects following approval by the Food and Drug Administration (FDA).

Power The ability to detect a statistical difference between study groups. Power is dependent on sample size and mathematically is calculated as 1 – beta.

Preferred drug product Specific drug product within a specific therapeutic class selected as the most appropriate to treat a specific disease or condition as determined by a pharmacy and therapeutics committee.

Preferred therapeutic class Specific drug class selected as the most appropriate to treat a specific disease or condition as determined by a pharmacy and therapeutics committee.

Prescribability The ability of a drug to be prescribed for the first time.

Prevalence Measures the number of people in the population who have the disease at a given time.

Primary author The author listed first on a publication. Sometimes referred to as the first author.

Primary literature Original research published in biomedical journals.

Principles In ethical analysis, a principle is relatively broad and fundamental in scope, and guides ethical decision-making or actions.

Prior authorization Authorization from the health plan or pharmacy benefit manager in conjunction with the Pharmacy and Therapeutics Committee for specified medications or specified quantities of medications. The request is reviewed against preestablished criteria, which are based on evidence-based medicine.

Procedures Specific actions to be taken.

Process indicators Quality assurance indicators based on the presence or absence of policies and procedures. These assume that if policies and procedures are appropriate they will be effective and be properly performed.

Professional ethics Rules of conduct or standards by which a particular group in society regulates its actions and sets standards for its members.

Professional writing Any written communication prepared in the fulfillment of the practice of a profession.

Programmatic research Research focused on the impact and economic value of programs and services provided by pharmacists in community and institutional settings.

Prospective indicator An indicator used in any quality assurance program that determines whether quality is acceptable before an action is taken or care is given.

Prospective study A study where data are collected forward in timefrom date of study initiation.

Publication bias The situation where research demonstrating favorable results is more likely to be published than that showing negative results.

Pure technical style A writing style used by professionals addressing other professionals in the same field. It tends to be formal and avoids use of the first person (e.g., I and us). Technical jargon can be used in this writing style.

Push technology A method by which information is actively sent to users' computers with little, if any, effort required by the user. The information may be displayed as a screen saver or the computer may in some way let the user know that the information is available to be displayed (e.g., pop-up notification).

P&T Committee See pharmacy and therapeutics committee.

Qualitative systematic review See systematic review.

Qualitative systematic review See meta-analysis.

Quality A degree or grade of excellence which and can be applied to goods, services, processes, or even people.

Quality assessment and assurance committee A committee found in long-term care facilities to evaluate quality of care, including drug usage evaluation.

Quality assurance A process used to ensure that something is done or made well enough. It is usually retrospective and focuses only on a particular component within a process, not the entire process.

Quality of life This is an evaluation of a patient's living situation based on the patient's environment, family life, financial situation, education, and health. It is used in quality assurance programs when developing indicators. In some cases, quality of life aspects will take precedence over the absolute best treatment. For example, a quick cure to a disease state may not be desirable when it costs so much that a family is bankrupted in the process.

Quantitative systematic review See meta-analysis.

Quantity limits Set quantity of drug that can be prescribed that is set by the health plan in conjunction with a pharmacy and therapeutics committee that is usually based on FDA prescribing guidelines.

Random error See sampling error.

Randomization The process used to ensure that subjects in a study have an equal and independent chance of being assigned to the intervention or control groups in a study.

Randomized clinical trial See controlled clinical trial.

Range The difference between the highest data value and the lowest data value.

Ratio data Data in which each measurement has an equal distance between points and also an absolute zero (e.g., temperature in Kelvin).

Rechallenge In relation to adverse drug reaction (ADR) this indicates that the drug was taken away and, after the ADR abates, the patient is given the same medication in an attempt to illicit the same response a second time.

Referee   An expert in a particular area who reviews a written document to determine whether it is appropriate for publication. Also, referred to as a reviewer.

Refereed publication   A publication in which the editors have experts in the appropriate field review items submitted for possible publication to determine whether those items are of suitable quality.

Relative risk   A statistical technique used in follow-up studies to determine the risk associated with exposure to a certain factor on disease state development. Relative risk estimates how many times greater the risk of disease state development is in patients exposed to a certain factor compared to those who are not exposed.

Research hypothesis   See hypothesis.

Response bias   See measurement error.

Respondeat Superior   Refers to the proposition that the employer is responsible for the negligent acts of its agents or employees.

Restatement (Second) of Torts   "An attempt by the American Law Institute to present an orderly statement of the general common law of the United States, including in that term not only the law developed solely by judicial decision, but also the law that has grown from the application by the courts of statutes...." It takes into account other factors, such as the modern trend of the law according to influential jurisdictions and well-thought out opinions.

Retrospective indicator   An indicator used in any quality assurance program that determines whether quality was acceptable after an action was taken or care was given.

Retrospective study   A study that analyzes historical data (e.g., previously collected data such as medical records or insurance information).

Reviewer   See referee.

RSS   This acronym has multiple meanings, but is usually defined as Really Simple Syndication. It is a method by which an aggregator program collects information from websites and weblogs (blog), which is then displayed as a collation. This allows individuals to monitor new or additional information on the Internet without having to use a browser to go to multiple websites.

Rule   In ethical analysis, a rule guides ethical decision-making or actions, but is relatively specific in context and restricted in scope.

Run-in phase   A phase of a clinical trial prior to randomization in which all subjects complete to determine the incidence of a prespecified outcome determined by the investigators (e.g., medication compliance and adverse effects).

Sample   A group of subjects chosen as representatives of a population to participate in a study.

Sample size   The number of subjects in a study.

Sampling bias   See sampling error.

Sampling error   Error that occurs when the research surveys only a subset (sample) of all possible subjects within the population of interest.

SD   See standard deviation.

Secondary literature   Resources that index and/or abstract literature from biomedical journals.

Selection bias   A problem with the way subjects are entered into a study. It can be of two primary types. In the first, subjects meeting the inclusion and exclusion criteria are not randomized into the study. The other type is the recruiting of unique subjects not completely representative of the population (i.e., those with a gastrointestinal bleed taking aspirin).

SEM   See standard error of the mean.

Sensitivity   The probability that a diseased individual will have a positive test result. It is the true positive rate of the test. The ability of a test to correctly identify those with the disease.

Sensitivity analysis   Tests that are undertaken to determine the influence of various criteria or conditions on study results. Sensitivity analyses are commonly used in meta-analyses and pharmacoeconomic research.

Skewness   The measure of symmetry of a curve.

Specificity   The probability that a disease-free individual will have a negative test result. Specificity is the true negative rate of the test. The ability of a test to correctly identify those without the disease.

Sponsor   An organization (or individual) that takes responsibility for and initiates a clinical investigation. The sponsor may be an individual or pharmaceutical company, government agency, academic institution, private organization, or other organization.

Sponsor-investigator   An individual who both initiates and conducts a clinical investigation, i.e., submits the INDA and directly supervises administration of the drug, as well as performing other investigator responsibilities.

Stability study   A study designed to determine the stability of drugs in various preparations.

Standard   A term used in quality assurance program that indicates how often an indicator must be complied with. The level of compliance will be set at either 0% (i.e., never done) or 100% (i.e., always done). A threshold, which allows compliance of between 0 and 100%, has sometimes been used instead of a standard.

Standard deviation (SD)   (1) A measurement of the range of data values (i.e., variability) around the mean. (2) The measure of the average amount by which each observation in a series of data points differs from the mean. In other words, how far away is each data point from the mean (dispersion or variability) or the average deviation from the mean.

Standard error of the mean (SEM)   An estimate of the true mean of the population from the mean of the sample. Mathematically, SEM is calculated as the standard deviation divided by the square root of the sample size. Ninety-five percent of the time, true mean of the population lies within ±2 standard errors of the sample mean.

Statistic   A measurement that describes part of a sample.

Statistical significance The impact of a study in terms of the outcome of statistical tests conducted on the data. A study is said to be statistically significant when statistical tests demonstrate a difference between treatment groups.

Statute Written law enacted by a legislature other than that of a municipality.

Step therapy Prescribing guidelines set by the health plan in conjunction with a pharmacy and therapeutics committee that specify which drugs should be prescribed first before more expensive drugs will be covered. Guidelines are based on evidence-based medicine.

Strict liability Liability without fault. Defendant is liable even though not lacking in care. Negligence despite proof of prudence.

Structure indicators Quality assurance indicators based on the presence or absence of items, such as staffing patterns, available space, equipment, resources, or administrative organization.

Study objective A brief statement of the goals and purpose of a research study.

Subgroup analysis Evaluation of study results within a subset of subjects enrolled in the study according to specific demographics (e.g., age, gender, and disease state).

Subject An individual who participates in a clinical investigation (either as the recipient of the investigational drug or as a member of the control group).

Surrogate endpoint A study measurement that serves as a substitute for a clinical outcome.

Survey research Research where responses to questions asked of subjects are analyzed to determine the incidence, distribution and relationships of sociologic and psychologic variables.

Switchability The ability to exchange one drug for another.

Symposium A meeting focused on a particular topic.

Systematic review A summary of previously conducted studies where the research to be included in the review is systematically identified; however, the results are not statistically combined as would occur with a quantitative systematic review or meta-analysis. Also, called a qualitative systematic review.

Target drug program A program that evaluates the use of a medication or group of medications on an ongoing basis. Within these programs, interventions are usually made at the time of discovery based on established criteria or guidelines.

Telnet A program for microcomputers that causes the computer to mimic a dumb terminal, so that it can run programs on other computers (usually minicomputers or mainframes) over the Internet or other computer networks.

Teratogenicity Toxicity of drugs to the unborn fetus.

Tertiary literature Textbooks and drug compendia (includes fulltext computer databases) that consists of established knowledge.

Third-party payer Organization that pays for or underwrites coverage for health care expenses for another entity.

Third-party plan A method of reimbursement for medical care in which neither the care provider or patient are charged. Third-party payers include insurance, health maintenance organizations, and government entities.

Threshold A term used in quality assurance programs that indicates how often an indicator must be complied with. Unlike standards, thresholds can be set at any level of compliance from 0 to 100%.

Tiered copayment benefit A pharmacy benefit design that encourages patients to use generic and formulary drugs, by requiring the patient to pay progressively higher copayments for brand name and nonformulary drugs.

Total quality management (TQM) A management concept dealing with the implementation of continuous quality improvement.

TQM See total quality management.

Trohoc study See case-control study.

True experiment A study where researchers apply a treatment and determine its effects on subjects.

True negatives Individuals without the disease that were correctly identified as being disease-free by the test.

True positives Individuals with the disease that were correctly identified as diseased by the test.

Type I error The probability of a false positive result. The probability of a Type I error is equal to alpha and occurs when the null hypothesis is rejected when it is in fact true.

Type II error The probability of a false negative result. The probability of a Type II error is equal to beta and occurs when the null hypothesis is accepted when it is in fact false.

Unexpected drug reaction The Food and Drug Administration defines this as "one that is not listed in the current labeling for the drug as having been reported or associated with the use of the drug. This includes an ADR that may be symptomatically or pathophysiologically related to an ADR listed in the labeling but may differ from the labeled ADR because of greater severity or specificity (e.g., abnormal liver function vs. hepatic necrosis)".

Uniform resource locator (URL) An Internet address (e.g., http://www.cdc.gov).

USENET news A large number of discussion groups that are replicated in numerous places on the Internet. Users can read items posted on a topic and can contribute their own items to be posted.

Validity The truthfulness of study results. Internal validity refers to the extent to which the study results reflect what actually happened in the study (i.e., appropriate and sound study methods). External validity is the degree to which the study results can be applied to patients routinely encountered in clinical practice.

Variables Factors (characteristics that are being observed or measured) that are the focus of a study. The independent variable (e.g., treatment) causes change in the dependent variable (e.g., outcome).

Variance A measurement of the range of data values (i.e., variability) about the mean. Variance is the square of the standard deviation.

Virtual private network (VPN) A method to connect computers over a distance, for example over the Internet that allows secure transmission of confidential data.

Warranty An assurance by one party to a contract of the existence of a fact on which the other party may rely, intended to relieve the promisee of any duty to ascertain the fact for himself or herself. Amounts to a promise to indemnify the promisee for any loss if the fact warranted proves untrue. Warranties may be express (made overtly) or implied (by implication).

Weblog (also known as blog) This is a public website where a person maintains a journal that is open to viewers.

Web browser A computer program used to access information on the World Wide Web. The most popular program is Microsoft® Internet Explorer.

Web portal A website that acts as an interface to the Internet for users. Many Internet search engines are considered to be web portals. A variation on this, the enterprise portal, can also be used by an institution to help guide employees to necessary information within the institution or out on the Internet.

Website A group of web pages that will provide information to the person requesting that information. These pages are generally grouped under one main Internet address (URL).

Wide area network (WAN) A group of computers connected in a way that they may share data, programs, and or equipment over a distance (e.g., connection between computers owned by an institution that are scattered in clinics around a city).

World Wide Web (WWW) Computers connected to the Internet that provide a graphical interface to a variety of information that is available as text, pictures, sounds, databases, and other electronic files. Generally accessed using a web browser, such as Internet Explorer.

XHTML—Extensible HTML A combination of HTML and Extensible Markup Language.

XML—Extensible Markup Language A superset of HTML that provides information on the content of a web page, presentation of the information (how it looks), and semantics (what it means). This is designed to make it easier to find more relevant information using search engines.

Index

Page numbers followed by italic *f* or *t* indicate figures or tables, respectively.